T0213852

Respiratory Medicine

Respiratory Medicine offers clinical and research-oriented resources for pulmonologists and other practitioners and researchers interested in respiratory care. Spanning a broad range of clinical and research issues in respiratory medicine, the series covers such topics as COPD, asthma and allergy, pulmonary problems in pregnancy, molecular basis of lung disease, sleep disordered breathing, and others.

The series editors are Sharon Rounds, MD, Professor of Medicine and of Pathology and Laboratory Medicine at the Alpert Medical School at Brown University, Anne Dixon, MD, Professor of Medicine and Director of the Division of Pulmonary and Critical Care at Robert Larner, MD College of Medicine at the University of Vermont, and Lynn M. Schnapp, MD, George R. And Elaine Love Professor and Chair of Medicine at the University of Wisconsin-Madison School of Medicine and Public Health.

More information about this series at https://link.springer.com/bookseries/7665

M. Safwan Badr • Jennifer L. Martin
Editors

Essentials of Sleep Medicine

A Practical Approach to Patients with Sleep
Complaints

Second Edition

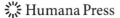 Humana Press

Editors
M. Safwan Badr
Department of Internal Medicine
Wayne State University School of Medicine
John D. Dingell VA Medical Center
Detroit, MI, USA

Jennifer L. Martin
Geriatric Research Education and Clinical
Center, Veteran Affairs Greater Los Angeles
Healthcare System
Department of Medicine
David Geffen School of Medicine
University of California, Los Angeles
Los Angeles, CA, USA

ISSN 2197-7372   ISSN 2197-7380   (electronic)
Respiratory Medicine
ISBN 978-3-030-93741-6   ISBN 978-3-030-93739-3   (eBook)
https://doi.org/10.1007/978-3-030-93739-3

This Humana imprint is published by the registered company Springer Nature Switzerland AG
The registered company address is: Gewerbestrasse 11, 6330 Cham, Switzerland

Foreword

In the last few decades, we have learned more and more about how important sleep is for our physical health, our mental health, and our general well-being. And yet, sleep problems continue to become more prevalent. The was a time when patients with problems sleeping would neglect to mention it to their health care professional. But those times are changing. As more and more research is done, as more and more articles are written about the importance of sleep, the general public has become more and more aware and better educated. And now they are not hesitating to talk about this major issue.

Which means that more general healthcare professionals and specialists, such as physicians, psychologists, nurse practitioners, and nurses, will be faced with dealing and treating these sleep problems. And that is where this book comes in.

But it is not just those first entering the field who will benefit from this book. As someone with over 40 years' experience in sleep medicine, I can attest to the fact that even those of us with loads of experience have new things to learn, and this book can help us all do just that.

The editors, Drs. Jennifer Martin and Safwan Badr, are internationally recognized and highly respected sleep medicine specialists, each with a long list of credentials. In *Introduction to Sleep Medicine*, they have assembled other experts in the field to cover everything from normal sleep, health disparity, and models of caring to descriptions of and treatment of specific sleep disorders, such as obstructive sleep apnea, insomnia, and circadian rhythm disorders, to name just a few. There are also chapters on special populations such as hospitalized patients, pregnant women, and older patients. And each chapter represents the very latest in research and clinical findings. In other words, everything a professional dealing with sleep problems needs to know.

No one book can be everything to everyone. But this book is an excellent addition to any private or public library collection, whether it be one filled with other books on sleep or a new collection of sleep books that is just beginning. Having a resource book such as this one can only help healthcare professionals better understand their patients.

Introduction to Sleep Medicine, in summary, is an extremely masterful and scholarly book that can be used by all professionals wanting to help their patients with sleep problems. I commend Drs. Martin and Badr on this comprehensive introduction to sleep medicine.

November 8, 2021   Sonia Ancoli-Israel
University of California
San Diego, CA, USA

Preface

Sleep has fascinated poets, lovers, and philosophers since time immemorial. It was a metaphor for rest, rejuvenation, and restoration. Physicians viewed sleep and thought of sleep as a "safe harbor" keeping illness away, and as a cuddly "teddy bear" giving warmth and serenity. Few physicians appreciated sleep complexity beyond the elemental aspects: patients need rest and sleep. Disorders of sleep were the subject of interesting discussions at teaching conferences, but the only condition worthy of discussion was lack of sleep, and it was often due to tension, anxiety, or stress.

The image of sleep as a quiescent period changed dramatically when scientists began to uncover the mysteries of sleep: the good, the bad, and the ugly! The discovery of REM sleep altered the popular image of sleep as a somewhat meaningless state of rest and revealed a fascinating constellation of active processes throughout the body and brain. However, it was the discovery of sleep apnea that propelled sleep into mainstream medicine. This is a condition where sleep is anything but rest. We learned that sleep can be seen as a "grizzly bear" as we discovered that sleep apnea (broadly referred to as sleep disordered breathing) can have significant adverse consequences and may contribute to mortality and to traffic fatalities.

The initial phase of sleep medicine was marked by different specialties providing care for conditions deemed within their domain. Neurologists, psychiatrists, and pulmonologists focused on different disorders and different approaches to diagnosis and treatment. Fortunately, we soon discovered that sleep is an interdisciplinary field, transcending traditional, system-based specialties, and that other health care providers and public health experts are needed to address the modern epidemic of sleep disorders.

Patients present with complaints and not diagnoses, and any one sleep disorder accounts for only a small proportion of patients with sleep-related complaints. We learned that snoring may represent a serious condition, that daytime sleepiness is not always a sign of narcolepsy, and that insomnia is not typically accounted for by co-occurring anxiety or depression. Therefore, healthcare providers who care for any sleep disorder must learn about all sleep disorders.

The focus of this book is practical; relevant facts help busy practicing clinicians provide better care for sleep disorders as part of a comprehensive approach to patient care. It is intended to equally address the needs of all clinicians who care for patients with sleep disorders. Residents and fellows may find the focused description and practical approach beneficial. This revised edition includes new chapters to address a broad range of considerations in delivering high quality care across the spectrum of sleep disorders.

This book represents the collective effort of a team of professionals. Each chapter was written by experts in the field, blending seasoned experts with emerging leaders.

Editing a book is a challenging process as one tries to keep a group of busy academicians, many of whom crafted their chapter during the COVID-19 pandemic, on schedule. We are grateful to Margaret Moore and Swathiga Karthikeyan of Springer for their support, guidance, and superb organizational skills. We would like to thank Springer Science and Business Media for supporting this project.

Detroit, MI, USA   M. Safwan Badr
North Hills, CA, USA   Jennifer L. Martin

Contents

Contributors

Sabra M. Abbott Northwestern University Feinberg School of Medicine, Department of Neurology, Chicago, IL, USA

Imran Ahmed Sleep-Wake Disorders Center, Montefiore Medical Center, and Albert Einstein College of Medicine, Bronx, NY, USA

Cathy Alessi David Geffen School of Medicine at University of California, Los Angeles, Los Angeles, CA, USA

Geriatric Research, Education and Clinical Center, Veterans Affairs Greater Los Angeles Healthcare System, Los Angeles, CA, USA

Vineet M. Arora Department of Medicine, University of Chicago Medical Center, Chicago, IL, USA

Rachel Atkinson University of Toledo College of Medicine and Life Sciences, Toledo, OH, USA

M. Safwan Badr Division of Pulmonary, Critical Care and Sleep Medicine, Department of Internal Medicine, Harper University Hospital, Wayne State University School of Medicine, Detroit, MI, USA

Judite Blanc University of Miami, Miller School of Medicine, Miami, FL, USA

Mia Y. Bothwell University of Illinois at Urbana-Champaign Medical Scholars Program, Champaign, IL, USA

Anthony Q. Briggs New York University Langone Health, Department of Population Health, New York, NY, USA

New York University Langone Health, Department of Psychiatry, New York, NY, USA

Gwendolyn C. Carlson Department of Mental Health, VA Greater Los Angeles Healthcare System, VA Health Services Research and Development Service (HSR&D) Center for the Study of Healthcare Innovation, Implementation and Policy, Los Angeles, CA, USA

Department of Psychiatry and Biobehavioral Sciences, David Geffen School of Medicine, University of California, Los Angeles, Los Angeles, CA, USA

Nishant Chaudhary Division of Pulmonary, Critical Care, and Sleep Medicine, Department of Medicine, University Hospitals of Cleveland, Case Western Reserve University, Cleveland, OH, USA

Susmita Chowdhuri Sleep Medicine Section, Medical Service John D. Dingell VA Medical Center, Detroit, MI, USA

Department of Medicine, Wayne State University, Detroit, MI, USA

Alicia Chung New York University Langone Health, Department of Population Health, New York, NY, USA

Nancy Collop Emory Sleep Center, Emory University School of Medicine, Atlanta, GA, USA

Janet H. Dailey Pharmacy Benefits Management Services, Veterans Health Administration, Washington, DC, USA

Christopher Drake Henry Ford Sleep Disorders and Research Center, Detroit, MI, USA

Kara L. Dupuy-McCauley Center for Sleep Medicine, Mayo Clinic, Rochester, MN, USA

Erica Feldman University of California, San Diego, Department of Medicine, Internal Medicine, La Jolla, CA, USA

Barry G. Fields Emory University, Division of Pulmonary, Allergy and Critical Care Medicine, Atlanta, GA, USA

Peter C. Gay Department of Medicine, Mayo Clinic, Rochester, MN, USA

Geoffrey Ginter Department of Internal Medicine, Harper University Hospital, Wayne State University School of Medicine, Detroit, MI, USA

Scott Hoff Emory Sleep Center, Emory University School of Medicine, Atlanta, GA, USA

Girardin Jean-Louis University of Miami, Miller School of Medicine, Miami, FL, USA

Biren B. Kamdar Department of Medicine, Division of Pulmonary, Critical Care and Sleep Medicine, University of California San Diego Health, La Jolla, CA, USA

Margaret A. Kay-Stacey Northwestern University Feinberg School of Medicine, Department of Neurology, Chicago, IL, USA

Jamie Nicole LaBuzetta Department of Neurosciences, Division of Neurocritical Care, University of California San Diego Health, La Jolla, CA, USA

Michael T. Y. Lam Department of Medicine, Division of Pulmonary, Critical Care, Sleep Medicine and Physiology, University of California San Diego Health, La Jolla, CA, USA

Atul Malhotra Department of Medicine, Division of Pulmonary, Critical Care, Sleep Medicine and Physiology, University of California San Diego Health, La Jolla, CA, USA

Haven R. Malish Sleep Medicine, Mayo Clinic, Rochester, MN, USA

Jennifer L. Martin Geriatric Research, Education and Clinical Center, Veteran Affairs Greater Los Angeles Healthcare System, Department of Medicine, David Geffen School of Medicine, University of California, Los Angeles, Los Angeles, CA, USA

Jesse Moore New York University Langone Health, Department of Population Health, New York, NY, USA

Louise M. O'Brien Division of Sleep Medicine, Department of Neurology, Michigan Medicine, Ann Arbor, MI, USA

Department of Obstetrics & Gynecology, Michigan Medicine, Ann Arbor, MI, USA

Amanda J. Piper Department of Respiratory and Sleep Medicine, Royal Prince Alfred Hospital, Camperdown, NSW, Australia

Faculty of Medicine and Health, University of Sydney, Camperdown, NSW, Australia

Janna Raphelson University of California, San Diego, Department of Medicine, Internal Medicine, La Jolla, CA, USA

April Rogers St. John's University, New York, NY, USA

Carol L. Rosen Department of Pediatrics, Case Western Reserve University School of Medicine, Cleveland, OH, USA

Ilene M. Rosen Division of Sleep Medicine, Perelman School of Medicine at the University of Pennsylvania PCAM, Philadelphia, PA, USA

James A. Rowley Division of Pulmonary, Critical Care and Sleep Medicine, Department of Internal Medicine, Harper University Hospital, Wayne State University School of Medicine, Detroit, MI, USA

Armand Michael Ryden Pulmonary, Critical Care and Sleep Medicine Division, Veterans Affairs Greater Los Angeles Healthcare System, Los Angeles, CA, USA

David Geffen School of Medicine at University of California, Los Angeles, Los Angeles, CA, USA

Azizi A. Seixas University of Miami, Miller School of Medicine, Miami, FL, USA

Jordan Taylor Standlee Northwestern University Feinberg School of Medicine, Department of Neurology, Chicago, IL, USA

Nancy H. Stewart Department of Medicine, University of Kansas Medical Center, Kansas City, KS, USA

Kingman P. Strohl Division of Pulmonary, Critical Care, and Sleep Medicine, Department of Medicine, University Hospitals of Cleveland, Case Western Reserve University, Cleveland, OH, USA

Michael Thorpy Sleep-Wake Disorders Center, Montefiore Medical Center, and Albert Einstein College of Medicine, Bronx, NY, USA

Arlener Turner University of Miami, Miller School of Medicine, Miami, FL, USA

Nidhi S. Undevia Department of Medicine, Division of Pulmonary and Critical Care Medicine, Loyola Center for Sleep Disorders, Loyola University Medical Center, Maywood, IL, USA

Bradley V. Vaughn Department of Neurology, University of North Carolina, Chapel Hill, NC, USA

Nathan A. Walker Department of Neurology, University of North Carolina, Chapel Hill, NC, USA

Ellita Williams New York University Langone Health, Department of Population Health, New York, NY, USA

Eric Yeh Division of Pulmonary, Critical Care, and Sleep Medicine, Department of Medicine, University Hospitals of Cleveland, Case Western Reserve University, Cleveland, OH, USA

Michelle R. Zeidler Sleep Disorders Center, VA Greater Los Angeles VA Healthcare System, Department of Medicine, David Geffen School of Medicine, University of California, Los Angeles, Los Angeles, CA, USA

Salam Zeineddine Department of Medicine, John D. Dingell VA Medical Center and Wayne State University School of Medicine, Detroit, MI, USA

Part I
Introduction to Sleep Medicine

Chapter 1
Normal Sleep

James A. Rowley and M. Safwan Badr

Keywords NREM sleep · REM sleep · EEG · Upper airway resistance · Hypocapnic apneic threshold · Critical closing pressure (Pcrit) · Heart rate variability · Esophageal sphincter

Normal Sleep Stages and Architecture

Normal human sleep is generally divided into four stages. Consensus definitions for the visual scoring of sleep were published in 2007 and the reader is referred to the American Academy of Sleep Medicine Scoring Manual for full definitions and criteria for the scoring of sleep on polysomnograms as these are periodically updated [1, 2]. The following will provide a brief overview of the electroencephalographic (EEG) characteristics of the different sleep stages (see also Fig. 1.1).

Full wakefulness is characterized by mixed-frequency, low-amplitude EEG activity, often in association with high chin muscle tone, eye blinks, and rapid eye movements. As the patient transitions to sleep with eyes closed, wakefulness is characterized by a 8–13 Hz sinusoidal activity called alpha sleep. Alpha sleep is best recorded over the occipital region and is attenuated by eye opening.

Non-rapid eye movement (NREM) sleep composes the majority of the night and is characterized by the predominance of homeostatic mechanisms for breathing, cardiovascular and gastrointestinal function, and normal thermoregulation. NREM sleep is divided into 3 stages. N1 sleep is a transitional period during which the individual still usually has some awareness of his/her environment. N1 sleep is characterized by a slowing of the background wake EEG frequencies with

J. A. Rowley (✉) · M. S. Badr
Division of Pulmonary, Critical Care and Sleep Medicine, Department of Internal Medicine, Harper University Hospital, Wayne State University School of Medicine, Detroit, MI, USA
e-mail: jrowley@med.wayne.edu; sbadr@med.wayne.edu

© Springer Nature Switzerland AG 2022
M. S. Badr, J. L. Martin (eds.), *Essentials of Sleep Medicine*,
Respiratory Medicine, https://doi.org/10.1007/978-3-030-93739-3_1

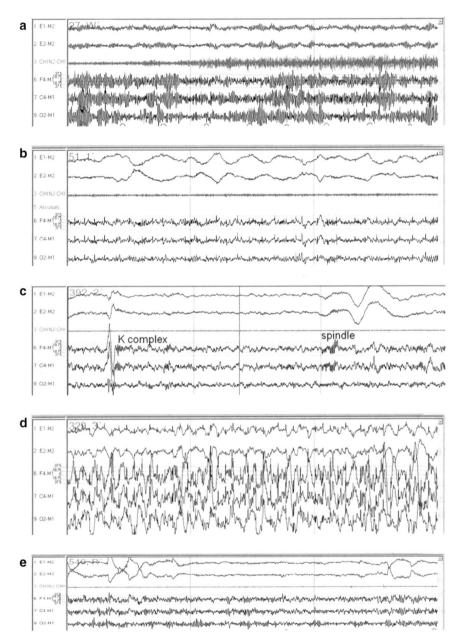

Fig. 1.1 Representative 30-second epochs of sleep stages. (**a**) Wakefulness with alpha rhythm; (**b**) Stage N1; (**c**) Stage N2 with K-complex and spindle; (**d**) Stage N3 (slow-wave sleep); and (**e**) Stage R. For all epochs: E1-M2: left electro-oculogram; E2-M2: right electro-oculogram; Chin 2: chin EMG; F4-M1: right frontal EEG; C4-M1: right central EEG; O2-M1: right occipital EEG

a predominance of low amplitude activity in 4–7 Hz (often referred to as theta activity). Slow eye movements are commonly observed during N1 sleep. N2 sleep, at which time the individual generally is no longer aware of his/her environment, is characterized by the appearance of sleep spindles and K complexes superimposed on a background of theta activity. Sleep spindles are rhythmic sinusoidal waves of 12–14 Hz, usually best recorded on central EEG leads. K complexes are diphasic waves having a well-delineated sharp negative component followed by a slow positive component. N3 sleep, commonly known as slow-wave sleep, is scored when slow-wave activity is recorded on >20% of an epoch. By definition, slow waves are of low frequency (generally 0.5–2 Hz) and have large amplitude (>75 μV).

As opposed to NREM sleep, rapid eye movement (REM or Stage R) is characterized by variations and instability in cardiopulmonary function and instability of body temperature control. In addition, Stage R is characterized by dreaming, relative atonia of all muscle groups except the diaphragm and in men, erections. On EEG, Stage R is characterized by a low-amplitude, mixed-frequency EEG, similar to that seen in Stage N1 sleep. In addition, Stage R is characterized by the presence of rapid eye movements and decreased chin muscle tone. Stage R is a unique time of the night in that dreaming occurs during Stage R sleep.

Sleep architecture describes the organization of the sleep stages over the course of the night (Fig. 1.2). The normal sleep cycle in a young adult (generally considered the standard) begins with transitioning from wakefulness to N1 sleep and then quickly transitioning to N2 and N3 sleep. The first occurrence of Stage R sleep is generally at about 90 minutes and individuals then cycle between NREM and REM sleep every 90–110 minutes throughout the night. In general, N3 sleep predominates in the first half of the night while Stage R predominates in the second half of the night. For an average individual in their second decade, Stage N1 is 2–5% of the total sleep time, Stage N2 is 45–55%, Stage N3 13–23%, and Stage R is 20–25% [3].

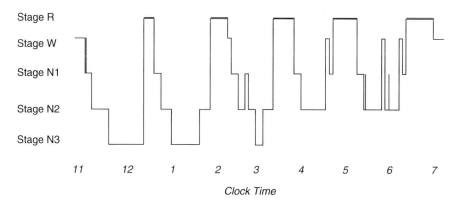

Fig. 1.2 Representative hypnogram showing normal sleep architecture

Overall sleep architecture is dependent upon stage of development and aging (Fig. 1.3). For instance, infants generally spend up to 50% of the night in Stage R sleep and often have a cycle of REM sleep prior to NREM sleep. In addition, the duration of the NREM-REM cycle is 60 minutes through most of childhood. Over the span of time between young adulthood to elderly, there are changes in most sleep stages, including decreased total sleep time and sleep efficiency, increased percentage of Stages N1 and N2, decreased percentage of Stage N3 and R. These changes with aging have been shown to be more prominent in men than women [3, 4].

Breathing During Sleep: Ventilation and the Upper Airway

Summary of Normal Breathing and Ventilation During Sleep

Ventilatory motor output during sleep decreases from its normal levels in wakefulness, leading to decreased tidal volume and minute ventilation. The decreased ventilation is accompanied by reduced upper-airway dilator muscle activity resulting in decreased upper-airways caliber and increased airflow resistance. These biological

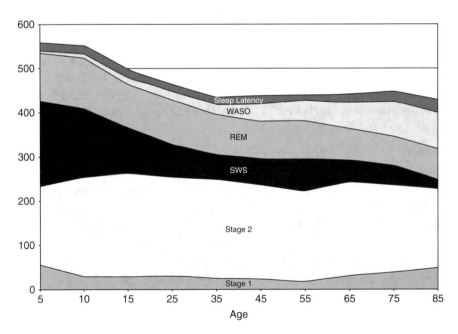

Fig. 1.3 Changes in sleep stages as a percentage of sleep time across the age span. WASO = wake after sleep onset; REM = rapid eye movement sleep; SWS = slow-wave sleep. See text for details

changes may account for the observed increase in Pa_{CO_2} and decrease in Pa_{O_2} during sleep, despite the diminished overall metabolic rate. A decrease in chemoresponsiveness during sleep may also explain the increased Pa_{CO_2}. Overall, breathing becomes more dependent on chemical stimuli, especially $PaCO_2$.

In contrast to NREM sleep, REM sleep is characterized by variability in ventilation. This variability consists of sudden changes in respiratory amplitude and frequency associated with the periods of phasic rapid eye movements. Because of this variability, minute ventilation in REM sleep has been shown to be the same, increased, or decreased compared with NREM sleep. Upper-airway resistance has also been reported variably as either the same or increased compared to wakefulness and NREM sleep. Finally, hypercapnic and hypoxic ventilatory chemoresponsiveness is decreased in REM sleep compared to wakefulness and possibly even NREM sleep.

Effect of Sleep on Control of Breathing

Chemoresponsiveness refers to changing ventilation in response to changes in chemical stimuli. Chemosensitivity is influenced by changes in neural activity during sleep. Thus, hypoxic and hypercapnic chemoresponsiveness contribute to maintaining ventilation during sleep. Conversely, hypocapnia is a potent inhibitor of ventilation during NREM sleep and is a key mechanism of central apnea [5].

The sleep state is characterized by decreased ventilatory response to hypercapnia (HCVR) in human adults compared to wakefulness [6–12]. While the sensitivity to Pa_{CO_2} does not appear to differ within NREM sleep stages, the HCVR during REM stage is depressed further compared with NREM sleep [6, 8]. Similarly, hypoxic ventilatory responsiveness (HVR) is also diminished during NREM sleep compared to wakefulness, with a further decrease in REM sleep [10, 13–15]. Nevertheless, the effect of sleep on chemoresponsiveness is confounded by the sleep effect on upper airway mechanics and associated decrease in ventilation.

The loss of wakefulness stimulus to breathe renders ventilation during NREM sleep critically dependent on chemoreceptor stimuli (Pa_{O_2} and Pa_{CO_2}). Reduced Pa_{CO_2} is a powerful inhibitory factor of ventilation during sleep. Therefore, central apnea develops when Pa_{CO_2} is reduced below a highly reproducible hypocapnic apneic threshold, unmasked by NREM sleep (Fig. 1.4) [5]. Hypocapnia is probably the most important inhibitory factor during NREM sleep. Hypocapnia, secondary to hyperventilation, is key to the genesis of central sleep apnea in congestive heart failure [16], and idiopathic central sleep apnea [17, 18], and may be relevant to the pathogenesis of obstructive sleep apnea (OSA) as well [19–21].

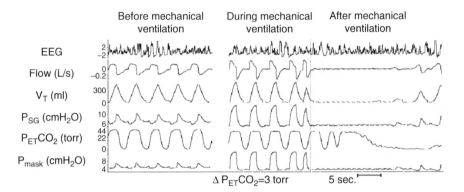

Fig. 1.4 Induced hypocapnic central apnea during NREM sleep. Nasal mechanical ventilation was used to decrease end-tidal P_{CO_2} ($P_{ET}CO_2$). Cessation of mechanical ventilation caused central apnea. P_{sg}, supraglottic pressure; P_{mask}, mask pressure

Effect of Sleep on Upper-Airway Structure and Function

The sleep state is a challenge, rather than a rest period, for the ventilatory system. Consequences of loss of wakefulness include reduced activity of upper-airway dilators, reduced upper-airway caliber, increased upper-airway resistance, loss of load compensation, and increased pharyngeal compliance and collapsibility. Ultimately, these changes lead to reduced tidal volume and hypoventilation.

The musculature of the upper airway consists of 24 pairs of striated muscles extending from the nares to the larynx [22, 23]. There are at least 10 muscles that are classified as pharyngeal dilators. There are two patterns of electrical discharge from these muscles: tonic (constant) activity, independent of phase of respiration, and phasic activity, occurring during one part of the respiratory cycle. It is widely accepted that upper-airway narrowing during sleep is due to a sleep-related decrease in upper-airway muscle activity. During NREM sleep, available evidence indicates a reduction in either the tonic or phasic activity during NREM sleep for a variety of upper-airway muscles [23], including the levator palatini [24], tensor palatini [25], palatoglossus [24], and geniohyoid [26]. The effect of REM sleep on upper-airway muscle activity is more compelling, with strong evidence that activity of phasic upper-airway dilating muscles, such as the genioglossus, is greatly attenuated during REM sleep [27, 28], particularly during periods of phasic rapid eye movements [29, 30].

The response of upper-airway muscle to chemical and mechanical perturbations may be more relevant physiologically than reduced baseline activity. Pharyngeal muscles display an attenuated response to negative pressure during NREM [31–33] and REM sleep [34] compared to wakefulness. Similarly, responsiveness of the genioglossus muscle to hypercapnia is also attenuated during sleep [35]. Decreased responsiveness to challenges indicates that upper-airway muscles are less able to maintain upper-airway patency in the face of chemical or mechanical perturbations.

The evidence for increased upper-airway resistance during sleep is compelling, even in normal subjects [36–39]. The preponderance of evidence is that there are no further increases in upper-airway resistance as subjects transition from NREM to REM sleep [38–40]. However, it is important to note that upper-airway resistance provides only a partial picture of the dynamic behavior of the pharyngeal airway during sleep. Specifically, upper-airway resistance is generally expressed as a single number representing the slope of pressure-flow relationship during inspiration. This computation is predicated on a constant relationship between driving pressure and inspiratory flow, which is true during normal breathing in normal subjects. However, many subjects exhibit inspiratory-flow limitation, in which the pressure-flow graph demonstrates a changing relationship culminating in complete dissociation between pressure and flow (pressure continues to decrease with no further increase in flow). While many authors equate increased upper airway resistance to increased collapsibility, it is in reality a rather limited surrogate for susceptibility to pharyngeal closure during sleep [41].

Using nasopharyngoscopy during naturally occurring sleep in normal subjects, Rowley et al. have shown that pharyngeal cross-sectional area is decreased during sleep at both the retropalatal and retroglossal levels [38, 39]. During NREM sleep, both retropalatal cross-sectional area and retroglossal cross-sectional area decreased to ~70% of the awake baseline cross-sectional area. The decreased cross-sectional area is consistent with a decrease in upper-airway dilator activity with the onset of NREM sleep. In REM sleep, retropalatal cross-sectional area did not decrease further compared to NREM sleep [38]. In contrast, retroglossal cross-sectional area did decrease further during REM compared to NREM sleep [39].

The ability of the ventilatory control system to compensate for changes in resistance is essential for the preservation of alveolar ventilation. Increased resistance is an example of resistive load, leading, during wakefulness, to increased effort to maintain ventilation and $Paco_2$. In contrast, hypoventilation occurs immediately upon imposing a resistive load during NREM sleep, perhaps implying that loads are not perceived during sleep [42]. Therefore, resistive loading results in decreased tidal volume and minute ventilation and, hence, alveolar hypoventilation. The ensuing elevation of arterial $Paco_2$ restores ventilation toward normal levels. Teleologically, failure to respond to loads preserves sleep continuity. The cost of allowing sleep continuity is a mild elevation of $Paco_2$. In fact, elevated $Paco_2$ during sleep is one of few physiologic situations where hypercapnia is tolerated.

The walls of the pharyngeal airway consist of compliant soft tissue structures, amenable to changes in pressure during the respiratory cycle. During wakefulness, upper-airway caliber is constant during inspiration, with a decreased caliber during expiration, returning to inspiratory values at end-expiration. This finding has been observed in both normal subjects [43, 44] and patients with sleep apnea [44] using either computerized tomographic (CT) scanning or nasopharyngoscopy. Using nasopharyngoscopy, NREM sleep was associated with significant dynamic within-breath changes in cross-sectional area, reaching a nadir at midinspiration [44], with a rapid increase in cross-sectional area during expiration [20].

The dynamic changes in upper-airway patency during sleep can be best investigated using compliance as a measurement. Traditionally, compliance is the change in volume for a given change in pressure. Compliance of the pharyngeal wall is an important modulator of the effect of pressure changes on upper-airway patency. Traditionally, upper-airway compliance has been measured in a static fashion by measuring changes in cross-sectional area at different levels of pressure applied to the upper airway [45–47]. Use of this technique has demonstrated that compliance is increased as the pharyngeal caliber decreases [45, 46, 48]. In contrast, we have combined measurement of cross-sectional area via fiberoptic nasopharyngoscopy and measurement of intraluminal pressure at the same level during NREM and REM sleep. These studies have confirmed that retropalatal compliance is increased during NREM sleep compared to wakefulness; in contrast, retropalatal compliance during REM sleep is similar to that in wakefulness [39]. At the retroglossal level, however, compliance was not increased during either NREM or REM sleep compared to wakefulness [38]. Thus, pharyngeal compliance was not increased, despite the known absence of upper-airway muscle activity during REM sleep.

Collapsibility refers to the propensity of the upper airway to collapse or obstruct under certain conditions. While often used interchangeably with compliance, it differs from compliance in that compliance measures the changes in upper-airway area for given changes in pressure and not the propensity to collapse. Upper-airway collapsibility has been primarily measured using the critical closing pressure or P_{crit}.

Measurement of critical closing pressure or P_{crit} is based upon the concept of the Starling resistor (Fig. 1.5) [49]. In a Starling resistor, maximal flow through the resistor is dependent upon the resistance of the segment upstream and the pressure surrounding the collapsible segment. In normal subjects, the application of progressively negative nasal pressure (upstream pressure) results in inspiratory-flow limitation, followed by complete upper-airway obstruction [50]. Thus, this model of upper-airway mechanics has several advantages as a method to study upper-airway collapsibility. First, it most closely approximates the inspiratory-flow limitation that characterizes the breathing of many subjects with snoring. Second, the model allows a functional approach to the upper airway, which is key, given the complicated anatomy of the upper airway.

Applying this model to humans, it has been shown that across the spectrum of sleep-disordered breathing, active P_{crit} becomes progressively more positive, indicative of increased propensity for airway collapse [50–52]. For instance, Pcrit in normal subjects is generally <10 cmH$_2$O while in patients with predominant hypopneas it is between 0 and −5 cmH$_2$O and in patients with predominant apneas it is >0 cmH$_2$O. Kirkness et al. found that in a group of 166 men and women with and without sleep-disordered breathing, passive Pcrit is higher in men and increases with increasing age and BMI [53]. In addition, in these studies sleep apnea was largely absent in subjects with a passive or active Pcrit more negative than −5 cmH$_2$O [53, 54].

Since gender and aging are important influences on the prevalence of obstructive sleep apnea, the influence of gender and aging on upper airway function has been explored. With regard to upper airway reflexes, no gender differences in the upper

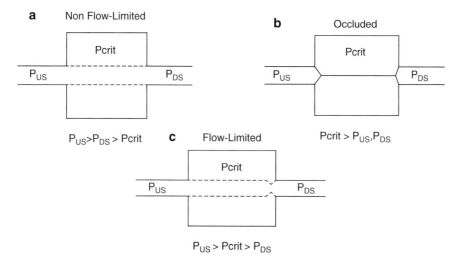

Fig. 1.5 Starling resistor model of the upper airway. In a Starling resistor there is a collapsible segment surrounded by an upstream and downstream non-collapsible segments. In this model, P_{crit} is assumed to be equal to the pressure surrounding airway. P_{US}, upstream (nasopharyngeal) pressure; P_{DS}: downstream (hypopharyngeal) pressure. In A, both the P_{US} and P_{DS} are greater than Pcrit, the airway is wide open and flow will be proportional to the difference between P_{US} and P_{DS}. In B, the Pcrit is greater than both P_{US} and P_{DS}, the airway is closed, and there is no flow. In C, P_{US} is greater than Pcrit but Pcrit is greater than P_{DS}, creating a condition of flow limitation; flow is proportional to the difference between P_{US} and Pcrit

airway negative pressure reflex were found during wakefulness [55]. However, the influence of gender on this reflex during sleep has not been studied. With regard to inspiratory loading, Pillar et al. performed a study comparing the inspiratory loading response during sleep in 16 normal men and women that were matched for age and body mass index [56]. They found that pharyngeal resistance increased more in men than women, suggesting increased upper airway collapse. However, there was no difference in the activity of the genioglossus or tensor palatini muscles to inspiratory loading. There was also no gender difference in central drive, suggesting that gender differences in upper airway anatomy or tissue characteristics, rather than upper airway reflexes, better explain changes in upper airway resistance during sleep. Finally, gender differences in Pcrit have been studied by two groups. Rowley et al. found no difference in Pcrit in a group of young, healthy men and women without sleep-disordered breathing. In contrast, Kirkness et al. found, in a group that included individuals with and without sleep-disordered breathing, that men had a higher Pcrit than women, suggesting a higher propensity for upper airway collapse.

There are a limited number of studies on the influence of aging on upper airway physiology. With regard to reflexes, the genioglossal reflex to negative pressure was studied in a group of 38 men and women during wakefulness and found that the reflex response decreased with age in the total group [57]. However, this effect of aging was only significant in men, not in women. The influence of aging on this reflex has not been studied during sleep. Another group compared the genioglossus EMG response to hypoxia in a group of younger (20–40 years) compared to older (41–60 years) subjects and found that the genioglossus response to hypoxia was decreased in the older subjects [58]. These studies show that upper airway reflexes are decreased in older subjects than younger subjects and could explain, in part, age-related changes in upper airway collapsibility. With regard to collapsibility, the aforementioned Kirkness study included an analysis of aging and found that Pcrit increased with increasing age. However, this change in Pcrit with aging was seen only in post-menopausal women, not men or pre-menopausal women.

Cardiovascular Function During Sleep

NREM sleep is characterized by autonomic stability, driven by increased vagal nerve activity and parasympathetic tone when compared to wakefulness. The increased vagal activity results in an overall decrease in heart rate during NREM sleep and frequent sinus arrhythmia coupled to respiratory variation. In sinus arrhythmia, there is an increase in heart rate during inspiration to accommodate increased venous return with a decrease in heart rate during expiration. Because of the increased vagal tone, NREM sleep is associated with an decrease in heart rate variability compared to wakefulness [59, 60]. In addition, NREM sleep is associated with a decrease in cardiac output and an ~10% decrease in blood pressure [61, 62]. Loss of the usual nocturnal decrease in blood pressure is frequently seen in patients with obstructive sleep apnea [62, 63]. Finally, NREM sleep is associated with decrements in both global cerebral blood flow and metabolism, both of which are particularly decreased during slow-wave sleep [64–66].

In contrast, during REM sleep, heart rate becomes increasingly variable with transient increases in heart rate in association with the rapid eye movements. These transient increases in heart rate are not observed following interruption of sympathetic neural output to the heart in animals, suggesting that the surges in heart rate are sympathetically driven [67]. In addition, heart rate variability is increased in REM sleep compared to NREM sleep [60, 68]. In association with the transient increases in heart rate, there are also transient increases in blood pressure. Both the heart rate and blood pressure may approach those observed during wakefulness. Finally, in contrast to NREM sleep, global cerebral blood flow and metabolism are unchanged compared to wakefulness in REM sleep [66]. However, there is evidence that there are significant regional differences in cerebral blood flow during REM sleep, with increased blood flow to areas of the brain associated with the generation of REM sleep such as the brainstem and thalamus with continued decreased blood flow to other areas such as the pre-frontal and fronto-parietal cortices [64, 69].

Endocrine Function During Sleep

The levels of circulating endocrine hormones are generally influenced either by circadian rhythms or the sleep-wake cycle [70, 71]. Growth hormone and prolactin are examples of hormones whose circulating levels are related to the sleep-wake cycle. Growth hormone secretion is tightly related to the sleep-wake cycle; when the sleep period is shifted, the major growth hormone pulse is also shifted and the growth hormone secretion is absent in sleep deprivation. Maximal growth hormone secretion is during slow-wave sleep, though this pattern is more generally observed in men than women. While prolactin levels generally increase in the afternoon after the usual nadir at noon, there is a major elevation in prolactin levels shortly after sleep onset. In addition, during naps, there is a generally a pulse of prolactin activity irrespective of the time of day.

Adreno-corticotrophic hormone and cortisol follow a circadian pattern. Levels of these hormones are generally increased in the later part of the night and are maximal in the early morning; levels then decline through the day with minimal levels generally around midnight.

Circulating levels of thyroid-stimulating hormone (TSH) are influenced by both circadian rhythms and the sleep-wake cycle. TSH levels are low during the day and increase in the evening under circadian influences. With sleep onset, levels decrease with the inhibitory influence primarily noted during slow-wave sleep. Consistent with the sleep-wake cycle influence, TSH levels continue to increase during sleep deprivation.

Gonadotrophic hormones, including both luteinizing hormone (LH) and follicular stimulating hormone (FHS), appear to be influenced by both circadian rhythm and sleep-wake state. However, the secretion of these hormones also vary by gender and stage of life. Both LH and FSH demonstrate pulsatile increases in children at sleep onset. The amplitude of these pulses increases at puberty; however, the daytime pulse amplitude also increases, and the diurnal rhythm is diminished during puberty. In men, this leads to a diurnal rhythm in testosterone, with minimal levels in late evening and maximal levels in early morning (with the increases possibly linked to REM sleep as well). In older men, the LH pulses decrease further but the circadian variation of testosterone remains, though dampened. In women, the 24-hour variation in plasma LH varies during the menstrual cycle. While levels are elevated in post-menopausal women, there is no clear circadian rhythm.

Leptin and ghrelin are hormones important to energy balance with leptin promoting satiety while ghrelin stimulates appetite. Ghrelin appears to be related to sleep-wake state with levels typically increasing in the first half of the night while decreasing in the second half. Leptin also peaks during the night with a nadir in early afternoon. Increases in both hormones have been linked to increases in slow-wave sleep.

Gastrointestinal Function During Sleep

The effects of sleep on the gastrointestinal system are driven by a variety of processes, including increased parasympathetic activity and circadian rhythms [72]. An example of decreased parasympathetic activity is the observed decrease in salivation during sleep. In contrast, basal gastric acid secretion follows a circadian rhythm, with peak secretion between 10 pm and 2 am and relative absence of basal secretion in the absence of meal simulation [73]. However, there is evidence that the increased gastric acid secretion is not associated with nadirs in gastric pH, which has been shown to be lower in awake patients than during NREM and REM sleep [74].

Sleep also effects the mobility of the gastrointestinal tract. The frequency of swallowing decreases significantly during sleep while there is also evidence of decreased esophageal peristaltic waves during NREM sleep [72, 75]. Traditionally, it has been believed that upper esophageal sphincter tone is unchanged during sleep while lower esophageal sphincter tone is decreased. However, recent data indicate that upper sphincter tone is more vulnerable to decreased tone during sleep with a smaller change in the lower esophageal sphincter tone, which generally stays greater than intragastric pressure [75–77]. Finally, there is evidence that the phasic myoelectrical activity and motor function of the stomach and intestines is decreased during sleep, with some evidence that the decrease could be in part circadian in origin [72, 75, 78, 79].

One of the major effects of the changes in gastrointestinal function during sleep is increased acid contact time [80]. Generally, during wakefulness, gastroesophageal reflux is a post-prandial event and acid is rapidly cleared from the esophagus because of increased salivary gland secretion, increased swallowing and primary peristalsis. While GER events are less frequent during sleep, events are associated with decreased acid clearance and increased acid contact time because of the sleep-related decreases in salivation, swallowing, and peristalsis. In addition, heartburn is a waking conscious phenomenon and this sensation is generally absent during sleep. Increased acid contact time has been shown to be related to proximal migration of refluxed gastric contents [81] and is a potential mechanism for the development of esophagitis, chronic cough, and exacerbations of bronchial asthma [82].

Renal Function During Sleep

Urine formation decreases during sleep compared to wakefulness. Both glomerular filtration rate and effective renal plasma flow [83, 84] and the urinary excretion of sodium and potassium [84, 85] have been found to be maximal during wakefulness with decreases during sleep; however, this is not a universal finding [86]. Water reabsorption also increases during sleep, likely due to changes in the renin-aldosterone levels. Studies have shown that both renin and aldosterone are increased during sleep, with a shift in the peak increase with a shift in the sleep schedule [87, 88]. In addition, cortisol appears to exert a circadian rhythm effect on aldosterone, as daytime oscillations in aldosterone are associated with daytime oscillations in cortisol [88]. The importance of sleep to urinary function is becoming increasingly evident as studies have shown that sleep deprivation is associated with larger declines in renal function in both normal subjects [89] and patients with chronic kidney disease [90].

References

1. Silber MH, Ancoli-Israel S, Bonnet MH, Chokroverty S, Grigg-Damberger MM, Hirshkowitz M, Kapen S, Keenan SA, Kryger MH, Penzel T, Pressman MR, Iber C. The visual scoring of sleep in adults. J Clin Sleep Med. 2007;3:121–31.
2. Berry RB, Quan SF, Abreu AR, Del Rosso L, Mao M, Plante D, Pressman MR, Troester D, Vaughn BV. The AASM manual for the scoring of sleep and associated events: rules, terminology and technical specifications. Darien: American Academy of Sleep Medicine; 2020.
3. Ohayon MM, Carskadon MA, Guilleminault C, Vitiello MV. Meta-analysis of quantitative sleep parameters from childhood to old age in healthy individuals: developing normative sleep values across the human lifespan. Sleep. 2004;27:1255–73.
4. Redline S, Kirchner HL, Quan SF, Gottlieb DJ, Kapur V, Newman A. The effects of age, sex, ethnicity, and sleep-disordered breathing on sleep architecture. Arch Intern Med. 2004;164:406–18.
5. Skatrud JB, Dempsey JA. Interaction of sleep state and chemical stimuli in sustaining rhythmic ventilation. J Appl Physiol. 1983;55:813–22.
6. Berthon-Jones M, Sullivan CE. Ventilation and arousal responses to hypercapnia in normal sleeping humans. J Appl Physiol. 1984;57:59–67.
7. Davis JN, Loh L, Nodal J, Charnock M. Effects of sleep on the pattern of CO2 stimulated breathing in males and females. Adv Exp Med Biol. 1978;99:79–83.
8. Douglas NJ, White DP, Weil JV, Pickett CK, Zwillich CW. Hypercapnic ventilatory response in sleeping adults. Am Rev Respir Dis. 1982;126:758–62.
9. Gothe B, Altose MD, Goldman MD, Cherniack NS. Effect of quiet sleep on resting and CO2-stimulated breathing in humans. J Appl Physiol. 1981;50:724–30.
10. Hedemark LL, Kronenberg RS. Ventilatory and heart rate responses to hypoxia and hypercapnia during sleep in adults. J Appl Physiol. 1982;53:307–12.
11. Browne HA, Adams L, Simonds AK, Morrell MJ. Ageing does not influence the sleep-related decrease in the hypercapnic ventilatory response. Eur Respir J. 2003;21:523–9.
12. Morrell MJ, Harty HR, Adams L, Guz A. Changes in total pulmonary resistance and PCO2 between wakefulness and sleep in normal human subjects. J Appl Physiol. 1995;78:1339–49.
13. Berthon-Jones M, Sullivan CE. Ventilatory and arousal responses to hypoxia in sleeping humans. Am Rev Respir Dis. 1982;125:632–9.
14. Douglas NJ, White DP, Weil JV, Pickett CK, Martin RJ, Hudgel DW, Zwillich CW. Hypoxic ventilatory response decreases during sleep in normal men. Am Rev Respir Dis. 1982;125:286–9.
15. White DP, Douglas NJ, Pickett CK, Weil JV, Zwillich CW. Hypoxic ventilatory response during sleep in normal premenopausal women. Am Rev Respir Dis. 1982;126:530–3.
16. Xie A, Skatrud JB, Puleo DS, Rahko PS, Dempsey JA. Apnea-hypopnea threshold for CO2 in patients with congestive heart failure. Am J Respir Crit Care Med. 2002;165:1245–50.
17. Xie A, Rutherford R, Rankin F, Wong B, Bradley TD. Hypocapnia and increased ventilatory responsiveness in patients with idiopathic central sleep apnea. Am J Respir Crit Care Med. 1995;152:1950–5.

18. Xie A, Wong B, Phillipson EA, Slutsky AS, Bradley TD. Interaction of hyperventilation and arousal in the pathogenesis of idiopathic central sleep apnea. Am J Respir Crit Care Med. 1994;150:489–95.
19. Badr MS, Toiber F, Skatrud JB, Dempsey J. Pharyngeal narrowing/occlusion during central sleep apnea. J Appl Physiol. 1995;78:1806–15.
20. Sankri-Tarbichi AG, Rowley JA, Badr MS. Expiratory pharyngeal narrowing during central hypocapnic hypopnea. Am J Respir Crit Care Med. 2009;179:313–9.
21. Salloum A, Rowley JA, Mateika JH, Chowdhuri S, Omran Q, Badr MS. Increased propensity for central apnea in patients with obstructive sleep apnea: effect of nCPAP. Am J Respir Crit Care Med. 2010;181(2):189–93.
22. van Lunteren E, Strohl KP. The muscles of the upper airways. Clin Chest Med. 1986;7:171–88.
23. Horner RL. Motor control of the pharyngeal musculature and implications for the pathogenesis of obstructive sleep apnea. Sleep. 1996;19:827–53.
24. Tangel DJ, Mezzanotte WS, White DP. Influences of NREM sleep on activity of palatoglossus and levator palatini muscles in normal men. J Appl Physiol. 1995;78:689–95.
25. Tangel DJ, Mezzanotte WS, White DP. Influence of sleep on tensor palatini EMG and upper airway resistance in normal men. J Appl Physiol. 1991;70:2574–81.
26. Wiegand DA, Latz B, Zwillich CW, Wiegand L. Geniohyoid muscle activity in normal men during wakefulness and sleep. J Appl Physiol. 1990;69:1262–9.
27. Sauerland EK, Harper RM. The human tongue during sleep: electromyographic activity of the genioglossus muscle. Exp Neurol. 1976;51:160–70.
28. Sauerland EK, Orr WC, Hairston LE. EMG patterns of oropharyngeal muscles during respiration in wakefulness and sleep. Electromyogr Clin Neurophysiol. 1981;21:307–16.
29. Wiegand L, Zwillich CW, Wiegand D, White DP. Changes in upper airway muscle activation and ventilation during phasic REM sleep in normal men. J Appl Physiol. 1991;71:488–97.
30. Eckert DJ, Malhotra A, Lo YL, White DP, Jordan AS. The influence of obstructive sleep apnea and gender on genioglossus activity during rapid eye movement sleep. Chest. 2009;135:957–64.
31. Horner RL, Innes JA, Murphy K, Guz A. Evidence for reflex upper airway dilator muscle activation by sudden negative airway pressure in man. J Physiol. 1991;436:15–29.
32. Wheatley JR, Mezzanotte WS, Tangel DJ, White DP. Influence of sleep on genioglossus muscle activation by negative pressure in normal men. Am Rev Respir Dis. 1993;148:597–605.
33. Wheatley JR, Tangel DJ, Mezzanotte WS, White DP. Influence of sleep on response to negative airway pressure of tensor palatini muscle and retropalatal airway. J Appl Physiol. 1993;75:2117–24.
34. Shea SA, Edwards JK, White DP. Effect of wake-sleep transitions and rapid eye movement sleep on pharyngeal muscle response to negative pressure in humans. J Physiol. 1999;520(Pt 3):897–908.
35. Stanchina ML, Malhotra A, Fogel RB, Ayas N, Edwards JK, Schory K, White DP. Genioglossus muscle responsiveness to chemical and mechanical stimuli during non-rapid eye movement sleep. Am J Respir Crit Care Med. 2002;165:945–9.
36. Kay A, Trinder J, Bowes G, Kim Y. Changes in airway resistance during sleep onset. J Appl Physiol. 1994;76:1600–7.
37. Kay A, Trinder J, Kim Y. Progressive changes in airway resistance during sleep. J Appl Physiol. 1996;81:282–92.
38. Rowley JA, Sanders CS, Zahn BR, Badr MS. Effect of REM sleep on retroglossal cross-sectional area and compliance in normal subjects. J Appl Physiol. 2001;91:239–48.
39. Rowley JA, Zahn BR, Babcock MA, Badr MS. The effect of rapid eye movement (REM) sleep on upper airway mechanics in normal human subjects. J Physiol. 1998;510(Pt 3):963–76.
40. Thurnheer R, Wraith PK, Douglas NJ. Influence of age and gender on upper airway resistance in NREM and REM sleep. J Appl Physiol. 2001;90:981–8.
41. Rowley JA, Deebajah I, Parikh S, Najar A, Saha R, Badr MS. The influence of episodic hypoxia on upper airway collapsibility in subjects with obstructive sleep apnea. J Appl Physiol. 2007;103:911–6.

42. Wiegand L, Zwillich CW, White DP. Sleep and the ventilatory response to resistive loading in normal men. J Appl Physiol. 1988;64:1186–95.
43. Schwab RJ, Gefter WB, Hoffman EA, Gupta KB, Pack AI. Dynamic upper airway imaging during awake respiration in normal subjects and patients with sleep disordered breathing. Am Rev Respir Dis. 1993;148:1385–400.
44. Morrell MJ, Badr MS. Effects of NREM sleep on dynamic within-breath changes in upper airway patency in humans. J Appl Physiol. 1998;84:190–9.
45. Isono S, Morrison DL, Launois SH, Feroah TR, Whitelaw WA, Remmers JE. Static mechanics of the velopharynx of patients with obstructive sleep apnea. J Appl Physiol. 1993;75:148–54.
46. Isono S, Remmers JE, Tanaka A, Sho Y, Sato J, Nishino T. Anatomy of pharynx in patients with obstructive sleep apnea and in normal subjects. J Appl Physiol. 1997;82:1319–26.
47. Kuna ST, Bedi DG, Ryckman C. Effect of nasal airway positive pressure on upper airway size and configuration. Am Rev Respir Dis. 1988;138:969–75.
48. Isono S, Feroah TR, Hajduk EA, Brant R, Whitelaw WA, Remmers JE. Interaction of cross-sectional area, driving pressure, and airflow of passive velopharynx. J Appl Physiol. 1997;83:851–9.
49. Gold AR, Schwartz AR. The pharyngeal critical pressure. The whys and hows of using nasal continuous positive airway pressure diagnostically. Chest. 1996;110:1077–88.
50. Schwartz AR, Smith PL, Wise RA, Gold AR, Permutt S. Induction of upper airway occlusion in sleeping individuals with subatmospheric nasal pressure. J Appl Physiol. 1988;64:535–42.
51. Gold AR, Marcus CL, Dipalo F, Gold MS. Upper airway collapsibility during sleep in upper airway resistance syndrome. Chest. 2002;121:1531–40.
52. Gleadhill IC, Schwartz AR, Schubert N, Wise RA, Permutt S, Smith PL. Upper airway collapsibility in snorers and in patients with obstructive hypopnea and apnea. Am Rev Respir Dis. 1991;143:1300–3.
53. Kirkness JP, Schwartz AR, Schneider H, Punjabi NM, Maly JJ, Laffan AM, McGinley BM, Magnuson T, Schweitzer M, Smith PL, Patil SP. Contribution of male sex, age, and obesity to mechanical instability of the upper airway during sleep. J Appl Physiol. 2008;104:1618–24.
54. Patil SP, Schneider H, Marx JJ, Gladmon E, Schwartz AR, Smith PL. Neuromechanical control of upper airway patency during sleep. J Appl Physiol. 2007;102:547–56.
55. White DP, Edwards JK, Shea SA. Local reflex mechanisms: influence on basal genioglossal muscle activation in normal subjects. Sleep. 1998;21:719–28.
56. Pillar G, Malhotra A, Fogel R, Beauregard J, Schnall R, White DP. Airway mechanics and ventilation in response to resistive loading during sleep: influence of gender. Am J Respir Crit Care Med. 2000;162:1627–32.
57. Malhotra A, Huang Y, Fogel R, Lazic S, Pillar G, Jakab M, Kikinis R, White DP. Aging influences on pharyngeal anatomy and physiology: the predisposition to pharyngeal collapse. Am J Med. 2006;119:72–14.
58. Klawe JJ, Tafil-Klawe M. Age-related response of the genioglossus muscle EMG-activity to hypoxia in humans. J Physiol Pharmacol. 2003;54(Suppl 1):14–9.
59. Penzel T, Kantelhardt JW, Grote L, Peter JH, Bunde A. Comparison of detrended fluctuation analysis and spectral analysis for heart rate variability in sleep and sleep apnea. IEEE Trans Biomed Eng. 2003;50:1143–51.
60. Vanoli E, Adamson PB, Ba L, Pinna GD, Lazzara R, Orr WC. Heart rate variability during specific sleep stages. A comparison of healthy subjects with patients after myocardial infarction. Circulation. 1995;91:1918–22.
61. Veerman DP, Imholz BP, Wieling W, Wesseling KH, van Montfrans GA. Circadian profile of systemic hemodynamics. Hypertension. 1995;26:55–9.
62. Suzuki M, Guilleminault C, Otsuka K, Shiomi T. Blood pressure "dipping" and "non-dipping" in obstructive sleep apnea syndrome patients. Sleep. 1996;19:382–7.
63. Loredo JS, ncoli-Israel S, Dimsdale JE. Sleep quality and blood pressure dipping in obstructive sleep apnea. Am J Hypertens. 2001;14:887–92.

64. Braun AR, Balkin TJ, Wesenten NJ, Carson RE, Varga M, Baldwin P, Selbie S, Belenky G, Herscovitch P. Regional cerebral blood flow throughout the sleep-wake cycle. An H2(15)O PET study. Brain. 1997;120(Pt 7):1173–97.

65. Madsen PL, Schmidt JF, Holm S, Vorstrup S, Lassen NA, Wildschiodtz G. Cerebral oxygen metabolism and cerebral blood flow in man during light sleep (stage 2). Brain Res. 1991;557:217–20.

66. Madsen PL, Schmidt JF, Wildschiodtz G, Friberg L, Holm S, Vorstrup S, Lassen NA. Cerebral O2 metabolism and cerebral blood flow in humans during deep and rapid-eye-movement sleep. J Appl Physiol. 1991;70:2597–601.

67. Kirby DA, Verrier RL. Differential effects of sleep stage on coronary hemodynamic function. Am J Physiol. 1989;256:H1378–83.

68. Cajochen C, Pischke J, Aeschbach D, Borbely AA. Heart rate dynamics during human sleep. Physiol Behav. 1994;55:769–74.

69. Madsen PL, Holm S, Vorstrup S, Friberg L, Lassen NA, Wildschiodtz G. Human regional cerebral blood flow during rapid-eye-movement sleep. J Cereb Blood Flow Metab. 1991;11:502–7.

70. Collop NA, Salas RE, Delayo M, Gamaldo C. Normal sleep and circadian processes. Crit Care Clin. 2008;24:449–60, v.

71. Leproult R, Spiegel K, van Cauter E. Sleep and endocrinology. In: Amlaner CJ, Fuller PM, editors. Basics of sleep guide. 2nd ed. Westchester: Sleep Research Society; 2009. p. 157–63.

72. Orr WC, Fass R, Sundaram SS, Scheimann AO. The effect of sleep on gastrointestinal functioning in common digestive diseases. Lancet Gastroenterol Hepatol. 2020;5:616–24.

73. Moore JG Jr, EE. Circadian rhythm of gastric acid secretion in man. Nature. 1970;226:1261–2.

74. Khanijow V, Prakash P, Emsellem HA, Borum ML, Doman DB. Sleep dysfunction and gastrointestinal diseases. Gastroenterol Hepatol (N Y). 2015;11:817–25.

75. Kanaly T, Shaheen NJ, Vaughn BV. Gastrointestinal physiology and digestive disorders in sleep. Curr Opin Pulm Med. 2009;15:571–7.

76. Bajaj JS, Bajaj S, Dua KS, Jaradeh S, Rittmann T, Hofmann C, Shaker R. Influence of sleep stages on esophago-upper esophageal sphincter contractile reflex and secondary esophageal peristalsis. Gastroenterology. 2006;130:17–25.

77. Eastwood PR, Katagiri S, Shepherd KL, Hillman DR. Modulation of upper and lower esophageal sphincter tone during sleep. Sleep Med. 2007;8:135–43.

78. Kumar D, Idzikowski C, Wingate DL, Soffer EE, Thompson P, Siderfin C. Relationship between enteric migrating motor complex and the sleep cycle. Am J Physiol. 1990;259:G983–90.

79. Soffer EE, Adrian TE, Launspach J, Zimmerman B. Meal-induced secretion of gastrointestinal regulatory peptides is not affected by sleep. Neurogastroenterol Motil. 1997;9:7–12.

80. Orr WC. Esophageal function during sleep: another danger in the night. Sleep Med. 2007;8:105–6.

81. Orr WC, Elsenbruch S, Harnish MJ, Johnson LF. Proximal migration of esophageal acid perfusions during waking and sleep. Am J Gastroenterol. 2000;95:37–42.

82. Orr WC, Chen CL. Sleep and the gastrointestinal tract. Neurol Clin. 2005;23:1007–24.

83. Voogel AJ, Koopman MG, Hart AA, van Montfrans GA, Arisz L. Circadian rhythms in systemic hemodynamics and renal function in healthy subjects and patients with nephrotic syndrome. Kidney Int. 2001;59:1873–80.

84. Koopman MG, Koomen GC, Krediet RT, de Moor EA, Hoek FJ, Arisz L. Circadian rhythm of glomerular filtration rate in normal individuals. Clin Sci (Lond). 1989;77:105–11.

85. Staessen JA, Birkenhager W, Bulpitt CJ, Fagard R, Fletcher AE, Lijnen P, Thijs L, Amery A. The relationship between blood pressure and sodium and potassium excretion during the day and at night. J Hypertens. 1993;11:443–7.

86. Pechere-Bertschi A, Nussberger J, Biollaz J, Fahti M, Grouzmann E, Morgan T, Brunner HR, Burnier M. Circadian variations of renal sodium handling in patients with orthostatic hypotension. Kidney Int. 1998;54:1276–82.

87. Brandenberger G, Charifi C, Muzet A, Saini J, Simon C, Follenius M. Renin as a biological marker of the NREM-REM sleep cycle: effect of REM sleep suppression. J Sleep Res. 1994;3:30–5.
88. Charloux A, Gronfier C, Lonsdorfer-Wolf E, Piquard F, Brandenberger G. Aldosterone release during the sleep-wake cycle in humans. Am J Physiol. 1999;276:E43–9.
89. McMullan CJ, Curhan GC, Forman JP. Association of short sleep duration and rapid decline in renal function. Kidney Int. 2016;89:1324–30.
90. Ricardo AC, Knutson K, Chen J, Appel LJ, Bazzano L, Carmona-Powell E, Cohan J, Kurella Tamura M, Steigerwalt S, Thornton JD, Weir M, Turek NF, Rahman M, Van Cauter E, Lash JP, Chronic Renal Insufficiency Cohort Study Investigators. The association of sleep duration and quality with CKD progression. J Am Soc Nephrol. 2017;28:3708–15.

Chapter 2
Pharmacology of Sleep

Janet H. Dailey and Susmita Chowdhuri

Keywords GABA γ(gamma)-aminobutyric acid · Histamine-3 inverse agonist · Benzodiazepines · Nonbenzodiazepine receptor agonists · Melatonin and melatonin receptor agonist: ramelteon · Orexin antagonists: suvorexant and lemborexant · Antidepressants, low-dose doxepin · Antipsychotics · Antihistamines · Amphetamines · Methylphenidate · Modafinil · Armodafinil · Sodium oxybate · Solriamfetol · Pitolisant

Introduction

Drugs that modulate sleep and wakefulness operate by modifying a complex network of sleep–wake neurotransmitters and neuromodulators in multiple locations in the brain. The pharmacologic agents used to treat two common sleep disorders, chronic insomnia and disorders of central hypersomnia, i.e., narcolepsy and idiopathic hypersomnia, are reviewed with emphasis on current updates. Several drugs target one or more of the sleep or wake–sleep-promoting neurotransmitters and neuromodulators [1], to treat insomnia and excessive daytime sleepiness, respectively.

J. H. Dailey
Pharmacy Benefits Management Services, Veterans Health Administration, Washington, D.C, USA
e-mail: Janet.Dailey@va.gov

S. Chowdhuri (✉)
Sleep Medicine Section, Medical Service John D. Dingell VA Medical Center, Detroit, MI, USA

Department of Medicine, Wayne State University, Detroit, MI, USA
e-mail: schowdh@med.wayne.edu

© Springer Nature Switzerland AG 2022
M. S. Badr, J. L. Martin (eds.), *Essentials of Sleep Medicine*,
Respiratory Medicine, https://doi.org/10.1007/978-3-030-93739-3_2

Nonpharmacologic therapies of these disorders and drugs indicated for other sleep disorders and recreational drugs that affect sleep will not be reviewed.

Sleep-promoting Drugs

Overall, drugs that are *agonistic* to the sleep-promoting GABA (γ(gamma)-aminobutyric acid) receptor or *antagonistic* to the wake-promoting neurotransmitters, norepinephrine, serotonin, histamine, acetylcholine, dopamine, and orexin are potentially sleep promoting. The major sleep-promoting region is located in the GABAergic ventrolateral preoptic (VLPO) nucleus of the hypothalamus. Conversely, inhibition of the wake-promoting regions of the brain, including the orexinergic lateral hypothalamus, histaminergic tuberomammillary nucleus, cholinergic pedunculopontine, lateral dorsal tegmental nuclei, noradrenergic locus coeruleus, serotonergic raphe nuclei, and the dopaminergic ventral tegmental area, could potentially promote sleep onset and maintenance [1].

Most hypnotics potentiate sleep via GABA by binding to the $GABA_A$ receptor [2] while others antagonize monoaminergic and/or orexin neurons or are agnostic to melatonin receptors (Fig. 2.1). An ideal drug for insomnia aims to enhance sleep onset and/or sleep maintenance without significant residual hangover, tolerance, dependence, or rebound insomnia upon discontinuation.

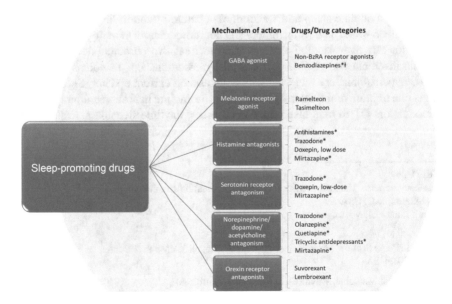

Fig. 2.1 Demonstrates the potential sites of action of sleep-promoting drugs. *Off label use; flurazepam, quazepam, estazolam, temazepam and triazolam are FDA approved for insomnia

Benzodiazepines

Benzodiazepines (BDZs) had been the pharmacotherapy mainstay for insomnia for decades, and despite current recommendations for short-term use, persistent inappropriately prolonged use of BDZs continues. Perhaps due to the established dependence level of patients chronically taking BDZs and/or the lack of knowledge or resources to implement non-pharmacological insomnia management, continuing BDZs versus discontinuing them for treating insomnia is deemed the path of least resistance. Benzodiazepines bind non-selectively to the $GABA_A$ receptor, and in addition to sedation, also mediate antianxiety, anticonvulsant, anterograde amnesia, and myorelaxant effects. They increase sleep duration and modify the sleep architecture by increasing slow-wave sleep (SWS) and decreasing rapid-eye movement (REM) sleep [3–5]. Table 2.1 includes the FDA-approved hypnotic agents for the treatment of insomnia; however, other BDZs are routinely used off-label despite inadequate efficacy and safety data.

Efficacy A meta-analysis [6] of 52 randomized controlled trials (RCTs) in adults treated with BDZs for chronic insomnia (4 weeks or more) decreased sleep onset latency (SOL) and wake after sleep onset (WASO), with increased total sleep time (TST) and sleep efficiency (SE) versus placebo. Compared with placebo, BDZs (≤4 weeks of therapy in most studies) significantly decreased SOL by polysomnography (PSG) weighted mean difference (WMD): −10.0 minutes or by sleep diary, WMD: −19.6 minutes, respectively. Additionally, objective WASO was decreased −16.7 minutes, or subjectively using a sleep diary −39.9 minutes; SE was

Table 2.1 Pharmacokinetics and dosing of oral benzodiazepines[a] in adults [71, 72]

Generic name	Trade name	Daily dose (mg)	Half-life range (h)	Longest active metabolites half-life (h)	Peak effect (h)
Long acting (>24) h					
Flurazepam[b]	Dalmane	15-30 mg	2.3	47–100	1.5–4.5
Quazepam[b]	Doral	7.5–15	39	73	2
Diazepam	Valium	2–10	20–80	40–120	1–2
Intermediate acting (6–24 h)					
Estazolam[b]	ProSom	1–2	10–24	2 major metabolites; minimal hypnotic effect	~2
Temazepam[b]	Restoril	7.5–30	8-15	None	1–2
Lorazepam	Ativan	0.5–2	10–20	None	1–6
Oxazepam	Serax	10–15	5–15	None	1–4
Short acting (<6 h)					
Triazolam[b]	Halcion	0.125–0.5	2–6	None	1–5

h hours

[a]Pregnancy: All BDZs cross the placenta. Symptoms of withdrawal occurring in newborns if exposed in utero have been reported

[b]FDA-approved agents for treatment of insomnia

Table 2.2 Effects on sleep parameters of FDA-approved sleep-promoting agents [2, 72–75]

	Sleep continuity parameters			NREM sleep parameters			REM sleep parameters	
Drugs	SL	SE	TST	Stage N1	Stage N2	Stage N3 (SWS)	REM onset latency	REM
BDZs	↓	↑	↑	↓	↑	↓	↑	↓
Z-drugs	↓	↑	↑	↔	↑	↔	↔	↔
Ramelteon	↓	↑	↑	↔	↑	↔	↔	↔
Suvorexant	↓	↑	↑	↓	↓	↔↓	↓	↑
Low-dose doxepin	↓	↑	↑	↔	↑	↔	↔	↔

BDZs benzodiazepines, *Z-drugs* zolpidem, zaleplon, eszopiclone; ↓ decreased, ↑ increased, ↔ minimal change, arrows do not represent the same degree of weight for each category. *SL* sleep latency, *SE* sleep efficiency, *TST* total sleep time, *SWS* slow-wave sleep, *NREM* non-rapid eye movement, *REM* rapid eye movement

increased 7.4% by PSG and 7.9% by sleep diary, and TST (by PSG) and sTST (by sleep diary) increased 32.7 and 52.6 minutes, respectively. In a separate meta-analysis [7] of 24 RTCs in the elderly with insomnia for at least 5 consecutive nights, significant improvement in sleep quality (SQ) and TST along with decreased nighttime awakening were experienced by those taking BDZs compared to placebo, although the authors reported the benefits may not outweigh the increased risk of adverse events (AEs). In one systematic review (SR) [8], BDZs were favored over placebo in many outcomes including SE, SOL, SQ, TST, and WASO (Table 2.2).

Safety The pharmacokinetics and pharmacodynamics differences of BDZs can often predict the potential incidence of AEs. Benzodiazepines are categorized into short-, intermediate-, and long-acting agents based on the duration of action (Table 2.1). Agents with longer duration of action are often associated with more dose-dependent AEs, including daytime drowsiness due to hangover effect, dizziness, anterograde amnesia, tolerance, drug dependence, withdrawal, rebound insomnia, and REM rebound [3–5]. Gradual dose reduction of BDZs, if taken chronically for the treatment of insomnia, is recommended versus abrupt discontinuation to avoid physical and psychological withdrawal effects [9].

Ingesting BDZs with opioid medicines, alcohol, or other CNS depressants can cause severe drowsiness, breathing problems, coma, and death. Many BDZs are identified as potentially inappropriate medications in patients 65 years and older due to an increased risk of impaired cognition, delirium, falls, fractures, and motor vehicle accidents.

Summary *Treating insomnia with FDA-approved BDZs has demonstrated favorable short-term sleep outcomes. However, the increased risk of potential AEs precludes BDZs from being the ideal first-line therapy for treating insomnia especially in the elderly and a limited role in treating individuals with chronic insomnia.*

Nonbenzodiazepine Receptor Agonists (Non-BzRAs)

The non-BzRAs have no anxiolytic, myorelaxant, and anticonvulsant properties but have strong hypnotic properties due to their selective binding to the $GABA_A$ receptor [2]. The three non-BzRA agents available in the United States, zolpidem, zaleplon, and eszopiclone are FDA-approved for treating insomnia. Zolpidem is currently available as immediate-release (IR) tablets, oral spray, sublingual (SL) tablets, and controlled/extended-release (ER) tablets. Zolpidem IR is indicated for short-term treatment of insomnia characterized by difficulties with sleep onset. Two zolpidem tartrate SL formulations are available. One SL product (Intermezzo IR®) is used for middle-of-the-night awakening followed by difficulty returning to sleep and only if >4 hours of bedtime remain. Edluar™ is a second sublingual zolpidem product approved for sleep initiation and should only be taken if 7–8 hours remain before arising. Agents with shorter-acting half-life such as zolpidem mist and zaleplon should be administered immediately before bedtime.

The non-BzRAs used mostly for sleep maintenance insomnia, zolpidem ER, and eszopiclone have been studied in clinical trials >6 months in duration. With many of these agents, the recommended initial doses in women compared to men are different because the non-BzRA clearance is lower in women. For faster sleep onset, all zolpidem products including eszopiclone should not be administered with or immediately after a meal.

Efficacy There are few head-to-head trials comparing the three U.S. available non-BzRAs. A SR [8] reviewed 31 RCTs in adults with insomnia disorder. Because the trials evaluated included various formulations, doses, and different frequency of administration including short duration (i.e., <6 weeks), comparisons were difficult. Four non-BzRAs (zolpidem, zaleplon, eszopiclone, and zopiclone) were objectively evaluated to placebo and efficacy data were compiled. About one-half of studies deemed of moderate quality, non-BzRAs were favored over placebo for objective SE. In addition, SOL, SQ, TST, and WASO were improved with non-BzRAs compared to placebo (Table 2.3).

Safety Despite non-BzRAs being effective in treating many sleep outcomes, all these agents especially those with longer half-lives have the potential to cause next-day impairment including residual sedation, somnolence, memory impairment, confusion, lethargy, and dizziness. Several FDA warnings exist about rebound insomnia, complex sleep behaviors including sleepwalking, and in some cases, sleep-driving resulting in death. Falls and withdrawals have also been reported. Adverse events (AEs) may occur even at the lowest dose and after one dose, and if so, the drug should be discontinued immediately [10]. The risk of AEs can compound when co-administered with other CNS depressants, alcohol, or with other drugs that increase the blood levels. Eszopiclone can cause unpleasant taste and dry mouth. Rare cases of anaphylactic and anaphylactoid reactions have been reported. These agents should only be used during pregnancy if the potential benefit outweighs the risk to the fetus as no adequate and well-controlled studies in pregnant

Table 2.3 Characteristics of non-BzRAs [10, 76, 77]

Generic/trade name	FDA indication(s)	Onset of action (min)	Duration of action	Usual adult daily dose (mg)	Dose in elderly[a]	Use in pregnancy	Controlled substance
Zolpidem IR Ambien®	Sleep onset	< 30	Short	Men: 5–10 Women: 5	5	Zolpidem crosses the placenta; reports of severe neonatal respiratory depression and sedation with other CNS depressants concurrently.	C-IV
Zolpidem ER Ambien CR®	Sleep onset/ maintenance	<30	Intermediate	Men: 12.5 Women: 6.25	6.25		
Zolpidem sublingual							
Edular®	Sleep initiation	<30	Short	Men: 5–10 Women: 5	5		
Intermezzo®	MOTN	20	Ultra-short	Men: 3.5 Women: 1.75	1.75		
Zolpidem oral spray Zolpimist™	Sleep initiation	20	Short	10 (2 sprays)	5	No adequate and well-controlled studies in pregnant women.	
Eszopiclone Lunesta®	Sleep onset/ maintenance	<30	Intermediate	2–3	1–2		
Zaleplon Sonata®	Sleep onset	< 30	Ultra-short	10	5	Not recommended	

IR intermediate release, ER extended release, CR controlled release, MOTN middle-of-the-night

[a]Or in mild-moderate hepatic impairment

women exists. Drugs that increase levels of all these non-BZRA agents include the CYP3A4 inhibitors.

Summary *Despite the strong evidence base that non-BzRAs have favorable sleep outcomes, treating insomnia chronically with non-BZRAs may have a limited role due to potential AEs. If prescribed, the lowest dose for the shortest period of time possible should be exercised.*

Melatonin

Melatonin is a neurohormone of the pineal gland that is modulated by the suprachiasmatic nucleus (SCN) of the hypothalamus. Regulation of melatonin synthesis by the SCN determines the circadian rhythm of sleep and wakefulness.

Efficacy Clinical guidelines do not support the use of melatonin for insomnia [11]. In a meta-analysis [12] including 19 studies ($n = 1683$) in adults and children, the study durations (average 50 days, range 7–182), dosing strategies (0.1 mg – 5 mg), and formulations varied, making comparison of the results impossible. Although a ~7-minute SOL reduction, an 8-minute TST increase, and a very small improvement in SQ favoring melatonin over placebo were seen, the clinical significance of these findings was unclear. However, strategically timed melatonin is effective for treating intrinsic circadian rhythm sleep-wake disorders such as delayed sleep phase disorders, non-24-hour sleep-wake disorder, and also REM sleep behavior disorders (RBD) [13]. In treating circadian rhythm sleep disorders with melatonin, optimal administration at the proper circadian time, based on an individual's circadian timing, is essential. If not administered correctly, melatonin may fail to produce the desired results or even produce opposite effects and perpetuate sleep disorders and important to remember when treating elderly due to a decreased production of endogenous melatonin during aging.

Melatonin is often used to treat insomnia because of its availability over-the-counter (OTC). While marketed as a "nutritional supplement", no proof of safety and effectiveness is required for OTCs, thus composition of melatonin varies and may have impurities [14]. To minimize potential differences in compositions, consumers and healthcare systems should always purchase melatonin that bears a Good Manufacturing Practices (GMP) seal as proof that the product is prepared, manufactured, and properly stored to the highest standards.

Safety Overall, when reported, most studies report minimal side effects to melatonin. However, in a recent review, 50% of the melatonin trials reported AEs including psychomotor and neurocognitive dysfunction, fatigue, or excessive sedation [15]. A few AEs impacting the phase-shifting circadian rhythms of other physiological functions besides sleep including endocrine/reproductive and cardiovascular parameters were reported. Other AEs attributed to dosage, dose timing, and drug-drug interactions were seen.

Summary *Providers and consumers often try melatonin first-line in treating insomnia due to its availability. However, melatonin is not recommended for treating chronic insomnia due to inadequate supporting data with low quality of evidence and potential for mild AEs.*

Melatonin Receptor Agonist: Ramelteon

Ramelteon is a synthetic analog of melatonin. It is a melatonin receptor agonist and acts by binding selectivity to the MT1 > MT2 receptors, two G-protein-coupled receptors [16].

Efficacy A SR [17] determined the efficacy of short-term use of ramelteon ($n = 5812$) for treating insomnia in mostly female individuals (62%) between 18 and 93 years old. The dose range of ramelteon was 4–32 mg/day (although the FDA-approved dose is 8 mg/day) and mean duration of therapy was 38 days. Relative to placebo, ramelteon significantly improved sSL and SQ, but not sTST. Ramelteon improved secondary outcomes SE, SOL, and TST.

Safety The incidence of AEs with ramelteon was low. Somnolence was the only significant AE. Angioedema and anaphylaxis, complex sleep-related behavior, hyperprolactinemia, and lower testosterone levels have been reported in post-marketing reports [16]. Ramelteon does not produce dependence and has no abuse potential unlike the GABAergic drugs. There was no tolerance, rebound insomnia on discontinuation, psychomotor, cognitive, or balance impairment [16].

Summary *Ramelteon had a favorable safety profile and responses on many sleep parameters. However, its clinical efficacy was small, therefore, is not an efficacious agent for the treatment of chronic insomnia.*

Orexin Antagonists: Suvorexant and Lemborexant

Orexin A and B (also called hypocretin-1 and 2) are neuropeptides located in the perifornical regions of the lateral hypothalamus and project to the brain stem and forebrain areas, innervating monoaminergic and cholinergic cells. While these neuropeptides influence numerous functions such as food intake, appetite, autonomic regulation, and endocrine function, they also serve to promote wakefulness and inhibit REM sleep [18]. Suvorexant and lemborexant are dual orexin receptor antagonist agents (DORAs) and bind selectively to the G-protein-coupled receptors,

OX1R and OX2R thus, altering the action of orexin in the brain and suppressing the sleep-wake drive. (See Table 2.4 for comparisons) [19, 20].

Efficacy Suvorexant was evaluated using dose ranges exceeding the current approved doses; 5 mg – 20 mg daily. A two-period cross-over efficacy study [21] examining suvorexant 10 and 20 mg versus placebo for 1 month included 254 patients with primary insomnia. The primary endpoint was SE. Secondary endpoints were WASO and latency to persistent sleep (LPS). After 4 weeks of therapy, compared to placebo, the 10 and 20 mg doses improved SE (4.7% and 10.4%), decreased WASO (−21.4 and −28.1 minutes) and LPS (−2.3 and −22.3 minutes), and improved the exploratory endpoint TST (22.3 and 49.9 minutes), respectively [21, 22]. To date, no head-to-head trials comparing suvorexant to other sedative hypnotics exist.

One SR [23] reported patients responding to suvorexant 15 or 20 mg at 3 months, a number to treat (NNT) of 13 and 16 would be required to achieve a ≥15% improvement in mean sTST and mean sWASO versus placebo, respectively. Other authors reported a NNT of eight to achieve a ≥6-point improvement in the patient-rated insomnia severity index (ISI) at 3 months with suvorexant 15/20 mg doses versus placebo [24].

The efficacy of lemborexant was shown in two Phase 3 RCTs [25, 26]. SUNRISE-1 trial [25] compared lemborexant 5 and 10 mg to placebo and active comparator, zolpidem ER 6.25 mg for 1 month in adults ($n = 1006$) aged ≥55 years with insomnia. Patients had a mean ISI score of 19 upon randomization and 86%

Table 2.4 Characteristics of orexin antagonists in adults[a] [19, 20]

Generic name	Suvorexant	Lemborexant
Trade name	Belsomra	Dayvigo
Onset of action (min)	30	<30
Tmax, hrs (range)	2 (0.5–6)	1–3
Elimination half-life; hrs. (range)	12	17–19
Duration	Intermediate	Intermediate
Metabolism	CYP3A4 (major); CYP2C19 (minor)	CYP3A4 (major); CYP3A5 (minor)
Recommended daily dose, adults; initial; maximum (mg)[a]	10; 20	5; 10
Exposure	Higher in women versus men and in obesity (>30 kg/m2) vs. non-obesity	N/A
Use in pregnancy	AEs observed in some animal reproduction studies. No adequate studies in women during the use in pregnancy for either agents.	
Controlled substance	IV	

N/A not applicable; *AE* adverse events
[a]Both agents are dosed ≥7 hours before planned time of awakening

were women. The primary endpoint was the mean change from baseline (CFB) in LPS versus placebo on days 29/30. Pre-specified key secondary outcomes included mean CFB in SE and WASO compared to placebo and WASO in the second half of the night (WASO2H) compared to zolpidem ER 6.25 mg on days 29/30. Lemborexant 5 and 10 mg improved LPS 11.6 and 13.6 minutes versus placebo at 1 month, respectively. The treatment effect of lemborexant 5 and 10 mg versus placebo at 6 months for SE was 3.9% and 4.9%; and for WASO was −7.7 and −9.1 minutes, respectively.

SUNRISE-2 [26] trial compared lemborexant 5 and 10 mg versus placebo for 6 months (Period 1) ($n = 959$) followed by 6 months active-treatment only period (Period 2-https://doi.org/10.1016/j.sleep.2021.01.048). The primary outcome of Period 1 was a mean CFB in sSL and the pre-specified key secondary efficacy endpoints were CFB for sSE and sWASO using electronic sleep diaries. At 6 months, both lemborexant doses demonstrated statistically significant superiority to placebo for all primary and key secondary outcomes. Lemborexant 5 and 10 mg improved LPS 11.2 and 14.1 minutes from placebo at 1 month, respectively. The treatment effect of lemborexant 5 and 10 mg compared to placebo at 6 months for sSE was 4.6% and 4.7% and for sWASO, −17.5 and −12.7 minutes, respectively.

A SR and network meta-analysis [27] evaluated the efficacy and safety outcomes between lemborexant and suvorexant. It included 4 double-blind, RCTs ($n = 3237$, mean age 58 years). Treatment arms included lemborexant 10 mg/day ($n = 592$); lemborexant 5 mg/day ($n = 589$); suvorexant 20/15 mg/day ($n = 493$); zolpidem ER 6.25 mg/day ($n = 263$); and placebo ($n = 1300$). The quality of evidence was rated low or very low. The analysis suggests that at 1 month, lemborexant 10 mg performed better compared to other agents and doses including placebo for subjective time to sleep onset (primary outcome), sTST and sWASO (secondary outcomes from sleep diaries) but was associated with a higher discontinuation rate due to AEs and a higher incidence of somnolence compared to zolpidem ER 6.25 mg/day.

Safety Both DORAs are contraindicated in patients with narcolepsy. The most common AEs with suvorexant during 1 year of treatment were somnolence, fatigue, and dry mouth [28]. A dose-related increase of AEs is seen [24–26]. The incidence of somnolence with suvorexant was 0.4%, 1.6%, and 4.9% for placebo, 10 and 20 mg/day, respectively [21]. The number needed to harm (NNH) using suvorexant 15 or 20 mg/day versus placebo was 28 [24]. Next-day somnolence, CNS depression, and sleep-related activities including sleepwalking, sleep-driving, and making phone calls while asleep without patients remembering have been reported. Suvorexant can impair next-day performance of activities that require mental alertness and motor coordination as did some patients taking lemborexant 10 mg/day. Of note, performance on some memory and attention tests was reduced with lemborexant 10 mg dose compared to placebo; 5 mg dose did not differ significantly from placebo in any of these measures.

No clinically significant respiratory depression in mild-to-moderate obstructive sleep apnea (OSA) and mild-to-moderate chronic obstructive pulmonary disease were noted with suvorexant. There were no cases of severe cataplexy, although some reports of "weaknesses" were noted. In patients with mild OSA, lemborexant did not increase the frequency of apneic events or cause oxygen desaturation. Symptoms similar to mild cataplexy can occur with lemborexant. No evidence of rebound insomnia, physical dependence, or withdrawal symptoms were seen with either agents. The incidence of somnolence or fatigue in a combined analysis pool (first 30 days) for SUNRISE-1 and SUNRISE-2 trials [22] for placebo, lemborexant 5 and 10 mg, was 1.3%, 6.9% (NNH = 18), 9.6% (NNH = 12), respectively. In SUNRISE-2 trial [23], the incidence of somnolence was higher in patients ≥65 years of age (19%) vs. subjects <65 years (10.9%) with lemborexant 10 mg (data on file, Eisai Inc.).

Summary *The DORAs are indicated for sleep onset and maintenance insomnia. No comparative trials between these two agents exist. Long-term outcomes are not known. Lemborexant 10 mg compared to zolpidem 6.25 ER had better outcomes in many of the subjective sleep parameters, however with more somnolence. The incidence of AEs is dose-dependent for both agents.*

Antidepressants

Several antidepressants are used off-label to treat insomnia although few controlled, short- or long-term studies to validate their efficacy and safety in patients with primary insomnia exists. The tolerability and safety of these agents used in high-quality trials long term is lacking. Patients with depression or anxiety disorders treated with SSRI (serotonin reuptake inhibitor) and SNRI (serotonin and norepinephrine reuptake inhibitor) antidepressants often complain of insomnia or daytime somnolence occurring with long-term treatment [29].

Low-dose doxepin Low-dose doxepin due to its antihistamine effects is FDA-approved for the treatment of sleep maintenance insomnia. One SR [30] comprised of 6 RCTs of low-quality evidence compared the efficacy of low-dose doxepin versus placebo in individuals with insomnia disorder diagnosis with treatment duration varying from 1 day to 12 weeks. The outcome, ISI, significantly improved at week four in 2 RCTs in older adults, favoring doxepin 3 or 6 mg dose over placebo.

None of the RCTs found significant differences in AE rates between low-dose doxepin and placebo treatment, although the SR did not combine AEs from different RCTs. Headache and somnolence were the most common AEs reported with low-dose doxepin with no significant next-day residual effects or withdrawal effects. Doxepin may potentially be an inappropriate medication in geriatric patients [31], and should be avoided when used in doses >6 mg/day due to the possible orthostatic hypotension, anticholinergic effects, or toxicity [32].

Antidepressants Used Off-Label

Trazodone Trazodone produces sedation by blocking the 5HT-2a/2c receptor. Trazodone continues to be a highly prescribed drug for insomnia even though the efficacy for treating insomnia has been studied in only small populations in depressed individuals, usually with limited subjective sleep evaluations and without objective PSG data.

In an SR, [33] three of 7 trazodone trials ($n = 379$) used doses between 25 and 150 mg. Moderate improvement in subjective sleep outcomes over placebo was seen. Two PSG trazodone studies resulted in little or no difference in SE (low-quality evidence). Two studies with low-quality evidence had more AEs with trazodone than placebo. Another SR [34] included seven trazadone trials of which only one trial included patients with primary insomnia ($n = 306$). The trial of 2 weeks in duration included three arms: trazodone 50 mg, zolpidem 10 mg, and placebo. Patients self-reported that both trazodone and zolpidem had shorter sleep latency than placebo, but similar in sleep duration.

Rates of AE were low in two of the trials; the other five studies did not present this data [34]. Trazodone has an FDA blackbox warning for the possibility of increasing suicidal thoughts and behaviors in pediatric and young adult patients [35]. Due to numerous other AEs and drug-drug interactions, trazodone is not considered a treatment of choice for chronic insomnia.

Summary *Only low-dose doxepin is FDA-approved for treatment of sleep maintenance insomnia. There is limited clinical evidence for using other antidepressants for managing insomnia.*

Antipsychotic Agents

Traditional and atypical antipsychotics are sedating due to their antagonism of dopaminergic, histaminergic, serotonergic, α(alpha)1-adrenergic systems. Anticholinergic effects, including sedating and hypotensive effects, occur with all antipsychotics in varying frequency and severity.

A SR [36] evaluated the benefits and AEs of atypical antipsychotics used to treat insomnia. Only one low-quality study using quetiapine met the inclusion criteria, and reported no statistically significant differences from baseline between quetiapine and placebo for TST, SL reduction, or sleep satisfaction improvement. No AEs were reported in the placebo group, but dry mouth and daytime drowsiness were found in the quetiapine with undetermined frequency. Quetiapine has a blackbox warning indicating a 1.6 to 1.7-fold increase in mortality in elderly populations with dementia-related psychosis and increased suicidal tendencies in children, adolescents, and young adults [37]. In addition, all atypical antipsychotics carry a strong recommendation to avoid their use in the elderly except in schizophrenia or bipolar disorders due to an increased risk of cerebrovascular accident and a greater rate of cognitive decline and mortality in persons with dementia [31].

Summary *The atypical antipsychotic used off-label most commonly to treat insomnia is quetiapine. There are limited number of studies with small sizes regarding efficacy of antipsychotics for treating insomnia and the drugs have risk for AEs in the elderly.*

OTC Drugs

Off-label use of antihistamines such as diphenhydramine and doxylamine produces subjective drowsiness and reduced SL but tolerance develops within 2 weeks of use [11]. The use of these agents and other antihistamines is *not* supported by rigorous data for treating chronic insomnia [11]. Valerian available as OTC is a plant extract with GABA activity and shortens SL and improves SE; however, evidence for its efficacy for treatment of insomnia is limited [11].

Wake-promoting Drugs

Drugs that are agonistic to the wake-promoting nuclei can potentially increase alertness. Thus, wake-promoting agents used to treat excessive daytime sleepiness (EDS) act via the activation of the noradrenergic, dopaminergic, serotonergic systems, and/or histamine [1] (Fig. 2.2). Agents treat narcolepsy symptoms, primarily EDS, but also REM sleep dysregulation symptoms (i.e., cataplexy, hypnagogic/

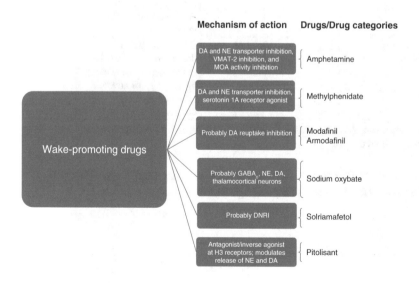

Fig. 2.2 Demonstrates the potential sites of action of wake-promoting drugs. *DA* dopamine, *NE* norepinephrine, *MAO* monoamine oxidase, *DNRI* dopamine and norepinephrine reuptake inhibitor, *H3* histamine 3, *VMAT-2* vesicular monoamine transporter, *GABA* gamma aminobutyric acid

Table 2.5 Pharmacology of wake-promoting agents [67, 78]

Generic/ (trade name)	Half-life (h)	Usual daily dose range (mg)	Use in pregnancy	Controlled substance
CNS stimulants (e.g., amphetamines; detroamphetamine) Desoxyn®; Dexedrine®)	Varies, depending on the formulation	5–60 (divided doses)	The safety of CNS stimulants during human pregnancy has not been established. There may be risks to the fetus associated with the use of CNS stimulants.	II
Methylphenidates (Concerta®; Ritalin®)	1.5–3	20–30		
Modafinil (Provigil®)	15	200–400 (narcolepsy; divided doses) 200 (OSA)	Registry data suggest potentially a higher rate of major congenital malformations than in the general population exposed within 6 weeks prior to conception or pregnancy.	IV
Armodafinil (Nuvigil®)	15	150–250		
Sodium oxybate (Xyrem®)	0.5–1	4.5–9 g/night divided into 2 doses	Insufficient data to determine developmental risk.	III
Calcium, magnesium, potassium, and sodium oxybates[a] (Xywav™)	0.5–1	Same as Xyrem	Insufficient data to determine developmental risk.	III
Pitolisant (Wakix®)	~20	8.9–35.6	Pre-clinical studies have shown reproductive toxicity. Insufficient human data to establish toxicity.	N/A
Solriamefetol (Sunosi®)	2–3	75–150 (narcolepsy) 37.5–150 (OSA)	Insufficient data to determine drug-associated risk of major birth defects, miscarriage, or adverse maternal or fetal outcomes.	IV

CNS central nervous system; *N/A* not applicable; *OSA* obstructive sleep apnea
[a]Low-dose sodium oxybate

hypnopompic hallucinations, sleep paralysis) and disrupted nighttime sleep. The pharmacology and dosing of the wake agents are described in Table 2.5.

Amphetamines and Methylphenidate

Amphetamines and methylphenidate are controlled substances that act by blocking the reuptake and enhancing the release of norepinephrine, dopamine, and serotonin [38]. Amphetamines reduce REM (rapid eye-movement) sleep, prolong REM latency, increase SL, and reduce TST [39].

Efficacy Efficacy data for the wake-promoting drugs are limited. Methylphenidate, methamphetamine, and dextroamphetamine are FDA-approved for EDS, but are not considered first-line therapy due to lack of evidence on benefit-to-risk ratios [40].

Safety Adverse events include headaches, irritability, nervousness or tremors, psychosis, anorexia, insomnia, gastrointestinal complaints, dyskinesias, and palpitations. The drugs are contraindicated in patients with advanced arteriosclerosis, symptomatic cardiovascular disease, moderate to severe hypertension, hyperthyroidism, history of drug abuse, or with administration of MAO inhibitors. Labeling for amphetamines includes a "black box" warning due to the high potential for abuse.

Summary Amphetamines and related medications have been used to improve alertness in patients with narcolepsy for decades but are not first-line therapy for EDS. The drugs have significant AEs and potential for abuse in specific situations.

Modafinil and Armodafinil

Modafinil is a nonamphetamine indicated for treatment of EDS for patients with narcolepsy and shift-work disorder, and with obstructive sleep apnea (OSA) with residual daytime sleepiness on adequate positive airway pressure therapy (PAP). Modafinil's mechanism of action (MOA) is not well understood but may be dopamine reuptake inhibition [41, 42].

Modafinil is comprised of two enantiomers, the S-isomer with a half-life of 3–4 hours and the R-isomer with a half-life of ~15 hours. Armodafinil is the R-enantiomer of modafinil. Modafinil's elimination half-life is almost 13 hours for single dosing and up to 15 hours after multiple dosing; the maximum concentration is achieved in 2–4 hours.

Modafinil Efficacy

Narcolepsy A meta-analysis pooled data from nine double-blind RCTs [43] in patients with narcolepsy ($n = 1054$) with or without cataplexy and with 2–9 weeks follow-up at daily doses of 200-, 300-, and 400 mg. Modafinil versus placebo significantly decreased EDS assessed by Epworth Sleepiness Scale (ESS) with WMD of −2.73 points, improved multiple sleep latency test (MSLT) and maintenance of wakefulness test (MWT) results, WMD of 1.11 and 2.82 minutes, respectively. Daytime sleepiness and the number of sleep attacks and naps per day decreased. There were no changes in sleep architecture. Following 9 weeks of treatment with 200 or 400 mg/day, modafinil improved quality of life on the SF-36 questionnaire and on a validated narcolepsy-specific questionnaire. Performance and clinical global impression (CGI) scores also improved. The likelihood of falling asleep increased after withdrawing modafinil [44]. Modafinil had a similar effect on EDS as sodium oxybate [45] with no difference in the change in ESS scores and mean sleep latency (MSL) on MWT. There are no RCTs comparing modafinil with methylphenidate or other amphetamine-like stimulants. Withdrawal symptoms such as those noted with amphetamines were absent, suggesting that modafinil is not "addictive" and has a lower potential for abuse. Modafinil 400 mg once daily or as a split dose in the morning and at midday improved wakefulness than modafinil 200 mg taken once daily in the morning [46]. Modafinil had no effect on cataplexy.

Obstructive Sleep Apnea

In one SR of 10 RCTs [47], modafinil/armodafinil used for the treatment of residual daytime sleepiness in OSA after adequate PAP therapy improved ESS score by 2.2 points over placebo (effect size 0.55), MWT by 3 minutes (effect size 0.41), and MSLT by 1.3 minutes (effect size 0.33).

Shift work disorder In shift work studies [48], the objective MSL increase was small (approximately, 2 minutes at both 200- and 400 mg); however, patients' subjective assessment of sleepiness was much improved, with an ESS score reduction by approximately 4 points and 6 points at 200 and 400 mg dosage, respectively.

Armodafinil Efficacy Armodafinil resulted in a small (2.3 minutes) but statistically significant increase from baseline MSL versus placebo on the first four 30 minutes MWT sessions in OSA patients with residual EDS [49, 50]. Armodafinil significantly increased the MSL on MWT in narcoleptic patients [51]. In patients with EDS associated with chronic shift-work disorder, armodafinil significantly improved wakefulness during scheduled night work, raising mean nighttime SL from 2.3 minutes at baseline, to 5.3 minutes over a period of 12 weeks [52]. The effectiveness of armodafinil lasted after long-term use ($\geq$12 month) and was well tolerated in open-label trials in patients with EDS associated with treated OSA, shift work disorder, or narcolepsy [52–54]. Armodafinil was also effective in reducing sleepiness due to jet lag following eastward travel through 6 time zones [55].

Safety Data compiled from six double-blind, RCTs demonstrated that modafinil has a good safety profile with low potential for abuse [42, 56]. The most common side effect is headache and anxiety. It does not affect the sleep architecture by PSG or any cardiovascular parameters (blood pressure or heart rate). A serious but rare side effect is drug rash. Psychiatric alterations have been noted in patients under combined treatment with sodium oxybate and modafinil [57] and should be monitored accordingly. These drugs induce cytochrome P450 enzyme, leading to reduced levels of oral contraceptives. Hence, female patients should use another form of contraception while on these medications. Neither modafinil nor armodafinil is FDA-approved for use in pediatric patients for any indication.

Summary *Modafinil and armodafinil are effective and safe agents in treating EDS associated with narcolepsy, shift work disorder, and in OSA treated with PAP.*

Sodium Oxybate

Sodium oxybate (Xyrem®) (SXB) and lower-sodium version (Xywav®) are oxybate salts of the recreational drug, gamma-hydroxybutyric acid (GHB). Both agents are FDA-approved for the treatment of cataplexy and EDS in patients with narcolepsy ≥7 years of age. While the MOA is unknown, both agents probably act by binding to $GABA_B$ receptors. Given the abuse potential and CNS depressant effects, the drugs are scheduled III controlled substances and available only through a restricted distribution program. Both agents are rapidly absorbed with a high first-pass metabolism; absorption is slowed by fatty meals, so should be taken a few hours after a meal. The agents are metabolized to water and carbon dioxide and eliminated rapidly from the circulation in 20–53 minutes, necessitating twice-nightly administration, taken at bedtime while in bed and again 2.5–4 hours later [58]

Efficacy In one meta-analysis, 2 RCTs measured the improvement of EDS with SXB using different MWT protocols ($n = 192$). At SXB doses, usually at 9 g/night for 4–8 weeks, SXB was significantly superior to placebo for increasing MSL (MD (mean difference): 5.18), and reducing mean sleep attacks (MD: −9.65) and increased CGI scores. When compared with placebo, cataplexy attacks were statistically significantly decreased with 4.5 g/night dose (pooled results: MD: −8.5, https://doi.org/10.5664/jcsm.2048)

In another meta-analysis of 9 RCTs ($n = 1154$), SXB also significantly reduced subjective daytime sleepiness (WMD −2.81) and sleep stage shifts (WMD −9.69, [59]). In one of the RCTs, there was a significant reduction of 20% and 27% in the ESS scores in the SXB monotherapy and SXB + modafinil combined therapy groups, respectively [45]. After 8 weeks, significant changes in sleep architecture among patients receiving SXB and SXB + modafinil included a median increase in Stage 3 and 4 sleep (43.5 and 24.25 minutes, respectively) and delta power and a median decrease in nocturnal awakenings (6.0 and 9.5, respectively) [60]. It did not significantly increase REM sleep versus placebo.

The efficacy of lower-sodium oxybate was established in Phase 3 trial, 16 weeks in duration with 2 weeks of data comparing it to placebo ($n = 201$, [61]). The sodium content in a 6–9 g dose SXB and lower-sodium oxybate is 1100–1640 mg vs. 87–131 mg, respectively. The primary outcome was the change in weekly number of cataplexy attacks from during the stable dose period (2 weeks) to withdrawal period (2 weeks). The key secondary outcome was a change in EES score. Weekly cataplexy scores and EES scores were significantly reduced compared to placebo. Most patients randomized to lower-sodium oxybate reported better PGIc (Patient Global Impression of Change) ratings, Short Form (SF)-36 physical component summary scores, and SF-36 mental component summary scores than the placebo group.

Safety SXB was well tolerated but patients had statistically more AEs versus placebo, including nausea (relative risk [RR]: 7.74), vomiting (RR:11.8), and dizziness (RR: 4.3). Enuresis was not significantly different from placebo [62]. Sleepwalking was reported in 4% of 717 patients treated in clinical trials with SXB [63]. Post-marketing data indicate a very low risk of abuse/misuse of SXB. Serious AEs, reported in ~6% of patients, included depression, angina, and suicide attempt. No acute withdrawal symptoms were observed after 2 weeks of discontinuation following an average of 21 months of therapy. The abrupt cessation of SXB did not cause acute rebound in cataplexy [64]. Caution is advised when treating narcoleptics with concurrent SXB, and to ensure adherence to positive pressure therapy before starting SXB. The overall safety profile including potential drug interactions of SXB is expected to be similar to lower-sodium oxybate [61].

Synergistic interactions of SXB with alcohol or other CNS depressants may increase the risk of intoxication or overdose. The agents should not be taken in combination with sedative hypnotics or in patients with succinic semialdehyde dehydrogenase deficiency. Patients with compromised liver function should have their starting dose decreased by one-half and response to dose increments monitored [58]. Most patients can be effectively transitioned from SXB to lower-sodium oxybate without any difficulties.

Summary *SXB is used in combination with other therapies to adequately control all symptoms of narcolepsy. A lower-sodium oxybate offers another treatment option for treating cataplexy in patients with narcolepsy and cardiovascular/renal disease or other health condition/valid medical reason requiring a lower daily sodium consumption.*

Solriamfetol

Solriamfetol is a dopamine and norepinephrine reuptake inhibitor (DNRI) indicated to improve wakefulness in adult patients with EDS. Solriamfetol was approved based on two 12-week RCTs, in patients with narcolepsy [65] and OSA [66], respectively. It is not approved for treating cataplexy.

Efficacy *Narcolepsy*: Treatment of Obstructive Sleep Apnea and Narcolepsy Excessive Sleepiness (TONES 2 and 3) were double-blind randomized, placebo-controlled parallel-group trials. In TONES 2 [65], patients with narcolepsy type 1 or 2 ($n = 231$) with baseline ESS of ≥ 10 (mean, 17.2) and a baseline mean SL of <25 minutes based on 4-naps MWT were randomized to receive placebo, solriamfetol 75, 150, or 300 mg daily. The co-primary endpoints were change from baseline to 12 weeks in MWT and ESS. The PGI-C at 12 weeks was the key secondary endpoint. At week 12, solriamfetol 150 and 300 mg significantly increased the mean change of SL versus placebo from baseline on MWT of 7.7 and 10.1 minutes, respectively. Significant decreases of −2.2, −3.8, and −4.7 in ESS scores were found with solriamfetol 75, 150, and 300 mg compared to placebo, respectively. The NNT to achieve an ESS ≤ 10 using solriamfetol 150 and 75 mg versus placebo at 12 weeks was calculated to be 4 and 7 in a post-hoc analysis, respectively. Improvements in MWT and EES scores were sustained throughout the trial's duration. The improvement in PGI-C (Patient Global Impression scale) was dose-dependent and significant at 150 and 300 mg doses versus placebo. However, the recommended doses for patients with narcolepsy are 75 and 150 mg once daily. Dosages above 150 mg increased dose-related AEs without additional benefit. No trials comparing solriamfetol with other agents used for the treatment of EDS are available.

OSA The TONES-3 trial randomized 476 adults with OSA and evaluated the efficacy and safety of solriamfetol 37.5, 75, 150, and 300 mg, with placebo over 12 weeks [66]. The participants had a mean baseline ESS score of ~15 and a mean MSL on MWT between 12 and 13 minutes. The participants had to either currently use or had prior use of a primary OSA therapy including PAP, mandibular advancement device, or surgical intervention. The severity of OSA was not specified. The trial did not specify whether surgery was effective in treating OSA or the required hours of PAP use. At baseline, primary OSA therapy was used by 69.7% of participants on placebo and 73.5% randomized to solriamfetol, of which ~90% were on PAP. The primary OSA therapy nonadherence ranged from 27.1% - 31.6% in the study. The inclusion criteria of baseline ESS score and endpoints were the same as in TONES-2 trial, and the baseline SL for MWT was ≤30 minutes.

All solriamfetol doses increased wakefulness significantly relative to placebo in patients with OSA. The SL mean change from baseline per MWT was 13.0, 11.0, 9.1, 4.7 minutes with 300, 150, 75, and 37.5 mg at 12 weeks, respectively. The dose-dependent effects were sustained over the study duration. All solriamfetol doses resulted in a decrease in sleepiness as indicated by the ESS score compared to placebo at 12 weeks. The ESS decrease was dose-dependent and ranged from −3.3 to −7.9 with solriamfetol 37.5–300 mg daily. The key secondary endpoint of PGI-C was met at all doses except for the 37.5 mg dose.

Safety In TONES 2, AEs incidence (≥5%) with all doses of solriamfetol included headache (21.5%), nausea (10.7%), decreased appetite (10.7%), nasopharyngitis (9%), dry mouth (7.3%), and anxiety (5.1%) [65]. Patients with previous history of headache or migraines had a higher incidence of headache. Of note, blood pressure (BP) taken 9 hours post dose showed an increase from baseline in systolic and diastolic BP (1–2 mmHg) and heart rate (2–4 beats per minutes) for solriamfetol 150 and 300 mg doses compared to placebo. The discontinuation rate was higher in the solriamfetol 300 mg group (27.1%), solriamfetol 75 mg (16.9%), placebo (10.3%), and solriamfetol 150 mg (7.3%). The NNH in TONES 2 for any or all treatment-emergent AEs was 8 and 3 for solriamfetol 75 mg and 150 mg, respectively, compared to placebo at 12 weeks.

In TONES 3, AEs and discontinuations caused by AEs were dose-dependent [66]. The most frequent AEs with solriamfetol occurring ≥5% were similar to what was seen in TONES-2 trial. At week 12, BP was increased compared to baseline with the highest increase noted when 300 mg dose was used; 2.5 and 1.5 mmHg systolic and diastolic, respectively. Small mean increase in heart rate was also seen with solriamfetol 150 and 300 mg doses. Long-term cardiovascular consequences are not available. The dose should be adjusted in patients with renal disease. There is potential for abuse of this drug. It is unknown whether solriamfetol in combination with other medications for the treatment of narcolepsy is safe and tolerated and whether this therapy can be extrapolated to those that refuse primary OSA therapy.

Summary *Solriamfetol is effective in reducing EDS in patients with narcolepsy and OSA treated with PAP, but there is risk for dose-dependent AEs.*

Pitolisant

Pitolisant is indicated for the treatment of EDS or cataplexy in adult patients with narcolepsy. Pitolisant is a histamine-3 (H3) receptor antagonist/inverse agonist that blocks the inhibitory effect of the H3 receptors and increases the synthesis and release of histamine into the brain synapse, so the locus coeruleus NE neurons are activated. The antagonism of the H3 receptors with pitolisant can increase the release of other neurotransmitters such as acetylcholine, norepinephrine, and dopamine levels in the prefrontal cortex [67].

Efficacy The efficacy of pitolisant in narcolepsy was established in two 8-week Phase 3 RCT studies involving narcoleptic adults ($n = 258$) with EDS [68, 69]. Randomized patients received pitolisant, placebo, or the active comparator agent, modafinil. In the first RCT ($n = 95$), 81% of narcoleptics had cataplexy upon entry. Pitolisant 9–36 mg/day demonstrated a significant improvement in EDS assessed by ESS compared to placebo at 8 weeks. The treatment effect changes from baseline EES score between pitolisant and placebo was −3.1. The improvement in objective test of wakefulness and attention tests with pitolisant versus placebo was confirmed but were not significantly different with modafinil 100–400 mg daily. The SL increased 32% with pitolisant and decreased 10% with placebo. Responder rates in the post-hoc analyses (defined as an EES score ≤10) for pitolisant were significantly greater compared to placebo (45% vs. 13%, respectively) but not compared with modafinil. Similarly, for the daily cataplexy rates in the post-hoc analyses, in which 35% of the patients continued their usual anticataleptic drugs (sodium oxybate, ($n = 8$); or antidepressants, ($n = 25$)), pitolisant was superior to placebo in decreasing the number of daily cataplexy attacks from baseline assessed by sleep diary entries but was not non-inferior to modafinil [68].

The second RCT (n = 164) studied a lower daily dose range of pitolisant of 4.5–17.8 mg [69]. The maximum dose was reached by 76% of the patients and ~78% of the patients had cataplexy upon randomization. Pitolisant had a treatment effect of −2.12 in the ESS score versus placebo after 8 weeks but there was no significant improvement in EDS. Non-inferiority test between pitolisant and modafinil 200 or 400 mg daily could not be concluded. On the objective tests MWT and SART (sustained attention to response task), pitolisant was significantly greater compared to placebo but not different from modafinil. In a post-hoc analyses, responder rate (defined as an ESS score ≤10 or ESS score reduction ≥3), pitolisant was significantly greater (64%) compared to placebo (35%). No significant difference between the responder rate for pitolisant and modafinil groups was seen and there was no reduction in cataplexy rates compared to placebo at this lower dose [69].

Safety The AEs most frequently reported for pitolisant from pooled studies (8 weeks) versus placebo were headache (18.7% vs. 14.9%), nausea (5.9 vs. 2.7%), and insomnia (5.8% vs. 2.3%). The neuropsychiatric AEs seen were insomnia (8.4%); dizziness (1.4%), depression (1.3%), tremor (1.2%), sleep disorders (1.1%), and vertigo (1.0%) [69].

Pitolisant is contraindicated in patients with Child-Pugh C. Clinically relevant interactions are expected with strong CYP2D6 inhibitors and CYP3A4 inducers. Concomitant administration of antihistamine-1 receptor antagonists and sedating antihistamines may impair the efficacy of pitolisant [69] and lower the efficacy of hormonal contraception. Supratherapeutic doses of pitolisant have been associated with QTc interval prolongation and drug monitoring is required in patients with cardiac disease. Pitolisant has no abuse, tolerance, rebound or withdrawal potential and it is not a scheduled controlled substance nor a stimulant.

Summary Pitolisant is an alternate agent that is not a scheduled controlled substance, effective in the treatment of EDS and cataplexy in narcolepsy, and to be used with caution in patients with cardiac disease.

Novel Drugs in Pipeline

Several drugs for either insomnia or EDS are undergoing clinical trials or have shown promise in animal studies and are awaiting clinical trials. These drugs and their potential site(s) of action are presented in Table 2.6 [70].

Table 2.6 Novel drugs in development [79]

Compound/ NTC number	Mechanism of action	Target indication
Daridorexant 02839200	Dual orexin receptor antagonist	Insomnia
Seltorexant 03682380	Selective orexin-2 receptor antagonist	Insomnia and related mood disorders (MDD)
SKP-1041 00878553	$GABA_A$ receptor enhancer- (experimental formulation of zaleplon)	Insomnia with middle of the night awakening
Lorediplon (unknown)	$GABA_A$ receptor enhancer: (longer acting non-BDZ)	Insomnia
EVT-201 00380003	$GABA_A$ receptor enhancer	Sleep initiation and maintenance
Esmirtazapine 00631657	Antidepressant	Sleep initiation and maintenance, mental disorders
LY2624803 000784875	Histamine H1 receptor serotonin2A (5HT-2A) receptor modulator	Insomnia
Piromelatine 02615002	NT1/2/3/5-HT1A/D receptor agonist	Cognitive and sleep effects in Alzheimer's disease
Pentetrazol BTD-001 03542851	Non-competitive $GABA_A$ receptor antagonist	Narcolepsy
FT218 02720744	Sodium oxybate ER	Long-acting sodium oxybate for narcolepsy
THN102 03624920	Combination of modafinil and flecainide	Parkinson's disease and EDS
Reboxetine (AXS-12) 03881852	A selective norepinephrine reuptake inhibitor	Narcolepsy and cataplexy
TAK-925 03332784	Hypocretin 2 receptor agonist	Narcolepsy

Conclusion

In summary, the drugs promoting sleep and wakefulness have evolved over the years to precisely target the sleep and wake-related neurons and neurotransmitters in the brain. These agents are meant for use in conjunction with non-pharmacologic therapies. Unlike the older pharmacologic agents, the newer medications for these disorders have been studied in well-designed placebo-controlled RCTs, albeit mostly industry-sponsored, with evaluation for efficacy and AEs. Many of the agents reviewed are indicated in adults with limited or ongoing studies in pediatric age groups. Personalized medicine has become increasingly important in effective patient care, and the future of sleep pharmacology rests with developing agents that target specific wake/sleep-promoting receptors, tailored for subpopulations of patients suffering from these disorders.

Acknowledgments Merit Review Award, Department of Veterans Affairs, Grant #1I01CX001938-01.

References

1. Eban-Rothschild A, Appelbaum L, de Lecea L. Neuronal mechanisms for sleep/wake regulation and modulatory drive. Neuropsychopharmacology. 2018;43(5):937–52.
2. Atkin T, Comai S, Gobbi G. Drugs for insomnia beyond benzodiazepines: pharmacology, clinical applications, and discovery. Pharmacol Rev. 2018;70(2):197–245.
3. Wagner J, Wagner ML, Hening WA. Beyond benzodiazepines: alternative pharmacologic agents for the treatment of insomnia. Ann Pharmacother. 1998;32(6):680–91.
4. Roth T, Roehrs TA. A review of the safety profiles of benzodiazepine hypnotics. J Clin Psychiatry. 1991;52(Suppl):38–41.
5. Mendelson WB. Clinical distinctions between long-acting and short-acting benzodiazepines. J Clin Psychiatry. 1992;53(Suppl):4–7; discussion 8–9.
6. Buscemi N, Vandermeer B, Friesen C, et al. The efficacy and safety of drug treatments for chronic insomnia in adults: a meta-analysis of RCTs. J Gen Intern Med. 2007;22(9):1335–50.
7. Glass J, Lanctôt KL, Herrmann N, Sproule BA, Busto UE. Sedative hypnotics in older people with insomnia: meta-analysis of risks and benefits. BMJ. 2005;331(7526):1169.
8. Winkler A, Auer C, Doering BK, Rief W. Drug treatment of primary insomnia: a meta-analysis of polysomnographic randomized controlled trials. CNS Drugs. 2014;28(9):799–816.
9. Baandrup L, Ebdrup BH, Rasmussen J, et al. Pharmacological interventions for benzodiazepine discontinuation in chronic benzodiazepine users. Cochrane Database Syst Rev. 2018;3:CD011481.
10. Prescribers' digital reference [Internet]. Whippany: PDR, L.L.C; 2020. zolpidem tartrate-Drug Summary; [cited 2020 July 31]; [about 1 page]. Available from: https://www.pdr.net/drug-summary/Ambien-zolpidem-tartrate-2515.
11. VA/DoD Clinical Practice Guideline. The Management of Chronic Insomnia Disorder and Obstructive Sleep Apnea. Washington, DC: U.S. Government Printing Office; 2019. https://www.healthquality.va.gov/guidelines/CD/insomnia/index.asp.
12. Ferracioli-Oda E, Qawasmi A, Bloch MH. Meta-analysis: melatonin for the treatment of primary sleep disorders. PLoS One. 2013;8(5):e63773.
13. Auger RR, Burgess HJ, Emens JS, Deriy LV, Thomas SM, Sharkey KM. Clinical practice guideline for the treatment of intrinsic circadian rhythm sleep-wake disorders: advanced sleep-wake phase disorder (ASWPD), delayed sleep-wake phase disorder (DSWPD), non-24-hour sleep-wake rhythm disorder (N24SWD), and irregular sleep-wake rhythm disorder (ISWRD). An update for 2015: an American Academy of Sleep Medicine clinical practice guideline. J Clin Sleep Med. 2015;11(10):1199–236.
14. Erland LA, Saxena PK. Melatonin natural health products and supplements: presence of serotonin and significant variability of melatonin content. J Clin Sleep Med. 2017;13(2):275–81.
15. Foley HM, Steel AE. Adverse events associated with oral administration of melatonin: A critical systematic review of clinical evidence. Complement Ther Med. 2019;42:65–81.
16. Prescribers' digital reference [Internet]. Whippany: PDR, L.L.C; 2020. ramelteon-Drug Summary; [cited 2020 July 31]; [about 1 page]. Available from: https://www.pdr.net/drug-summary/Rozerem-ramelteon-562.
17. Kuriyama A, Honda M, Hayashino Y. Ramelteon for the treatment of insomnia in adults: a systematic review and meta-analysis. Sleep Med. 2014;15(4):385–92.
18. Liu L, Wang Q, Liu A, Lan X, Huang Y, Zhao Z, et al. Physiological implications of orexins/Hypocretins on energy metabolism and adipose tissue development. ACS Omega. 2020;5(1):547–55.
19. Prescribers' digital reference [Internet]. Whippany: PDR, L.L.C; 2020. suvorexant -Drug Summary cited 2020 July 31]; Available from: https://www.pdr.net/drug-summary/Belsomra-suvorexant-3605
20. Lemborexant. https://www.accessdata.fda.gov/drugsatfda_docs/label/2019/212028s000lbl.pdf.
21. Herring WJ, Snyder E, Budd K, et al. Orexin receptor antagonism for treatment of insomnia: a randomized clinical trial of suvorexant. Neurology. 2012;79(23):2265–74.

22. Patel KV, Aspesi AV, Evoy KE. Suvorexant: a dual orexin receptor antagonist for the treatment of sleep onset and sleep maintenance insomnia. Ann Pharmacother. 2015;49(4):477–83.
23. Kuriyama A, Tabata H. Suvorexant for the treatment of primary insomnia: A systematic review and meta-analysis. Sleep Med Rev. 2017;35:1–7.
24. Citrome L. Suvorexant for insomnia: a systematic review of the efficacy and safety profile for this newly approved hypnotic - what is the number needed to treat, number needed to harm and likelihood to be helped or harmed? Int J Clin Pract. 2014;68(12):1429–41.
25. Rosenberg R, Murphy P, Zammit G, et al. Comparison of lemborexant with placebo and zolpidem tartrate extended release for the treatment of older adults with insomnia disorder: A phase 3 randomized clinical trial. JAMA Netw Open. 2019;2(12):e1918254.
26. Kärppä M, Yardley J, Pinner K, et al. Long-term efficacy and tolerability of lemborexant compared with placebo in adults with insomnia disorder: results from the phase 3 randomized clinical trial SUNRISE 2. Sleep. 2020;43(3)
27. Kishi T, Nomura I, Matsuda Y, et al. Lemborexant vs suvorexant for insomnia: A systematic review and network meta-analysis. J Psychiatr Res. 2020;128:68–74.
28. Michelson D, Snyder E, Paradis E, et al. Safety and efficacy of suvorexant during 1-year treatment of insomnia with subsequent abrupt treatment discontinuation: a phase 3 randomised, double-blind, placebo-controlled trial. Lancet Neurol. 2014;13(5):461–71.
29. Thompson C. Onset of action of antidepressants: results of different analyses. Hum Psychopharmacol. 2002;17(Suppl 1):S27–32.
30. Yeung WF, Chung KF, Yung KP, Ng TH. Doxepin for insomnia: a systematic review of randomized placebo-controlled trials. Sleep Med Rev. 2015;19:75–83.
31. American Geriatrics Society Beers Criteria® Update Expert Panel. American Geriatric Society 2019 Update AGS Beers Critieria® for potentially inappropriate medication use in older adults. J Am Geriatr Soc. 2019;67(4):674–94.
32. Fung SJ, Yamuy J, Sampogna S, Morales FR, Chase MH. Hypocretin (orexin) input to trigeminal and hypoglossal motoneurons in the cat: a double-labeling immunohistochemical study. Brain Res. 2001;903(1):257–62.
33. Everitt H, Baldwin DS, Stuart B, Lipinska G, Mayers A, Malizia AL, et al. Antidepressants for insomnia in adults. Cochrane Database Syst Rev. 2018;5:CD010753.
34. Yi XY, Ni SF, Ghadami MR, Meng HQ, Chen MY, Kuang L, et al. Trazodone for the treatment of insomnia: a meta-analysis of randomized placebo-controlled trials. Sleep Med. 2018;45:25–32.
35. Full prescribing information: Desyrel. U.S. Food and Drug Administration; 2017.
36. Thompson W, Quay TAW, Rojas-Fernandez C, Farrell B, Bjerre LM. Atypical antipsychotics for insomnia: a systematic review. Sleep Med. 2016;22:13–7.
37. Prescribers' digital reference [Internet]. Whippany: PDR, L.L.C; 2020. quetiapine -Drug Summary cited 2020 July 31]; Available from: https://www.pdr.net/drug-summary/Seroquel-quetiapine-fumarate-2185.
38. Raiteri M, Bertollini A, Angelini F, Levi G. d-Amphetamine as a relaeser of reuptake inhibitor of biogenic amines in SYnaptosomes. Eru J Pharmacol. 1975;34:189–95.
39. Nicholson A, Stone BM. Heterocyclic amphetamine derivatives and caffeine on sleep in man. Br J Clin Pharmacol. 1980;9(2):195–203.
40. Morgenthaler TI, Kapur VK, Brown T, et al. Practice parameters for the treatment of narcolepsy and other hypersomnias of central origin. Sleep. 2007;30(12):1705–11.
41. Lammers GJ. Drugs used in narcolepsy and other hypersomnias. Sleep Med Clin. 2018;13(2):183–9.
42. Murillo-Rodríguez E, Barciela Veras A, Barbosa Rocha N, et al. An overview of the clinical uses, pharmacology, and safety of modafinil. ACS Chem Neurosci. 2018;9(2):151–8.
43. Golicki D, Bala MM, Nieanda M, Wierzbika A. Modafinil for narcolepsy: systemic review and meta-analysis. Med Sci Monit. 2010;16(8):177–86.
44. Moldofsky H, Broughton R, Hill J. A randomized trial of the ling-term, continued efficacy and safety of modafinil in marcolepsy. Sleep Med. 2000;1:109–16.

45. Black J, Houghton WC. Sodium oxybate improves excessive daytime sleepiness in narcolepsy. Sleep. 2006;29(7):939–46.
46. Schwartz J, Feldman N, Bogan R, Nelson M, Huges R. Dosing regimen effects of modafinil for improving daytime wakefulness in patients with narcolepsy. Clin Neurpharmacol. 2003;164(9):252–7.
47. Chapman JL, Vakulin A, Hedner J, Yee BJ, Marshall NS. Modafinil/armodafinil in obstructive sleep apnoea: a systematic review and meta-analysis. Eur Respir J. 2016;47(5):1420–8.
48. Czeisler CA, Walsh JK, Roth T, et al. Modafinil for excessive sleepiness associated with shift-work sleep disorder. N Engl J Med. 2005;353(5):476–86.
49. Hirshkowitz M, Black J, Wesnes K, et al. Adjunct armodafinil improves wakefulness and memory in obstructive sleep apnea/hypopnea syndrome. Respir Med. 2007;101(3):616–27.
50. Roth T, White D, Schmidt-Nowara W, et al. Effects of armodafinil in the treatment of residual excessive sleepiness associated with obsturctive sleep apnea/hypopnea syndrome: A 12-week, mulitcenter, double-blind, randomized, placebo-controlled study in nCPAP-adherent adults. Clin Ther. 2006;28(5):689–706.
51. Harsh J, Hayduk R, Rosenberg R, et al. The efficacy and safety of armodafinil as treatment for adults with excessive sleepiness associated with narcolepsy. Curr Med Res Opin. 2006;22(4):761–74.
52. Czeisler C, Walsh J, Wesnes K, Arora S, Roth T. Armodafinil for treatment of excessive sleepiness associated with shift-work disorder: a randomized controlled study. Mayo Clin Proc. 2009;84(11):958–72.
53. Black J, Hull S, Tiller J, Yng R, Harsh J. The long-term tolerability and efficacy of armodafinil in patients with excessive sleepiness associated with treated obstructive sleep apnea, shift work disorder, or narcolepsy: and open-label extension study. J Clin Sleep Med. 2010;6(5):458–66.
54. Schwartz J, Kahn A, McCall W, Weintraub J, Tiller J. Tolerability and efficacy of armodafinil in naive patients with excessive sleepiness associated with obsturctive sleep apnea, shift work, disorder, or narcolepsy: a 12-month, open-label, flexiable-does study with an extension period. J Clin Sleep Med. 2010;6(5):450–7.
55. Rosenberg R, Bogan R, Tiller J, et al. A phase 3, double-blind, randomized, placebo-controlled study of armodafinil for excessive sleepiness associated with jet lag disorder. Mayo Clin Proc. 2010;85(7):630–8.
56. Roth T, Schwartz J, Hirshkowitz M, et al. Evaluation of the safety of modafinil for treatment of excessive sleepiness. J Clin Sleep Med. 2007;75(20):595–602.
57. Rossetti A, Heinzer R, Tafti M, Buclin T. Rapic occurance of depression following addition of sodium oxybate. Sleep Med. 2010;11:500–1.
58. Xyrem (sodium oxybate) [prescribing information]. Palo Alto: Jazz Pharmaceuticals; September 2020. Xywav (calcium, magnesium, potassium, and sodium oxybates) October 2020.
59. Boscolo-Berto R, Viel G, Montagnese S, et al. Narcolepsy and effectiveness of gamma-hydroxybutyrate (GHB): a systematic review and meta-analysis of randomized controlled trials. Sleep Med Rev. 2012;16(5):431–43.
60. Black J, Pardi D, Hornfeldt C, Inhaber N. The nightly administration of sodium oxybate results in significant reduction in the nocturnal sleep disruption of patients with narcolepsy. Sleep Med. 2009;10(8):829–35.
61. Bogan RK, Thorpy MJ, Dauvilliers Y, et al. Efficacy and safety of calcium, magnesium, potassium, and sodium oxybates (lower-sodium oxybate [LXB]; JZP-258) in a placebo-controlled, double-blind, randomized withdrawal study in adults with narcolepsy with cataplexy. Sleep. 2021;44(3)
62. Alshaikh MK, Tricco AC, Tashkandi M, et al. Sodium oxybate for narcolepsy with cataplexy: systematic review and meta-analysis. J Clin Sleep Med. 2012;8(4):451–8.
63. Xyrem International Study Group. A double-blind, placebo-controlled study demonstrates sodium oxybate is effective for the treatment of excessive daytime sleepiness in narcolepsy. J Clin Sleep Med. 2005;1(4):391–7.
64. The abrupt cessation of therapeutically administered sodium oxybate (GHB) does not cause withdrawl symptoms. J Toxicol Clin Toxicol 2003;41:131–5.

65. Thorpy MJ, Shapiro C, Mayer G, et al. A randomized study of solriamfetol for excessive sleepiness in narcolepsy. Ann Neurol. 2019;85(3):359–70.
66. Schweitzer PK, Rosenberg R, Zammit GK, et al. Solriamfetol for excessive sleepiness in obstructive sleep apnea (TONES 3). A RCT. Am J Respir Crit Care Med. 2019;199(11):1421–31.
67. Thorpy MJ, Bogan RK. Update on the pharmacologic management of narcolepsy: mechanisms of action and clinical implications. Sleep Med. 2020;68:97–109.
68. Dauviliers Y, Bassetti C, Lammers GJ, Amulf I, Mayer G, Rodenbeck A, Lehert P, Ding CL, Lecomte JM, Schwartz JC, HARMONY I Study Group. Pitolisant versus placebo or Modafinil in patients with narcolepsy: a double-blind, randomised trial. Lancet Neurol. 2013;12(11):1068–75.
69. Kollb-Sielecka M, Demolis P, Emmerich J, Markey G, Salmonson T, Haas M. The European medicines agency review of pitolisant for treatment of narcolepsy. Sleep Med. 2017;33:125–9.
70. Bouryi VA, Lewis DI. The modulation by 5-HT of glutamatergic inputs from the raphe pallidus to rat hypoglossal motoneurones, in vitro. J Physiol. 2003;553(3):1019–31.
71. Griffin CE 3rd, Kaye AM, Bueno FR, Kaye AD. Benzodiazepine pharmacology and central nervous system-mediated effects. Ochsner J. 2013;13(2):214–23.
72. Janto K, Prichard JR, Pusalavidyasagar S. An update on dual orexin receptor antagonists and their potential role in insomnia therapeutics. J Clin Sleep Med. 2018;14(8):1399–408.
73. Reynolds AP, Adams R. Treatment of sleep disturbance in older adults. J Pharm Pract Res. 2019;49(3):296–304.
74. Wichniak A, Wierzbicka A, Walęcka M, et al. Effects of antidepressants on sleep. Curr Psychiatry Rep. 2017;19:63.
75. Snyder E, Ma J, Svetnik V, Connor KM, et al. Effects of suvorexant on sleep architecture and power spectral profile in patients with insomnia: analysis of pooled phase 3 data. Sleep Med. 2016;19:93–100.
76. Prescribers' digital reference [Internet]. Whippany: PDR, L.L.C; 2020. zaleplon -Drug Summary cited 2020 July 31]; Available from: https://www.pdr.net/drug-summary/Sonata-zaleplon-1491.
77. Prescribers' digital reference [Internet]. Whippany: PDR, L.L.C; 2020. eszopiclone -Drug Summary cited 2020 July 31]; Available from: https://www.pdr.net/drug-summary/Lunesta-eszopiclone-2082.
78. Ghaffari N, Robertson PA. Caution in prescribing modafinil and armodafinil to individuals who could become pregnant. JAMA Intern Med. 2021;181(2):277–8.
79. U.S. National Library of Medicine. ClinicalTrials.gov [Internet]. Bethesda. MD. [cited 2020 July 30.] Available from: https://clinicaltrials.gov/.

Chapter 3
Sleep Health among Racial/Ethnic groups and Strategies to achieve Sleep Health Equity

Azizi A. Seixas, Anthony Q. Briggs, Judite Blanc, Jesse Moore, Alicia Chung, Ellita Williams, April Rogers, Arlener Turner, and Girardin Jean-Louis

Keywords Sleep quality · Rapid eye movement · Insomnia · Circadian rhythms · Social jetlag · Non-rapid eye movement (NREM) · Sleep architecture · Thyromental angle

Introduction

Relative to Whites, racial/ethnic minorities are more likely to experience a higher burden of poor health, chronic disease, accelerated aging, and premature/excess deaths [1–6]. These health burdens can be attributed to several biological, psycho-social, and environmental factors and mechanisms. Notable biological explanations include, but are not limited to, advanced cell aging, DNA methylation, telomerization of cells, and multimorbidity [2, 7–14]. However, the pathogenesis of poor health, accelerated aging, and disease burden among racial/ethnic minorities is not solely a biological process; it also occurs epigenetically where chronic exposure to

---

Azizi A. Seixas (AS) and Anthony Q. Briggs (AB) are co-first authors.

A. A. Seixas (✉) · J. Blanc · A. Turner · G. Jean-Louis
University of Miami, Miller School of Medicine, Miami, FL, USA
e-mail: azizi.seixas@nyulangone.org; azizi.seixas@nyumc.org

A. Q. Briggs
New York University Langone Health, Department of Population Health, New York, NY, USA

New York University Langone Health, Department of Psychiatry, New York, NY, USA

J. Moore · A. Chung · E. Williams
New York University Langone Health, Department of Population Health, New York, NY, USA

A. Rogers
St. John's University, New York, NY, USA

© Springer Nature Switzerland AG 2022
M. S. Badr, J. L. Martin (eds.), *Essentials of Sleep Medicine*,
Respiratory Medicine, https://doi.org/10.1007/978-3-030-93739-3_3

noxious exogenous factors cause disease by introducing heritable changes in genetic expression or chromosomal function into the biology of individuals to cause disease [11, 12, 15–17]. Growing evidence highlights that the burden of poor health, chronic disease, and accelerated cellular aging among racial/ ethnic minorities is observed across the lifespan, suggesting that the roots of poor health begin as early as the in-utero period and childhood [18]. However, extant etiological frameworks to explain the burden of poor health, chronic disease, accelerated aging, and premature/excess deaths heavily emphasize proximal and exogenous effects of life stressors and exclude potential distal and upstream factors such as the cumulative effect of prejudice and discrimination, as well as environmental (noxious noise, light, and air quality), political (taxes, policies, governmental programs, and nativity/citizen status) [19], and social determinants of health (poor access to health services, socioeconomic status, neighborhoods, and education) [20].

Although it is difficult to identify a single cause for the burden of poor health outcomes, chronic disease, accelerated aging, and premature/excess deaths, there are some factors that may offer upstream (etiology) and downstream (consequences) insights into the chronicity, pervasiveness, and ubiquity of poor health among racial/ ethnic minorities. Growing evidence points to sleep health (duration, sleep disorders, efficiency, sleep quality, sleepiness (alertness), and timing/chronotype) as being one such factor that might provide a unique upstream and downstream explanation for the life-course burden of poor health, chronic disease, accelerated aging, and premature/excess deaths among racial/ethnic minorities [21–25].

Sleep disruptions represent both a cause and consequence of poor health outcomes in racial/ethnic minorities. Mounting evidence indicates that racial/ethnic groups are unequally burdened by a wide range of sleep disruptions and poor sleep health outcomes, which lead to further disparities in cardiovascular disease, cancer, dementia, and mental health outcomes [21–28]. Although the burden of poor sleep health outcomes affects most racial/ethnic groups, relative to Whites, their manifestation and causes at the population level are specific to each group. For example, Black and Latino children and adults alike have a predominantly higher risk for poor sleep health (inconsistent sleep schedules, insufficient sleep duration, sleep-disordered breathing problems, and daytime sleepiness) compared to their White counterparts. It is likely that poor sleep health, experienced as a child, has residual and insidious effects on later life, thus increasing likelihood of debilitating poor sleep and adverse functional and health outcomes, such as poor cognitive performance, car accidents and occupational accidents, cardiovascular disease, diabetes, and mental health, all of which are higher among racial/ethnic minorities compared to Whites [29, 30].

To better understanding sleep health burden among racial/ethnic groups, we will describe the prevalence and burden of sleep health parameters: (1) sleep duration, (2) sleep disorders, (3) sleep timing/chronotype, (4) sleep architecture, (5) sleep quality, (6) sleepiness/alertness, and (7) sleep efficiency (See Fig. 3.1). Then, we will describe upstream processes and causes of poor sleep health parameters among racial/ethnic groups, which can be attributed to a variety of biological (circadian rhythm), behavioral (diet and exercise mental health), psychosocial (stress, mental

Fig. 3.1 Sleep health
components diagram

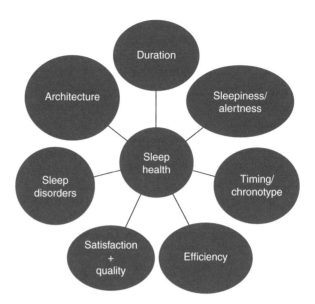

health, poverty, social demands), and environmental factors (noise and light), which we describe in detail. Lastly, we will describe the downstream processes and consequences of poor sleep health among racial/ethnic groups, which include but are not limited to a variety of adverse health outcomes, chronic diseases (cardiovascular disease, diabetes, and mental health), and poor functional and performance outcomes.

Prevalence and Burden of Poor Sleep Health

Sleep health is characterized by seven sleep parameters: (1) sleep duration, (2) sleep disorders, (3) sleep timing/chronotype, (4) sleep architecture (sleep stages divided into rapid eye movement (REM) and non-REM sleep), (5) sleep quality, (6) sleepiness, and (7) sleep efficiency [31]. Mounting evidence highlight an alarming trend of sleep health disparities across certain demographic groups, most notably among racial/ethnic minorities who compared to their White counterparts experience significant burden in all seven sleep parameters which have been attributed to several adverse health and functional outcomes and provide some explanation for elevated and high burden of certain chronic diseases, such as cardiovascular disease, mental health, and dementia. From this growing and heterogenous evidence, there is an emerging coalescing definition of sleep health disparity, which the NIH describes as any difference in one or more dimensions of sleep health (regularity, quality, alertness, timing, efficiency, and duration)—on a consistent basis—that adversely affects designated disadvantaged populations [29]. Although this definition of sleep health disparity is not final or comprehensive, it represents an excellent start and working definition that provides the critical lens through which one can identify, define, measure, and study the drivers and consequences of sleep health disparity. Therefore, we use this definition of sleep health disparity as the lens to identify sleep health disparities among racial/ethnic groups for the current book chapter. However, to better understand sleep health disparity, it is important to go beyond identifying differences (which is often restricted to numerical difference), and seek to understand the fundamental causes and consequences of these differences.

Therefore, for the current chapter, we define sleep health disparity as differences that are due to deeply entrenched cause[s] (biological, psychosocial, and environmental) and downstream consequences that even the counterfactual cannot escape. For example, sleep health disparity exists because both poor and wealthy racial/ethnic minorities are more burdened by poor sleep health outcomes, compared to their poor and wealthy White counterparts (even when comparing a wealthy minority with a poor White individual). This evidence should not be misunderstood as a positing and privileging of ontogeny/biological causes over social causes but rather an acknowledgment of the syndemic and epigenetic etiology of sleep health disparity. In fact, sleep health disparity may be due to omni-directional relationships among latent hard-wired biological factors, noxious psychosocial and environmental terroir and contexts, and defunct system-level factors that would normally ameliorate health risk (such as the inability of our poor healthcare system to address sleep health disparities and its consequences or poor labor policies that prevent individuals from earning a living wage causing poorer populations to work multiple jobs that induce stress and disrupt sleep health). For the sections below, we establish: (1) sleep health disparities by describing numerical differences across all sleep health parameters (highlighting higher burden, prevalence rates, and likelihoods among racial/ethnic minorities compared to their counterfactual counterparts), (2) biological, psychosocial, and environmental antecedents and causes of sleep health differences, and (3) functional and health consequences of sleep health differences among racial/ethnic minorities (See Table 3.1).

Sleep Duration

There are significant differences in sleep duration and total sleep time among several demographic groups (sex, geographic, and socioeconomic status). The most compelling and robust evidence for group-based differences in sleep duration are observed among racial/ethnic minorities and so for the current chapter we focus only on racial/ethnic groups. Racial/ethnic differences in sleep duration have been noticed as early as childhood and persist throughout the lifespan to adulthood. Regardless of age group, racial/ethnic minorities do not receive adequate sleep duration for their age sleep. Although the American Academy of Sleep Medicine recommends that 3–5-year-old children receive on average 10–13 hours (including naps) daily, 9–12 hours for 9–12-year-old children, and 7–9 hours for adults, racial/ethnic minorities consistently experience insufficient sleep duration (See Table 3.1).

Table 3.1 Racial-ethnic disparities in health outcomes in selected sleep dimensions compared to White adults

	Sleep duration	Sleep disorders	Chrono type- circadian rhythm	Sleep architecture	Social jet lag- excessive sleepiness	Sleep quality
African-American/ Black	⬇ 12–14,29,30–33	⬇ 6,19,31,32,44–46	⬇ 50,52,53	⬇ 64,21	⬇ 23,43	⬇ 44,57,58,59
Hispanics-Latinos	⬇ 17,26,38	⬇ 20,31,35,47,49	⬇ IES	⬇ 64	⬇ 43	⬇ 57
Asian	⬇ 12	31,20	IES	IES	IES	IES
Native Hawaiian and Pacific Islander	⬇ 12	44	IES	64	26	IES

Note: The direction of the arrow refers to the direction of how these groups are more at risk to experience sleep disparities in the selected categories (e.g., lower or higher)
Abbreviations: *MR* mixed results, IES insufficient evidence in sleep

Chronic insufficient sleep duration (such as short sleep duration <7 hours) has been linked with increased risk for cognitive impairment, occupational hazards, mistakes, poor cardiovascular health and disease, mental illness, dementia, and cancer [32–36].

Based on data from the National Health and Nutrition Examination Survey (NHANES), short sleep duration is highly prevalent in the United States with a conservative overall estimate of 37.1% across the lifespan. However, these same data reveal that the greatest burden of short sleep duration is experienced among middle age individuals: (1) 20–39 years of age (37.0%); (2) 40–59 years (40.3%); and 60 years and older (32.0%), highlighting severe sleep deprivation across all age groups [37]. Stratifying these results by race/ethnicity highlights the fact that among children 6 months and 2 years old, only 6% of Black children slept the recommended amount of 12 hours daily, while 83% of White children slept at least 12 hours daily. Similar trends have been observed among adolescents, where Asians (76%) and Blacks (71%) had the highest rates of short sleep duration/insufficient sleep relative to Whites (68%), except Latinx (67%). Similarly among adults, Native Hawaiian-Pacific Islanders (46.3%); Blacks (45.8%); Other Multiracial (44.3%); American Indian-Alaska Native (40.4%); Asian (37.5%); and Latins (34.5%) all have higher prevalence of short/insufficient sleep relative to Whites (33.4%).

Sleep health disparities among minorities are not limited to adult populations only. A review of 23 studies investigated racial/ethnic sleep health disparities among American minority youth between the ages of 6–19 years and found that white youth (adolescents) had more sufficient sleep compared to racial/ethnic minorities, most notably Blacks and Hispanics/Latinos. Blacks had overall shorter sleep duration and later bedtimes than Hispanics/Latinos [38]. Black and Hispanic youth also spent more time traveling to school, had earlier start times, and spent more time watching television, more likely to share a bedroom and partake in regular naps. Evidently, napping decreased with age, and some studies have shown that Blacks and Hispanics/Latino are more likely to nap on the weekday while other researchers have suggested that naps are more likely to happen on the weekends [39]. In other studies, Black and Hispanics slept an hour less than Whites [40–47].

Outside of epidemiological data, community-based findings with similar trends further validate the notion that sleep health differences do exist across the lifespan. In a cross-sectional community study of children, 39.1% of Black children reported poorer sleep duration and more naps compared to 4.9% White children. To explain this twin phenomenon of sleep deprivation and napping, it is likely that Black children who are sleep deprived try to catch up on lost sleep, through napping, and extended sleep duration over the weekend than weekday [44, 48, 49]. Further stratification by sex also shows race-sex differences in sleep duration. In a community study in Chicago, Illinois White men (6.7 hours) have the highest average sleep (actigraphy), then White women (6.1 hours), then Black women (5.9 hours), and then Black men (5.1 hours) [36], a trend observed across other studies [47, 50–53]. The burden of short sleep duration and sleep deprivation, among racial ethnic minorities, is consequential as they are linked with several chronic health conditions [46, 54–58].

Sleep Disorders

It is estimated that 50–70 million people have a sleep disorder, with obstructive sleep apnea (OSA) and insomnia being the two most prevalent in the United States. OSA is a sleep breathing disorder characterized by partial or complete blockage of the upper airway, resulting in reflexive awakenings and transient cessation in breathing patterns (apneas and hypopneas). Apnea and hypopnea events cause oxygen desaturation and physiological stress, thus affecting key homeostatic physiological processes. Key OSA symptoms include: sleep-related pauses in respiration, arousals, unrefreshing sleep, snoring, restlessness, poor concentration, fatigue, and excessive daytime sleepiness [34]. OSA is considered one of the most common sleep disorders, among middle and older aged adults, affecting around 24% and 49.7% of the US population [52]. Obesity, large neck size, instability in respiratory control system, and craniofacial structures are key OSA risk factors. OSA is associated with cardiovascular disease, cardiometabolic conditions, cerebrovascular, low and worsen cognitive performance, and dementia [34, 59, 60].

The burden of OSA risk and disease is high among racial-ethnic minorities (among pediatric and adult populations), specifically Blacks (See Table 3.1). Blacks children aged 2–18 were more likely to experience sleep-disordered breathing (SDB), even after controlling for specific variables, obesity, respiratory problems, smoking, and neighborhood of residence. Even racial and ethnic parents have reported that their child snores more than non-ethnic parents. Other estimates indicate that Black children are 4–6 times more likely to have OSA, Hispanic/Latinx children have a greater severity, Native American children are 1.7 times more likely to have moderate to severe OSA, and Asian Americans have similar or lower OSA prevalence compared to White children [59]. In an adult population using data from the Jackson Heart sleep study ($n = 852$), approximately 24% of the sample had moderate to severe OSA based on apnea-hypopnea index (a measure of severity), but only 5% had a diagnosis, indicating that the overwhelming majority of participants were undiagnosed (95%). Black men had a higher prevalence of OSA compared with Black women [61]. The foregoing evidence suggests that even when Blacks experience OSA symptoms, they were less likely to be diagnosed and treated. Similar trends are observed among Latinx and Asian popualtions [34], with 49.4% of Latinos and 43.1% of Asians reporting significant snoring, a major OSA symptom and risk factor. Although population estimates are high, community-level estimates indicate even higher burden among racial/ethnic minorities. In a study conducted in primary care community-based clinics in Brooklyn NY, almost half of Black patients (45%) reported debilitating snoring and about one-third reported excessive daytime sleepiness (33%) and difficulty maintaining sleep, a sign of insomnia (34%) [6]. However, for Latinx population being overweight/obese was the strongest marker and predictor of OSA risk, while for Asians craniofacial features and not body adiposity was most predictive of OSA risk [62]. The heterogeneity in OSA risk across racial/ethnic groups has proved difficult for adequate screening, assessment, and treatment, often leading to high rates of untreated individuals. The consequence of untreated OSA has proved consequential, especially among Blacks, as it is linked to elevated, uncontrolled, and resistant blood pressure and stroke [34, 59, 60].

OSA burden and disparity are not just observed and confined to differential estimates of the disease but also rooted in the uneven distribution of upstream and downstream consequences of OSA, as well as the lack of system level infrastructures to attenuate or buffer these burdens. Adherence to OSA treatments is a major problem among racial and ethnic minority groups as Blacks have one of the poorest OSA treatment (positive airway pressure [PAP]) adherence rates [63]. Poor treatment adherence is credited more to system-level barriers in the healthcare system such as poor insurance coverage, under-resourced sleep clinics in predominantly low-income and minority neighborhoods, and the limited amount of board-certified minority clinicians and providers.

Insomnia is another prevalent sleep disorder among racial/ethnic minorities. Although the prevalence of an insomnia diagnosis is mixed among minority groups, the prevalence of insomnia symptoms such as involuntary early morning awakenings, difficulty falling asleep, and issues with staying asleep are high. For racial and ethnic groups, insomnia is one of the most common sleep complaints and disorders, with approximately 30% reporting at least one insomnia symptom, 5–10% meeting threshold for an insomnia disorder, and approximately 6% with an actual diagnosis [51, 64, 65]. Insomnia's nocturnal symptoms and daytime consequences include lack of energy, difficulty concentrating, fatigue, tiredness, irritability, and moodiness. Insomnia disorder increases the risk of stress, anxiety, depression, and decreased quality of life.

Several population studies show that Blacks are more likely to be affected by insomnia symptoms compared to other racial/ethnic groups. In a US National Institute of Health (NIH) study with 825 Black Americans (both men and women), 1 in 5 participants had insomnia and 6.7% an insomnia diagnosis. Another study demonstrated that Blacks reported greater nighttime insomnia relative to their other racial/ethnic counterparts.

Chronotype and Circadian Rhythms

Observed differences in circadian rhythms, chronotype, and sleep timing (irregular sleep time between weekdays and weekends such as social jetlag) among racial/ethnic minorities relative to Whites is well-documented (See Table 3.1). Circadian rhythms is the 24-hour internal clock that regulates the scheduling of important bio-behavioral activities such as eating, metabolizing food, sleep and rest, and when a person is most active or stressed. The circadian master clock, the superchiasmatic nucleus, coordinates, and synchronizes with peripheral clocks in the body (i.e., heart, cells) to ensure all biological and functional processes are aligned, synchronized, and working optimally. Circadian rhythms are influenced by exogenous cues and stimuli such as light, darkness, and sound that help punctuate the day and signal shifts that help the body regulate itself. However, desynchronized and chronic exposure to these cues and stimuli can result in circadian dysregulation and possible misalignment. Circadian misalignment occurs when an individual's central and peripheral biological clocks become misaligned from their daily behavioral clock, such as the time an individual the routine sleep, meal, and activity [45, 57, 66–69]. The desynchrony of exogenous, endogenous, and behavioral clocks can occur as early as childhood and is linked to poor emotion regulation and obesity across the lifespan [57, 70].

Chronotype among minorities Persons with evening chronotype are less likely to have regular exercise and more likely to partake in unhealthy diets and lifestyle choices that increase their cardiovascular risk. In a study made up of 61.5% of racially and ethnically diverse women in the United States (N = 506) greater morningness was associated with a more favorable cardiovascular profile which included BMI, blood pressure, cholesterol, and glucose levels compared to their white counterparts. Conversely, compared to the morning chronotype, evening persons had a greater than two-fold higher odds of having a poor cardiovascular profile and sleep duration of less than 7 hours per night [71]. Among adults in the Southern region of the United States, obesity was significantly associated with evening chronotype in whites, but not blacks even after adjusting for important covariates like shift work, physical activity, and sleep duration which could suggest the need for more pointed research exploring the multidimensional nature of racial and ethnic chrono-types [71].

Circadian rhythms among minorities Several studies show that Blacks have shorter free-running circadian periods (tau) than Whites (24.07 hours vs 24.33 hours). Shorter free-running circadian periods make it more difficult to adjust to night-shift work and delayed (daytime) sleep schedule [67–69]. The health consequences of shifts in circadian rhythms can be grave, as studies indicate that Black night shift workers are more likely to have elevated blood pressure and hypertensive compared to Black day workers. In a community sample of Blacks in New York City, Black shift workers had 35% increased odds of having hypertension among Blacks [OR = 1.35, CI: 1.06–1.72. $P < 0.05$], compared to their White counterparts. Circadian rhythm disruption among Blacks who work non-traditional hours leads to sleep deprivation and shorter sleep duration and 80% increased cardiovascular disease risk such as hypertension [OR = 1.81, CI: 1.29–2.54, $P < 0.01$] [67]. Blacks who have shorter circadian periods and live closer to the equator with longer exposure to sunlight were less likely to have disrupted circadian rhythms.

Social jetlag among minorities A prevalent phenomenon that may impact sleep habits is the concept of "social jetlag". Social jetlag occurs when an individual's weekday and weekend sleep time is significantly different from their body's endogenous circadian clock. This results in poorer sleep quality, sleep time in deep sleep, and may result in other adverse functional and health outcomes. Disruptions in sleep timing can have ripple effects on the timing of other key social and biological activities such as eating. It is highly likely that disruptions in sleep timing due to social jetlag may also result in eating jet lag. Eating jetlag occurs when an individual's meal timing is misaligned with their endogenous metabolic circadian clock. Combined, irregular sleep, physical activity, and mealtimes are key contributors to circadian misalignment and has been linked to adverse functional and health outcomes. Social jetlag can have severe and adverse health consequences. For example, the New Hoorn study cohort ($n = 1585$) investigated the association between social jet lag, metabolic syndrome, cardiovascular health and found that individuals younger than 61 years of age who reported social jetlag (1–2 hours) had approximately a two-fold greater risk of metabolic syndrome and prediabetes/diabetes compared to their counterparts who reported less than 1 hour of social jetlag [72].

Sleep Architecture

Sleep architecture represents the cyclical pattern of sleep as it shifts between the different sleep stages, non-rapid eye movement (NREM) and rapid eye movement (REM) sleep. An individual's sleep architecture is made up of sleep cycles and stages marked by unique neurological, autonomic, and physiological signals that correspond to the stage of sleep or wake an individual is experiencing [61, 73]. Each full cycle of NREM and REM sleep lasts about 90 to 120 minutes. NREM sleep is characterized by 3 stages of sleep (N1, N2, and N3). Stage 1 of NREM is the lightest form of sleep marked by low amplitude alpha brain waves, Stage 2 is marked by sleep spindles and K complexes, and Stage 3 is marked by higher amplitude delta waves signifying deeper more restorative sleep. A normal pattern of sleep cycles (as shown in the hypnogram) includes a greater portion of time spent in Stages 2 and 3 sleep at the beginning of the night and more REM sleep at the second half of the night, with a few possible brief awakenings scattered throughout the sleep stages.

Racial/ethnic differences, in the quantity and quality of sleep architecture, are well documented, where Blacks tend to get more light sleep and less deep sleep compared to Whites (See Table 3.1) [48]. In the Outcomes of Sleep Disorders in Older Men (Mr OS Sleep) Study with Black, Asian American, Hispanic and White men ($n = 2823$), Black men relative to other races/ethnicities had the lowest percentage of Stage 1 non-REM sleep (6.59%) and slow-wave sleep Stage 3 sleep (7.99%). However, Blacks had the highest percentage of Stage 2 non-REM sleep (64.79%) and REM sleep (20.71%) [74]. Overall, Blacks spend less time in slow-wave sleep and spend greater time in REM relative to Whites. Therefore, it is likely that sleep-deprived Blacks are more likely to experience daytime sleepiness and physical fatigue.

Sleep Efficiency

Sleep efficiency is another sleep health parameter that racial/ethnic differences can be observed. Overall, sleep efficiency captures how much sleep an individual actually experiences and is predicated on several sleep characteristics, such as sleep latency and wake after sleep onset. In a population-based study, Black men had lower sleep efficiency (79.7%), due to longer sleep latency (29.4 minutes) and greater WASO (90.4%) relative to Whites, Hispanic/Latinx, and Asian Americans [74]. These results suggest that Blacks took a longer time to fall asleep, had less efficient sleep (meaning that they spent less time sleeping while in bed), and had the greatest levels of awakenings after sleep was initiated.

Sleep Quality and Sleepiness

Racial/ethnic minorities have a higher burden of daytime sleepiness and poor sleep quality compared to Whites (See Table 3.1). In the Multi-Ethnic Study of Atherosclerosis (MESA) study, Blacks had the highest rates of excessive daytime sleepiness (using the Epworth Sleepiness Scale [ESS] score > 12) at 13.1%, compared to Hispanic/Latinx at 9.2%, Whites at 8.0%, and Chinese at 7.5% [75]. However, Whites reported highest rate of being sleepy for more than 5 days of the month (18.6%) compared to the other racial/ethnic groups (Black = 14.4%, Hispanic/

Latinx = 16.9%, and Chinese = 12.3%). Compared to Whites, Blacks, Hispanic/ Latinx, and Chinese Americans had lower odds of excessive sleepiness ≤5 days/ month, after adjusting for demographic factors. However, after adjusting for physical health and psychosocial variables, differences in sleepiness between Whites and Chinese Americans decreased suggesting that these factors play a crucial role in the estimates on the amount of sleepy days among Chinese Americans. Relative to Whites, Black Americans had the highest odds (and only, as Hispanic/Latinx and Chinese were not significant) of excessive daytime sleepiness (ESS scale >12) (ORs range across 4 adjusted models 1.43–1.74, adjusting for sociodemographic, psychosocial, physical health, and sleep duration and disorders). The greatest attenuation in the differential estimates of daytime sleepiness between Blacks and Whites was observed when controlling for physical health and sleep variables, but not for psychosocial factors.

Causes of Poor Sleep Health

The root cause of sleep health disparities among racial/ethnic minorities is multifarious and complex, as several biological, psychosocial, and environmental factors may explain the burden of poor sleep health.

Biological Causes

Empirical studies highlight several biological causes of racial/ethnic differences on sleep health parameters. Biological explanations for sleep health disparities include genetic, circadian, and anthropometric. Although genetic causes of differential sleep health estimates are intricate and inconclusive, initial evidence from large genetic studies indicate a possible ancestry link. For example, in a study that investigated 1698 ancestry genetic markers, individuals with higher percentage of African ancestry had lower percentage of slow-wave sleep SWS and explained 11% of the variability in slow-wave sleep, a marker of sleep depth [76]. As indicated above, Blacks or individual with African Ancestry have shortened free-running circadian period (tau) compared with their White counterparts [68]. Anthropometric causes may also explain differential estimates of sleep health outcomes. In a study comparing the link between craniofacial features and risk for sleep apnea among Asian and White Americans, neck circumference, body mass index, mallampati score (MS) (measurement of tongue and mouth during a breath hold at end-tidal inspiration with the mouth wide open and tongue fully protruded), thyromental distance (TMD), and thyromental angle (TMA) (angle between the soft tissue of backside of neck, the soft tissue mentum, and the thyroid) were the best predictors of OSA risk and severity [77]. Asians had different MS, TMD and TMA compared to Whites which was associated with greater sleep apnea severity and had higher MS, smaller

TMD, and larger TMA. In another study, obesity explained sleep apnea risk among Whites, while skeletal restriction explained sleep apnea risk among Chinese. Despite this difference, the ratio between obesity to craniofacial bone size, a determinant of upper airway volume and OSA risk, was not statistically different between Chinese and Whites [78].

Psychosocial Causes

There are several psychosocial factors that might explain sleep health disparities among racial/ethnic minorities. These factors include but are not limited to social stressors, beliefs, and attitudes and behaviors.

Social stressors Several researchers suggest that racial inequalities and social inequities developed through racial segregation, food desserts, lack of resources, educational attainment, employment status, and limited to no access to health care system care can be linked to psychological distress, anxiety, depression and poor sleep and unhealthy sleep behaviors [46, 79, 80].

In a sample of 4863 Black adults, psychosocial stressors such as perceived stress, major life events stress, and weekly stress were associated with short sleep duration and poorer sleep quality. The effects of weekly stress on sleep duration was most pronounced among younger (<60 hears old) and college-educated Blacks [81]. Similar trends can be observed for the Latinx population, where depressive symptoms, employment status, and low education level were independently associated with short sleep duration, while unemployment, low household income, and low level of education were independently associated with long sleep [82]. In a study that explored the influence of perceived racial discrimination and the risk of insomnia on middle-age elderly Black women ($N = 26,139$), participants with higher perceived levels of discrimination had higher insomnia symptoms and shorter sleep duration (<7 hours) [83]. While in another study, economic disadvantage and poor physical and mental health were statistically were associated with insomnia among older Blacks ($N = 398$) in Southern Los Angeles [35].

Beliefs and attitudes Racial ethnic minorities' beliefs and attitudes about sleep and sleep health play crucial roles in the amount of sleep an individual receives and the quality of their sleep. The association beliefs and attitudes have on sleep outcomes is likely to be indirect and reflects a mediated association between inadequate sleep health literacy, unhealthy sleep behavior, and poor sleep health outcomes. Individuals may not know or appreciate the importance of sleep and how it impacts their health and functional outcomes. For example, some racial/ethnic minorities have considered deep habitual snoring or snoring as relatively good sleep and are unaware that it may portend something more ominous such as a sleep breathing disorder like sleep apnea. In a study of community-dwelling Black men, participants with elevated and high risk for OSA were more likely to report false and maladaptive beliefs about sleep [84]. In another study, Blacks reported using napping and consuming caffeine to cope with sleep deprivation and sleepiness. In the same study, participants reported using electronic devices (such as TV and phone) to blunt racing and ruminative thoughts that prevented them from falling asleep [85].

Behaviors There are a number of behaviors that can affect differential sleep estimates across racial/ethnic groups. These include but are not limited to mental health, diet, and physical activity. For example, studies have shown that Blacks with elevated emotional distress are more likely to report short or long sleep durations [86]. In a nationally representative study, insufficient sleep (<7 hours) was associated with unhealthy diets, suggesting a potential bi-directional relationship where poor sleep leads to poor diet and food choices and poor food choices, such as night eating and consumption of high-calorie foods close to bedtime may lead to later bedtime, late sleep onset, and disrupted sleep [87]. Other studies have found that Blacks and Whites respond differently to food stimulants like caffeine when they found that Blacks who consume caffeinated drinks were more likely to have disrupted sleep compared to Whites [50]. Physical activity/exercise is another behavior that might cause differential sleep health estimates between racial/ethnic groups and Whites. In a sample of 246 Black adolescents, physical activity protected against short sleep duration [88]. Specifically, race and sleep duration appeared to be only significant at lower levels of physical activity and Black adolescents who reported shorter sleep durations had lower physical activity.

Physical and Built Environment Causes

There is growing evidence that environment, physical and built, can affect sleep health outcomes. Patterns of Insufficient sleep is more prevalent in poor urban and rural settings relative to their more affluent counterparts [89]. These findings highlight that geographical effect on sleep health outcomes may traverse race/ethnicity, as majority of the region is White, although the amount of Black (4%), Asian (26%), and Hispanic (37%) residents have been increasing, according to a 2019 Pew Trust research poll. Outside of geographic patterns of and effects on sleep health outcomes, more granular evidence highlight the contribution of noxious noise, light and temperature have on sleep health outcomes, as well as physical environment of an individual's community influences their sleep. For example, social cohesion, safety, light, traffic, air quality and pollution, noise, greenspace, and neighborhood cohesion/disorder and walkability may impact sleep health outcomes. Data shows that racial/ethnic minorities might be particularly vulnerable to the effects of environmental factors on sleep health outcomes.

Of the environmental factors listed above, the role of light on sleep has the most robust evidence to date explaining racial/ethnic differences in sleep health outcomes. The proliferation and exposure to artificial light presents the clearest and most present danger to sleep health. Artificial light (ALAN) during the day and mostly at night is harmful, and evidence points the unfortunate burden and vulnerability among racial/ethnic minorities [90]. Blacks and Hispanics when exposed to ALAN 2 times greater than Whites [56]. Dominant artificial light exposure from in-house sources such as laptops, individual's computer, cellphones, televisions, and outside sources including street lights are more likely to disrupt an individual's natural sleep-wake cycles causing circadian misalignment and sleep disruption.

Noise levels from several sources such as train, industrial activity, traffic, nocturnal noise can have deleterious effects on sleep health outcomes such as sleep disturbances, daytime sleepiness, irritated, frustrated, annoyance, inconsistent mood changes, and adverse to long-term effects on cardiometabolic outcomes. Excessive noise pollution may trigger stress hormones that can increase blood pressure, heart rate during sleep times, and autonomic arousals thus leading to microarousal that lead to shallow, fragmented, and unrestorative sleep. A study funded by Robert Wood Johnson and National Cancer Institute found that neighborhoods with predominantly Asians, Blacks, and Hispanics residents had higher levels of noxious noise levels during the day and at night (approximately 4 decibels higher on average) compared to neighborhoods without racial and ethnic groups [65].

Health Consequences of Poor Sleep Health

The third set of evidence to establish a health disparity is the higher burden of downstream consequences as a result of poor sleep health experienced by racial/ethnic minorities. Racial/ethnic minorities as at significantly higher risk for a host of adverse functional and health outcomes, such as cardiovascular disease, cardiometabolic conditions, and poor brain health (mental health and dementia).

First, poor sleep health, which includes sleep deprivation, shorter sleep duration, sleep disorders (sleep apnea and insomnia), and poor sleep quality, is directly linked to increased cardiovascular risks such as heart disease, high blood pressure, stroke, diabetes, and cardiovascular health and disease, among racial/ethnic minorities [36, 37, 86, 91–94]. For example, in the CARDIA study ($n = 578$; ages 33–45), shorter sleep duration predicted hypertension (OR 1.37, 95% CI: 1.05, 1.78) [95]. The direct association between poor sleep and adverse health outcomes among racial/ethnic minorities is due to high prevalence of sleep deprivation, where they are twice as likely to sleep less than their white counterparts.

Second, poor sleep health parameters are indirectly linked to adverse health outcomes among racial/ethnic minorities. Evidence of these indirect associations include the mediated role of shift work, where racial/ethnic minorities working night shift are at increased risk for circadian misalignment and cardiometabolic disease and poor mental health outcomes [25, 96–99]. The indirect association between sleep and adverse health outcomes is significant and consequential because Blacks and Latina/os are more likely to work non-traditional work shifts compared to their White counterparts. Blacks who work night shifts are at greater risk and burden for hypertension compared to Blacks that work day shifts, whereas, for Whites no differences between day and night shift work were observed [50]. These racial/ethnic differences in shift work may partly explain the burden of hypertension in Blacks, as night shift workers have lower blood pressure dipping at night than day shift workers at the same time causing a prolonged elevated blood pressure. Prolonged elevated blood pressure can cause hypertension, resistant hypertension, and elevated risk for stroke, all health conditions highly prevalent among Blacks [53, 98, 100, 101].

The indirect and mediated relationships between sleep and adverse health outcomes are not solely due to social determinants of health or psychosocial factors but also may be engendered by biological, physiological, and anatomical factors [40]. Individuals who report insufficient sleep over a period of time have a higher caloric intake (+30% of daily caloric requirement), compared to Whites. Insufficient sleep and sleep deprivation may induce poor eating habits, thus increasing the higher caloric intake of carbohydrates, snacks, unhealthy foods, age, gender, and BMI, which can promote weight gain [102]. A meta-analysis of 72 studies found that in restricted sleep short and long sleep durations were associated with cardiovascular inflammatory markers such as: C-reactive protein and interleukin (IL)-6, factors linked with cardio-metabolic conditions (obesity and type 2 diabetes), neurodegenerative and pulmonary disease [79].

Several studies note significant brain health consequences – cognitive decline, cognition impairment, and neurodegenerative disease like dementia –as a result of poor sleep health among racial/ethnic groups. For example, excessive daytime sleepiness is associated with cognitive decline, impaired cognition, mood, executive decisions, minimal attention span, memory and emotionally memory, and inflammation of the brain [9, 10, 56–62]. Race stratified analyses indicate that the associations between sleep health parameters (notably daytime sleepiness, short sleep duration, and long sleep duration) and cognitive impairment/decline are most pronounced in Blacks and Hispanics compared to other racial/ethnic groups [43, 47].

In one population-based study ($n = 28,756$), the majority of participants with extreme sleep deprivation (less than 4 hours or more than 10 hours per night) experienced greater cognitive decline than individuals with at least 7 hours of sleep per night, [62] with racial ethnic minorities appearing to be most affected. In another study with middle-age adults, inconsistent sleep time had a negative impact on cognitive functioning as individuals showed clinically significant signs of cognitive decline after 3 weeks [103]. The adverse effects of poor sleep can have long-term effects on cognition. In a sample of Japanese-Americans, individuals with high levels of daytime sleepiness had a greater odds of dementia and cognitive decline in a three-year follow-up [104]. Findings from these studies highlight that two possibilities. First, poor sleep health may be a risk factor for acute and chronic cognitive decline. Second, sleep may serve as an early sign of cognitive decline, which may portend the onset of dementia.

Conclusion

The aim of this chapter was to describe extant estimates of poor sleep health among racial/ethnic minorities, multilevel determinants of sleep health disparities among racial/ethnic minorities, including biological, environmental, and psychosocial factors, and associated downstream health outcomes among racial/ethnic minorities. Over the past decades, important efforts have been made by health disparities clinicians and researchers to raise awareness about new approaches to tackle disparities in sleep health. However, data highlighted in this book chapter indicates that there is still a long road to travel until we arrive at sleep health equity in the United States [44, 49, 57, 59, 60, 63, 83, 105–108]. Building upon the sleep health framework, we suggest that one of the first crucial steps in addressing racial/ethnic disparities in sleep health is to define the concept of sleep health equity that we conceptualized as the equal opportunity to experience and obtain healthy sleep regardless of age, sex, race/ethnicity, geographical location, and socioeconomic status to obtain satisfactory sleep that promotes physical and mental well-being [28]. We also argue that achieving sleep health equity requires a multi-level and multisystem approach that includes patients, providers, payers, and the entire healthcare ecosystem. To achieve sleep health equity involves the following five steps and initiatives [28]:

1. We encourage implementation of sleep health literacy programs for all ages – from early screening and treatment for sleep disorders starting in preschool, elementary schools, high schools, and university. This will provide sleep health literacy modules, workshops, webinars, throughout websites, social media outlets, and mobile apps.
2. This awareness and sleep health access for ethnic and racial minorities could be achieved through the creation and multilingual sleep centers in vulnerable communities. Such multi-ethnic and multi-lingual initiatives could also be replicated in additional health centers located in vulnerable communities.
3. Culturally tailored behavioral sleep health interventions may increase adherence to physician's recommendations among racial and ethnic minorities. For instance, this could be achieved through required, culturally sensitive training in sleep medicine programs where physicians are better equipped in administering sleep health medicine and interventions for vulnerable populations.
4. We need training programs across all educational levels from high school to university (Ex: the New York University's PRIDE and COMRADE programs), which aims to increase diversity in the sleep health medicine workforce.
5. Public health policies to address and reduce the burden of environmental (ex: noise and light) exposures that are underpinning poor sleep health among racial/ethnic minorities are strongly encouraged. This is very important because Blacks and other minorities experience a higher rate of environmental risk living in disfranchised neighborhoods and communities.

References

1. Geronimus AT, Hicken MT, Pearson JA, Seashols SJ, Brown KL, Cruz TD. Do US black women experience stress-related accelerated biological aging? Hum Nat. 2010; https://doi.org/10.1007/s12110-010-9078-0.
2. Geronimus AT, Hicken M, Keene D, Bound J. "Weathering" and age patterns of allostatic load scores among blacks and whites in the United States. Am J Public Health. 2006; https://doi.org/10.2105/AJPH.2004.060749.
3. Kaestner R, Pearson JA, Keene D, Geronimus AT. Stress, allostatic load, and health of Mexican immigrants. Soc Sci Q. 2009; https://doi.org/10.1111/j.1540-6237.2009.00648.x.
4. Duru OK, Harawa NT, Kermah D, Norris KC. Allostatic load burden and racial disparities in mortality. J Natl Med Assoc. 2012; https://doi.org/10.1016/S0027-9684(15)30120-6.
5. Levine ME, Crimmins EM. Evidence of accelerated aging among African Americans and its implications for mortality. Soc Sci Med. 2014; https://doi.org/10.1016/j.socscimed.2014.07.022.
6. Wei MY, Levine DA, Zahodne LB, Kabeto MU, Langa KM. Multimorbidity and cognitive decline over 14 years in older Americans. J Gerontol A Biol Sci Med Sci. 2020; https://doi.org/10.1093/gerona/glz147.
7. Jung M, Pfeifer GP. Aging and DNA methylation. BMC Biol. 2015; https://doi.org/10.1186/s12915-015-0118-4.
8. Lu AT, Quach A, Wilson JG, et al. DNA methylation GrimAge strongly predicts lifespan and healthspan. Aging (Albany NY). 2019; https://doi.org/10.18632/aging.101684.
9. Horvath S. DNA methylation age of human tissues and cell types. Genome Biol. 2013; https://doi.org/10.1186/gb-2013-14-10-r115.
10. Richardson B. Impact of aging on DNA methylation. Ageing Res Rev. 2003; https://doi.org/10.1016/S1568-1637(03)00010-2.
11. Unnikrishnan A, Freeman WM, Jackson J, Wren JD, Porter H, Richardson A. The role of DNA methylation in epigenetics of aging. Pharmacol Ther. 2019; https://doi.org/10.1016/j.pharmthera.2018.11.001.
12. Ciccarone F, Tagliatesta S, Caiafa P, Zampieri M. DNA methylation dynamics in aging: how far are we from understanding the mechanisms? Mech Ageing Dev. 2018; https://doi.org/10.1016/j.mad.2017.12.002.
13. Oeseburg H, De Boer RA, Van Gilst WH, Van Der Harst P. Telomere biology in healthy aging and disease. Pflugers Arch Eur J Physiol. 2010; https://doi.org/10.1007/s00424-009-0728-1.
14. Marengoni A, Angleman S, Melis R, et al. Aging with multimorbidity: a systematic review of the literature. Ageing Res Rev. 2011; https://doi.org/10.1016/j.arr.2011.03.003.
15. Horvath S, Gurven M, Levine ME, et al. An epigenetic clock analysis of race/ethnicity, sex, and coronary heart disease. Genome Biol. 2016; https://doi.org/10.1186/s13059-016-1030-0.
16. Tajuddin SM, Hernandez DG, Chen BH, et al. Novel age-associated DNA methylation changes and epigenetic age acceleration in middle-aged African Americans and whites. Clin Epigenetics. 2019; https://doi.org/10.1186/s13148-019-0722-1.
17. Dhingra R, Nwanaji-Enwerem JC, Samet M, Ward-Caviness CK. DNA methylation age—environmental influences, health impacts, and its role in environmental epidemiology. Curr Environ Heal Rep. 2018; https://doi.org/10.1007/s40572-018-0203-2.
18. Javed R, Chen W, Lin F, Liang H. Infant's DNA methylation age at birth and epigenetic aging accelerators. Biomed Res Int. 2016; https://doi.org/10.1155/2016/4515928.
19. Mackenbach JP. Political determinants of health. Eur J Pub Health. 2013; https://doi.org/10.1093/eurpub/ckt183.
20. Braveman P, Gottlieb L. The social determinants of health: it's time to consider the causes of the causes. Public Health Rep. 2014; https://doi.org/10.1177/00333549141291s206.
21. Grandner MA, Williams NJ, Knutson KL, Roberts D, Jean-Louis G. Sleep disparity, race/ethnicity, and socioeconomic position. Sleep Med. 2016;18:7–18. https://doi.org/10.1016/j.sleep.2015.01.020.

22. Dietch JR, Taylor DJ, Smyth JM, et al. Gender and racial/ethnic differences in sleep duration in the North Texas heart study. Sleep Heal. 2017; https://doi.org/10.1016/j.sleh.2017.07.002.

23. Patel NP, Grandner MA, Xie D, Branas CC, Gooneratne N. "Sleep disparity" in the population: poor sleep quality is strongly associated with poverty and ethnicity. BMC Public Health. 2010; https://doi.org/10.1186/1471-2458-10-475.

24. Grandner MA, Patel NP, Gehrman PR, et al. Who gets the best sleep? Ethnic and socio-economic factors related to sleep complaints. Sleep Med. 2010; https://doi.org/10.1016/j.sleep.2009.10.006.

25. Carnethon MR, De Chavez PJ, Zee PC, et al. Disparities in sleep characteristics by race/ethnicity in a population-based sample: Chicago Area Sleep Study. Sleep Med. 2016;18:50–5. https://doi.org/10.1016/j.sleep.2015.07.005.

26. Redline S, Tishler PV, Hans MG, Tosteson TD, Strohl KP, Spry K. Racial differences in sleep-disordered breathing in African-Americans and Caucasians. Am J Respir Crit Care Med. 1997; https://doi.org/10.1164/ajrccm.155.1.9001310.

27. Loredo JS, Soler X, Bardwell W, Ancoli-Israel S, Dimsdale JE, Palinkas LA. Sleep health in U.S. Hispanic population. Sleep. 2010; https://doi.org/10.1093/sleep/33.7.962.

28. Blanc J, Nunes J, Williams N, Robbins R, Seixas AA, Jean-Louis G. Sleep health equity. Sleep Health. Elsevier. 2019:473–80. https://doi.org/10.1016/b978-0-12-815373-4.00035-6.

29. Jackson CL, Walker JR, Brown MK, Das R, Jones NL. A workshop report on the causes and consequences of sleep health disparities. Sleep. 2020; https://doi.org/10.1093/sleep/zsaa037.

30. Reither EN, Krueger PM, Hale L, Reiter EM, Peppard PE. Ethnic variation in the association between sleep and body mass among US adolescents. Int J Obes. 2014; https://doi.org/10.1038/ijo.2014.18.

31. Buysse DJ. Sleep health: can we define it? Does it matter? Sleep. 2014; https://doi.org/10.5665/sleep.3298.

32. Anujuo K, Stronks K, Snijder MB, et al. Relationship between short sleep duration and cardiovascular risk factors in a multi-ethnic cohort – the Helius study. Sleep Med. 2015;16(12):1482–8. https://doi.org/10.1016/j.sleep.2015.08.014.

33. Wang Y-H, Wang J, Chen S-H, et al. Association of longitudinal patterns of habitual sleep duration with risk of cardiovascular events and all-cause mortality. JAMA Netw Open. 2020;3(5) https://doi.org/10.1001/jamanetworkopen.2020.5246.

34. He Z, Wallace DM, Barnes A, Tang X, Jean-Louis G, Williams NJ. Reporting results in U.S. clinical trials for obstructive sleep apnea and insomnia: how transparent are they? Sleep Heal. 2020; https://doi.org/10.1016/j.sleh.2019.11.009.

35. Bazargan M, Mian N, Cobb S, Vargas R, Assari S. Insomnia symptoms among African-American older adults in economically disadvantaged areas of South Los Angeles. Brain Sci. 2019; https://doi.org/10.3390/brainsci9110306.

36. Seixas AA, Chung DP, Richards SL, et al. The impact of short and long sleep duration on instrumental activities of daily living among stroke survivors. Neuropsychiatr Dis Treat. 2019;15 https://doi.org/10.2147/NDT.S177527.

37. Report MW. Effect of short sleep duration on daily activities--United States, 2005-2008. MMWR Morb Mortal Wkly Rep. 2011;60(8):239–42. http://www.ncbi.nlm.nih.gov/pubmed/21368739.

38. Knutson KL, Van Cauter E, Rathouz PJ, et al. Association between sleep and blood pressure in midlife: the CARDIA sleep study. Arch Intern Med. 2009;169(11):1055–61. https://doi.org/10.1001/archinternmed.2009.119.

39. Jackson CL, Patel SR, Jackson WB, et al. Agreement between self-reported and objectively measured sleep duration among white, black, Hispanic, and Chinese adults in the United States: Multi-Ethnic Study of Atherosclerosis. Sleep. 2018;41(6):1–12. https://doi.org/10.1093/sleep/zsy057.

40. Sehgal A, Mignot E. Genetics of sleep and sleep disorders. Cell. 2011;146(2) https://doi.org/10.1016/j.cell.2011.07.004.

41. Nevarez MD, Rifas-Shiman SL, Kleinman KP, Gillman MW, Taveras EM. Associations of early life risk factors with infant sleep duration. Acad Pediatr. 2010;10(3) https://doi.org/10.1016/j.acap.2010.01.007.
42. Williams NJ, Butler M, Roseus J, et al. 0373 blacks with obstructive sleep apnea Report greater nighttime insomnia symptoms than whites, but don't endorse daytime impairment. Sleep. 2020;43(Supplement_1) https://doi.org/10.1093/sleep/zsaa056.370.
43. Nadybal SM, Collins TW, Grineski SE. Light pollution inequities in the continental United States: a distributive environmental justice analysis. Environ Res. 2020;189:109959. https://doi.org/10.1016/j.envres.2020.109959.
44. Guglielmo D, Gazmararian JA, Chung J, Rogers AE, Hale L. Racial/ethnic sleep disparities in US school-aged children and adolescents: a review of the literature. Sleep Heal. 2018;4(1) https://doi.org/10.1016/j.sleh.2017.09.005.
45. Kantermann T, Eastman CI. Circadian phase, circadian period and chronotype are reproducible over months. Chronobiol Int. 2018;35(2) https://doi.org/10.1080/07420528.2017.1400979.
46. Redline S, Sotres-Alvarez D, Loredo J, et al. Sleep-disordered breathing in Hispanic/Latino individuals of diverse backgrounds. The Hispanic Community Health Study/Study of Latinos. Am J Respir Crit Care Med. 2014;189(3):335–44. https://doi.org/10.1164/rccm.201309-1735OC.
47. Rogers AJ, Kaplan I, Chung A, et al. Obstructive sleep apnea risk and stroke among blacks with metabolic syndrome: results from Metabolic Syndrome Outcome (MetSO) Registry. Int J Clin Res Trials. 2020;5(1):143. https://doi.org/10.15344/2456-8007/2020/143.
48. Crosby B, LeBourgeois MK, Harsh J. Racial differences in reported napping and nocturnal sleep in 2- to 8-year-old children. Pediatrics. 2005;115(1):225–32. https://doi.org/10.1542/peds.2004-0815D.
49. Smith JP, Hardy ST, Hale LE, Gazmararian JA. Racial disparities and sleep among preschool aged children: a systematic review. Sleep Heal. 2019;5(1) https://doi.org/10.1016/j.sleh.2018.09.010.
50. Grandner MA, Knutson KL, Troxel W, Hale L, Jean-Louis G, Miller KE. Implications of sleep and energy drink use for health disparities. Nutr Rev. 2014; https://doi.org/10.1111/nure.12137.
51. Grandner MA, Patel NP, Jean-Louis G, et al. Sleep-related behaviors and beliefs associated with race/ethnicity in women. J Natl Med Assoc. 2013;105(1):4–16. https://doi.org/10.1016/s0027-9684(15)30080-8.
52. Zizi F, Jean-Louis G, Fernandez S, von Gizycki H, Lazar JM, Nunes JBC, Zizi F, Jean-Louis G, et al. Symptoms of obstructive sleep apnea in a Caribbean sample. Sleep Breath. 2008;12(4):317–22. https://doi.org/10.1007/s11325-008-0190-x.
53. Ceïde ME, Pandey A, Ravenell J, Donat M, Ogedegbe G, Jean-Louis G. Associations of short sleep and shift work status with hypertension among black and white Americans. Int J Hypertens. 2015;2015 https://doi.org/10.1155/2015/697275.
54. Irwin MR, Olmstead R, Carroll JE. Sleep disturbance, sleep duration, and inflammation: a systematic review and meta-analysis of cohort studies and experimental sleep deprivation. Biol Psychiatry. 2016;80(1):40–52. https://doi.org/10.1016/j.biopsych.2015.05.014.
55. Knutson KL, Van Cauter E, Rathouz PJ, et al. Association between sleep and blood pressure in midlife. Arch Intern Med. 2009;169(11) https://doi.org/10.1001/archinternmed.2009.119.
56. Jackson CL, Agénor M, Johnson DA, Austin SB, Kawachi I. Sexual orientation identity disparities in health behaviors, outcomes, and services use among men and women in the United States: a cross-sectional study. BMC Public Health. 2016; https://doi.org/10.1186/s12889-016-3467-1.
57. Moreno JP, Crowley SJ, Alfano CA, Hannay KM, Thompson D, Baranowski T. Potential circadian and circannual rhythm contributions to the obesity epidemic in elementary school age children. Int J Behav Nutr Phys Act. https://doi.org/10.1186/s12966-019-0784-7.

58. Malone SK, Patterson F, Lu Y, Lozano A, Hanlon A. Ethnic differences in sleep duration and morning–evening type in a population sample. Chronobiol Int. 2016;33(1) https://doi.org/1 0.3109/07420528.2015.1107729.
59. Dudley KA, Patel SR. Disparities and genetic risk factors in obstructive sleep apnea. Sleep Med. 2016;18 https://doi.org/10.1016/j.sleep.2015.01.015.
60. Wallace DM, Williams NJ, Sawyer AM, et al. Adherence to positive airway pressure treatment among minority populations in the US: a scoping review. Sleep Med Rev. 2018;38:56–69. https://doi.org/10.1016/j.smrv.2017.04.002.
61. Profant J, Ancoli-Israel S, Dimsdale JE. Are there ethnic differences in sleep architecture? Am J Hum Biol. 2002; https://doi.org/10.1002/ajhb.10032.
62. Ma Y, Liang L, Zheng F, Shi L, Zhong B, Xie W. Association between sleep duration and cognitive decline. JAMA Netw Open. 2020;3(9):–e2013573. https://doi.org/10.1001/jamanetworkopen.2020.13573.
63. Zerón-Rugerio M, Hernáez Á, Porras-Loaiza A, et al. Eating jet lag: a marker of the variability in meal timing and its association with body mass index. Nutrients. 2019;11(12) https://doi.org/10.3390/nu11122980.
64. Petrov ME, Lichstein KL. Differences in sleep between black and white adults: an update and future directions. Sleep Med. 2016;18 https://doi.org/10.1016/j.sleep.2015.01.011.
65. Shaw R, McKenzie S, Taylor T, et al. Beliefs and attitudes toward obstructive sleep apnea evaluation and treatment among blacks. J Natl Med Assoc. 2012;104(11–12):510–9. https://doi.org/10.1016/S0027-9684(15)30217-0.
66. Bauducco S, Richardson C, Gradisar M. Chronotype, circadian rhythms and mood. Curr Opin Psychol. 2020;34 https://doi.org/10.1016/j.copsyc.2019.09.002.
67. Eastman CI, Suh C, Tomaka VA, Crowley SJ. Circadian rhythm phase shifts and endogenous free-running circadian period differ between African-Americans and European-Americans. Sci Rep. 2015;5(1) https://doi.org/10.1038/srep08381.
68. Eastman CI, Molina TA, Dziepak ME, Smith MR. Blacks (African Americans) have shorter free-running circadian periods than whites (Caucasian Americans). Chronobiol Int. 2012;29(8) https://doi.org/10.3109/07420528.2012.700670.
69. Eastman CI, Tomaka VA, Crowley SJ. Circadian rhythms of European and African-Americans after a large delay of sleep as in jet lag and night work. Sci Rep. 2016;6(1) https://doi.org/10.1038/srep36716.
70. Reyes AN, Molina ML, Jansen K, et al. Biological rhythm and emotional and behavioral problems among schoolchildren in Southern Brazil. Chronobiol Int. 2019;36(3) https://doi.org/10.1080/07420528.2018.1545781.
71. Makarem N, Paul J, Giardina E-GV, Liao M, Aggarwal B. Evening chronotype is associated with poor cardiovascular health and adverse health behaviors in a diverse population of women. Chronobiol Int. 2020; https://doi.org/10.1080/07420528.2020.1732403.
72. Wong PM, Hasler BP, Kamarck TW, Muldoon MF, Manuck SB. Social jetlag, chronotype, and cardiometabolic risk. J Clin Endocrinol Metab. 2015;100(12) https://doi.org/10.1210/jc.2015-2923.
73. Tomfohr L, Pung MA, Edwards KM, Dimsdale JE. Racial differences in sleep architecture: the role of ethnic discrimination. Biol Psychol. 2012;89(1):34–8. https://doi.org/10.1016/j.biopsycho.2011.09.002.
74. Song Y, Ancoli-Israel S, Lewis CE, Redline S, Harrison SLSK. The association of race/ethnicity with objectively measured sleep characteristics in older men. Behav Sleep Med. 2011;10(1):54–69. https://doi.org/10.1080/15402002.2012.636276.
75. Baron KG, Liu K, Chan C, Shahar E, Hasnain-Wynia R, Zee P. Race and ethnic variation in excessive daytime sleepiness: the multi-ethnic study of atherosclerosis. Behav Sleep Med. 2010; https://doi.org/10.1080/15402002.2010.509247.
76. Halder I, Matthews KA, Buysse DJ, et al. African genetic ancestry is associated with sleep depth in older African Americans. Sleep. 2015; https://doi.org/10.5665/sleep.4888.

77. Lam B, Ip MSM, Tench E, Ryan CF. Craniofacial profile in Asian and white subjects with obstructive sleep apnoea. Thorax. 2005; https://doi.org/10.1136/thx.2004.031591.
78. Sutherland K, Lee RWW, Cistulli PA. Obesity and craniofacial structure as risk factors for obstructive sleep apnoea: impact of ethnicity. Respirology. 2012; https://doi.org/10.1111/j.1440-1843.2011.02082.x.
79. Li W, Youssef G, Procter-Gray E, et al. Racial differences in eating patterns and food purchasing behaviors among urban older women. J Nutr Health Aging. 2017;21(10) https://doi.org/10.1007/s12603-016-0834-7.
80. Jasani FS, Seixas AA, Madondo K, Li Y, Jean-Louis G, Pagán JA. Sleep duration and health care expenditures in the United States. Med Care. 2020;58(9) https://journals.lww.com/lww-medicalcare/Fulltext/2020/09000/Sleep_Duration_and_Health_Care_Expenditures_in_the.3.aspx.
81. Johnson DA, Lisabeth L, Lewis TT, et al. The contribution of psychosocial stressors to sleep among African Americans in the Jackson heart study. Sleep. 2016; https://doi.org/10.5665/sleep.5974.
82. Patel SR, Sotres-Alvarez D, Castañeda SF, et al. Social and health correlates of sleep duration in a US Hispanic population: results from the Hispanic Community Health Study/Study of Latinos. Sleep. 2015; https://doi.org/10.5665/sleep.5036.
83. Bethea TN, Zhou ES, Schernhammer ES, et al. Perceived racial discrimination and risk of insomnia among middle-aged and elderly Black women. Sleep. 2020;43(1):1–10. https://doi.org/10.1093/sleep/zsz208.
84. Williams NJ, Jean Louis G, Ceide ME, et al. Effect of maladaptive beliefs and attitudes about sleep among community dwelling African American men at risk for obstructive sleep apnea. J Sleep Disord Ther. 2017; https://doi.org/10.4172/2167-0277.1000269.
85. Baron KG, Gilyard SG, Williams JL, Lindich D, Koralnik L, Lynch EB. Sleep-related attitudes, beliefs, and practices among an urban-dwelling African American community: a qualitative study. Sleep Heal. 2019; https://doi.org/10.1016/j.sleh.2019.06.004.
86. Seixas AA, Auguste E, Butler M, et al. Differences in short and long sleep durations between blacks and whites attributed to emotional distress: analysis of the National Health Interview Survey in the United States. Sleep Heal. 2017;3(1) https://doi.org/10.1016/j.sleh.2016.11.003.
87. Grandner MA, Jackson NJ, Izci-Balserak B, et al. Social and behavioral determinants of perceived insufficient sleep. Front Neurol. 2015; https://doi.org/10.3389/fneur.2015.00112.
88. Gillis BT, Shimizu M, Philbrook LE, El-Sheikh M. Racial disparities in adolescent sleep duration: physical activity as a protective factor. Cult Divers Ethn Minor Psychol. 2020; https://doi.org/10.1037/cdp0000422.
89. Grandner MA, Smith TE, Jackson N, Jackson T, Burgard S, Branas C. Geographic distribution of insufficient sleep across the United States: a county-level hotspot analysis. Sleep Heal. 2015; https://doi.org/10.1016/j.sleh.2015.06.003.
90. Johnson DA, Billings ME, Hale L. Environmental determinants of insufficient sleep and sleep disorders: implications for population health. Curr Epidemiol Rep. 2018; https://doi.org/10.1007/s40471-018-0139-y.
91. Piccolo RS, Yang M, Bliwise DL, Yaggi HK, Araujo AB. Racial and socioeconomic disparities in sleep and chronic disease: results of a longitudinal investigation. Ethn Dis. 2013;
92. Sabanayagam C, Shankar A. Sleep duration and cardiovascular disease: results from the National Health Interview Survey. Sleep. 2010; https://doi.org/10.1093/sleep/33.8.1037.
93. Ramos AR, Wallace DM, Pandi-Perumal SR, et al. Associations between sleep disturbances and diabetes mellitus among blacks with metabolic syndrome: results from the Metabolic Syndrome Outcome Study (MetSO). Ann Med. 2015; https://doi.org/10.3109/07853890.2015.1015601.
94. Grandner MA, Buxton OM, Jackson N, Sands-Lincoln M, Pandey A, Jean-Louis G. Extreme sleep durations and increased C-reactive protein: effects of sex and ethnoracial group. Sleep. 2013; https://doi.org/10.5665/sleep.2646.

95. Williams N, Jean-Louis G, Pandey A, Ravenell J, Boutin-Foster C, Ogedegbe G. Excessive daytime sleepiness and adherence to antihypertensive medications among Blacks: analysis of the counseling African Americans to control hypertension (CAATCH) trial. Patient Prefer Adherence. 2014; https://doi.org/10.2147/PPA.S53617.

96. Ceïde ME, Williams NJ, Seixas A, Longman-Mills SK, Jean-Louis G. Obstructive sleep apnea risk and psychological health among non-Hispanic blacks in the Metabolic Syndrome Outcome (MetSO) cohort study. Ann Med. 2015; https://doi.org/10.3109/07853890.2015.1107186.

97. Presser HB. Race-ethnic and gender differences in nonstandard work shifts. Work Occup. 2003; https://doi.org/10.1177/0730888403256055.

98. Yamasaki F, Schwartz JE, Gerber LM, Warren K, Pickering TG. Impact of shift work and race/ethnicity on the diurnal rhythm of blood pressure and catecholamines. Hypertension. 1998; https://doi.org/10.1161/01.HYP.32.3.417.

99. Smith MR, Burgess HJ, Fogg LF, Eastman CI. Racial differences in the human endogenous circadian period. PLoS One. 2009; https://doi.org/10.1371/journal.pone.0006014.

100. Suzuki M, Guilleminault C, Otsuka K, Shiomi T. Blood pressure "dipping" and "non-dipping" in obstructive sleep apnea syndrome patients. Sleep. 1996; https://doi.org/10.1093/sleep/19.5.382.

101. Esquirol Y, Perret B, Ruidavets JB, et al. Shift work and cardiovascular risk factors: new knowledge from the past decade. Arch Cardiovasc Dis. 2011; https://doi.org/10.1016/j.acvd.2011.09.004.

102. Thomas SAH, et al. Benefits of community-based approaches in assessing and addressing sleep health and sleep-related cardiovascular disease risk: a precision and personalized population health approach. Curr Hypertens Rep. 1906; https://doi.org/10.1007/s11906-020-01051-3.

103. Jean-Louis G, Kripke DF, Ancoli-Israel S, Klauber MR, Sepulveda RS. Sleep duration, illumination, and activity patterns in a population sample: effects of gender and ethnicity. Biol Psychiatry. 2000;47(10) https://doi.org/10.1016/S0006-3223(99)00169-9.

104. Foley D, Monjan A, Masaki K, et al. Daytime sleepiness is associated with 3-year incident dementia and cognitive decline in older Japanese-American men. J Am Geriatr Soc. 2001; https://doi.org/10.1046/j.1532-5415.2001.t01-1-49271.x.

105. Lucassen EA, Rother KICG. Interacting epidemics? Sleep curtailment, insulin resistance, and obesity. Ann N Y Acad Sci. 2012;1264(1):110–34. https://doi.org/10.1111/j.1749-6632.2012.06655.x.

106. Partonen T. Chronotype and health outcomes. Curr Sleep Med Rep. https://doi.org/10.1007/s40675-015-0022-z.

107. Taveras EM, Gillman MW, Kleinman KP, Rich-Edwards JW, Rifas-Shiman SL. Reducing racial/ethnic disparities in childhood obesity: the role of early life risk factors. JAMA Pediatr. 2013;167(8):731–8. https://doi.org/10.1001/jamapediatrics.2013.85.

108. Sun X, Gustat J, Bertisch SM, Redline S, Bazzano L. The association between sleep chronotype and obesity among black and white participants of the Bogalusa Heart Study. Chronobiol Int. 2020;37(1) https://doi.org/10.1080/07420528.2019.1689398.

Chapter 4
The Future of Sleep Medicine: A Patient-Centered Model of Care

Barry G. Fields and Ilene M. Rosen

Keywords Future of sleep medicine · Patient-centered care · Collaborative care · Sleep telemedicine · Artificial intelligence

Nearly 70 years ago, Nathaniel Kleitman, a professor of physiology at the University of Chicago, and his graduate student, Eugene Aserinksy, studied eye movements leading to a seminal paper in 1953 describing a new sleep state, rapid eye movement (REM) sleep. In 1957, Kleitman and William Dement, another graduate student, described the human sleep cycle of NREM sleep stages of increasing depth followed by periods of REM sleep, with the cycles repeating through the night [1]. These discoveries established sleep as a scientific discipline. Over the next 30 years, sleep medicine developed as its own clinical discipline with development of American Academy Sleep Medicine (AASM)-accredited clinical training pathways starting in 1988 and certification available through the American Board of Sleep Medicine (ABSM) from 1991 to 2006. During this time, 3500 physicians were ABSM certified in sleep medicine. In 2005, Sleep Medicine training was officially recognized by the Accreditation Council of Graduate Medical Education (ACGME) with approval by the American Board of Medical Specialties (ABMS) to offer a certification examination.

Currently, there are approximately 200 positions available for one-year subspecialty training in sleep medicine nationwide [2] and approximately 175–180 are

B. G. Fields
Emory University, Division of Pulmonary, Allergy and Critical Care Medicine, Atlanta, GA, USA

I. M. Rosen (✉)
Division of Sleep Medicine, Perelman School of Medicine at the University of Pennsylvania PCAM, Philadelphia, PA, USA
e-mail: ilene.rosen@pennmedicine.upenn.edu; Ilene.Rosen@uphs.upenn.edu

© Springer Nature Switzerland AG 2022
M. S. Badr, J. L. Martin (eds.), *Essentials of Sleep Medicine*,
Respiratory Medicine, https://doi.org/10.1007/978-3-030-93739-3_4

trained each year. In the last decade, there were 3500 first-time takers of the ABMS-certification exam in sleep medicine; this number is down 1500 since 2018 [3]. In the early years, many physicians practicing sleep medicine took the exam based on a clinical-experience waiver; these physicians, along with those who were still only certified by the ABSM, led to a peak number of nearly 6000 Board-Certified Sleep Medicine Physicians (BCSMPs) in 2018. Since that time, those numbers have waned. Starting in 2013, physicians needed to complete an ACGME-accredited sleep fellowship in order to sit for the certification exam. Furthermore, the total number of retired sleep physicians from 2013 to 2018 was 7 times the number of new BCSMPs during the same time period (AASM, email communication, October 2018).

As a result, the BCSMP workforce is insufficient to meet the demands of the enormous population of patients who have a sleep disease, including an estimated 23.5 million U.S. adults with undiagnosed OSA and the 24.2 million individuals with chronic insomnia [4]. This shortfall results from some unintended consequences of recognition of sleep medicine as a specialty by the ACGME and ABMS. First, there are now a limited number of ACGME-accredited training spots that allow physicians to sit for the certification examination. Second, interest in those slots has varied in recent years, perhaps because of the need for a full extra year of training along with concerns regarding reduced reimbursements as home sleep apnea testing becomes the norm [5].

These workforce pipeline issues interact with known factors at the individual (e.g., race), family (e.g., beliefs), and broader socio-cultural (e.g., insurance coverage) levels to limit access to sleep medicine care [6]. Pre-existing geographic barriers and accredited sleep centers' clustering in more highly populated areas further exacerbate these disparities. This situation highlights the need for shared responsibility among BCSMPs and other providers for treating patients with sleep disorders. Given the magnitude of individuals who suffer with a sleep disorder and the benefits associated with treatment, patients deserve a collective response from our healthcare system. There are six feeder specialties including Anesthesia, Family Medicine, Internal Medicine, Neurology, Otorhinolaryngology (Ear, Nose & Throat/ENT), and Pediatrics. Unfortunately, there has been a disconnect between the magnitude of the disease burden, the broad relevance across many specialties, and the lack of success of the efforts to infuse sleep education at all levels [7]. Not only is it difficult to gain traction for sleep medicine curricula in medical schools, but also in the feeder specialties into sleep medicine; only ENT has specific program requirements about education in sleep beyond the general ACGME requirements of fatigue mitigation strategies.

Re-centering the spotlight on patient-centered care requires reconsideration of the current model of care which presently involves nearly automatic referral of patients with a sleep complaint to a sleep specialist or to a sleep center for testing. Unfortunately, long waits and fragmented care have been the norm. Although the spread of telemedicine during the COVID-19 pandemic has potentially improved access to care by removing geographic barriers, the sleep field still suffers from a conundrum: As the general public increasingly recognizes importance of sleep health, there is a scarcity of providers to ensure it. Thus, we propose a patient-centered point of care model that facilitates the patient receiving the best possible care for their sleep complaints to promote sleep health which utilizes patient, provider, educational, and technological resources.

A Patient-Centered Model of Sleep Care

Figures 4.1 and 4.2 outline our proposed integrated model for the future of sleep care, and they will be referenced throughout the rest of this chapter. The emphasis is on a patient-centered approach, so that a patient can get the sleep care they need at a time and place that is convenient for them, regardless of the availability of a one-on-one appointment with a sleep specialist. Figure 4.1 traces a patient's evaluation and diagnosis pathway from left to right, starting with their symptomatic concerns and finishing with patient-centered education and treatment. This intervention may occur through a referral to sleep specialist or non-sleep specialist workup. Figure 4.2 follows a patient from treatment initiation through ongoing management. Here, the stress is on ongoing *collaboration* between non-sleep medicine specialists and sleep medicine specialists. Points A–F indicated throughout Figs. 4.1 and 4.2 refer to topics presented in each of the next five sections.

Primary Care and Broader Medical Community Collaboration (Point A)

Existing Paradigms   There is a growing body of evidence that espouses primary care provider involvement in the care of patients with a sleep complaint. Internationally, there have been randomized controlled trials that support primary care physicians and nurses in the management of OSA [8–11]. Additionally, identi-

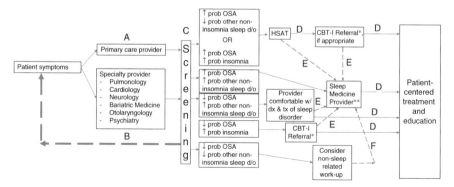

Fig. 4.1 Patient-centered access to sleep care: entry, diagnosis, and initiation of treatment. A Primary care and broader medical community collaboration, B Non-sleep specialty care collaboration, C Development of sound screening protocols, D Leveraging telemedicine, E Provider-to-provider interaction, F Ongoing sleep concerns requiring sleep medicine referral. *In person, telemedicine, or online. **In person or telemedicine

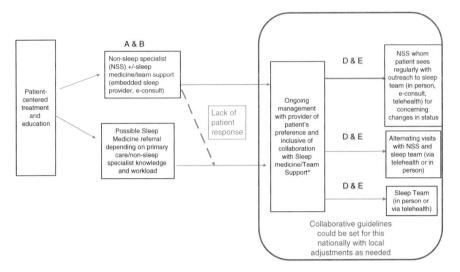

Fig. 4.2 Patient-centered access to sleep care: long-term care management, patient and provider education and collaboration. A Primary care and broader medical community collaboration, B Non-sleep specialty care collaboration, D Leveraging telemedicine, E Provider-to-provider interaction. *In person, telemedicine, or online

fication of OSA has been augmented by community pharmacist involvement in screening and appropriate communication with primary care providers [12, 13]. In the United States, similar models have been employed in family practice clinics, the Wisconsin Department of Corrections [14], and the Veterans Health Administration, as well as at Kaiser Permanente. However, the success of these programs has not been systematically studied. Newer models involve healthcare businesses, such as CVS Health, utilizing direct-to-consumer marketing and treatment [15].

Although the majority of these models have a primary focus on obstructive sleep apnea, more recently there has been attention to models to treat insomnia outside of sleep specialists and accredited-sleep centers [16–18]. A majority of patients with insomnia present to their primary care provider with complaints of insomnia [19, 20], but primary care has a shortage of treatment options [21]. Many primary care providers recognize the limitations of the use of prescription hypnotic medications; they may or may not share sleep hygiene recommendations depending on their knowledge of and comfort with such suggestions. Despite the recommendations for non-pharmacologic treatments such as cognitive behavioral therapy for insomnia (CBTi), [22–24] many non-sleep providers rarely provide such therapies likely due to a lack of knowledge [25–27], training [25, 27, 28], and time [25, 29]. Despite these barriers, improvement in important sleep variables has been noted when nurses in primary care deliver strictly manual-based cognitive behavioral therapy for insomnia (CBTi), [16, 17] mental health nurse practitioners provide brief behavioral therapy for insomnia to elderly patients in a primary care practice [30], and health district nurses offer cognitive-behavioral therapy for insomnia to patients in primary health care center [21]. Additionally, it has been recognized that primary care providers play an important role in the diagnosis and initial treatment of restless leg syndrome [31].

We propose the integration of primary care into the paradigm of evaluation and treatment of common sleep disorders including a combination of both stepped care and hub and spoke models [32]. If the hub is the BSCMP, the Sleep Team and the accredited sleep center, the spokes are primary care providers and non-sleep specialists. A stepped care model would outline patient populations and tasks that could be shifted to these non-sleep medicine providers and appropriate team members in the spokes that may not ever require interaction with the hub. Such models have been proposed for obstructive sleep apnea [32] and chronic insomnia [33]. Accounting for the high prevalence of OSA and insomnia as well as the reality of OSA with significant comorbid insomnia [34, 35], a truly patient-centered care model would consider the management of both of these disorders. Given the known barriers which typically limit access to the specialist in the stepped model, clear delineations of hubs and the leveraging of telemedicine will need to be considered [14, 18, 32, 36]. Additionally, identification of barriers and facilitators of care with relevant stakeholders, inclusive of providers and patients, is required to ensure optimal sleep care delivery [37].

Project ECHO   To support the "proof of concept" programs described above, educational opportunities are needed for practicing primary care providers in sleep medicine management (Fig. 4.1, Point A). One strategy utilized in the Veterans Administration (VA) system has been Specialty Care Access Network-Extension for Community Healthcare Outcomes (Scan-ECHO), subsequently re-labeled Project ECHO. The program, developed at the University of New Mexico in 2003, was implemented to better serve rural patients with limited access to specialty care. Frequently, their challenge is not actually *seeing* a specialist; clinical video telehealth is filling this role more and more. Rather, the challenge is the limited number of specialists available. Project ECHO seeks to involve more primary care providers in specialty care through education, thereby improving access to that care.

The VA-based program (VA-ECHO) leverages telehealth (described more below) to drive educational outcomes. Specialists present short didactic sessions to primary care clinicians through real-time video over the course of months. As the program progresses, the generalists may engage in case discussions with the specialists. Other professionals such as nurses, pharmacists, and technicians are often involved on both sides of the camera to enhance a team-based approach to patient care [38]. VA-ECHO has been deployed in many specialties, with positive outcomes published in hepatology, [39] geriatrics [40], and pain management [41]. Sleep VA-ECHO has also emerged. A pilot program at the VA Puget Sound Health Care System (VAPSHCS) found rural providers receptive to its curriculum over the 3-month course. Participants reported enhanced comfort managing common sleep complaints (e.g., sleep-disordered breathing, insomnia, PTSD-related sleep problems) and providing appropriate patient education [42].

Programs like Project ECHO could enhance current sleep medicine care models by expanding the number of providers from which that care can be delivered, even if they are not BCSMPs. However, challenges remain. The authors at the VAPSHCS surveyed rural providers who had *not* taken part in the training; lack of protected time was the most common reason [42]. For already-overburdened providers, it can be difficult to fit regular specialty training into their day. Another challenge is one of generalizability. That is, how well does VA ECHO translate outside of a single-payer health system? Significant investment is needed, in both time and money, for any health system to implement the program. Strong business cases are required to show that patient health and their healthcare expenditures could be optimized if more non-subspecialist providers could integrate sleep medicine care into that which they already provide. Data on the success of non-VA ECHO type programs is lacking.

Non-Sleep Specialty Care Collaboration (Point B)

As noted above, a collaborative sleep care model involving non-BCSMPs hinges on non-specialty trained providers' sufficient education in the specialty. While board certification in sleep medicine requires both completion of a 1-year Accreditation Council for Graduate Medical Education (ACGME)-accredited fellowship and passing a certification examination, many non-BCSMPs can participate substantively in patients' care. Opportunities for this education may come either during professional training (i.e., medical school, residency, non-sleep medicine fellowship) or after that training as part of continuing medical education (CME).

American medical schools allot just 2–4 hours to sleep education, 0.06% of their preclinical curriculum [43]. There have been pilot projects aimed at increasing that proportion. In one study, faculty presented 87 Johns Hopkins University medical students with online learning modules. These students showed significant improvement in sleep-related knowledge after viewing these 20- to 30-minute modules compared to "sham" modules [44]. Nevertheless, similar efforts have not gained a wide-scale footing. A frequently cited challenge is time; medical school faculty are increasingly challenged to fit the breadth of human medicine into a limited schedule while attending to other needs such as students' wellness and early clinical exposure. Neurology educators have suggested including sleep medicine content into medical students' neuroscience curriculum. They propose this content be presented for 2–4 hours per year as flipped-classroom sessions, didactics, and clinical opportunities depending on the year of training [45]. This dovetailing of sleep content with existing curriculum blocks offers another strategy to expose medical students to more substantive sleep education throughout their undergraduate medical training.

To augment these efforts, many non-BCSMPs would benefit from sleep medicine exposure during their post-graduate training years (i.e., residency and fellowship). While otolaryngology (ENT) residents are eligible for sleep medicine fellowship training upon completion of their residency, they could also serve a unique role in sleep disorders management without that subspecialty training. A recent survey revealed that ENT attendings vary widely in their sleep surgical practice and, therefore, the amount of sleep training they provide to their residents. An ENT surgeon having obtained sleep medicine board certification predicted the extent of trainee exposure to the subspecialty [46]. Another survey used consensus among academic otolaryngologists involved in sleep disorder treatment to create sleep-related learning objectives for ENT residencies. These objectives form the basis of online learning modules, enhancing the level of sleep education even among non-sleep-focused otolaryngologists [47]. Such strategies may also help widen the pipeline of ENT trainees entering sleep medicine fellowships. Neurologists found that residency programs investing more heavily in sleep education report more program graduates entering the subspecialty [48].

In addition to ENT and neurology trainees, pulmonary medicine fellows are uniquely positioned to participate in collaborative sleep care whether or not they subspecialize in sleep medicine. Indeed, sleep content accounts for about 10% of the American Board of Internal Medicine's pulmonary medicine examination [49]. A multi-society panel was convened to develop sleep-related curricular recommendations for pulmonary medicine fellowships. After 5 rounds of voting, they created 52 elements, ranging from recognizing central apnea on sleep testing to insomnia and narcolepsy evaluation. Therefore, they advocate pulmonologists not only be well-versed in sleep-disordered breathing, but also in more psychologically and neurologically based sleep disorders. Threshold for referral to a sleep medicine specialist is left to the individual provider based on self-perception of knowledge base and local availability of such subspecialization [50]. Of course, as in undergraduate medical education, time in a pulmonary medicine fellowship is limited. Program directors could integrate sleep content with training modules that already exist to enhance efficiency of its delivery (e.g., nocturnal PAP therapy for severe COPD) [51].

Development of Sound Screening Protocols (Point C)

Questionnaires Point of care interventions to further facilitate screening and management of sleep disorders have included clinician chart reminders [52] and efforts to promote shared decision making [53] including patient decision aids [54–57] and patient educational websites [58–60]. The promotion of screeners for sleepiness [61] and questionnaires such as the STOP-BANG for OSA, [62–64] Insomnia Severity Index for insomnia, [61, 65] and several for restless leg syndrome [66–69] with appropriate clinical nudges [70] have been shown to facilitate appropriate diagnosis and access to care for patients with these sleep disorders. Additionally, there are several questionnaires that screen for multiple sleep disorders at one time which may be suitable as a general sleep disorders screener [71].

Despite such available tools, a majority of the screening initiatives have focused narrowly on OSA. While increased screening, evaluation, and treatment for OSA alone will undoubtedly have a significant impact, broader consideration of sleep disorders will better facilitate access to care in a patient-centered fashion. To our knowledge, the only trans-sleep-disorders approach to be adopted exists in the Veterans Health Administration (VHA) [72]. The VHA TeleSleep system utilizes non-sleep specialists to increase patient screening with subsequent referral to a Sleep Center "Hub" for diagnosis and treatment. However, this model of relying on the provider to identify signs and symptoms of a sleep disorder has been noted to be an inconsistent and unreliable paradigm [73]. Adding patient-administered screeners, which then serves as a chart-based "nudge" to the busy primary care provider, is an innovation that fundamentally changes sleep-care paradigms by leveraging technology and patient empowerment [74].

Artificial Intelligence/Machine Learning Despite sleep disorders' prevalence and a myriad of available screening tools, sleep problems can be challenging to screen for and identify in busy, non-sleep specialized clinical environments. Robust, accessible tools are needed to guide the clinicians who work in them without disruption to their other duties. Artificial intelligence (AI) holds promise to fill this vital role. AI refers to computers' ability to perform tasks traditionally completed by humans [75]. Machine learning (ML) is a term often used interchangeably with AI; instead of relying on direct computer programming for each action, ML algorithms "learn" from previous experience to enhance future performance on tasks such as disease classification. A recent American Academy of Sleep Medicine (AASM) Position Statement on AI suggests that multi-channel polysomnographic (PSG) data lends itself particularly well to this type of ML analyses [75]. However, the opportunity for AI in sleep medicine care goes far beyond the sleep laboratory.

There are many opportunities for AI utilization throughout sleep medicine and other specialties that interface with it. Patients possess a wealth of symptomatic, demographic, and comorbidity-based data "channels" even at their initial presentation to primary care providers and non-sleep specialists (Fig. 4.1, Points A & B). It is likely that AI will leverage ML using electronic medical record (EMR) data and patients' symptomatic reports to identify individuals at risk for a sleep disorder who may benefit from a thorough sleep evaluation. For instance, there is growing evidence that obstructive sleep apnea (OSA) symptom phenotypes can be clustered into disturbed sleep, slightly sleepy, moderately sleepy, and excessively sleepy subtypes [76, 77] Identifying patients with sleepier subtypes is important given these subtypes' association with worsened CVD, CHF, and CAD [78]. An ML system integrated into the EMR could function in this manner, alerting providers that a patient's objective (e.g., age, gender, and BMI) and subjective (e.g., sleepiness) phenotype places that individual into a high-risk group if found to have OSA. More detailed OSA screening could be prioritized for such a subset of patients.

The importance of AI-based phenotypic subtyping may also extend to OSA treatment initiation. A more nuanced, personalized treatment plan could develop as more is learned about etiologic OSA subtypes. Emerging data suggest that this disorder is the final common endpoint of diverse, sleep-induced pathophysiological processes such as impaired pharyngeal dilator muscle function, increased sensitivity to airway narrowing (low arousal threshold), and respiratory control instability from the central nervous system. ML that incorporates these parameters could reveal more targeted and personalized treatment options a given patient may tolerate best [79]. If more conventional positive airway pressure (PAP) is the chosen intervention, AI would once again have a role. Although some studies have cast doubt on the cardiovascular disease benefits of PAP, many of the sleepiest patients were excluded from these analyses [80, 81]. Given the increased CVD implications in OSA patients with excessive sleepiness, AI may help identify those patients who could benefit most from PAP use [82]. Providers would be better informed as to whom to focus cloud-based PAP adherence monitoring, and patients could experience enhanced motivation to continue with that therapy.

AI's involvement in sleep medicine may also extend to other disorders, such as narcolepsy. Multiple sleep latency testing (MSLT) has limited specificity (73.3% at the <8 minute mean sleep onset latency cutoff), due at least in part to suboptimal interrater reliability among epochs scored [83]. Researchers have leveraged ML to stage as little as 5 seconds of sleep, a level of precision much greater than the conventional 30-second epoch scoring. They demonstrated 96% sensitivity and 91% specificity for narcolepsy Type 1, a specificity that rises to 99% when adding HLA-DQB1*06:02 typing to their model [84]. As the authors state, AI-guided diagnosis should not supplant BCSMP review and judgment. On the contrary, AI can be utilized as another type of twenty-first century "physician extender," allowing them to focus more efficiently on the most complex patient management issues while reaching a larger population. Reviewing Fig. 4.1, one can foresee AI assisting both sleep clinicians and non-clinicians at each step in the initial symptom presentation and evaluation process. Indeed, even non-sleep clinicians could be guided to order home sleep apnea testing (HSAT) in the higher risk patients for OSA (Fig. 4.1, Point D). AI could then assist BCSMPs in interpreting the studies, prescribing the most effective therapies, and assisting clinicians with ongoing follow up (e.g., anticipate needed changes in PAP settings or to other modes of treatment).

Patient and Provider Portals Whether it is a nudge from AI or from clinical judgment that leads a provider to suspect a sleep disorder, further symptom-based screening is typically indicated (Fig. 4.1). This screening is essential to gauge potential sleep disorder severity, delineate among potential disorders, and create a symptomatic baseline with which to compare symptoms after any treatment has commenced. Screening tools can also help primary care physicians and non-sleep providers triage this group of patients; as noted above, some clinicians may choose to order HSAT for patients with a high probability of OSA but a low probability of other sleep disorders (Fig. 4.1, Point D).

One strategy to expedite and streamline patients' symptomatic information flow to providers (both at initial presentation and during follow-up) has been through dual-facing, internet-based patient and provider portals. Although there are no published clinical trials utilizing such a portal, one is currently being conducted using the Remote Veteran Apnea Management Platform (REVAMP). REVAMP has been designed with input from veterans and clinicians throughout the VA system, under the direction of the VA Office of Connected Care and the Office of Rural Health. Now available at over 50 VA medical centers, REVAMP provides users with the 7 core elements of internet-based portals above. Veterans are offered REVAMP access upon their initial referral to the sleep center. They complete several validated sleep screening questionnaires, and sleep clinicians utilize those responses to help guide patients to their next stage of testing. Patients started on PAP can view their night-to-night PAP machine adherence and efficacy data through REVAMP, where they can also complete follow-up questionnaires, access educational materials, and send a message to their provider. Clinicians access REVAMP through a designated provider-facing portal. There, they can view all pertinent data, offer the patient additional questionnaires to complete, and incorporate all patient- and PAP-machine entered data into a comprehensive clinic note [85].

Leverage Telemedicine (Point D)

Of course, some patients cannot access such tools independently due to lack of internet connectivity and physical challenges. Healthcare models should always account for these situations, offering patients as diverse an array of modalities as possible (e.g., telephone visits, clinical video telehealth, or in-person visits) [72]. As noted above, potential strategies to improve patient access to sleep care include better training for primary care providers and specialists, bringing more BCSMPs through the training pipeline, and promoting the development of sleep teams. Nevertheless, the AASM asserts "None of these solutions has more immediate potential to overcome these challenges than telemedicine, which can dramatically increase sleep medicine accessibility and clinical efficacy" [36].

Terminology Sharing a common language is important when considering telemedicine's impact on future sleep medicine paradigms. According to the Health Resources and Services Administration, "telehealth" is a broad term implying "the use of electronic information and telecommunication technologies to support and promote long-distance clinical health care [86], patient and professional health-related education, public health and health administration." In contrast, "telemedicine" specifically refers to patient-provider interactions. The Federation of State Medical Boards defines telemedicine as "the practice of medicine using electronic communication, information technology, or other means between a physician in one location, and a patient in another location, with or without an intervening health care provider" [87]. Since the focus of this chapter is on patient care, we favor the term "sleep telemedicine." Sleep telemedicine can be categorized as either synchronous or asynchronous, a key distinction with implications described below. (See Feasibility section). Asynchronous telemedicine includes patient-provider messaging through a secure email-style system and store-and-forward technologies such as the patient- and provider-facing online platforms now available from most PAP machine manufacturers. Figure 4.1 illustrates another use for asynchronous telemedicine: provider-to-provider interaction (Point E). As shown, there can be many decision points for non-BCSMPs once screening and initial work-up are complete. Collaboration with a BCSMP or team member through secure email systems, portals, or a common electronic medical record (EMR) can be crucial to streamlined patient management. For example, the VA health care system has employed provider-to-provider asynchronous telemedicine through its use of "e-consults." Non-BCSMPs place relatively straightforward clinical questions directly into the EMR; BCSMPs and their team members may answer those questions and guide further work-up. Therefore, many veterans may begin their work-up and treatment without waiting for, or traveling to, the sleep center [72].

As opposed to asynchronous telemedicine, synchronous telemedicine is real-time communication between patients and providers. Telephone calls are one example, as are the audio-visual interactions used for Clinical Video Telehealth (CVT). CVT visits are currently accepted for initial visits, ongoing patient follow-up, and encounter reimbursement, and they closely emulate a traditional in-person visit. Long the CVT standard, Center-to-Center (C2C) telemedicine implies a provider (at a *distant* site) and a patient (at an *originating* site) are both in clinical locations. Emerging CVT modalities include Center-to-Home (C2H) telemedicine where the patient is in a non-clinical location and Out-of-Center (OOC) telemedicine where both patient and provider are at non-clinical locations. C2H and OOC telemedicine provide progressive levels of patient-centered flexibility but also come with their own complexities since distant-site providers are more reliant on originating site patients' technical savviness and troubleshooting.

Feasibility of Communication via Telemedicine Represented by Point D in Figs. 4.1 and 4.2, telemedicine can be employed for many initial and follow-up encounters. Sleep patients' receptiveness to telemedicine has been demonstrated for at least the past decade [88]. Nevertheless, questions persist as to how feasible it really is to include telemedicine in future sleep care models. The COVID-19 pandemic brought with it a rapid migration to telemedicine [89], forcing many sleep providers to reckon with several aspects of its feasibility presently and moving forward: technology, privacy and security, reimbursement, licensing, and clinical outcomes.

Sleep telemedicine (specifically CVT) is technically feasible, and CVT visits have been conducted for more than a decade. Various platforms allow real-time audiovisual communication and several of them also offer tele-stethoscope and portable camera options; these physical exam tools are typically utilized only for C2C telemedicine. The AASM recommends up-to-date software with a minimum connection speed of 384 kbps and 640×480 video resolution transmitted at 30 frames per second [90]. Sleep telemedicine is also feasible from a privacy and security perspective, with the AASM making further recommendations that any CVT platform be patched with the latest security updates, encrypted, and only accessible by authorized users [90].

Financial feasibility has long been an impediment to sleep telemedicine's proliferation, though changes just before and during the Covid-19 pandemic have been quite impactful. Most states now have "parity laws" that require private insurers to reimburse providers the same for a telemedicine visit as for an in-person visit. States' Medicaid reimbursement has also become more favorable toward telemedicine, but knowing terminology is key; "telemedicine" is typically limited to CVT-style visits whether seeking private or Medicaid reimbursement. Researching guidelines at both the distant and the originating site is key to understanding whether reimbursement can occur [91]. Federal reimbursement from the Centers for Medicare and Medicaid Services (CMS) has also been fraught with complexity. Prior to the Covid-19 pandemic, C2C sleep telemedicine reimbursement was available only for the most rural originating sites, and it was not available at all for C2H or OOC sleep telemedicine models. The Covid-19-associated public health emergency loosened those restrictions at least temporarily. The CMS website should be consulted for the latest guidance [92].

Sleep telemedicine's feasibility from a licensing perspective has also been complex. Providers must generally be licensed in the patient's state (originating site) for them to practice. The Federation of State Medical Boards has developed an Interstate Medical Licensure Compact that now includes most states. The Compact allows a physician in one state to have licensure facilitated in another state as long as both states are part of the Compact. Additional strategies to facilitate interstate medical licensing, and even to develop a unified national medical license, have been proposed [93]. Further progress in this area will continue to lower the hurdles toward telemedicine's wider adoption.

The most important measure of sleep telemedicine's feasibility may come through the lens of clinical outcomes. That is, can we maintain the same level of clinical care in the Fig. 4.1 model, or any model, using sleep telemedicine? Previous work has suggested that OSA patients' functional outcomes, PAP adherence, and satisfaction do not differ when assessed and followed through telemedicine (CVT) versus traditional in-person care [94, 95]. Those findings, especially in light of the AASM's OSA Quality Measures, [96] suggest that sleep telemedicine for OSA *is* feasible from a clinical outcomes perspective assuming the other elements of feasibility above are fulfilled (adequate technology, etc.). Similar results have emerged recently from insomnia research. Cognitive behavioral therapy for insomnia (CBT-I) provided through CVT produces similar improvements in Insomnia Severity Index as CBT-I provided in-person [97]. CVT-based treatment outcome studies in other sleep disorders remain lacking.

Special Considerations Sleep telemedicine is still a relatively nascent and developing field. Though its utilization appears more and more essential to the future of sleep telemedicine paradigms (Figs. 4.1 and 4.2, Point D), its deployment remains complex. Providers should consider carefully not only the feasibility issues above, but also specific laws and regulations pertaining to their specific state(s) of practice. As of the writing of this chapter, there has been no successful litigation of a sleep provider simply due to the use of telemedicine. However, standards of care should be upheld, and it is up to that provider to ensure that all applicable rules are followed (e.g., interstate medication prescribing, licensing). The AASM provides a "checklist" of regulatory issues to aid new and more experienced sleep telemedicine providers [98].

A discussion of sleep telemedicine must also address technology the *patient* brings to the visit. Wearable consumer sleep technologies will undoubtedly play an increasing role in sleep medicine as newer devices become more advanced and fulfill the broad definition of asynchronous, store-and-forward sleep telemedicine. Though their accuracy and reliability in data reporting has long been suspect, current device algorithms more closely mimic established tools such as home sleep apnea testing (HSAT) and actigraphy [99]. Indeed, the evolution of sleep medicine may rely increasingly upon the most patient-centered data of all: that which these patients collect themselves in their natural environment. It will be up to the provider, whether BCSMP or non-BCSMP, to integrate that information with evolving clinical guidelines to devise collaborative sleep disorder management plans.

Putting It All Together

Ideally, given the importance of sleep health and how ubiquitous sleep complaints are, a patient should be able to access sleep medical care in a way that is patient-centered. Care should be convenient, timely, and evidenced based. We propose a model of care that starts with the identification of a patient who has a sleep complaint (Fig. 4.1, Point A–C). This identification could be based on provider inquiry and/or patient self-screening. Artificial intelligence would also leverage information in the electronic health record, and chart nudges would prompt formal screening questionnaires and/or provider inquiry to the patient. If a patient is determined to have a high pretest probability for obstructive sleep apnea with or without comorbid insomnia, the involved provider would order a home sleep apnea test and place a referral for CBT-I, if appropriate (Fig. 4.1, Point D). If the HSAT was positive for OSA, the ordering provider would initiate treatment with CPAP and follow the patient to ensure symptom improvement as well as ongoing adherence to CPAP as part of routine care. If the patient is not responsive to usual therapy, a referral would be made to a sleep medicine specialty team (Fig. 4.1, Point E). The guidelines for and facilitation of such a referral should be predetermined, similar to how a provider would refer a patient with difficulty to control diabetes or hypertension would be referred to an endocrinologist or cardiologist, respectively. Importantly, patients with concern or high risk for sleep-disordered breathing that is not straightforwad OSA should be referred to a sleep medicine provider directly to expedite evaluation and treatment.

Alternatively, if a patient is noted to have insomnia or another sleep disorder that the engaged provider is comfortable diagnosing treating (e.g., restless leg syndrome), a treatment plan can be initiated by the non-sleep specialist, as appropriate (Fig. 4.1,

Point E; Fig. 4.2, Point D). Again, if the patient is not responsive to usual therapy or if the provider is not comfortable or feels uncertain with any aspect of diagnosis or treatment, a referral would be made to a sleep medicine specialty team (Fig. 4.1, Point E; Fig. 4.2, Point D). A patient who has a sleep complaint but who does not screen positive for a sleep disorder should be evaluated for the appropriate non-sleep disorders related to their complaint (e.g., mood disturbance, thyroid disease, asthma). If no obvious cause is determined and ongoing concerns about sleep remain, a referral to a sleep medicine physician could be considered. (Fig. 4.1, Point F).

The model we propose identifies several areas for future development. These fall under the categories of telemedicine, education, industry partners, and guidelines. Leveraging telemedicine to facilitate patient identification, screening and provider response is critical. Non-sleep provider education along with easy access to treatment guidelines and pathways is vitally important as well. All primary care providers (e.g., internal medicine, family medicine, pediatrics, OB/GYN, and general surgery) and relevant specialties (e.g., cardiology, pulmonary, and ENT) should have ACGME and ABMS mandates to learn about basic sleep disorders as part of their training. Similarly, advanced practice providers should be expected to learn this as part of their specialty training. Providers who have already completed their training could be encouraged to learn about important sleep disorders via state-mandated licensure requirements, maintenance of certification, CME, and/or CNE offerings. Additionally, we believe industry should be called upon to leverage artificial intelligence to facilitate initial patient identification (i.e., EHR vendors) as well as those who would benefit from stepped up care. For example, PAP vendors could create a dashboard that alerts a provider to all patients in their panel who are not adherent to PAP or whose PAP is not effectively treating their sleep apnea, as opposed to requiring a provider to log into a specific patient's PAP data.

Last but not least, we enthusiastically support the development of national guidelines to further articulate the collaboration between sleep medicine specialists and non-sleep trained providers. Such guidelines should have input from a diverse set of applicable stakeholders, inclusive of patients, relevant industry and business partners, leaders from appropriate professional organizations familiar with clinical guideline development, and sleep and non-sleep providers. Insurers and self-insured businesses should be called upon to work together as stakeholders to test these guidelines and demonstrate value. Once such collaborative guidelines are outlined, adjustments can be made locally between the spoke and hub providers, as needed, to further facilitate access to patient-centered sleep care.

References

1. Shepard JW, Buysse DJ, Chesson AL, Dement WC, Goldberg R, Guilleminault C, et al. History of the development of sleep medicine in the United States. J Clin Sleep Med. 2005;1(1):61–82.
2. FREIDA. AMA program results 2021. Available from: https://freida.ama-assn.org/search/list?spec=43391%20Put%20out%20by%20the%20AMA.

3. American Board of Medical Specialties. ABMS board certification report 2021. Available from: https://www.abms.org/board-certification/abms-board-certification-report/.
4. Frost & Sullivan; American Academy of Sleep Medicine. Medicine Hidden health crisis costing America billions: underdiagnosing and undertreating obstructive sleep apnea draining health care system. 2016. Available from: http://aasm.org/wp-content/uploads/2017/10/sleep-apnea-economic-crisis.pdf.
5. Quan SF. Graduate medical education in sleep medicine: did the canary just die? J Clin Sleep Med. 2013;09(02):101–2.
6. Billings ME, Cohen RT, Baldwin CM, Johnson DA, Palen BN, Parthasarathy S, et al. Disparities in sleep health and potential intervention models: a focused review. Chest. 2021;159(3):1232–40.
7. Owens J. Introduction to special section: NIH sleep academic award program. Sleep Med. 2005;6(1):45–6.
8. Chai-Coetzer CL, Antic NA, Rowland LS, Reed RL, Esterman A, Catcheside PG, et al. Primary care vs specialist sleep center management of obstructive sleep apnea and daytime sleepiness and quality of life: a randomized trial. JAMA. 2013;309(10):997–1004.
9. Sánchez-de-la-Torre M, Nadal N, Cortijo A, Masa JF, Duran-Cantolla J, Valls J, et al. Role of primary care in the follow-up of patients with obstructive sleep apnoea undergoing CPAP treatment: a randomised controlled trial. Thorax. 2015;70(4):346.
10. Sánchez-Quiroga MÁ, Corral J, Gómez-de-Terreros FJ, Carmona-Bernal C, Asensio-Cruz MI, Cabello M, et al. Primary care physicians can comprehensively manage patients with sleep apnea. A noninferiority randomized controlled trial. Am J Respir Crit Care Med. 2018;198(5):648–56.
11. Tarraubella N, Sánchez-de-la-Torre M, Nadal N, De Batlle J, Benítez I, Cortijo A, et al. Management of obstructive sleep apnoea in a primary care vs sleep unit setting: a randomised controlled trial. Thorax. 2018;73(12):1152.
12. Fuller JM, Wong KK, Grunstein R, Krass I, Patel J, Saini B. A comparison of screening methods for sleep disorders in Australian community pharmacies: a randomized controlled trial. PLoS One. 2014;9(6):e101003.
13. Perraudin C, Fleury B, Pelletier-Fleury N. Effectiveness of intervention led by a community pharmacist for improving recognition of sleep apnea in primary care – a cohort study. J Sleep Res. 2015;24(2):167–73.
14. Rosen IM, Rowley JA, Malhotra RK, Kristo DA, Carden KA, Kirsch DB. Strategies to improve patient care for obstructive sleep apnea: a report from the American Academy of Sleep Medicine Sleep-Disordered Breathing Collaboration Summit. J Clin Sleep Med. 2020;16(11):1933–7.
15. Brennan T. A new approach to sleep apnea 2021. Available from: https://payorsolutions.cvshealth.com/insights/new-approach-sleep-apnea.
16. Espie CA, MacMahon KMA, Kelly H-L, Broomfield NM, Douglas NJ, Engleman HM, et al. Randomized clinical effectiveness trial of nurse-administered small-group cognitive behavior therapy for persistent insomnia in general practice. Sleep. 2007;30(5):574–84.
17. Bothelius K, Kyhle K, Espie CA, Broman JE. Manual-guided cognitive-behavioural therapy for insomnia delivered by ordinary primary care personnel in general medical practice: a randomized controlled effectiveness trial. J Sleep Res. 2013;22(6):688–96.
18. Chai-Coetzer CL, Antic NA, McEvoy RD. Identifying and managing sleep disorders in primary care. Lancet Respir Med. 2015;3(5):337–9.
19. Morin CM, LeBlanc M, Daley M, Gregoire JP, Mérette C. Epidemiology of insomnia: prevalence, self-help treatments, consultations, and determinants of help-seeking behaviors. Sleep Med. 2006;7(2):123–30.
20. The Physicians Foundation. The Physicians Foundation 2016 Physician Survey 2016. Available from: http://www.physiciansfoundation.org/healthcare-research/physiciansurvey.
21. Sandlund C, Hetta J, Nilsson GH, Ekstedt M, Westman J. Improving insomnia in primary care patients: a randomized controlled trial of nurse-led group treatment. Int J Nurs Stud. 2017;72:30–41.

22. Morgenthaler TI, Owens J, Alessi C, Boehlecke B, Brown TM, Coleman J Jr, et al. Practice parameters for behavioral treatment of bedtime problems and night wakings in infants and young children. Sleep. 2006;29(10):1277–81.
23. Qaseem A, Kansagara D, Forciea MA, Cooke M, Denberg TD. Management of chronic insomnia disorder in adults: a clinical practice guideline from the American College of Physicians. Ann Intern Med. 2016;165(2):125–33.
24. Rios P, Cardoso R, Morra D, Nincic V, Goodarzi Z, Farah B, et al. Comparative effectiveness and safety of pharmacological and non-pharmacological interventions for insomnia: an overview of reviews. Syst Rev. 2019;8(1):281.
25. Koffel E, Bramoweth AD, Ulmer CS. Increasing access to and utilization of cognitive behavioral therapy for insomnia (CBT-I): a narrative review. J Gen Intern Med. 2018;33(6):955–62.
26. Maire M, Linder S, Dvořák C, Merlo C, Essig S, Tal K, et al. Prevalence and management of chronic insomnia in Swiss primary care: cross-sectional data from the "Sentinella" practice-based research network. J Sleep Res. 2020;29(5):e13121.
27. Ulmer CS, Bosworth HB, Beckham JC, Germain A, Jeffreys AS, Edelman D, et al. Veterans affairs primary care provider perceptions of insomnia treatment. J Clin Sleep Med. 2017;13(8):991–9.
28. Davy Z, Middlemass J, Siriwardena AN. Patients' and clinicians' experiences and perceptions of the primary care management of insomnia: qualitative study. Health Expect. 2015;18(5):1371–83.
29. Cheung JM, Atternäs K, Melchior M, Marshall NS, Fois RA, Saini B. Primary health care practitioner perspectives on the management of insomnia: a pilot study. Aust J Prim Health. 2014;20(1):103–12.
30. Buysse DJ, Germain A, Moul DE, Franzen PL, Brar LK, Fletcher ME, et al. Efficacy of brief behavioral treatment for chronic insomnia in older adults. Arch Intern Med. 2011;171(10):887–95.
31. Smallheer BA. Evaluation and treatment of restless legs syndrome in the primary care environment. Nurs Clin North Am. 2018;53(3):433–45.
32. Donovan LM, Yu L, Bertisch SM, Buysse DJ, Rueschman M, Patel SR. Responsiveness of patient-reported outcomes to treatment among patients with type 2 diabetes mellitus and OSA. Chest. 2020;157(3):665–72.
33. Espie CA. "Stepped care": a health technology solution for delivering cognitive behavioral therapy as a first line insomnia treatment. Sleep. 2009;32(12):1549–58.
34. Sweetman A, Lack L, Catcheside PG, Antic NA, Smith S, Chai-Coetzer CL, et al. Cognitive and behavioral therapy for insomnia increases the use of continuous positive airway pressure therapy in obstructive sleep apnea participants with comorbid insomnia: a randomized clinical trial. Sleep. 2019;42(12):zsz178.
35. Sweetman AM, Lack LC, Catcheside PG, Antic NA, Chai-Coetzer CL, Smith SS, et al. Developing a successful treatment for co-morbid insomnia and sleep apnoea. Sleep Med Rev. 2017;33:28–38.
36. Watson NF, Rosen IM, Chervin RD. The past is prologue: the future of sleep medicine. J Clin Sleep Med. 2017;13(1):127–35.
37. Pendharkar S, Blades K, Kelly J, et al. Perspectives on primary care management of obstructive sleep apnea: a qualitative study of patients and health care providers. J Clin Sleep Med. 2021;17(1):89–98.
38. Stevenson L, Ball S, Haverhals LM, Aron DC, Lowery J. Evaluation of a national telemedicine initiative in the Veterans Health Administration: factors associated with successful implementation. J Telemed Telecare. 2018;24(3):168–78.
39. Su GL, Glass L, Tapper EB, Van T, Waljee AK, Sales AE. Virtual consultations through the veterans administration SCAN-ECHO project improves survival for veterans with liver disease. Hepatology. 2018;68(6):2317–24.
40. Guzman-Clark J, Harrell K, Leff A, Henriques D, Ines E, Rofail M, et al. Implementation of an ECHO-based program to provide geriatric specialty care consultation and education to remote primary care teams. Fed Pract. 2016;33(4):40–5.

41. Ball S, Wilson B, Ober S, McHaourab A. SCAN-ECHO for pain management: implementing a regional telementoring training for primary care providers. Pain Med. 2018;19(2):262–8.
42. Parsons EC, Mattox EA, Beste LA, Au DH, Young BA, Chang MF, et al. Development of a sleep telementorship program for rural Department of Veterans Affairs primary care providers: sleep veterans affairs extension for community healthcare outcomes. Ann Am Thorac Soc. 2017;14(2):267–74.
43. Smith AG. A sleep medicine medical school curriculum: time for us to wake up. Neurology. 2018;91(13):587–8.
44. Salas RE, Gamaldo A, Collop NA, Gulyani S, Hsu M, David PM, et al. A step out of the dark: improving the sleep medicine knowledge of trainees. Sleep Med. 2013;14(1):105–8.
45. Salas RME, Strowd RE, Ali I, Soni M, Schneider L, Safdieh J, et al. Incorporating sleep medicine content into medical school through neuroscience core curricula. Neurology. 2018;91(13):597–610.
46. Lam AS, Wise SK, Dedhia RC. Practice patterns of sleep otolaryngologists at training institutions in the United States. Otolaryngol Head Neck Surg. 2017;156(6):1025–31.
47. Cass N, Kominsky A, Cabrera-Muffly C. Otolaryngology sleep medicine curriculum objectives as determined by sleep experts. Am J Otolaryngol. 2017;38(2):139–42.
48. Avidan AY, Vaughn BV, Silber MH. The current state of sleep medicine education in US neurology residency training programs: where do we go from here? J Clin Sleep Med. 2013;9(3):281–6.
49. American Board of Internal Medicine. Pulmonary disease certification examination blueprint 2021. Available from: https://www.abim.org/~/media/ABIM%20Public/Files/pdf/exam-blueprints/certification/pulmonary-disease.pdf.
50. Schulman DA, Piquette CA, Alikhan MM, Freedman N, Kumar S, McCallister J, et al. A sleep medicine curriculum for pulmonary and pulmonary/critical care fellowship programs: a multi-society expert panel report. Chest. 2019;155(3):554–64.
51. Mehra R, Rosen IM. Clarifying requisite sleep medicine content for the pulmonary and critical care medicine fellow: a key step forward, but where do we go from here? Chest. 2019;155(3):460–2.
52. Namen AM, Wymer A, Case D, Haponik EF. Performance of sleep histories in an ambulatory medicine clinic: impact of simple chart reminders. Chest. 1999;116(6):1558–63.
53. Sepucha KR, Simmons LH, Barry MJ, Edgman-Levitan S, Licurse AM, Chaguturu SK. Ten years, forty decision aids, and thousands of patient uses: shared decision making at Massachusetts General Hospital 2016. Available from: https://www.healthaffairs.org/doi/10.1377/hlthaff.2015.1376.
54. Maguire E, Hong P, Ritchie K, Meier J, Archibald K, Chorney J. Decision aid prototype development for parents considering adenotonsillectomy for their children with sleep disordered breathing. J Otolaryngol Head Neck Surg. 2016;45(1):57.
55. Fung CH, Martin JL, Liang LJ, Hays RD, Col N, Patterson ES, et al. Efficacy of a patient decision aid for improving person-centered decision-making by older adults with obstructive sleep apnea. J Clin Sleep Med. 2021;17(2):121–8.
56. Chai-Coetzer CL, Antic NA, Rowland LS, Catcheside PG, Esterman A, Reed RL, et al. A simplified model of screening questionnaire and home monitoring for obstructive sleep apnoea in primary care. Thorax. 2011;66(3):213–9.
57. Epton MJ, Kelly PT, Shand BI, Powell SV, Jones JN, McGeoch GRB, et al. Development and outcomes of a primary care-based sleep assessment service in Canterbury, New Zealand. NPJ Prim Care Respir Med. 2017;27(1):26.
58. McPherson CJ, Higginson IJ, Hearn J. Effective methods of giving information in cancer: a systematic literature review of randomized controlled trials. J Public Health Med. 2001;23(3):227–34.
59. Mills ME, Sullivan K. The importance of information giving for patients newly diagnosed with cancer: a review of the literature. J Clin Nurs. 1999;8(6):631–42.
60. Saunders CH, Petersen CL, Durand MA, Bagley PJ, Elwyn G. Bring on the machines: could machine learning improve the quality of patient education materials? A systematic search and rapid review. JCO Clin Cancer Inform. 2018;2:1–16.

61. Luyster FS, Choi J, Yeh CH, Imes CC, Johansson AE, Chasens ER. Screening and evaluation tools for sleep disorders in older adults. Appl Nurs Res. 2015;28(4):334–40.

62. Chung F, Abdullah HR, Liao P. STOP-Bang questionnaire: a practical approach to screen for obstructive sleep apnea. Chest. 2016;149(3):631–8.

63. Nagappa M, Liao P, Wong J, Auckley D, Ramachandran SK, Memtsoudis S, et al. Validation of the STOP-Bang questionnaire as a screening tool for obstructive sleep apnea among different populations: a systematic review and meta-analysis. PLoS One. 2015;10(12):e0143697.

64. Tan A, Yin JD, Tan LW, van Dam RM, Cheung YY, Lee CH. Predicting obstructive sleep apnea using the STOP-Bang questionnaire in the general population. Sleep Med. 2016;27-28:66–71.

65. Martin JL, Song Y, Hughes J, Jouldjian S, Dzierzewski JM, Fung CH, et al. A four-session sleep intervention program improves sleep for older adult day health care participants: results of a randomized controlled trial. Sleep. 2017;40(8):zsx079.

66. Allen RP, Walters AS, Montplaisir J, Hening W, Myers A, Bell TJ, et al. Restless legs syndrome prevalence and impact: REST general population study. Arch Intern Med. 2005;165(11):1286–92.

67. Ferri R, Lanuzza B, Cosentino FI, Iero I, Tripodi M, Spada RS, et al. A single question for the rapid screening of restless legs syndrome in the neurological clinical practice. Eur J Neurol. 2007;14(9):1016–21.

68. Nichols DA, Allen RP, Grauke JH, Brown JB, Rice ML, Hyde PR, et al. Restless legs syndrome symptoms in primary care: a prevalence study. Arch Intern Med. 2003;163(19):2323–9.

69. Walters AS, Frauscher B, Allen R, Benes H, Chaudhuri KR, Garcia-Borreguero D, et al. Review of diagnostic instruments for the restless legs syndrome/Willis-Ekbom Disease (RLS/WED): critique and recommendations. J Clin Sleep Med. 2014;10(12):1343–9.

70. Harrison JD, Patel MS. Designing nudges for success in health care. AMA J Ethics. 2020;22(9):E796–801.

71. Klingman KJ, Jungquist CR, Perlis ML. Questionnaires that screen for multiple sleep disorders. Sleep Med Rev. 2017;32:37–44.

72. Sarmiento KF, Folmer RL, Stepnowsky CJ, Whooley MA, Boudreau EA, Kuna ST, et al. National expansion of sleep telemedicine for veterans: the TeleSleep program. J Clin Sleep Med. 2019;15(9):1355–64.

73. Senthilvel E, Auckley D, Dasarathy J. Evaluation of sleep disorders in the primary care setting: history taking compared to questionnaires. J Clin Sleep Med. 2011;07(01):41–8.

74. Hwang D, Woodrum R. Inadequacy of current solutions to address provider shortage. Chest J. 2020;157(5):1055–7.

75. Goldstein CA, Berry RB, Kent DT, Kristo DA, Seixas AA, Redline S, et al. Artificial intelligence in sleep medicine: an American Academy of Sleep Medicine position statement. J Clin Sleep Med. 2020;16(4):605–7.

76. Keenan BT, Kim J, Singh B, Bittencourt L, Chen NH, Cistulli PA, et al. Recognizable clinical subtypes of obstructive sleep apnea across international sleep centers: a cluster analysis. Sleep. 2018;41(3):zsx214.

77. Kim J, Keenan BT, Lim DC, Lee SK, Pack AI, Shin C. Symptom-based subgroups of Koreans with obstructive sleep apnea. J Clin Sleep Med. 2018;14(3):437–43.

78. Mazzotti DR, Keenan BT, Lim DC, Gottlieb DJ, Kim J, Pack AI. Symptom subtypes of obstructive sleep apnea predict incidence of cardiovascular outcomes. Am J Respir Crit Care Med. 2019;200(4):493–506.

79. Eckert DJ. Phenotypic approaches to obstructive sleep apnoea – new pathways for targeted therapy. Sleep Med Rev. 2018;37:45–59.

80. McEvoy RD, Antic NA, Heeley E, Luo Y, Ou Q, Zhang X, et al. CPAP for prevention of cardiovascular events in obstructive sleep apnea. N Engl J Med. 2016;375(10):919–31.

81. Peker Y, Glantz H, Eulenburg C, Wegscheider K, Herlitz J, Thunström E. Effect of positive airway pressure on cardiovascular outcomes in coronary artery disease patients with nonsleepy obstructive sleep apnea. The RICCADSA randomized controlled trial. Am J Respir Crit Care Med. 2016;194(5):613–20.

82. Zinchuk A, Yaggi HK. Sleep apnea heterogeneity, phenotypes, and cardiovascular risk. Implications for trial design and precision sleep medicine. Am J Respir Crit Care Med. 2019;200(4):412–3.

83. Johns MW. Sensitivity and specificity of the multiple sleep latency test (MSLT), the maintenance of wakefulness test and the epworth sleepiness scale: failure of the MSLT as a gold standard. J Sleep Res. 2000;9(1):5–11.

84. Stephansen JB, Olesen AN, Olsen M, Ambati A, Leary EB, Moore HE, et al. Neural network analysis of sleep stages enables efficient diagnosis of narcolepsy. Nat Commun. 2018;9(1):5229.

85. Kuna ST. The MISSION act: challenges to sleep medicine and other specialties in the veterans health administration. Am J Respir Crit Care Med. 2019;200(6):663–4.

86. Health Resources & Services Administration. Telehealth programs 2021. Available from: https://www.hrsa.gov/rural-health/telehealth.

87. The Federation of State Medical Boards. House of delegates annual business meeting 2018. Available from: https://www.fsmb.org/siteassets/annual-meeting/hod/april-28-2018-fsmb-hod-book.pdf.

88. Kelly JM, Schwamm LH, Bianchi MT. Sleep telemedicine: a survey study of patient preferences. ISRN Neurol. 2012;2012:135329.

89. Johnson KG, Sullivan SS, Nti A, Rastegar V, Gurubhagavatula I. The impact of the COVID-19 pandemic on sleep medicine practices. J Clin Sleep Med. 2021;17(1):79–87.

90. Singh J, Badr MS, Diebert W, Epstein L, Hwang D, Karres V, et al. American Academy of Sleep Medicine (AASM) position paper for the use of telemedicine for the diagnosis and treatment of sleep disorders. J Clin Sleep Med. 2015;11(10):1187–98.

91. The Center for Connected Health Policy. Current state laws & reimbursement policies 2021. Available from: https://www.cchpca.org/telehealth-policy/current-state-laws-and-reimbursement-policies.

92. Centers for Medicare & Medicaid Services. Medicare telemedicine health care provider fact sheet 2020. Available from: https://www.cms.gov/newsroom/fact-sheets/medicare-telemedicine-health-care-provider-fact-sheet.

93. Mehrotra A, Nimgaonkar A, Richman B. Telemedicine and medical licensure — potential paths for reform. N Engl J Med. 2021;384(8):687–90.

94. Fields BG, Behari PP, McCloskey S, True G, Richardson D, Thomasson A, et al. Remote ambulatory management of veterans with obstructive sleep apnea. Sleep. 2016;39(3):501–9.

95. Parikh R, Touvelle MN, Wang H, Zallek SN. Sleep telemedicine: patient satisfaction and treatment adherence. Telemed J E Health. 2011;17(8):609–14.

96. Aurora RN, Collop NA, Jacobowitz O, Thomas SM, Quan SF, Aronsky AJ. Quality measures for the care of adult patients with obstructive sleep apnea. J Clin Sleep Med. 2015;11(3):357–83.

97. Arnedt JT, Conroy DA, Mooney A, Furgal A, Sen A, Eisenberg D. Telemedicine versus face-to-face delivery of cognitive behavioral therapy for insomnia: a randomized controlled noninferiority trial. Sleep. 2021;44(1):zsaa136.

98. American Academy of Sleep Medicine. Download the sleep telemedicine implementation guide – a FREE resource from AASM 2021 [February 28, 2021]. Available from: https://aasm.org/download-the-sleep-telemedicine-implementation-guide-a-free-resource-from-aasm/.

99. Goldstein C. Current and future roles of consumer sleep technologies in sleep medicine. Sleep Med Clin. 2020;15(3):391–408.

Part II
Sleep Disordered Breathing

Chapter 5
Obstructive Sleep Apnea: Clinical Epidemiology and Presenting Manifestations

Eric Yeh, Nishant Chaudhary, and Kingman P. Strohl

Keywords Epidemiology · Cardiovascular · OSA management · Pathogenesis
Obstructive sleep apnea · Renal disease · Psychiatric disease

Introduction

Obstructive sleep apnea (OSA) is a common chronic sleep condition. The clinical diagnosis is called obstructive sleep apnea hypopnea syndrome (OSAHS), defined by symptoms of unrefreshing and disturbed sleep, loud snorts and snoring, daytime impairment from sleepiness or a fatigue-like state and a certain number (usually >5/hour or an average of one every 12 minutes) of predominantly obstructive apneas and hypopnea per hour (referred to as apnea-hypopnea index or AHI). If one remains uncertain of the precise pathogenesis or risk, OSAHS is resolved of symptoms by treatment of upper airway obstruction during sleep. In that regard, two treatments are available where there is robust evidence for symptomatic and objective effectiveness are tracheostomy [41], and excellent adherence to continuous positive airway pressure (CPAP) [36]. OSA is found at all stages of life, in all races, and with all shapes and sizes of people, and can rise to the level of a disorder (OSAHS).

At this point in time, defining OSA and OSAHS are no longer the critical questions. Instead, the questions are how these conditions affect morbidity are chronic medical conditions. The concepts for this chapter are those that consider the prevalence of the clinically recognized disorder, concepts summarized in Fig. 5.1. OSA can be predicted on a sleep study to some degree by a constellation of risk factors and presenting classical complaints, like sleepiness, disrupted sleep, snoring and

E. Yeh · N. Chaudhary · K. P. Strohl (✉)
Division of Pulmonary, Critical Care, and Sleep Medicine, Department of Medicine,
University Hospitals of Cleveland, Case Western Reserve University, Cleveland, OH, USA
e-mail: kingman.strohl@uhhospitals.org

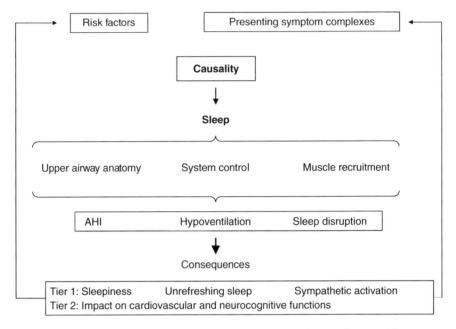

Fig. 5.1 Shown are the pathway relationships from risk factors and presenting complaints to consequences. The causal factors of sleep, upper airway anatomy, (ventilatory) system control, and muscle recruitment lead to the apneas and hypopneas (AHI), hypoventilation, and sleep disruptions leading to the Tier 1 (immediate) and Tier 2 (long term remodeling) of cardiovascular and neural physiology

obesity [12], but those non-obese with non-traditional symptoms like insomnia or parasomnia are also found to be enriched for OSA, compared to the general population. There are no tests or biologic markers. It is that OSA is a complex disease in which no one feature or genetic set point or biological marker alone sets it apart as a diagnosis.

Risk factors and complaints are not causal factors. Sleep precipitates disordered breathing in the otherwise healthy individual, and added to it are additional aspects – the ventilatory control system which is a source of instability over time, the tendency for the upper airway to close, and the degree of upper airway muscle activation in sleep or in response to upper airway closure [40]. All conspire to increase or decrease the measurable polysomnographic counts of sleep-disordered breathing [46].

The presence and severity of OSA is currently represented by the apnea-hypopnea index (AHI), hypoventilation assessed by measures of hypoxic stress by oximetry and of carbon dioxide excretion, and sleep disruption, often indicated by EEG arousals. The consequences of these events can be considered as short-term and chronic outcomes, and the associations with disease and treatment mitigation will inform medical practitioner about the rationale for clinical recognition and treatment. There is a feedback loop from consequences which over time can influence risk factors and presenting complaints. For instance, the effects of AHI sympathetic activation and hypoxia releases insulin which in turn promotes appetite and fat acquisition or heart failure which compromises upper airway patency or promotes breathing instability, respectively [39].

Other chapters will go into detail on the relationships shown in Fig. 5.1. For our purposes this schema sets the stage for our view of how the current body of knowledge in OSA epidemiology has led to current management and identification strategies. Thus, this chapter is designed less to provide facts and more to examine presentations and recognition of pathways of clinical importance that present in outpatient vs. inpatient care settings and consider potential policy changes or preventative medicine. The overall objectives are to introduce the scope of the epidemiology in each setting rather than review all datasets, which are addressed in several recent, more granular reviews. Finally, there is a goal for sleep medicine to provide individual OSA management (personalized medicine). The rationale and details of how disease evolves over time have now a body of literature that indicates a heterogeneity in outcomes depending upon various domains of symptom presentation, polysomnographic variables, and genetic predisposition to increase or decrease risk of the consequences. These will be reviewed in more detail in other chapters in this book. The epidemiology of OSA serves as an introduction to this approach.

There are a variety of terms and abbreviations in the epidemiology literature with the result that the one must notice definitions of OSA or OSAHS [47]. Conclusions, while internally consistent with the definitions, might differ with another definition making direct meta-comparisons among cohorts, even in the present time, problematic. Table 5.1 lists some of the more common metrics and groupings of illness severity that are generally used and inform many of the opinions in this review. There are other measures coming on line in clinical medicine that begin to define

Table 5.1 Conservative odds ratio (OR) for finding sleep apnea in each of several individual medical conditions and three reported behaviors, all other things being equal

Condition	OR
Systemic hypertension	1.5–4
Stroke	1.2–3
Myocardial infarction	1.3–2.5
Nocturnal angina	8–15
Hyperlipidemia	2–3
Asthma	1.5–2.0
Diabetes	2
Menopause	1.27
Depression	1.92
Pulmonary hypertension	1.2
Activity	
Regular physical exercise	0.5–0.9
Snoring	2–6
Obesity (BMI >30)	8–12

features of sleep hypoventilation (time > 55 mm Hg transcutaneous CO_2), and of features in sleep-disordered breathing (apnea time, cycle length, submental EMG recruitment); however, reporting is just beginning to appear in retrospective studies of cohorts.

Population Epidemiology

Figure 5.2 illustrates the OSA epidemiology regarding populations and prevalence, in particular, the perspectives that might influence decision making. The large box illustrates an unfiltered population, and the succession of boxes inside it represents a range of sub-populations. Among population cohorts, prevalence rates for self-proclaimed healthy individuals vary by gender and weight, and community as represented by race or ethnicity. The prevalence estimates in the community are lower than in clinical settings, because the ascertainment attempts to be random or at least a representative of the group living in any given region.

In the primary care population where the most common initial complaint for a new appointment is fatigue, and obesity (~BMI >30), the result is a pre-test probability of ~37% [27]. In heart failure clinics estimates are the same or higher. In the bariatric clinics, it does not make sense to even ask about sleep apnea, as the prevalence is generally greater than 60%; uncommon are the ~15% of patients who are

Fig. 5.2 This figure represents the greater population at lare (whole box) and the various subsets in the general population with estimates of prevalence of sleep-disordered breathing

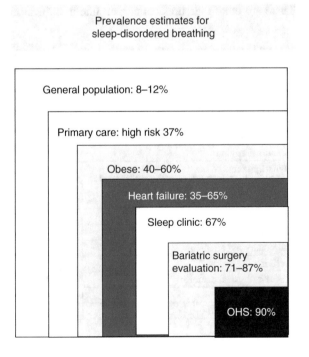

morbidly obese who do not have symptoms of sleep apnea and low AHI values (<10/h). A high prevalence of sleep apnea and obstructive apnea in particular is present in the hospital setting enriched for chronic cardiopulmonary disorders admitted for acute illness [34]. Obesity hypoventilation syndrome is more often found during a hospitalization for acute medical illness or in the setting of a poor recovery from a surgical procedure [24].

If a community prevalence is used as the standard, almost any adult clinical setting will have a prevalence is higher than in the community. In specialty samples, comparisons are made between clinical cohorts in which some have clinical symptoms of high risk, and those who do not, and this leads to interesting associations. For instance, sleep apnea prevalence is higher than the general population in floppy eyelid syndrome, nonarteritic anterior ischemic optic neuropathy, central serous retinopathy, retinal vein occlusion, and glaucoma, and post-hoc ascribed to vascular consequences of OSA [11, 35]. One is not really sure whether these reports represent a causal OSA factor, an epiphenomenon, or an ascertainment within an older population. Whether ascertainment for OSA should lead to a routine referral of floppy eyelid or other ophthalmologic condition should await data on whether identification and treatment of OSA makes sense. Likewise, a mandate to sleep specialists to assess ophthalmologic as well as cardiovascular conditions is not part of routine practice. The burden of OSAHS estimated at any one time is also confounded by the uncertainty about the latency to clinical detection, a subtle effect of co-morbidity, or susceptibility to other disorders.

The prevalence rate of OSA (AHI >5/h) in industrialized countries is 10–20% of middle-aged adults with a syndromic group estimated at 4–8% of men and 2–4% of women, and in the same cohort repeat testing some years later suggest prevalence increasing from 1993 to 1998 [30]. Worldwide estimates have come up with a sleep apnea prevalence of a little less than 1 billion individuals, with an AHI >5 cutoff, and a half billion with an AHI >15. This estimate is seriously flawed by ascertainment bias by study, selective reporting, differences in the methodology (testing, questionnaire, AHI criteria, or derivation from estimates from BMI or other measures of body habitus) [4]. The data do not indicate who needs treatment or might benefit from interventions. It does serve a purpose, however. While lower than hypertension, the estimate puts OSA as potentially significant as a driver of chronic illness; the estimate illustrates the population substrate out of which OSAHS is derived; and the estimate serves to drive further the attention of international health agencies to consider health policy initiatives and of industry to recognize market opportunities, similar to what is seen worldwide in cardiovascular disease and diabetes. Treatment in non-Western-oriented medical systems which are resource-limited may turn up inventive approaches that will in turn inform Western medicine.

In the US Wisconsin cohort, a group of employed state workers, the measurement of sleep-disordered breathing was the primary outcome and a sense of the impact of a report of snoring or the presence of obesity was demonstrated [50]. Shown in Fig. 5.3 is a graph of the cumulative percent of people with a given AHI when parsed into those who do not snore, those who are habitual snorers (4–7 times a week), and the obese (BMI >30). This graph does not indicate which patients

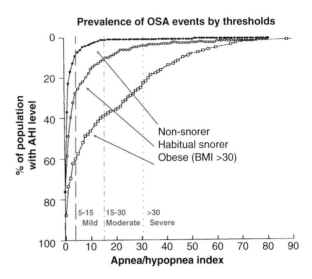

Fig. 5.3 This depicts the data from the 1993 and 2003 publications of the Wisconsin cohort to summarize the prevalence of OSA in regard to AHI categories and prevalence – percent (%) of the population – with a certain AHI level of mild, moderate, and severe as events/hour

would need or seek therapy given this information, but it does illustrate an instance where differences exist in population estimates if there are differences in reportable symptoms or BMI as a surrogate for weight.

High rates of community OSA have been recently published, albeit in the Western literature. The first is the population-based Study of Health in Pomerania which utilized objective measures to examine the prevalence and risk factors of obstructive sleep apnea in a German cohort between 20 and 81 years old [15]. The OSA prevalence was 46% (59% men and 33% women) for an AHI ≥5%, and 21% (30% men, 13% women) for an AHI ≥15. However, adding symptoms, OSAHS prevalence (apnea-hypopnea index ≥5; Epworth Sleepiness Scale >10) was 6%. Gender, age, body mass index, waist-to-hip ratio, snoring, alcohol consumption (for women only), and self-reported cardiovascular diseases were significantly positively associated with AHI >5. Diabetes, hypertension, and metabolic syndrome were positively associated with AHI >30. A second report from Switzerland, a country that one might think would have relatively low rates, included 3043 consecutive participants who underwent polysomnography [16]. About 50% were men, median age of 57 years with a median BMI of ~25·6. Participants underwent complete polysomnographic recordings at home. AHI >15 was ~23% in women and ~50% in men for AHI >15. Association for trend indicated hypertension (OR 1.6), diabetes (OR 2.0), metabolic syndrome (OR 1.8), and depression (OR 1.92). These two reports suggest a cross-sectional community burden of sleep apnea in Western populations, associated with other common chronic diseases.

The reports from Asian countries take advantage of universal health coverage and community-based health surveys. In the Taiwanese individuals, habitual snoring overall was ~52%, a bit higher in males at 61% than females at 43%. Corresponding rates for witnessed apnea during sleep was 2.6%, 3.4%, and 1.9%, respectively. The prevalence of having both traits was also higher in males than in females. Prevalence of hypertension, cardiovascular disease, diabetes mellitus, arthritis, and backache was higher in those who snored or had witnessed apnea [9]. In South Korea, a similar pattern emerges with high risk for OSA at 16% and risk for OSA being higher with age ≥70 years (OR 2.68) and body BMI ≥25 kg/m² (OR 10.75), even though the BMI range is lower than in Caucasians [42]. As in other samples, hypertension (OR 5.83), diabetes mellitus (OR 2.54), hyperlipidemia (OR 2.85), and anxiety (OR 1.63) were comorbid conditions. Interestingly, a report of regular physical activity (OR 0.70) had a protective effect, giving a clue to directions for policy to mitigate OSA.

The literature is clear in greater susceptibility of men to snoring and sleep apnea until the age where women experience menopause. The USA values generally cited are on the order of 17% of women and 22% of men, if the threshold is an AHI of ≥5 [49]. Recognition strategies for sleep apnea built on such risk factors, with male sex (1 point for male and 0 for female), reflect a greater positive predictive value, although the relative proportion of risk in a multivariate tool like the STOP-BANG is modest [10]. The obvious mechanism is a hormonal one and the potentially protective effects of progesterone and estrogen, opposed to testosterone in men.

In one large Chinese hypertensive population OSA prevalence is related to age in women but only to BMI in men [6]. Reports appear which explain this by an impact on hormonal milieu, for instance in the Nurses' Health Study II during 1995–2013, compared with natural menopause, surgical menopause by hysterectomy and/or oophorectomy, the hazard ratio for OSA was 1.27 (95% confidence interval (CI): 1.17, 1.38), even after accounting for age, risk was higher among non-obese women. Interestingly among women who never used hormone therapy AHI and hypertension risk was lower than those who had used some hormone therapy. Surgical as compared with natural menopause was independently associated with higher OSA risk in women in the postmenopausal phase of life [17]. These cohort studies start to define risk factors.

The presence of OSA in otherwise healthy people has an impact on subsequent health, as shown in the Wisconsin cohort where a dose-response association was uncovered between AHI levels at baseline and the clinical presence of hypertension 4 years later, independent of many of the known risk factors confounding factors including age, sex, and body weight [31]. Relative to a reference of 0/h, presence of hypertension at follow-up for an AHI 1 to <5 was 1.42, for 5–14.9/h 2.03, and for >15/h 2.89, significant at all levels [31]. These observations are consistent with sleep apnea being a modifiable risk factor for cardiovascular disease, given that hypertension is the greatest risk for heart failure, renal failure, and cardiac arrhythmias.

Community studies also suggest a complex, and bidirectional interaction of OSA with common respiratory disorders, one example of which is asthma. The Wisconsin Sleep Cohort Study has longitudinal data on respiratory status and overnight polysomnography studies at 4-year intervals [43]. The associations of presence and duration of asthma with OSA. Participants with incident asthma were found to experience incident OSA more than those without asthma; the corresponding adjusted relative risk was significant (RR 1.39), controlling for sex, age, baseline and change in body mass index, and other factors. Asthma was also associated with new-onset OSA with sleepiness, hallmarks of the development of OSAHS. Therefore, one may look at the better-developed asthma surveillance systems for clues as to the potential for new OSA cases.

Many suspect that the origins of disease start in childhood patterns of dietary intake, exercise need and habit, and changes in head form, followed by habitual alcohol and smoking, and in parallel risk of cardiovascular disease. There are few long-term observational studies of individuals spanning the ages of 18 to about 55 years of age, about the sixth decade being the most common mean or median age found in many cohorts including the initial reports from the Wisconsin Sleep Cohort [50] and the Sleep Heart Health Study [29, 37]. It is difficult to "look back" at the trajectory of disease, and consider which causal pathway drove the propagation of sleep apnea, as captured by AHI, over time. One modest study showed that over a five-year period the significant odds ratio for incident sleep-disordered breathing started with being male (OR ~ 2.29), and then age and waist-hip ratio (both OR ~ 1.5), and then BMI and cholesterol (at OR ~ 1.1) [44]. Over the past two decades, with the increasing prevalence of adult obesity in the Western world, the most important risk factor in sleep breathing disorders, the number of patient diagnosed as suffering from OSA has increased and it will increase over the coming years unless this obesity trend is mitigated.

Office Epidemiology

The early reports of sleep apnea in primary care population surprised those who believed that it would reflect community estimates. One such early study was a two-step survey of primary care practices where a questionnaire was used to assess risk and polygraphic study was used to measure suspected OSA [38]. Fifty percent of all primary care patients reported to snore while 31% of snorers reported to snore every night. Based on this first questionnaire algorithm 20% were at high risk for SDB, compared to 18.5% for PLMD and 25% with insomnia. Daytime sleepiness and fatigue were associated in patients with likelihood of any or all of these three suspected conditions. SDB was twice as common in men than in women.

In 1997, a Berlin, Germany, conference of primary care practitioners and sleep specialists resulted in a tool called the Berlin Questionnaire designed for primary care office use. Its intent was to use a predictive approach that three domains (snoring and disturbed sleep, sleepiness, and a combination of BMI >30 and/or hypertension) would constitute a high pre-test probability for OSA [28]. For the 100 patients who underwent sleep studies, risk grouping was generally useful in the prediction of the number of events. While it could not tell one whether high risk meant a need for therapy, it was useful for its negative predictive value. The value of the tool was explored in relation to its domains and risk in 8000 adults across primary care practices in the United States and Europe. One-third (32%) had a high pretest probability for OSA, with a higher rate in the

United States (36%) than in Europe (26%). Sleepiness (32% vs 12%) followed by obesity and/or hypertension (45% vs 37%, respectively; $p < 0.01$) contributed to the OSA risk difference between participants in the United States and Europe, as frequent snoring and breathing pauses were similarly reported (44%). A high pretest probability for OSA was more often present in men than in women (38% vs 28%) and in those that were obese, a condition more common in the United States (28% vs 17%). The conclusions were that primary care physicians would encounter a high demand for services to confirm or manage sleep apnea, sleepiness, and obesity (Fig. 5.4).

A similar survey 15 years later expanded on this theme [2]. The target was five different family medicine practice locations in North Carolina for assessment of the burden of sleep complaints in the system. More than 50% of the respondents reported excessive daytime sleepiness, one-third reported insomnia, 13–33% were dealing with symptoms consistent with OSA and OSAHS; in addition, more than one-quarter had clinical symptoms of restless legs syndrome. The correlation of poor health and sleep disturbance was high, and comorbidities such as hypertension, pain syndromes, and depression were also shown to be associated with more sleep complaints. Besides fatigue and excessive daytime sleepiness, complaints such as headache, nocturia, undesired awakening with or without inability to fall back to sleep, morning dry mouth, and nocturnal gastroesophageal reflux, and subjective reduced concentration and memory, and "mood disorder", were mapped to sleep complaints. Sleep was noted to be important in the assessment of isolated chief complaints like frequent nocturia particularly in older males that would before lead to a only work up for benign prostate hypertrophy, or heartburn in obese patients that lead to only GERD management, or dry mouth upon awakening being

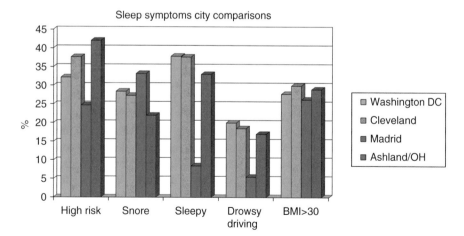

Fig. 5.4 Shown are unpublished data from the study published as Netzer et al. (2003) is graphed to compare among two large cities (Washington DC and Madrid Spain), a medium-sized city, Cleveland Ohio, and a small town, Ashland Ohio, the computation of High Risk in the Berlin Questionnaire and various factors including drowsy driving

attributed to medication side effects particularly if the sleep aid had anticholinergic action. Though many of these previously routine referrals are still reasonable, one should create a differential diagnosis that might include sleep apnea which has been associated with all these complaints.

Management of OSA and OSAHS has become increasingly common. In a review of annual stratified samples of patients identified as having sleep apnea in hospital-based and non-hospital-based physician office visits in the U.S. National Ambulatory Medical Care Survey database between 1993 and 2010, reports of a diagnosis of sleep apnea increased 14.6-fold [26]. Thirty-three percent were reported by primary care providers, 17% by pulmonologists, and 10% by otolaryngologists, with an increasing number of "other practitioners" listing a diagnosis of sleep apnea as new. Regions that reported a higher per capita rate of sleep apnea correlated with the rates of obesity and health insurance status.

In 2013, the American College of Physicians reported on their consensus as to the most effective therapy of obstructive sleep apnea and concluded that weight loss was the most supported therapy [33]; the fact that obesity is present in ~50% of patients did not deter the committee from their conclusions. Medicare by that time had endorsed requirements for continuous positive pressure therapy some time before [20]. It is time that practice pathways for the management of OSAHS will be designed with primary care tools and decision trees to know when and how to manage, engage sleep specialists and other providers, and provide value to patients. There is precedent for these to be developed and used in diabetes, but in this instance, there is a relatively simple blood marker to begin the process of prevention and treatment. Often primary care physicians are skeptical of patient-based sleep apnea risk assessments because of its subjective nature. Yet, offices deploy the PHQ-2 to collect a depression risk in those with a complaint of fatigue or low mood, and there are management guidelines. The prevalence of sleep disorders is higher than depression. However, even tools like the Berlin Questionnaire or the STOP-BANG require a decision about what to do next. If a test is ordered, like home sleep testing, what to do with the data are not embedded in practice guidelines. One can only compare the detailed directions for what to do when diabetes is suspected by the primary care physician and suspected by an elevated Hemoglobin A1c, to the lack of consensus we have as to when and how to assess at a primary care level a report of AHI and severity levels. Utilization of screening tools such as STOP-BANG and Berlin Questionnaire is useful but not diagnostic and skewed toward elimination of those without moderate or severe OSA, rather that suggest who should be treated or who might accept treatment or the preventive approach to managing sleep-disordered breathing. Reliance on testing and response to autotitration therapy could be useful as a primary action, but not without a recognition and management strategy for those who do not respond.

Sleep Medicine Practices

It is worthwhile to pause briefly to describe sleep medicine, as one other feature of clinical care. The specialty started as a collection of sleep laboratories in the United States and Europe when sleep disorders were considered rare and curious, OSAHS being defined in 1964 when the first tracheostomy was performed, and narcolepsy as a distinct syndrome described using symptoms and the combined use of a polysomnogram and Multiple Sleep Latency Test. Organizing a professional society in the 1980s, the leaders of the field pushed for standards, training, and medical codes for management of a host of sleep disorders. One measure of progress was a survey in 2000 undertaken to determine the spectrum of sleep-related disorders diagnosed in regional sleep centers and compare this information to a previous survey published in 1982, at the origin of the sleep center. In a two-month prospective point-prevalence survey, across 19 accredited regional sleep centers in the United States.

The major referrals in 2000 are similar to today with snoring, sleepiness, and other sleep-related reports as the presenting complaints (Fig. 5.5a). In 2000 most patients underwent polysomnography as similar to that done in 1982. In 2000, obstructive sleep apnea, narcolepsy, and restless legs syndrome were the top three reported primary diagnoses with a prevalence of ~69%, ~5%, and ~3%, respectively (Fig. 5.5b). The entire range of 93 sleep disorders, however, was represented in the 2000 survey. In this sample, true even today, when a sleep specialist interviews a patient, nearly a third of patient had either a primary or secondary diagnosis of a non-respiratory sleep disorder, and many had more than one sleep diagnosis. Compared to the previous survey from 1982, there has been an absolute increase in patient referrals/center with a two- to four-fold increase in the number of patients/center with a final diagnosis of a non-respiratory sleep-related problem. However, there had been a 20-fold increase in the diagnosis of obstructive sleep apnea.

Since 2000 there has been a further increase in sleep centers and diagnostic facilities, the creating of an American Board of Internal Medicine Sleep Medicine specialty examination, and a 1-year ACGME fellowship program. Sleep specialists are encountering increasing referrals from family internal medicine, pulmonary medicine, and otolaryngology, and a broad range of sleep-related disorders. Now, the now mandatory for sleep medicine board certification eligibility has had the unintended consequence of restricting the influx of young physicians to the field [45]. The number of sleep specialists who are retiring now exceeds the number that are trained through ACGME-accredited programs leading to a specialty certificate in Sleep Medicine. New training pathways are being developed to provide flexibility in high-quality, comprehensive, and multidisciplinary sleep medicine training to meet the sleep health needs of the present and future [32].

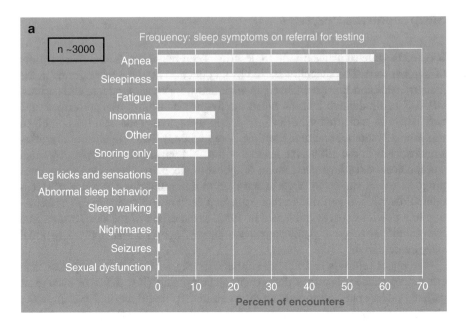

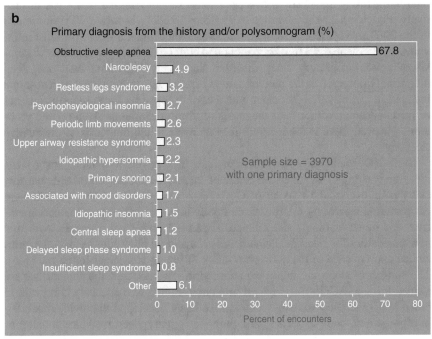

Fig. 5.5 (**a**) This is a graphical representation of the data in Punjabi et al. (2003) on the percent of encounters for referral for a polysomnography from 19 sleep centers in the United States over a 3-month period. (**b**) This is a graphical representation of the data in Punjabi et al. (2003) on the percent of encounters with a given diagnostic outcome from 19 sleep centers in the United States over a 3-month period

OSA in Medical, Neurologic, and Psychiatric Disorders

Diagnoses of sleep apnea during outpatient visits to hospital-based and non-hospital-based practices in the United States were much more frequent in 2010 than in 1993, as reported by outpatient practice clinicians participating in national surveys [26]. Although 60% of diagnoses of sleep apnea were reported by a combination of pulmonary and ENT specialty and primary care offices, there was a substantial increase in reports of sleep apnea by clinicians practicing other specialties during this period. This trend appears to continue. Discussed below are conditions selected for data availability of prevalence rates influencing outcome.

Pulmonary Clinics In a cross-sectional study from the US National Health and Nutrition Examination Survey (NHANES) data (year 2005–2008), subjects ≥20 years were identified who had no COPD or OSA, or only OSA, or had only COPD, or had OSA/COPD overlap syndrome [13]. The COPD and OSA/COPD overlap syndrome groups had significantly higher chance of all-cause mortality than the group of subjects who did not have OSA or COPD (adjusted hazard ratio [HR] =1.5 for the COPD group and 2.4 for the overlap syndrome group). OSA/COPD overlap syndrome was associated with a modest likelihood of death than COPD alone (HR =1.5; $P = 0.160$). Other factors associated with higher overall mortality were aging, poorer family status, current smoker, serum vitamin D deficiency, cardiovascular disease, history of cancer, diabetes, and impaired renal function. COPD and the combination of OSA and COPD leading to symptoms and signs of hypoventilation were markers of higher all-cause mortality compared to the control group. Interestingly simple OSA did not significantly increase mortality in patients with COPD. Hence the challenge in pulmonary clinics is to identify and manage OSA/COPD patients with a complex co-morbidity.

Endocrine Clinics Given the community correlations of OSA to obesity, it should come as no surprise that OSA and OSAHS are present in nearly all type 2 diabetes mellitus patients. In patients with metabolic syndrome, OSAS is an independent risk factor for the onset of type 2 diabetes and a worsening glycemic control [7]. In diabetics, the well-known clinical appearance of accumulation of adipose tissue in the neck and limited chest wall dynamics, hypoxia, and local micro-inflammation link visceral obesity closely with OSAS, with bidirectional effects. Promoting exercise, improving sleep habits, and diet weight loss can treat both metabolic syndrome and OSAS, especially in obese patients. There is also a high incidence of OSAS in acromegaly, although growth hormone treatments seem to be unrelated to the onset of apnea in GH-deficient individuals.

Neurology Clinics In patients with spinal cord injury, approaching 60% in motor complete persons with tetraplegia. Central apnea is more common in patients with tetraplegia than in patients with paraplegia [8]. In this population there is a lack of correlation between symptoms and SDB, and unfortunately there is insufficient evidence in the literature on the impact of treatment on morbidity, mortality, and quality of life outcomes.

Neuromuscular specialists encounter a common and predictable development of chronic sleep-disordered breathing in the neuromuscular syndromes which because of the patterning of respiratory muscle output during sleep and smaller lung volumes make patients particularly vulnerable to upper airway collapse, hypoventilation, and disturbed sleep that reduce the quality of life [1, 3]. Obstructive and central sleep apneas are common and noninvasive ventilation can improve survival and quality of sleep. Early detection with monitoring at home and polysomnography help guide therapy for sleep-disordered events, before and during non-invasive ventilation.

There is likely a bidirectional relationship between sleep apnea and stroke, resulting in close association between the two conditions. In addition, sleep apnea is a potentially modifiable risk factor in stroke and stroke rehabilitation. For instance, in a moderately sized group of stroke patients sleep apnea was determined by a validate algorithm and functional outcome was measured using Barthel score on day 7 and at third month following the onset of stroke. A high pre-test probability of sleep apnea was present in 31% patients, more in males (68%) and with advanced age [25]. Hypertension was present in 66.6% of patients with sleep apnea. Recovery scores at third month were somewhat better among patient with no apnea, but this was not statistically significant. Gain in functional independence in no apnea group was better than those in whom sleep apnea was strongly suspected. Sleep apnea is amenable to treatment and should be considered in patients with acute ischemic stroke to improve the chance of recovery, and to reduce the risk of recurrence.

Psychiatry Clinics Sleep disturbances have been associated with increased risk for suicidal thought and behavior. The literature regarding sleep and suicide, however, has focused predominantly on generalized sleep disturbance or insomnia. A secondary analysis of 2014 data from the National Survey on Drug Use and Health. Respondents from a random sample of US households 18 years or older is informative [5]. The prevalence of a diagnosis of sleep apnea was 3%. Prevalence of suicidality was ~10% for suicidal ideation, 3% for suicide planning, and 1% for suicide attempt compared with 5%, 2%, and 1%, respectively, for those without sleep apnea. Analyses revealed that sleep apnea was significantly but modestly associated with both suicidal ideation (OR = 1.50) and suicide planning (OR = 1.56) after controlling for age, sex, ethnicity, past-year substance use disorder, self-rated overall health, past-year sedative-hypnotic misuse, past-year depressive episode, heart disease, high blood pressure, stroke, diabetes, and body mass index. Sleep apnea was not significantly associated with report of past-year suicide attempt. A consideration of sleep apnea may represent an early opportunity for providers to discuss suicide and mental health with their patients.

Obstetric Clinics Sleep-disordered breathing (SDB) is recognized in pregnancy and may be a modifiable factor for adverse outcomes including pre-eclampsia and premature birth. Nulliparous women ($n = 3700$) completed validated questionnaires to assess for symptoms related to snoring, fatigue, excessive daytime sleepiness, insomnia, and restless leg syndrome, along with an at-home portable monitor [21]. The prevalence of risk for sleep-disordered breathing was 3.6% and 8.3%, for early and mid-pregnancy, respectively. At each time point in gestation, frequent snoring, chronic hypertension, greater maternal age, body mass index, neck circumference, and systolic blood pressure were associated most strongly with an increased risk of sleep-disordered breathing. Current age, body mass index, and frequent snoring predicted sleep-disordered breathing in early pregnancy, sleep-disordered breathing in mid pregnancy, and new-onset sleep-disordered breathing in mid pregnancy. In the follow-up analyses [14], the prevalence of preeclampsia was 6.0%, hypertensive disorders of pregnancy 13.1%, and GDM 4.1%. In early and mid-pregnancy the adjusted odds ratios for preeclampsia when sleep-disordered breathing was present were 1.94 (95% CI 1.07–3.51) and 1.95 (95% CI 1.18–3.23), respectively; hypertensive disorders of pregnancy 1.46 (95% CI 0.91–2.32) and 1.73 (95% CI 1.19–2.52); and GDM 3.47 (95% CI 1.95–6.19) and 2.79 (95% CI 1.63–4.77). Increasing exposure-response relationships were observed between apnea-hypopnea index and both hypertensive disorders and GDM. There appears a somewhat independent association between sleep-disordered breathing and preeclampsia, hypertensive disorders of pregnancy, and gestational diabetes mellitus. In a study from another group of 1345 women, the overall prevalence of high risk for OSA was 10.1% (95% confidence intervals [CIs] 8.5–11.7), associated with pre-pregnancy body mass index and stress [18]. An adjusted odds ratio (OR) for preeclampsia-eclampsia in women with high risk for OSA was 2.72 (95% CI 1.33–5.57).

Disability Assessments There are reported associations between sleep apnea and receipt of mortality or a disability pension [34]. In a prospective study of the Swedish Patient Register from 2000 to 2009 (74,543 sleep apnea cases: 60,125 outpatient, 14,418 inpatient), cases were matched to 5:1 non-cases and tracked from diagnosis/inclusion into the study. During ~5.1 years, 13% of men and 21% of women with inpatient sleep apnea received a disability pension. Inpatient sleep apnea was associated with higher total mortality (hazard ratio (HR) = for men 1.71, and for women, 2.33) with associations to ischemic heart disease (for men, HR = 2.27 and for women HR = 5.27), respiratory disorders (for men, HR = 3.29, and for women, HR = 5.24), and suicide (for men, HR 2.60 and for women, HR = 4.33). Notice that the HR was always higher in women. There were no associations to ascertainment for inpatient sleep apnea with cancer mortality. Outpatient sleep apnea was associated with a higher risk of receiving a disability pension but not higher total mortality. In conclusion, inpatient sleep apnea was higher risk of mortality and disability pension receipt, a decade after diagnosis.

Obesity Hypoventilation Syndrome (OHS) This condition is considered in more detail in other chapters of this book. While it is a diagnosis often made while the patient is awake, it is important in our Chapter as it is part of the spectrum of sleep-disordered breathing. It is defined as a combination of obesity (body mass index ≥ 30 kg·m(-2)), daytime hypercapnia (arterial carbon dioxide tension ≥ 45 mmHg), and sleep-disordered breathing, after ruling out other disorders that may cause alveolar hypoventilation. OHS prevalence has been estimated to be ~0.4% of the adult population [24], but becomes an important condition in acute hospitalizations. OHS is typically diagnosed during an episode of acute-on-chronic hypercapnic respiratory failure or when symptoms of dyspnea lead to pulmonary or sleep consultation in stable conditions. The most frequent comorbidities are heart failure, coronary disease, uncontrolled diabetes, and pulmonary hypertension. A recognition strategy and appropriate management with medications and rehabilitation programs are key issues for improving prognosis.

Medical Training A prospective cross-sectional study was performed among young doctors less than 40 years old, using questionnaires and home sleep apnea testing [48]. Mean age and mean body mass index (BMI) were 31 years and 23, respectively. The prevalence of OSA and OSAHS were 40.4 and 5.8%, respectively, with one-third having at least moderate OSA. History of snoring, being male, and perception of inadequate sleep were significant predictors for OSA with the odds ratio of 34.5, 18.8, and 7.4, respectively. Only observed apnea was a significant predictor for OSAS with odds ratio of 30.7 ($p = 0.012$, 95% CI = 2.12–442.6). Number of naps per week was a significant predictor for excessive daytime sleepiness. OSA and total number of call days per month were significant predictors for tiredness with the odds ratio of 4.8 and 1.3, respectively. OSA was the only significant predictor for perception of inadequate sleep. This is the only study that reports prevalence of OSA and OSAS among young doctors and emphasizes the need for detection at an earlier age. It is not that the subjects were doctors but the group in early adulthood with demanding jobs and long hours of work, likely present in many work settings.

Sleep Detection and Gaps in Knowledge

There are efforts to develop and validate a tool that does not rely on subjective reports so that estimates of the burden of sleep apnea may be made using electronic databases, relevant to both outpatient and inpatient settings. The symptomless Multi-Variable Apnea Prediction index (sMVAP) has three variables (age, sex, and weight) and was developed to identify OSA as a presumptive diagnosis and deployed to assess the relationship between sMVAP and adverse outcomes in patients having elective surgery for non-bariatric and bariatric procedures [22]. Using data from 40,432 elective inpatient surgeries, we used logistic regression to determine the relationship between sMVAP and previous OSA, current hypertension, and postoperative complications: extended length of stay (ELOS), intensive-care-unit-stay (ICU-stay), and respiratory complications (pulmonary embolism, acute respiratory distress syndrome, and/or aspiration pneumonia). Higher sMVAP was associated with increased likelihood of previous OSA, hypertension and all postoperative complications, and the top quintile had increased odds of postoperative complications compared to the bottom quintile. For ELOS, ICU-stay, and respiratory complications, respective significant odds ratios were 1.83, 1.44, and 1.85, respectively. With propensity matching in patients having bariatric surgery, sMVAP was more strongly associated with postoperative complications in non-Bariatric surgical groups. The idea is that OSA risk measured by a symptomless calculation correlates with higher risk for select postoperative complications. Interestingly, associations are stronger for non-Bariatric surgeries. The implications are that preoperative screening with variables collected from charted measures is sufficient to risk stratify for adverse postoperative outcomes. The sMVAP as a risk stratifier in the assessment of commercial motor vehicle operators was tested with and without the addition of symptoms and its accuracy was better with the additional information [23]. It should be noted that the use of this tool does not preclude more precise individual assessments [19] (Fig. 5.6).

The literature on the epidemiology has progressed from community surveys to an understanding of OSA as a common condition. We are however still in lacking information at early asymptomatic phases and from young adulthood, limiting the ability to detect what human features alone or collectively can produce a propagation of events during sleep, prospectively. This gap occurs in those with clinical collections, like obesity or neuromuscular disorders, where there is a high likelihood of progression of objective markers and symptomatic outcomes. Established,

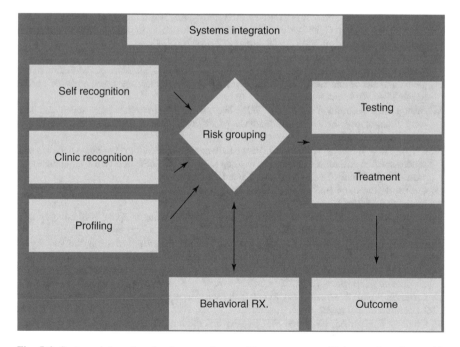

Fig. 5.6 Systems integration for the arc of recognition to outcome. Risk grouping along with individualized (personal) medicine would determine the manner of testing and therapy, but ultimately the outcome remains to be defined better

symptomatic patients must be present in many clinical systems, as OSA recognition can be triggered by events like stroke, myocardial infarction, or detection of hypoventilation. Some inroads are there in recognition profiling for perioperative patients, and in the current literature on profiling using the EMR. The high prevalence of OSA and OSAHS, limited information on management outcomes, and transparent costs of treating established disease justify research into more available and less costly, but comparably reliable, alternative treatments. To this end, all levels of medical care must be involved: (1) primary care or specialists not directly involved with sleep, (2) second-level hospitals, which should have the ability to perform simplified studies, and (3) tertiary hospitals with complex equipment and multidisciplinary environment have to be prepared to receive patients with complex sleep disorders of breathing as well as to solve the sleep-related diseases. Thus, there appears value in recognition and management of OSAHS and a rationale for prevention and early detection of OSA.

References

1. Aboussouan LS, Mireles-Cabodevila E. Sleep-disordered breathing in neuromuscular disease: diagnostic and therapeutic challenges. Chest. 2017;152:880–92.
2. Alattar M, Harring JJ, Mitchell M, Sloane P. Sleep problems in primary care: a North Carolina family practice research network (NC-FP-RN) study. J Am Board Fam Med. 2007;20:365–74.
3. Albdewi MA, Liistro G, El Tahry R. Sleep-disordered breathing in patients with neuromuscular disease. Sleep Breathing = Schlaf Atmung. 2018;22:277–86.
4. Benjafield AV, Ayas NT, Eastwood PR, Heinzer R, Ip MSM, Morrell MJ, Nunez CM, Patel SR, Penzel T, Pépin JL, Peppard PE, Sinha S, Tufik S, Valentine K, Malhotra A. Estimation of the global prevalence and burden of obstructive sleep apnoea: a literature-based analysis. Lancet Respir Med. 2019;7:687–98.
5. Bishop TM, Ashrafioun L, Pigeon WR. The association between sleep apnea and suicidal thought and behavior: an analysis of National Survey Data. J Clin Psychiatry. 2018;79:17m11480.
6. Cai A, Zhou Y, Zhang J, Zhong Q, Wang R, Wang L. Epidemiological characteristics and gender-specific differences of obstructive sleep apnea in a Chinese hypertensive population: a cross-sectional study. BMC Cardiovasc Disord. 2017;17:8.
7. Ceccato F, Bernkopf E, Scaroni C. Sleep apnea syndrome in endocrine clinics. J Endocrinol Investig. 2015;38:827–34.
8. Chiodo AE, Sitrin RG, Bauman KA. Sleep disordered breathing in spinal cord injury: a systematic review. J Spinal Cord Med. 2016;39:374–82.
9. Chuang LP, Hsu SC, Lin SW, Ko WS, Chen NH, Tsai YH. Prevalence of snoring and witnessed apnea in Taiwanese adults. Chang Gung Med J. 2008;31:175–81.
10. Chung F, Abdullah HR, Liao P. STOP-Bang questionnaire: a practical approach to screen for obstructive sleep apnea. Chest. 2016;149:631–8.
11. Cristescu Teodor R, Mihaltan FD. Eyelid laxity and sleep apnea syndrome: a review. Romanian J Ophthalmol. 2019;63:2–9.
12. Crummy F, Piper AJ, Naughton MT. Obesity and the lung: 2. Obesity and sleep-disordered breathing. Thorax. 2008;63:738–46.
13. Du W, Liu J, Zhou J, Ye D, OuYang Y, Deng Q. Obstructive sleep apnea, COPD, the overlap syndrome, and mortality: results from the 2005-2008 National Health and Nutrition Examination Survey. Int J Chron Obstruct Pulmon Dis. 2018;13:665–74.

14. Facco FL, Parker CB, Reddy UM, Silver RM, Koch MA, Louis JM, Basner RC, Chung JH, Nhan-Chang CL, Pien GW, Redline S, Grobman WA, Wing DA, Simhan HN, Haas DM, Mercer BM, Parry S, Mobley D, Hunter S, Saade GR, Schubert FP, Zee PC. Association between sleep-disordered breathing and hypertensive disorders of pregnancy and gestational diabetes mellitus. Obstet Gynecol. 2017;129:31–41.
15. Fietze I, Laharnar N, Obst A, Ewert R, Felix SB, Garcia C, Gläser S, Glos M, Schmidt CO, Stubbe B, Völzke H, Zimmermann S, Penzel T. Prevalence and association analysis of obstructive sleep apnea with gender and age differences – results of SHIP-trend. J Sleep Res. 2019;28:e12770.
16. Heinzer R, Vat S, Marques-Vidal P, Marti-Soler H, Andries D, Tobback N, Mooser V, Preisig M, Malhotra A, Waeber G, Vollenweider P, Tafti M, Haba-Rubio J. Prevalence of sleep-disordered breathing in the general population: the HypnoLaus study. Lancet Respir Med. 2015;3:310–8.
17. Huang T, Lin BM, Redline S, Curhan GC, Hu FB, Tworoger SS. Type of menopause, age at menopause, and risk of developing obstructive sleep apnea in postmenopausal women. Am J Epidemiol. 2018;187:1370–9.
18. Jaimchariyatam N, Na-Rungsri K, Tungsanga S, Lertmaharit S, Lohsoonthorn V, Totienchai S. Obstructive sleep apnea as a risk factor for preeclampsia-eclampsia. Sleep Breathing = Schlaf Atmung. 2019;23:687–93.
19. Jonas DE, Amick HR, Feltner C, Weber RP, Arvanitis M, Stine A, Lux L, Middleton JC, Voisin C, Harris RP. U.S. preventive services task force evidence syntheses, formerly systematic evidence reviews. In: Screening for obstructive sleep apnea in adults: an evidence review for the US preventive services task force. Rockville: Agency for Healthcare Research and Quality (US); 2017.
20. Loube DI, Gay PC, Strohl KP, Pack AI, White DP, Collop NA. Indications for positive airway pressure treatment of adult obstructive sleep apnea patients: a consensus statement. Chest. 1999;115:863–6.
21. Louis JM, Koch MA, Reddy UM, Silver RM, Parker CB, Facco FL, Redline S, Nhan-Chang CL, Chung JH, Pien GW, Basner RC, Grobman WA, Wing DA, Simhan HN, Haas DM, Mercer BM, Parry S, Mobley D, Carper B, Saade GR, Schubert FP, Zee PC. Predictors of sleep-disordered breathing in pregnancy. Am J Obstet Gynecol. 2018;218:521.e521–12.
22. Lyons MM, Keenan BT, Li J, Khan T, Elkassabany N, Walsh CM, Williams NN, Pack AI, Gurubhagavatula I. Symptomless multi-variable apnea prediction index assesses obstructive sleep apnea risk and adverse outcomes in elective surgery. Sleep. 2017;40:zsw081.
23. Lyons MM, Kraemer JF, Dhingra R, Keenan BT, Wessel N, Glos M, Penzel T, Gurubhagavatula I. Screening for obstructive sleep apnea in commercial drivers using EKG-derived respiratory power index. J Clin Sleep Med. 2019;15:23–32.
24. Masa JF, Pépin JL, Borel JC, Mokhlesi B, Murphy PB, Sánchez-Quiroga M. Obesity hypoventilation syndrome. Eur Respir Rev. 2019;28:180097.
25. Nair R, Radhakrishnan K, Chatterjee A, Gorthi SP, Prabhu VA. Sleep apnea-predictor of functional outcome in acute ischemic stroke. J Stroke Cerebrovasc Dis. 2019;28:807–14.
26. Namen AM, Chatterjee A, Huang KE, Feldman SR, Haponik EF. Recognition of sleep apnea is increasing. Analysis of trends in two large, representative databases of outpatient practice. Ann Am Thorac Soc. 2016;13:2027–34.
27. Netzer NC, Hoegel JJ, Loube D, Netzer CM, Hay B, Alvarez-Sala R, Strohl KP. Prevalence of symptoms and risk of sleep apnea in primary care. Chest. 2003;124:1406–14.
28. Netzer NC, Stoohs RA, Netzer CM, Clark K, Strohl KP. Using the Berlin questionnaire to identify patients at risk for the sleep apnea syndrome. Ann Intern Med. 1999;131:485–91.
29. Nieto FJ, Young TB, Lind BK, Shahar E, Samet JM, Redline S, D'Agostino RB, Newman AB, Lebowitz MD, Pickering TG. Association of sleep-disordered breathing, sleep apnea, and hypertension in a large community-based study. Sleep Heart Health Study. JAMA. 2000;283:1829–36.

30. Peppard PE, Young T, Barnet JH, Palta M, Hagen EW, Hla KM. Increased prevalence of sleep-disordered breathing in adults. Am J Epidemiol. 2013;177:1006–14.
31. Peppard PE, Young T, Palta M, Skatrud J. Prospective study of the association between sleep-disordered breathing and hypertension. N Engl J Med. 2000;342:1378–84.
32. Plante DT, Epstein LJ, Fields BG, Shelgikar AV, Rosen IM. Competency-based sleep medicine fellowships: addressing workforce needs and enhancing educational quality. J Clin Sleep Med. 2020;16:137–41.
33. Qaseem A, Holty JE, Owens DK, Dallas P, Starkey M, Shekelle P. Management of obstructive sleep apnea in adults: a clinical practice guideline from the American College of Physicians. Ann Intern Med. 2013;159:471–83.
34. Rod NH, Kjeldgård L, Åkerstedt T, Ferrie JE, Salo P, Vahtera J, Alexanderson K. Sleep apnea, disability pensions, and cause-specific mortality: a Swedish Nationwide Register Linkage Study. Am J Epidemiol. 2017;186:709–18.
35. Santos M, Hofmann RJ. Ocular manifestations of obstructive sleep apnea. J Clin Sleep Med. 2017;13:1345–8.
36. Schwab RJ, Badr SM, Epstein LJ, Gay PC, Gozal D, Kohler M, Levy P, Malhotra A, Phillips BA, Rosen IM, Strohl KP, Strollo PJ, Weaver EM, Weaver TE. An official American Thoracic Society statement: continuous positive airway pressure adherence tracking systems. The optimal monitoring strategies and outcome measures in adults. Am J Respir Crit Care Med. 2013;188:613–20.
37. Shahar E, Whitney CW, Redline S, Lee ET, Newman AB, Nieto FJ, O'Connor GT, Boland LL, Schwartz JE, Samet JM. Sleep-disordered breathing and cardiovascular disease: cross-sectional results of the Sleep Heart Health Study. Am Rev Respir Crit Care Med. 2001;163:19–25.
38. Stoohs RA, Barger K, Dement WC. Sleep disordered breathing in primary care medicine. Sleep Breathing = Schlaf Atmung. 1997;2:11–22.
39. Strohl KP. Diabetes and sleep apnea. Sleep. 1996;19(10 Suppl):S225–8.
40. Strohl KP, Butler JP, Malhotra A. Mechanical properties of the upper airway. Compr Physiol. 2012;2(3):1853–72.
41. Strohl KP, Cherniack NS, Gothe B. Physiologic basis of therapy for sleep apnea. Am Rev Respir Dis. 1986;134:791–802.
42. Sunwoo JS, Hwangbo Y, Kim WJ, Chu MK, Yun CH, Yang KI. Prevalence, sleep characteristics, and comorbidities in a population at high risk for obstructive sleep apnea: a nationwide questionnaire study in South Korea. PLoS One. 2018;13:e0193549.
43. Teodorescu M, Barnet JH, Hagen EW, Palta M, Young TB, Peppard PE. Association between asthma and risk of developing obstructive sleep apnea. JAMA. 2015;313:156–64.
44. Tishler PV, Larkin EK, Schluchter MD, Redline S. Incidence of sleep-disordered breathing in an urban adult population: the relative importance of risk factors in the development of sleep didordered breathing. JAMA. 2003;289:2230–7.
45. Watson NF, Rosen IM, Chervin RD. The past is prologue: the future of sleep medicine. J Clin Sleep Med. 2017;13:127–35.
46. Wellman A, Edwards BA, Sands SA, Owens RL, Nemati S, Butler J, Passaglia CL, Jackson AC, Malhotra A, White DP. A simplified method for determining phenotypic traits in patients with obstructive sleep apnea. J Appl Physiol. 1985;114:911–22, 2013.
47. Whyte KF, Allen MB, Fitzpatrick MF, Douglas NJ. Accuracy and significance of scoring hypopneas. Sleep. 1992;15:257–60.
48. Yasin R, Muntham D, Chirakalwasan N. Uncovering the sleep disorders among young doctors. Sleep Breathing = Schlaf Atmung. 2016;20:1137–44.
49. Young T, Palta M, Dempsey J, Skatrud J, Weber S, Bader S. The occurrence of sleep disordered breathing in middle-aged adults. New Engl J Med. 1993;328:1230–5.
50. Young T, Palta M, Dempsey J, Skatrud J, Weber S, Badr S. The occurrence of sleep-disordered breathing among middle-aged adults. N Engl J Med. 1993;328:1230–5.

Chapter 6
Obstructive Sleep Apnea: Diagnosis with Polysomnography and Portable Monitors

Janna Raphelson, Erica Feldman, and Atul Malhotra

Keywords Sleep · Apnea · Diagnosis · Lung · Monitoring · Breathing

Introduction

OSA is the leading cause of referral to sleep laboratories worldwide, accounting for at least 75–80% of diagnoses [1]. In the last few decades, there have been considerable advances in knowledge regarding the underlying mechanisms, diagnostic approaches, treatment options, and the impact of OSA on personal as well as public health of OSA. The global prevalence of OSA was recently estimated at up to 1 billion people worldwide. Even using a stricter definition (based on Apnea–Hypopnea Index AHI > 15/h) there are still up to 500 million estimated cases worldwide [2]. The current definitions of sleep apnea are not uniform, but most of them attempt to characterize the frequency of sleep-disordered breathing events (e.g., AHI "Apnea–Hypopnea Index" or RDI "Respiratory Disturbance Index") along with the severity (e.g., oxygen desaturation) of each event (e.g., complete (apnea) and partial (hypopnea) cessation of breathing during sleep). By convention, an apnea is defined as greater than 90% reduction of airflow for at least 10 s [3, 4]. A hypopnea is defined as a reduction in airflow that is followed by an arousal from sleep or a decrease in oxyhemoglobin saturation. While AHI is the most commonly used parameter to assess sleep apnea severity, several additional measures of sleep such as the degree of nocturnal oxyhemoglobin desaturation and the extent of carbon dioxide elevation have been used to characterize disease severity in clinical and research settings (Table 6.1).

J. Raphelson · E. Feldman
University of California, San Diego, Department of Medicine, Internal Medicine, La Jolla, CA, USA
e-mail: jraphelson@health.ucsd.edu

A. Malhotra (✉)
Department of Medicine, Division of Pulmonary, Critical Care, Sleep Medicine and Physiology, University of California, San Diego Health, La Jolla, CA, USA
e-mail: amalhotra@ucsd.edu

© Springer Nature Switzerland AG 2022
M. S. Badr, J. L. Martin (eds.), *Essentials of Sleep Medicine*,
Respiratory Medicine, https://doi.org/10.1007/978-3-030-93739-3_6

Table 6.1 Common OSA terminology

Apnea— Hypopnea Index (AHI)	The number of apneas and hypopneas a patient has per hour of sleep
Respiratory Disturbance Index (RDI)	A formula used in reporting polysomnography data: the number of apneas, hypopnea, and RERAs a patient has per hour of sleep
Apnea	Complete cessation of breathing during sleep, defined by greater than 90% reduction in airflow for at least 10 s, has no requirement for a desaturation or arousal
Hypopnea	Reduction in airflow that is followed by an arousal from sleep or a decrease in oxyhemoglobin saturation
Respiratory effort-related arousal (RERA)	A series of respiratory cycles of increase/decreasing effort or flattening for at least 10 s, recorded by nasal manometry and leading to an arousal that cannot be defined as an apnea or hypogea
Sleep-disordered breathing	Umbrella term for a constellation of sleep-related breathing disorders and abnormalities of respiration during sleep that does not meet criteria for a disorder

The mechanisms of sleep-disordered breathing are complex, but can involve either obstruction of the upper airways (OSA) in the presence of intact respiratory drive; the absence of ventilatory drive (CSA or central sleep apnea) in the presence of a patent airway; or mixed apnea, which has features of both OSA and CSA [5–7]. Pure CSA is much less common than OSA in the general population; CSA occurs most often in individuals with congestive heart failure (CHF) or occasionally with neurological compromise or chronic narcotic intake [8–10].

Patients with OSA can frequently experience sleep fragmentation, daytime somnolence, or suboptimal psychomotor function. Untreated OSA can also lead to common comorbidities such as hypertension, diabetes, stroke, and depression. Individuals with moderate and severe OSA have increased risks for hypertension, cerebrovascular accident (CVA), cardiovascular diseases, diabetes mellitus, depression, road traffic crashes, poor performance in school and work, and decreased productivity in the workplace [11–23].

Prevalence and Epidemiology

The estimated prevalence of symptomatic OSA in the United States in early 1990s by Young et al. was 4% among adult men and 2% among adult women [24]. Since then, prevalence data from other countries have emerged. The prevalence of OSA associated with daytime sleepiness is conservatively 3–7% in adult men and 2–5% in adult women. Subgroups of those populations have higher prevalence, including persons with older age, male gender, and obesity [25]. Though diagnostic methodologies vary, most available epidemiological data on prevalence of OSA confirm Young's finding across the globe. Interestingly, the prevalence of OSA in developing countries such as India and China is on the same order of magnitude as that in the developed countries, despite less obesity [2]. Therefore, OSA is not only a disease of more developed countries, but a common disease worldwide. Additionally, there are huge and growing individual and public health costs associated with OSA, whether from lost productivity at workplaces, motor vehicle accidents from drowsy driving, or the cardiovascular and metabolic comorbidities of OSA [26]. Because the obesity epidemic is spreading worldwide, we can only imagine an increasingly higher prevalence of OSA in the twenty-first century [27].

Risk Factors

Despite substantial research on OSA in the past several decades, OSA remains underdiagnosed. This finding is due in part by the lack of awareness of the disease by patients as well as the general public, and insufficient clinical suspicion on the part of providers. Therefore, it is important for clinicians to gain proper knowledge of OSA risk factors, so that timely diagnoses can be made and treatment can be initiated as appropriate.

OSA risk factors include obesity, older age, male gender, postmenopausal status, Asian/African American races, tobacco, and alcohol use [28]. Studies have shown that up to 70% of men and 56% of women between age 65 and 99 years have some form of OSA [29]. The mechanisms for age-related OSA include deposition of adipose tissue in the parapharyngeal area and anatomical changes surrounding the pharynx [30–32]. Disease prevalence for OSA is relatively low among premenopausal women and increases postmenopausally [33]. Obesity is the single most treatable factor predictive of OSA [34–36]. Data collected in Sleep Heart Health Study (SHHS) have shown that moderate and severe OSA is independently associated with BMI, neck circumference, as well as waist circumference. Individuals with OSA have significantly more visceral distribution of fat than central fat after controlling for BMI. Visceral fat is significantly correlated with AHI. Waist–hip ratio has also been shown in some studies to be more predictive of severe OSA than obesity in general. Only 10–15% of the population with diagnosis of OSA have body mass index (BMI) less than 25 kg/m^2. Individuals with large neck circumferences (men >17 in., women >16 in.) should raise the clinician's suspicion for OSA.

There are multiple theories as to why OSA prevalence in women is lower than that in men. One of them is that male bed partners of women are less likely to report bedtime symptoms of OSA than the female bed partners of men. Women with OSA also tend to have less "classic" daytime symptoms of OSA; instead of reporting daytime sleepiness they may report fatigue and lack of energy. Lastly, women have different anatomical and functional properties of their upper airways and differences in control of breathing. Thus, both diagnostic biases and biological factors contribute to the gender imbalance in sleep apnea prevalence [37–42].

Among different races, obesity plays a varying degree of importance. Middle-aged (age 25–65 years) African Americans have similar disease prevalence than the other racial groups, but adult African Americans younger than 25 years or older than 65 years have a higher prevalence than the others. Among the East Asian population, though the prevalence of obesity is less than the whites, the prevalence of OSA is not less than that in the West. Therefore, the relationship between obesity and OSA is less clear-cut among Asians. However, differences in adipose tissue distribution (i.e., peripheral vs. visceral) may play a more important role in Asians [43]. Table 6.2 risk factors for OSA.

Clinical History

A sleep history looking for OSA should be obtained either as a routine health maintenance evaluation, or as part of an assessment for potential OSA in symptomatic people. In addition, a comprehensive evaluation should be considered in those at high risk for OSA, and as a part of a screen for sleep disorders in commercial drivers, other transportation operators and persons involved in safety-sensitive work. A good sleep history should address both sleep and wakefulness. Because individuals with OSA often disrupt their bed partners' sleep, bed partners should be encouraged to participate in this part of the evaluation process. Loud snoring, awakenings due to choking and/or gasping, and witnessed apneic episodes during sleep are common symptoms reported by OSA patients or their bed partners. OSA can make falling asleep and maintaining sleep difficult. Excessive daytime sleepiness (EDS) is a common complaint, although many patients do not report sleepiness per se [44]. For an individual with OSA, EDS most likely will persist even after adequate amount of total sleep time (TST) is achieved. The Epworth Sleepiness Scale (ESS), a self-reported score, combines a series of answers for likelihood of dozing off in eight different scenarios. An ESS of greater than 12 (out of 24) is usually considered "sleepy." Though subjective, ESS is frequently used to quantify EDS and is useful as a reference scale for assessing future treatment effectiveness [27, 45, 46]. Questions on general sleep history such as TST, sleep fragmentation, sleep

Table 6.2 Common risk factors of obstructive sleep apnea (OSA)

Anthropometric measures	BMI >28 kg/m^2, neck circumference >17 in. (43 cm) for men, or >16 in.(41 cm) for women
Physical exam	Retrognathia, high modified Mallampati score (III/IV), large tonsils (>2), macroglossia
Age	Age 35 or greater
Ethnicity	Asian, African American, Hispanic ethnicities
Gender	Male gender
Hormone	Postmenopausal status in women
Habits	Alcohol, tobacco, physical inactivity

maintenance, as well as questions related to insomnia (difficulty falling asleep or going back to sleep) should also be asked to generate a differential diagnosis. Lack of concentration and/or cognitive abilities, decreased libido, risk of motor vehicle accidents, mood disorders, morning headaches, and dry mouth are other common complaints in OSA patients. History of common comorbidities such as hypertension, stroke, myocardial infarction, cor pulmonale, and arrhythmia should also be obtained. In pediatric populations, the complaint of excessive sleepiness is often replaced by hyperactivity, attention deficit, and mouth breathing. OSA is more frequently present among children of OSA subjects, suggesting the role of genetic factors in OSA [47, 48]. Table 6.3 lists questions that a healthcare provider should ask of an individual suspected of having OSA. Other questionnaires have been assessed in this context with variable predictive value, including the STOP-BANG and NO-OSAS [27]. These questionnaires may be preferable to ESS in certain populations, including bariatric surgery patients.

Taking a medical history from certain populations among whom symptoms and signs of OSA may affect their employment status may be challenging. For example, unlike the sleep clinic setting where patients are seeking diagnosis and treatment for sleep difficulties, it is common for commercial vehicle drivers, pilots, and train operators to avoid an OSA diagnosis because of its economic and occupational implications. Thus, relying on self-reported symptoms by commercial drivers for screening for OSA has a very low yield in these occupational settings. These groups often do not report any symptoms. Furthermore, drivers with previously diagnosed OSA initially have been reported to deny the presence of a sleep disorder until they are told that based on screening criteria they are required to obtain a sleep study. A 2006 study in Israel showed 78% of its commercial drivers with BMI greater or equal to 32 kg/m^2 had polysomnography (PSG)-confirmed OSA and almost half had objectively confirmed EDS as measured by a multiple sleep latency test (MSLT), but 100% of the affected drivers denied symptoms of OSA or EDS [49]. Likewise, most OSA-affected commercial motor vehicle (CMV) operators report very low ESS score at driver certifications exams (range 3–4 or 2–5 out of 24), which are markedly lower than average ESS scores among college and medical students (range 7–8). Therefore, at the present time, examiners must rely primarily upon anthropometric and other objective criteria when evaluating transportation operators.

A summary statement from the Joint Task Force (JTF) of American College of Occupational and Environmental Medicine/American College of Chest Physicians/National Sleep Foundation of screening criteria for OSA among CMV operators

Table 6.3 Five questions to screen patients for obstructive sleep apnea (OSA)

1.	"Do you have trouble falling asleep or maintaining asleep at night?"
2.	"Have you ever been told that you snore during sleep?"
3.	"Have you ever woken up choking or gasping for air when you are asleep?"
4.	"Has anyone ever witnessed you stop breathing during sleep?"
5.	"Do you have trouble staying awake during the day?" (Epworth sleepiness scale questionnaire)

was published in the journal *Chest* in 2006 [50]. The statement recommends a 3-month maximum certification, pending OSA evaluation, for the CMV operator if the operator falls into any one of the five major categories. Of note, the only objectively measurable major category in the JTF statement is the subject's anthropometric characteristics and blood pressure measured during the office visit. Therefore, in the setting of occupational certification, the suspicion for OSA should be elevated with or without a clear subjective reporting of symptoms of OSA (i.e., EDS). Timely referral for an OSA evaluation is warranted, if the examinee seeking certification has two of the following three objectives measurements in clinic:

1. BMI >35 kg/m^2
2. Neck circumference >17 in. in men or 16> in. in women
3. Hypertension

Patients with first-degree relatives with OSA are more likely to have OSA than those without first-degree relatives with OSA. Additionally, multiple medical conditions have been associated with OSA. In the field of endocrine disorders, type 2 diabetes, polycystic ovary syndrome (PCOS), and hypothyroidism are known to be associated with OSA. Congenital diseases such as Down's syndrome or microcephaly are associated with OSA. Pregnant women can present with OSA as gestational weight gain progresses. Occasionally, rare anatomical abnormalities of the airway such as Eagle Syndrome can cause OSA. Table 6.4 illustrates complications from OSA.

Physical Exam

Vital signs can frequently reveal hypertension in people with OSA. Neck circumference should be documented as it is an important anthropometric measurement. Obesity (BMI of ≥30 kg/m^2) is probably the most common finding among OSA patients. The rest of the physical exam should include head and neck, airway or respiratory, cardiac, neurologic exams. The head and neck exam of an OSA patient can present with crowded posterior pharyngeal space (i.e., modified Mallampati III or IV), large tongue with teeth mark (macroglossia), tonsillar hypertrophy, dental

Table 6.4 Complications of obstructive sleep apnea (OSA)

Cardiovascular	Hypertension, coronary artery disease, atrial fibrillation, cardiac arrhythmia, heart failure
Neurological	Stroke, depression, psychosis, sexual dysfunction, inattention, cognitive deficits
Pulmonary	Group 3 pulmonary hypertension
Endocrine	Metabolic syndrome, type 2 diabetes
Gastrointestinal	Nonalcoholic fatty liver disease
Rheumatologic	Gout
Trauma	Motor vehicle accidents

malocclusion (class II), retracted mandible relative to the maxilla (retrognathism or micrognathism), or deviated nasal septum. In children with OSA, hypertrophied adenoids or tonsils are common, and children often compensate by becoming obligatory mouth breathers. Nasopharyngeal fiberscope can be used in office to evaluate for the shape and size of the retropalatal/retroglossal airway, though there is no currently available evidence-based guidelines using this as a diagnostic tool. Internal jugular venous distension and peripheral edema should be assessed as part of the heart exam. Cardiac auscultation and pulse palpation can be helpful, particularly given the known association between atrial fibrillation and sleep apnea. Neurological examination should focus on muscle strength and presence of any focal deficits, since neuromuscular disease can present with sleep apnea and/or hypoventilation.

Diagnosis of OSA

There are currently two major methods to diagnose OSA: full in-lab PSG and portable monitoring (PM) or limited-channel testing (LCT) device. There is much ongoing debate as to the utility of each diagnostic tool. In general, PSG offers more thorough measurements of various aspects of sleep, but it is time-consuming, expensive, and performed outside the home. PM offers convenience to patients, but PM is limited by its reduced sensitivity, specificity, and measured information. Patient history and physical exam are key determinants for diagnostic route. Due to financial considerations, PM is becoming increasingly common in the USA and has been used with reasonable success worldwide. There are four types of PMs Type I–IV, in the order of decreasing measurements of sleep and respiratory variables (see Table 6.5).

Table 6.5 Summary characteristics of polysomnogram (type I) and portable monitor (type II–IV)

	Type I PSG	Type II PSG	Type III PSG	Type IV PSG
Monitoring personnel	Yes	No	No	No
Oximetry	Yes	Yes	Yes	Yes
Respiratory effort	Yes	Yes	Yes	No
Airflow	Yes	Yes	Yes	No
Body positions	Yes	Yes/No	Yes/No	No
EMG-AT	Yes	Yes	No	No
EEG	Yes	Yes	No	No
ECG-heart rate	Yes	Yes	Yes	No
EOG	Yes	Yes	No	No
Surface EMG	Yes	Yes	No	No
Video recording	Yes/No	No	No	No
Sound recording	Yes/No	No	No	No
Minimum number of channels for CMS* reimbursement	14–16	≥ 7	≥ 4	≥ 3

Overnight Polysomnography (PSG)

The current gold standard test for assessing the severity of OSA is in-laboratory, technician-monitored PSG. A full PSG (or type I monitor) has been performed since the 1960s. The initial uses of PSG were to assess sleep physiology in normal individuals and those with various neurologic or sleep disorders such as seizures, insomnia, narcolepsy, periodic limb movement, and the parasomnias, as well as to examine the effect of hypnotics and other drugs on sleep. The pulmonary components of the PSG were added later as OSA was becoming increasingly appreciated in the 1970s.

PSG, which is usually performed as an overnight study, typically assesses physiological parameters by recording sleep–wake stage, heart rhythm, skeletal muscle activities, respiratory patterns, sound of snoring, and oxygen saturation. Each of the above respective components is monitored by electroencephalogram (EEG), electrooculogram (EOG) or eye movement, heart rate and rhythm (ECG), electromyogram (EMG) of skeletal muscle activity (usually at the chin and tibialis anterior), respiratory effort, snoring (microphone), respiratory airflow, thermistor, and pulse oximetry. Nasal pressure technology is also commonly used to detect subtle respiratory events since it has been shown to be more sensitive than standard thermistor. However, the specificity of nasal pressure has been less well studied, i.e., the consequences of these subtle events (which are not observed in the thermistor) are unclear. Occasionally, sleep studies are done at different times of the day, depending on the suspected symptoms of the subjects (circadian rhythm disorder, etc.).

The definition of OSA currently involves the measured AHI, the average number of apnea and hypopnea episodes over an hour. RDI has also been used as an alternative scale for those measures. We can think of AHI as a subset of RDI, as the definition of RDI is less strict than AHI. During a full overnight PSG, an apnea is defined by AASM as cessation (more than 90% reduction) of air movement lasting 10 or more seconds. As stated previously, the distinction between RDI and AHI is related to "respiratory effort-related arousals" (RERA), which are subtle hypopneas. These RERAs are included in RDI but not in AHI. Apnea can be distinguished from hypopnea via a thermistor in PSGs, although the consequences of hypopneas vs. apneas are generally felt to be similar. While the definition of apnea has been less debated, the definition of hypopnea is far from settled. The ideal hypopnea definition is unknown. There are historically at least three different criteria to score hypopneas: the AASM recommended criteria, and AASM alternative criteria and the "Chicago Criteria" (see Table 6.6).

The "Chicago Criteria" was the 1999 version of the AASM recommended criteria for hypopnea. These criteria were designed mainly for clinical research rather than clinical practice. Nasal pressure was early in development at the time of Chicago criteria and was suggested but not strongly recommended. The lack of hypopnea criteria for clinical practice was further addressed by AASM in 2001. Via the Clinical Practices Review Committee, AASM defined hypopnea as having at least 30% reduction of airflow lasting at least 10 s, and with 4% reduction in

Table 6.6 Commonly used PSG criteria for scoring hypopnea

Criteria names	Definitions of hypopnea (at least one of the followings)
"Chicago criteria"	Reduction of airflow ≥50%
	Discernable decrement in airflow with either EEG arousal of oxyhemoglobin desaturation ≥3%.
AASM recommended or "Medicare criteria"	Reduction of nasal pressure ≥30%
	Oxyhemoglobin desaturation ≥4%
AASM alternative	Reduction of nasal pressure ≥50% and oxyhemoglobin desaturation ≥3%
	Reduction of nasal pressure signal ≥50% and EEG evidence of arousal

oxyhemoglobin saturation. Since then, the 2001 AASM definition has been adopted by Center for Medicare and Medicaid Services (CMS) as its criteria for AHI scoring. However, the 2007 Manual for Scoring of Sleep and Associated Events published by AASM introduced only two definitions: "recommended" and "alternative". The AASM Recommended Criteria is the same as the desaturation-based Medicare criteria, i.e., with no importance placed on arousal from sleep:

Reduction of Nasal Pressure Signal ≥30% and Oxygen Desaturation ≥4%

The alternative criteria by AASM defines hypopnea as one of the following two features:

1. Reduction of nasal pressure signal ≥50% and oxygen desaturation ≥3%
2. Reduction of nasal pressure signal ≥50% and associated arousal

A common obstacle in communications between sleep specialists and primary care physicians (PCPs) is that sleep reports often do not specify which criteria the sleep lab has adopted as a standard for scoring OSA. The same obstacle is magnified further in the case of diagnostic interpretation of OSA using PMs. Therefore, any sleep report should include not only the calculated AHI or RDI, but also an explanation of the criteria used for scoring.

The severity of sleep apnea is typically assessed by AHI, but AHI correlates only loosely with EDS and other outcomes. Different parameters measured by a sleep study are predictive of various outcomes of OSA. For example, the degree of oxyhemoglobin desaturation threshold may vary depending on the clinical or research outcome of interests (i.e., hypertension vs. insulin resistance vs. memory consolidation). Additional markers have been suggested as risk factors for disease severity; for example, the degree of nocturnal hypoxemia and the frequency of arousal from sleep. Therefore, when discussing sleep study findings, it is imperative for clinicians to integrate patient's initial chief compliant, unique history, risk factor, and lifestyle into the assessment. In addition, further data are required regarding which disease indices have the best predictive value for various outcome measures.

The limitations of in-lab PSG include the "first-night" effect where sleep is less than usual due to being in a foreign environment, night-to-night variability of the findings, effects of sleep position (which may be different in home, with a bed partner), and the effects of certain medications (i.e., selective serotonin receptor inhibitors, benzodiazepines, hypnotics/alcohol, and stimulants). In-house PSG is quite labor-intensive, requiring oversight by a skilled sleep technician. However, in-lab PSG remains the gold standard for diagnosis of OSA given the reliability and quantity of the data provided.

Split Night Study (Diagnosis Combined with Titration)

Frequently a "split-night" study can be done during a full in-laboratory PSG. In a "split-night" study, an initial impression of the severity of OSA undergoes a "real-time" assessment by a supervising technician. If the patient qualifies for moderate or severe OSA during the first half of the overnight study, a titration study is initiated in the second half of the night to determine an appropriate positive airway pressure (PAP) for treatment. A split-night study is theoretically less sensitive than a full nocturnal study because the AHI is assessed in half of the usual duration. A recent study, however, showed that the AHI derived from the first 2 or 3 h of a split-night study is of sufficient diagnostic accuracy to rule-in OSA at an AHI threshold of five in patients suspected of having OSA [56]. However, medical history is important in interpretation of the split-night study. For example, patient's underlying unusual circadian rhythm as well as sleep-onset/sleep-maintenance insomnia can alter the diagnostic impression of the study. All things considered, the need to extend the "split-night" study into a second nocturnal study is uncommon. Therefore, a "split-night" study not only brings convenience to the patient by avoiding an extra evening of titration study but also reduces the overall cost for the diagnosis and treatment of OSA. A split-night study has become the "default" study type for individuals suspected of OSA.

Portable Monitoring (PM)

PM, or LCTs, is a simple methodology to diagnose OSA. PM testing gives limited data (discussed in detail below) but perhaps is more comfortable for the subject and thus offers a more natural perspective for the severity of OSA at home. However, without a technician on site, the quality of PM studies is only as good as the technologies available.

Types of PMs (Type II–IV)

The American Academy of Sleep Medicine (AASM) has classified sleep studies into four types, depending on the channels they record and evaluate [57]. Type I PSG serves as a reference standard PSG, and it is usually a nocturnal, technician-attended, full in-laboratory sleep study with 14–16 channel monitoring. Type II–IV sleep studies are all simplified versions of Type I PSG. Type II records essentially the same information as full in-lab PSG, except that technician attendance is not present. SHHS, a large NIH-funded multiyear multicentered cohort study on the cardiovascular and other consequences of sleep-disordered breathing, used Type II portable monitors for diagnosis of OSA at home.

Type III PM has been the focus of an ongoing debate on the effectiveness and utility of PMs in diagnosing OSA. Type III PM includes oximetry, at least two respiratory channels (two airflow channels or one airflow plus one respiratory effort channel) and ECG-monitored heart rate, but it does not include EEG, EMG, and EOG. As a result, signals used to detect sleep stages and arousals from sleep (seen in Type I and II sleep studies) are missing in Type III PM. Therefore, Type III PM cannot calculate a true AHI, RDI, or sleep efficiency as it does not record the denominator, sleep time. Instead, Type III PM can only report a value defined by respiratory events divided by total recording time. However, the value reported by Type III PMs does not necessarily imply sleep was recorded. Given that not all study time is necessarily sleep time, reporting from Type III PM is a less sensitive method than values from Type I or II PSG. Another major problem for Type III PM is that without documenting sleep, an individual could wear the device (or give it to someone else) and stay awake yielding an artifactually low AHI. It is worthwhile to mention that "AHIs" or "RDIs" reported by different Type III PMs also vary with different device manufacturers. Therefore, exact definitions of "AHI" or "RDI" vary across different studies of Type III PMs.

The inability to detect respiratory event-related arousals (RERAs) may lead to underestimation of the RDI and underrecognition of upper airway resistance syndrome (UARS). Positional OSA can also be underdiagnosed by those Type III PMs that do not include body position. Naturally, a "split-night" study is not applicable for individuals who undergo Type III PM. A separate overnight in lab titration study will likely be necessary for CPAP set up should the individual be diagnosed of OSA by a Type III PM device.

Pulse oximetry and airflow are the physiological variables that are most commonly measured in Type IV PM. As a result, the frequency of apneas or hypopneas (AHI) as well as the baseline, mean, frequency, duration, and degree of oxyhemoglobin desaturation can be estimated. Naturally, Type IV PMs share at least the same shortcomings of Type III PM, and the current CMS requires a minimum of three channels to meet the reimbursement criteria. However, we emphasize the sensitivity and specificity of the various diagnostic techniques rather than the number of channels per se.

When Should PM Be Considered for Diagnosis of OSA?

While PM has an obvious advantage over PSG in its ease of use, the safety, reliability, and diagnostic accuracy of PMs have been controversial. Bodily injuries from loose wires, faulty oximeter, and monitor disconnection by PMs have been reported. Data loss in Type III and IV PMs has been estimated to be between 2 and 18%. Additionally, interrater and intrarater reliability as well as night-to-night variability of PM is greater than those of PSG. Currently, the scoring of apnea and hypopnea events can be done either manually by a technologist or sleep physician, automatically by the software of the PMs, or combined (manual correction on the automated scoring is allowed). However, subtle points such as positional severity of OSA are more difficult to characterize unattended PM than PSG. The lack of standardization of testing and scoring protocols for PM is of greater concern as there are greater differences in signals recorded by different PM devices. In a comprehensive literature review done by AASM, false-negative results in unattended PM studies could be as high as 15–17%. Likewise, false-positive results in unattended home PM studies could be as high as 30%.

The American Academy of Sleep Medicine published its first guidelines for usage of PM in the diagnosis and management of patients with OSA in 2007. The guidelines stated the following principles for clinicians who consider PM as an alternative to PSG. PM usage should only be considered as part of an integrative patient evaluation for OSA, under the direction of a sleep specialist board certified in sleep medicine.

The one-size-fits-all approach to screen for OSA in the general asymptomatic population is not only medically and ethically unsound but also expensive and inaccurate in terms of healthcare cost and clinical outcome. Whether an individual should undergo PM vs. PSG depends on the individual's OSA risk factors, physical exam, medical comorbidities, suspicion of non-OSA sleep disorders, suspicion of any secondary gain/loss from the test result, and an overall pretest probability for OSA. PM should only be used for screening in subpopulations in which there is substantial published knowledge on specificity and sensitivity of the test. PM can be considered an alternative to PSG for patients with high pretest probability for moderate to severe OSA. Furthermore, PM is not appropriate for diagnosis of OSA in patients with major comorbid medical conditions that would lower the accuracy of PM (i.e., severe pulmonary disease, neuromuscular disease, CHF, CSA). PM should not be used for the diagnostic evaluation of OSA in patients suspected of having other sleep disorders such as CSA, periodic limb movement disorder (PLMD), insomnia, parasomnias, circadian rhythm disorders, or narcolepsy. The utility and efficacy of Type III PM have not been adequately studied for use in the occupational setting in diagnosing at risk operators of motor vehicle operators, who, unlikely the general population, often avoid an OSA diagnosis. Figure 6.1 illustrates the decision-making diagram clinicians can use to decide if PSG or PM should be used to diagnose OSA in a patient.

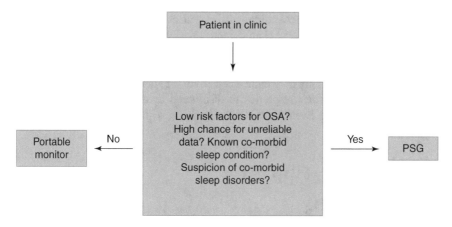

Fig. 6.1 Portable monitor vs. in-lab PSG decision-making diagram

The United States CMS in 2008 approved reimbursement for the uses of PMs, after Agency for Health Quality Research (AHQR) published a mostly positive review of the PMs, particularly pertaining to its comparable clinical utility to predict clinical outcomes (i.e., CPAP compliance rate) in a population with high pretest probability.

Recent advances in wearable technologies may lead to a change in diagnostic approach for sleep-disordered breathing. Although currently the data fall short of recommending these devices as diagnostic tools, the data and technology are rapidly evolving. Currently, some devices can provide a reasonable estimate of sleep architecture and sleep duration. However, estimation of the Apnea–Hypopnea Index and other metrics of sleep-disordered breathing will require further study.

Current Roles of Autotitrating Positive Airway Pressure (APAP)

Autotitrating positive airway pressure (APAP) devices have been increasingly used for titrating pressure and treating adult patients with OSA in the last decade. The devices can be used in place of in-lab continuous positive airway pressure (CPAP) titration study when attended CPAP titration is not possible or patient comfort is a great concern. They work by changing the treatment pressure based on patients' airflow, pressure fluctuations, or airway resistance.

As PMs are increasingly used as an initial diagnostic tool in populations with high likelihood of moderate to severe OSA, APAP has been identified as a partner strategy in the treatment phase to replace the more costly CPAP titration with in-lab PSG. We note here that the 2008 AASM Guidelines for APAP stated that APAP devices can only be used for unattended treatment of patients with moderate and severe OSA without significant comorbidities such as CHF, COPD, and CSA. Since then, a large VA study by Berry et al. demonstrated that diagnoses by PM followed by APAP titration resulted in comparable CPAP adherence and clinical outcomes to using traditional in-lab PSG. However, as APAP technology is fast evolving, different APAP devices differ not only in their sensitivities to detect severity of disordered breathing but also in their responses to disordered breathing. Therefore, overall assessment of cost-effectiveness of APAP combining with PMs is complicated.

Cost-effectiveness of PSG vs. PM

Although the cost of PM devices has seen a substantial drop in recent years, the total healthcare cost of evaluating and treating individuals with OSA using PM compared to PSG has not been studied adequately and is largely controversial. Though gross cost savings were frequently reported, the high false-negative rate of PMs along with the current guideline that all negative tests of PMs should be referred to a full in-lab PSG by a sleep specialist translates into high cost if the currently available PMs were to become the mainstream of screening tools. Furthermore, few cost analyses compared usage of PMs to increasingly popular use of split-night study protocols, in which both diagnostic PSG and titration studies are done in a single night. Further studies using a decision model are much needed to provide a theoretical framework as well as evidence to ascertain the pretest disease probability above which portable studies would be economically attractive as an initial test in the assessment of suspected OSA.

Utilities of Multiple Sleep Latency Test (MSLT) in OSA

MSLT is one of a few currently available de facto standard tests to measure physiological sleep tendency in the absence of external alerting factors. The test is based on the premise that the degree of sleepiness is correlated with and therefore reflected by sleep latency (the amount of time it takes for the individual to fall asleep). MSLT is usually ordered to diagnosis narcolepsy or other conditions of hypersomnia. The individuals with these conditions typically have reduced sleep-onset latency and early onset of REM sleep. However, MSLT is occasionally indicated to quantify objectively sleepiness, e.g., residual daytime sleepiness despite presumed adequate CPAP treatment of OSA. For example, professional drivers or pilots with OSA may at times be subjected to medicolegal actions in order to objectify whether their residual sleepiness is significant enough to keep them off the roads. The test is usually done immediately following an overnight in-lab PSG in order to control for the patient's sleep characteristics. The test asks the patient to have four or five naps (2 h between each) in a naturally dim-light environment during the day. The sleep onset latency is recorded for each nap. If the patient does not fall asleep within 20 min of each nap, the sleep onset latency is assumed to be 20 min. The average of the sleep onset latency is used as objective measure of sleepiness. With high test–retest reliability and inter-rater/intra-rater reliabilities, MSLT has demonstrated its ability to differentiate normal healthy subjects from those with pathologic sleepiness on both driving simulators as well as long-term road accidents. However, MSLT is not a reliable predictor of traffic accidents, emphasizing the need for more research in this area.

Future Outlook

One of the ongoing research goals in OSA is to identify a relatively easily assayed biomarker. For example, recent studies have shown that amylase in saliva (i.e., salivary amylase activity as well as amylase mRNA levels) are elevated in individuals with EDS and OSA. Among individuals with OSA, who are assumed to have higher sleep drive, systemic inflammation may be involved in the pathogenesis of OSA. Studies using microarrays looking at gene expression have shown that overnight expression of oxidative stress response genes such as antioxidant enzyme superoxidase dismutase 2 (SOD2) and catalase are up-regulated. Proteomic analyses of serum and urine may yield future techniques for identifying individuals with OSA. Even though there is a lack of data in the adult population, recent findings suggest that proteins such as gamma-carboxyglutamic acid, perlecan, and gelsolin are differentially expressed among children with OSA and the control. Specific subpopulations of leukocytes such as TNF-alpha, IL-6, and some T lymphocytes have been found to be elevated among patients with OSA. Brief paroxysmal bursts of alpha activity have been identified before serious driving errors in simulation studies. Similarly, a significant increase of eye blinks, in both number and duration, have been described before driving errors. Furthermore, an alteration of eyes blinking duration has been observed with increased driving time. With identification of more reliable biomarkers, the tasks of diagnosing OSA and sleepiness individuals will become less challenging.

   Given the recent appreciation that OSA is heterogeneous, there have been ongoing efforts to define underlying mechanisms (endotypes) of disease as well as variable clinical manifestations of disease (phenotypes). Recognition of the OSA endotypes may be important since mechanisms can inform therapeutic interventions or help predict response to various therapies. In addition, studies and clinical experience have shown phenotypic variability with some patients have sleepiness (with associated cardiovascular risk) whereas other OSA patients develop fragmented sleep (with insomnia) and other patients remain asymptomatic. Thus, future efforts with diagnostic testing will likely focus on assessing disease severity, but also prognosis and clinical guidance regarding response/need for various interventions.

Summary Outline

- In clinic pretest screening questions (symptoms of snoring, daytime sleepiness, and common comorbidities) for OSA are important to efficaciously diagnose OSA. In some special clinical scenarios (i.e., occupational clinic), screening for OSA should rely more on objective anthropometric measurements.
- OSA risk factors include obesity, older age, male gender, postmenopausal status, Asian/African American races, tobacco, and alcohol use.
- The diagnostic criteria of sleep apnea are not uniform, but most of them try to characterize the frequency of sleep-disordered breathing events along with the degree of oxygen desaturation of each event.
- Three most commonly used diagnostic criteria for OSA are the AASM "Recommended" Criteria (or the "Medicare" Criteria), AASM "Alternative" Criteria, and "the Chicago" Criteria.
- There are four types of sleep studies available. Both in-lab PSG, or Type I, and portable monitors (PM), or Type II–IV, are being used for diagnosis of OSA. PSG is the gold standard test for diagnosis of OSA. PM offer a less-expensive and in-home alternative, with limitations in both sensitivity and specificity.
- A "split-night" study not only brings convenience to the patient by avoiding an extra evening of titration study but also reduces the overall cost for the diagnosis and treatment of OSA. A split-night study has become the "default" study type for individuals suspected of OSA.
- Whether an individual should undergo PM vs. PSG depends on the individual's OSA risk factors, physical exam, medical comorbidities, suspicion of non-OSA sleep disorders, suspicion of any secondary gain/loss from the test result, and an overall pretest probability for OSA.

References

1. Gottlieb DJ, Punjabi NM. Diagnosis and management of obstructive sleep apnea: a review. JAMA. 2020;323(14):1389–400.
2. Benjafield AV, Ayas NT, Eastwood PR, et al. Estimation of the global prevalence and burden of obstructive sleep apnoea: a literature-based analysis. Lancet Respir Med. 2019;7(8):687–98.
3. AASM. Sleep-related breathing disorders in adults: recommendations for syndrome definition and measurement techniques in adults. Sleep. 1999;22(5):667–89.
4. AASM. International classification of sleep disorders, Diagnostic and coding manual. 2nd ed. Westchester: American Academy of Sleep Medicine; 2005.
5. Eckert DJ, Jordan AS, Merchia P, Malhotra A. Central sleep apnea: pathophysiology and treatment. Chest. 2007;131(2):595–607.
6. Morrell M, Arabi Y, Zahn B, Badr M. Progressive retropalatal narrowing preceding obstructive apnea. Am J Respir Crit Care Med. 1998;158:1974–81.
7. Badr MS, Dingell JD, Javaheri S. Central sleep apnea: a brief review. Curr Pulmonol Rep. 2019;8(1):14–21.
8. Javaheri S, Malik A, Smith J, Chung E. Adaptive pressure support servoventilation: a novel treatment for sleep apnea associated with use of opioids. J Clin Sleep Med. 2008;4(4):305–10.

9. Javaheri S, McKane SW, Cameron N, Germany RE, Malhotra A. In patients with heart failure the burden of central sleep apnea increases in the late sleep hours. Sleep. 2019;42(1):zsy195.
10. Javaheri S, Somers VK. Cardiovascular diseases and sleep apnea. Handb Clin Neurol. 2011;98:327–45.
11. Punjabi N, Sorkin J, Katzel L, Goldberg A, Schwartz A, Smith P. Sleep-disordered breathing and insulin resistance in middle-aged and overweight men. Am J Respir and Crit Care Med. 2002;165:677–82.
12. Punjabi NM, Ahmed MM, Polotsky VY, Beamer BA, O'Donnell CP. Sleep-disordered breathing, glucose intolerance, and insulin resistance. Respir Physiol Neurobiol. 2003;136(2–3):167–78.
13. Punjabi NM, Beamer BA. Alterations in glucose disposal in sleep-disordered breathing. Am J Respir Crit Care Med. 2009;179(3):235–40.
14. Punjabi NM, Caffo BS, Goodwin JL, et al. Sleep-disordered breathing and mortality: a prospective cohort study. PLoS Med. 2009;6(8):e1000132.
15. Punjabi NM, Newman AB, Young TB, Resnick HE, Sanders MH. Sleep-disordered breathing and cardiovascular disease: an outcome-based definition of hypopneas. Am J Respir Crit Care Med. 2008;177(10):1150–5.
16. Redline S, Yenokyan G, Gottlieb DJ, et al. Obstructive sleep apnea-hypopnea and incident stroke: the sleep heart health study. Am J Respir Crit Care Med. 2010;182(2):269–77.
17. Gottlieb DJ, Yenokyan G, Newman AB, et al. Prospective study of obstructive sleep apnea and incident coronary heart disease and heart failure: the sleep heart health study. Circulation. 2010;122(4):352–60.
18. Gottlieb JD, Schwartz AR, Marshall J, et al. Hypoxia, not the frequency of sleep apnea, induces acute hemodynamic stress in patients with chronic heart failure. J Am Coll Cardiol. 2009;54(18):1706–12.
19. Yaggi HK, Concato J, Kernan WN, Lichtman JH, Brass LM, Mohsenin V. Obstructive sleep apnea as a risk factor for stroke and death. N Engl J Med. 2005;353(19):2034–41.
20. Arzt M, Young T, Finn L, Skatrud JB, Bradley TD. Association of sleep-disordered breathing and the occurrence of stroke. Am J Respir Crit Care Med. 2005;172(11):1447–51.
21. Arzt M, Young T, Peppard PE, et al. Dissociation of obstructive sleep apnea from hypersomnolence and obesity in patients with stroke. Stroke. 2010;41(3):e129–34.
22. Leung RS, Bradley TD. Sleep apnea and cardiovascular disease. Am J Respir Crit Care Med. 2001;164(12):2147–65.
23. Raphelson JR, Kreitinger KY, Malhotra A. Positive airway pressure therapy in sleep-disordered breathing. Neurotherapeutics. 2021;18(1):75–80.
24. Young T, Palta M, Dempsey J, Skatrud J, Weber S, Badr S. The occurrence of sleep-disordered breathing among middle-aged adults. New Engl J Med. 1993;32:1230–5.
25. Young T, Peppard PE, Gottlieb DJ. Epidemiology of obstructive sleep apnea: a population health perspective. Am J Respir Crit Care Med. 2002;165(9):1217–39.
26. Teran-Santos J, Jimenez-Gomez A, Cordero-Guevara J. The association between sleep apnea and the risk of traffic accidents. Cooperative Group Burgos-Santander. N Engl J Med. 1999;340(11):847–51.
27. Kreitinger KY, Lui MMS, Owens RL, et al. Screening for obstructive sleep apnea in a diverse bariatric surgery population. Obesity (Silver Spring). 2020;28(11):2028–34.
28. Young T, Peppard P, Gottlieb D. The epidemiology of obstructive sleep apnea: a population health perspective. Am J Respir Crit Care Med. 2002;165:1217–39.
29. Heinzer R, Vat S, Marques-Vidal P, et al. Prevalence of sleep-disordered breathing in the general population: the HypnoLaus study. Lancet Respir Med. 2015;3(4):310–8.
30. Edwards BA, O'Driscoll DM, Ali A, Jordan AS, Trinder J, Malhotra A. Aging and sleep: physiology and pathophysiology. Semin Respir Crit Care Med. 2010;31(5):618–33.
31. Edwards BA, Wellman A, Sands SA, et al. Obstructive sleep apnea in older adults is a distinctly different physiological phenotype. Sleep. 2014;37(7):1227–36.
32. Malhotra A, Huang Y, Fogel R, et al. Aging influences on pharyngeal anatomy and physiology: the predisposition to pharyngeal collapse. Am J Med. 2006;119(1):72 e79–14.

33. Young T, Finn L, Austin D, Peterson A. Menopausal status and sleep-disordered breathing in the Wisconsin Sleep Cohort Study. Am J Respir Crit Care Med. 2003;167:1181–5.
34. Peppard PE, Young T, Palta M, Dempsey J, Skatrud J. Longitudinal study of moderate weight change and sleep-disordered breathing. JAMA. 2000;284(23):3015–21.
35. Foster GD, Borradaile KE, Sanders MH, et al. A randomized study on the effect of weight loss on obstructive sleep apnea among obese patients with type 2 diabetes: the sleep AHEAD study. Arch Intern Med. 2009;169(17):1619–26.
36. Foster GD, Sanders MH, Millman R, et al. Obstructive sleep apnea among obese patients with type 2 diabetes. Diabetes Care. 2009;32(6):1017–9.
37. Malhotra A, Huang Y, Fogel R, et al. The male predisposition to pharyngeal collapse: the importance of airway length. Am J Resp Crit Care Med. 2002;166:1388–95.
38. Malhotra A, Mesarwi O, Pepin JL, Owens RL. Endotypes and phenotypes in obstructive sleep apnea. Curr Opin Pulm Med. 2020;26(6):609–14.
39. Badr MS. Pathophysiology of upper airway obstruction during sleep. Clin Chest Med. 1998;19(1):21–32.
40. Badr MS. Pathogenesis of obstructive sleep apnea. Prog Cardiovasc Dis. 1999;41(5):323–30.
41. Rowley JA, Sanders CS, Zahn BR, Badr MS. Gender differences in upper airway compliance during NREM sleep: role of neck circumference. J Appl Physiol. 2002;92(6):2535–41.
42. Rowley JA, Zhou X, Vergine I, Shkoukani MA, Badr MS. Influence of gender on upper airway mechanics: upper airway resistance and Pcrit. J Appl Physiol. 2001;91(5):2248–54.
43. Lee YH, Johan A, Wong KK, Edwards N, Sullivan C. Prevalence and risk factors for obstructive sleep apnea in a multiethnic population of patients presenting for bariatric surgery in Singapore. Sleep Med. 2009;10(2):226–32.
44. Johns MW. A new method for measuring daytime sleepiness: the Epworth sleepiness scale. Sleep. 1991;14(6):540–5.
45. Patel SR, White DP, Malhotra A, Stanchina ML, Ayas NT. Continuous positive airway pressure therapy for treating sleepiness in a diverse population with obstructive sleep apnea: results of a meta-analysis. Arch Intern Med. 2003;163(5):565–71.
46. Jenkinson C, Davies RJ, Mullins R, Stradling JR. Comparison of therapeutic and subtherapeutic nasal continuous positive airway pressure for obstructive sleep apnoea: a randomised prospective parallel trial. Lancet. 1999;353(9170):2100–5.
47. Pack AI. Obstructive sleep apnea. Adv Intern Med. 1994;39:517–67.
48. Pack AI. Further development of P4 approach to obstructive sleep apnea. Sleep Med Clin. 2019;14(3):379–89.
49. Dagan Y, Doljansky JT, Green A, Weiner A. Body Mass Index (BMI) as a first-line screening criterion for detection of excessive daytime sleepiness among professional drivers. Traffic Inj Prev. 2006;7(1):44–8.
50. Hartenbaum N, Collop N, Rosen IM, et al. Sleep apnea and commercial motor vehicle operators: statement from the joint task force of the American College of Chest Physicians, the American College of Occupational and Environmental Medicine, and the National Sleep Foundation. Chest. 2006;130(3):902–5.

Chapter 7
A Brief Review of Treatment of Obstructive Sleep Apnea

Scott Hoff and Nancy Collop

Keywords Continuous positive airway pressure (CPAP) · Apnea hypopnea index (AHI) · critical closing pressure (Pcrit)

Obstructive sleep apnea (OSA) is a sleep-related breathing disorder characterized by repeated partial or complete collapse of segments of the upper airway compromising airflow to varying degrees. These recurrent episodes can be associated with transient activation of the sympathetic nervous system, intermittent hypoxemia, and a higher risk for adverse cardiovascular outcomes. Of a limited number of treatment options for OSA, continuous positive airway pressure (CPAP) remains the first choice in most circumstances. Rationale for use of CPAP is strong, however adherence to therapy remains suboptimal in many patients.

As with studies involving other biological conduits, pharyngeal collapsibility has been studied using a model of flow through a collapsible tube. Differences in pharyngeal collapsibility between normal subjects, snorers, and subjects with obstructive sleep apnea have been quantified using such a model [11]. The model depicts the upper airway as a tube with rigid segments at either end and a collapsible segment housed within a fixed pressure box in between [11]. When the pressure within the collapsible segment exceeds that surrounding it within the box, the collapsible segment will remain open; however, if the pressure within the collapsible segment falls below that surrounding it within the box, the segment will collapse. The *critical closing pressure* (Pcrit) is the pressure within the collapsible segment equaling the pressure surrounding it within the box at which collapse of the segment occurs halting the flow through it.

S. Hoff · N. Collop (✉)
Emory Sleep Center, Emory University School of Medicine, Atlanta, GA, USA
e-mail: nancy.collop@emory.edu

© Springer Nature Switzerland AG 2022
M. S. Badr, J. L. Martin (eds.), *Essentials of Sleep Medicine*,
Respiratory Medicine, https://doi.org/10.1007/978-3-030-93739-3_7

Flow through the collapsible segment is therefore dependent upon the differences between the pressure upstream (Pus) from the collapsible segment, Pcrit, and that downstream from the collapsible segment. When the upstream pressure is less than Pcrit, no flow occurs through the collapsible segment. If the upstream pressure exceeds Pcrit and the pressure in the rigid segment downstream from the collapsible segment does not, then there will be fluttering of the collapsible segment. When the upstream pressure exceeds Pcrit, it will drive the collapsible segment open; however, if the downstream segment is at a pressure lower than Pcrit then it will cause closure of the terminal point of the collapsible segment, which will be at Pcrit. The cessation of flow would allow the intraluminal pressure throughout the collapsible segment to equilibrate with that of the upstream segment again opening the collapsed part of the tube and restoring flow. When both the upstream and the downstream segments have a pressure exceeding Pcrit, then flow will continue unimpeded throughout the tube. Aspects of the upper airway behave in a manner described by the model.

Aberrations of airflow that comprise OSA result from the pressure-flow relationships described by the collapsible tube model. The upstream pressure in the human airway is usually represented by nasal pressure (Pn), which is generally around atmospheric pressure. Pcrit has been demonstrated to be based in the pharyngeal airway as a result of nasopharyngeal intubation studies, not the laryngeal airway as was originally speculated [30]. In the first instance described above, in which Pn is less than Pcrit, an obstructive apnea results. In the second instance, when Pn > Pcrit, but the downstream pressure is not, then hypopneas, flow limitation, and snoring occur. In this situation, the maximum flow through the system will be limited by the collapsible segment dynamics, and will be a function of the driving pressure (Pus – Pcrit) relative to the resistance of the upstream segment. The resistance of the upstream segment can be determined by measuring the flow through the system while different pressures are applied, and then taking the reciprocal of the slope of the plotted measures. The third instance reflects the normal functioning upper airway in which normal airflow is maintained throughout inspiration.

There are two main factors which contribute to collapsibility of the upper airway transmural pressure and pharyngeal compliance. The transmural pressure is the difference in forces acting across the wall of the collapsible segment of the upper airway. Forces tending to promote airway collapse include the intraluminal negative pressure generated by the respiratory apparatus during inspiration, and the pressure exerted by tissues, such as fat, extrinsic to the airway. Those forces are opposed by the pharyngeal dilator muscles, which act to expand the upper airway diameter. Pharyngeal compliance has an important influence on transmural pressure. Compliance is a function, in large part, of the intrinsic muscle activity of the upper airway, but may also be contributed to by blood volume perfusing the upper airway with greater perfusion associated with lower compliance.

Studies have demonstrated levels of Pcrit at which sleep-disordered breathing events may be predicted. When the Pcrit exceeds atmospheric pressure, then the patient will be prone to repeated obstructive apneas, and when the Pcrit remains negative relative to atmospheric pressure, then the upper airway remains patent. A

Pcrit in the middle results in hypopneas, flow limitation, and snoring. Pcrit therefore represents the susceptibility of the upper airway to collapse, and is different from one person to another.

The effects of sleep stages on Pcrit remain uncertain. Some data demonstrate a significant influence on upper airway closing pressure with a higher pressure, implying a more collapsible airway, noted during stage N1, N2, and REM sleep than during deep sleep [14]. Other data do not demonstrate a statistically significant association between sleep stage and collapsibility [26]. Ultimately, the activity of the genioglossus and other pharyngeal dilators must balance the negative intraluminal pressure generated by the muscles of inspiration for airway patency to be preserved [4].

During the time studies were intensely investigating the upper airway dynamics (the late 1970s and early 1980s), few options existed for the treatment of OSA aside from weight loss and tracheostomy. Armed with new knowledge regarding pharyngeal airway collapsibility, Sullivan et al. sought to demonstrate that CPAP applied through the nares would act as a "pneumatic splint" for the upper airway preventing occlusion [36]. Subsequently, in order to evaluate whether CPAP activates upper airway muscular reflexes, or acts passively via increasing intraluminal pressure, EMG recordings were made during sleep while CPAP was applied in patients with OSA. Use of 10–13 cm of water pressure resulted in elimination of apneas, improvement in oxygen saturation, and reduction or elimination of EMG activity, and when CPAP was abruptly lowered, EMG activity did not immediately return. The investigators concluded that CPAP was indeed a pneumatic splint acting passively to open the airway [34]. This was followed by another study in which application of positive airway pressure between 10 and 12 cm of water resulted in a significant increase in pharyngeal airway size demonstrated by computed tomography in awake, obese patients with OSA, and in patients without OSA; however, the change in airway size was smaller in patients with OSA. Concomitant EMG recordings of the genioglossus and alae nasi muscles with and without positive airway pressure demonstrated a decrease, or no change in activity associated with pressure [16].

It would appear that CPAP alleviates sleep-disordered breathing events through its effects on transmural pressure. Application of positive airway pressure raises intraluminal pressure counteracting the collapsing effects of external tissue pressure thereby favorably affecting transmural pressure, overcoming Pcrit. Also, even small enhancements of end-expiratory lung volume exert a caudal force on the trachea likely stiffening the upper airway to some degree favorably affecting pharyngeal compliance. In terms of the model of flow through a collapsible tube, as CPAP is gradually increased, Pus increases until reaching a level that exceeds Pcrit at which point apneas resolve. Further increases in pressure will gradually increase intraluminal pressure across the entire collapsible segment until the applied positive airway pressure is communicated to the downstream pressure at which point hypopneas, flow limitation, and snoring should be abolished.

Positive airway pressure therapy can be delivered in two major modalities, continuous and bilevel. Continuous positive airway pressure, CPAP, is a continuous stream of airflow unchanging throughout the respiratory cycle. Bilevel positive airway pressure (BPAP), consists of two independent airflows: inspiratory positive airway pressure (IPAP) and expiratory positive airway pressure (EPAP). Obviously, these distinct flows are state-dependent on the respiratory cycle. The difference between the IPAP and the EPAP describes the pressure support (PS), which can augment the inspired tidal volume improving ventilation.

Therapy with CPAP can be initiated by two methods, titration in the sleep lab, or using autotitrating devices in an out-of-center setting. Manual titration of CPAP in the sleep lab typically involves a night's stay in the sleep lab during which CPAP is initiated at a low level, typically 4 or 5 cm of water to overcome the resistance of the tubing, while the patient is monitored using polysomnography. As airflow events (apneas, hypopneas, respiratory effort-related arousals (RERAs), and snoring) occur, the pressure is increased in 1–2 cm of water increments and the patient is observed for recurrent airflow events for a minimum of 5 minutes of sleep time. Apneas will resolve first as the pressure reaches the minimum level necessary to stent the airway opened. Then, hypopneas, RERAs, and snoring will resolve as the luminal pressure increases with increasing delivered CPAP level. Optimal pressure will be recognized when snoring resolves and sleep remains continuous with minimal fragmentation. It should be noted that REM sleep, which is a sleep stage commonly associated with worsened OSA, and sleep in the supine position, a sleep position commonly associated with worsened OSA, ideally occur especially together in order to truly determine an optimal pressure. At times, additional titration steps are made as exploratory measures after airflow events have apparently resolved to determine whether sleep becomes better consolidated with fewer arousals and better architecture.

In instances in which manual titration of BPAP becomes necessary, the EPAP is typically started at the CPAP level when obstructive apneas resolved and the IPAP is initiated at 4 cm of water above the EPAP. Again, this EPAP will be the minimum pressure required to maintain the patency of the upper airway. The EPAP is left at this level as long as no obstructive apneas recur at which point both EPAP and IPAP are raised equally. Other persistent obstructive events are managed by further upward titration of the IPAP until hypopneas, RERAs, and snoring have resolved. The act of increasing the IPAP relative to the EPAP will increase pressure support. Titrations in which pressure support becomes necessary to manage hypercapnia can be performed with transcutaneous carbon dioxide monitoring, which may provide evidence of improvement in carbon dioxide levels with titration of PS.

Devices with autotitrating, or self-adjusting, algorithms are now the norm for treating most uncomplicated cases of OSA. These devices employ mechanisms through which airway patency assessments are made, and then adjustments to airflow are enacted using programmed responses. There are both autotitrating CPAP and BPAP devices on the market. The clinician programs a minimum pressure level and a maximum pressure level (either CPAP, or EPAP and IPAP), and the machine operates between these boundaries making adjustments to airflow throughout the night attempting to minimize generated upper airway pressure while maintaining airway patency. This could prove useful when lab titration studies fail to provide optimal pressure settings, or when specific situations occur that may lead to higher pressures during the situation resulting in possible over titration of pressure for the remainder of the sleep period. Examples of such situations may include a significant disparity in severity of OSA during REM sleep, or in the supine position. A 90th or 95th percentile pressure is reported by the device, depending on the manufacturer, which can then be used to prescribe a fixed pressure for therapy. Alternatively, the patient can be maintained on the autotitrating mode as a long-term therapy. Research has not demonstrated improved adherence to therapy or greater therapeutic efficacy on fixed pressure versus autotitrating modes. As there is a competitive marketplace for these therapeutic devices, machines can have different sensing mechanisms and different response characteristics both of which can result in different therapeutic efficacies for individual patients. Although an AHI is reported by the devices, the patient's reported symptoms, if any, should be carefully monitored as a measure of efficacy.

There may be factors that steer therapy to one modality of PAP therapy versus another. In most instances, CPAP suffices for treatment of OSA; however, some patients intolerant of CPAP may find BPAP to be a more comfortable experience and will acclimate better to BPAP. In cases involving hypoventilation, such as hypercapnic COPD, use of BPAP with the ability to titrate PS by increasing IPAP relative to EPAP can be highly advantageous. In patients with obesity hypoventilation syndrome (OHS), use of BPAP results in improvements in $PaCO_2$; however, use of CPAP may also result in $PaCO_2$ improvement, but only after adjustment for adherence with therapy. Use of both CPAP and BPAP can improve nocturnal oxygenation and sleep quality in OHS patients [21]. A separate analysis of CPAP and BPAP effects on PCO_2 in patients with OHS without severe CPAP-resistant nocturnal hypoxemia demonstrated no significant treatment effect difference with both positive airway pressure groups demonstrating significant improvements in PCO_2. The BPAP group experienced better improvements in sleep quality and psychomotor vigilance test performance than the CPAP group [28]. In patients with OHS followed up for a median of over 5 years, there was no difference in the change in PCO_2, or in cardiovascular outcomes or sleepiness between groups using CPAP or BPAP [22]. A systematic review comparing CPAP and BPAP treatment effects in patients with OSA found no differences in the improvement in either PCO_2, PO_2, sleepiness, quality of life, or healthcare resource use with either PAP modality after 3 months of treatment. Because BPAP use generally has higher costs involved, the authors recommended CPAP rather than BPAP for the initial treatment of patients with OHS although acknowledged that the evidence was weak [33].

BPAP with a programmed backup respiratory rate can also be trialed in patients who demonstrate emergence of central apneas while on CPAP, also known as complex sleep apnea. Data in patients with complex sleep apnea randomized to either non-invasive positive pressure ventilation (NPPV) or adaptive servoventilation, an advanced form of bilevel positive airway pressure ventilation in which the device's algorithm seeks to learn and maintain an averaged, consistent minute ventilation while eliminating apneas and hypopneas, demonstrated that NPPV with a backup respiratory rate initially improved the AHI measured on CPAP to the same degree as ASV did, after 6 weeks, the AHI in the NPPV group had crept up a little bit while that in the ASV group had slightly decreased further [6].

Positive airway pressure therapy must be delivered into the upper airway through the use of an interface applied to the nose, or nose and mouth. Nasal masks were the original interface and continue to enjoy widespread use. This type of interface generally covers the nares and the bridge of the nose; however, alternatives include a component under the nose bridging the nares with soft material that inflates to seal along the sides of the nose when air circulates through the mask. Nasal pillows consist of two soft prongs that sit on the perimeter of the nares to form a seal and airflow is delivered directly into the nares. Full face masks generally cover the external nose and mouth generating a pressure effect over both. As many people tend to breathe through their mouths while they sleep, nasal-focused interfaces may not maintain therapeutic efficacy as airflow intended to generate upper airway pressure may instead leak out of the mouth. These patients may consider use of a full face mask, or application of a chin strap, which runs from the top of the head to under the jaw in order to resist mouth opening, in conjunction with a nasal interface.

There are small but significant data indicating some benefits of nasal masks over full face, or oronasal masks. Oronasal masks have been demonstrated to have greater time in large leak when compared to nasal masks, and the residual AHI using an oronasal mask, while reduced when compared to baseline, was found to be higher than that achieved with the use of nasal masks. In addition, patients reported more restful sleep, overall higher satisfaction, and less mask noise with the use of a nasal mask compared to an oronasal one. However, despite all of these positive findings associated with nasal masks, there were no differences in adherence assessed after 4 weeks of use of each mask type [32]. Switching to an oronasal mask during the course of outpatient CPAP therapy after optimal titration of pressure in the sleep lab to an AHI less than 5 events/hour was associated with a higher residual AHI when compared to that using a nasal mask. However, again, adherence to CPAP therapy was no different between the groups [7]. Fewer patients may be successfully titrated with CPAP using oronasal masks than with nasal masks, and the pressures needed for a successful titration may be significantly higher with an oronasal mask. Titration using an oronasal mask has been shown to be successful only in nasal breathers [20]. Despite these findings, full face masks have remained in widespread use for CPAP therapy.

There are numerous facets involved in assessing the efficacy of positive airway pressure therapy. First, and foremost, improvement in the patient's symptoms should be considered. Snoring, awakenings associated with gasping, and other sleep-related breathing issues should resolve with application of adequate positive airway pressure. With improvement in arousals associated with respiratory events or flow limitation, the resulting sleep fragmentation should improve resulting in improvement in daytime fatigue, hypersomnolence, concentration lapses, and memory impairment that were attributable to the sleep-disordered breathing. Research has demonstrated improvement in sleepiness associated with use of CPAP in patients with OSA [10, 25]. Neurocognitive benefits have been demonstrated in executive and frontal lobe function domains with the use of CPAP [17]. Driving performance and reaction times have been demonstrated to improve after patients are started on CPAP [23].

Another category of assessment of positive airway pressure efficacy consists of PAP device-derived data. The data storage capabilities of current PAP machines provide useful information regarding machine use, residual airflow events, and system leak. Adherence to therapy can be measured as a percentage of time the device is used over the course of a specified time interval, the average hours of use of PAP therapy per night, or the percentage of nights with PAP use of at least 4 hours. The Centers for Medicare and Medicaid Services (CMS) defines adherence as the use of PAP therapy for at least 4 hours per night for an average of 70% of the audited time frame, typically 30 days. Adherence to therapy is a critical metric in both clinical practice and research studies; however, uncertainty exists regarding what represents the most important benchmark for adherence. Data indicate that longer use of CPAP on a nightly basis is generally associated with improved outcome measures; however, as CPAP use as a percentage of total sleep time increases, untreated sleep time decreases, and this may also be an important factor influencing outcome measures.

Many factors can influence a patient's adherence to PAP therapy. Mask-related issues can have a significant effect on adherence. Leakage from a mask can cause airflow into unintended places, such as the eyes, or can result in sleep-disrupting noise or vibrations. Mask leak can also have a significant impact on the efficacy of a level of pressure as well as on the ability of the PAP device to detect use and residual AHI accurately. As the length of time a particular mask is used increases, oils from the face can lead to a loss of integrity of the components contacting the face resulting in an increased tendency for the mask to leak. Improperly sized masks, or significant weight loss affecting the fit of a mask can be causes of mask leak. Rotating the head when one changes sleeping positions, or use of a soft pillow can result in dislodgment of the mask and significant mask leak. Intolerance of pressure can have a significant negative impact on a patient's adherence to therapy. Overtitration of pressure can cause uncomfortable sensations associated with both inhalation and exhalation, described as smothering, drowning, or increased work of breathing, leading to discontinuation of therapy. Overtitration can also be associated with the development of central apneas which can have a detrimental effect on sleep continuity and sleep quality. Under titration of pressure can similarly cause uncomfortable sensations of breathing akin to air hunger or starvation.

There can be many different types of side effects associated with use of PAP therapies. The most common complaint associated with PAP use is dry mouth. The delivery of continuous airflow across surfaces will have a drying effect. Leak from the system, be it from a poor sealing mask, or from an opened mouth, will result in augmentation of airflow from the device to compensate for the pressure loss further exacerbating the dryness. A poor sealing mask can also direct unintended airflow toward the eyes resulting in dry and irritated eyes. Swallowing of excess air from the upper airway, aerophagia, can cause abdominal cramps and excess eructation or flatulence. Aerophagia may improve with a slight drop in CPAP level.

PAP Alternatives

Oral Appliances

Oral appliances are often considered as the first choice CPAP alternative for management of OSA for patients who are intolerant of CPAP, or for those who prefer an alternative to CPAP, and are also effective as remedies for snoring in patients without OSA. The most widely used type of oral appliance are the mandibular advancement devices. The devices engage the maxillary and mandibular arches causing protrusion of the mandible [29]. Doing so increases the lateral diameter of the pharynx, provides stability to the hyoid bone and soft palate, stretches the tongue muscles, and opposes the tendency for posterior rotation of the mandible [1]. Oral appliances can consist of a single component that maintains the mandible in a fixed position, or they can have two components which allow adjustments to the mandibular position in different spatial planes. The devices can be prefabricated or custom-made. Prefabricated devices, or so-called "boil and bite plates," are widely available over-the-counter and are set up usually by immersing the device in hot water to make it soft followed by gently biting into the material with the jaw in a thrusted position to create an impression of the mandibular and maxillary arches. Custom-made devices are fabricated off of impressions of the patient's teeth made in a qualified dentist's office, and can then be progressively adjusted to maximize efficacy while minimizing side effects.

Oral appliances can be highly efficacious for OSA management. OA reduce the frequency and intensity of snoring, improve sleep quality for both patients who snore and their bed partners, and improve QOL measures [29]. Research has demonstrated no significant difference between the percentages of patients with mild OSA achieving the target AHI using an OA versus using CPAP; however, there was a statistically significantly greater odds for patients with moderate to severe OSA achieving the target AHI using CPAP than those who used an OA [13]. Data evaluating a population with an average AHI of 13.1 events/hour randomized to use of either a custom-made device, or a prefabricated device for a 3-month period. The percentage of patients reaching an AHI less than 5 events/hour was 64% in the custom-made device group versus 24% in the prefabricated device group. The number of patients failing to have at least a 50% drop in AHI also favored the custom device with 4% of the patients in the custom device group having a treatment failure, and 36% in the prefabricated group having one [15]. An earlier trial using a different prefabricated device demonstrated similar findings favoring the custom-made appliance with 60% patients in the custom-made device group achieving an AHI less than 5 events per hour, or at least a 50% reduction in AHI, compared to 31% of patients in the prefabricated device group. Treatment failure, again defined as a residual AHI greater than 50% of the baseline AHI, was not statistically significantly different between the groups (31% for the custom-made device group and 34% for the prefabricated device group); however, 63% of the patients who had treatment failure with the prefabricated device had treatment success with the custom-made device [37].

Positional Therapy

Positional therapy should be an option considered primarily for patients who demonstrate a supine preponderance with respect to their OSA. Positional OSA is often defined as an AHI of at least 5 events/hour with associated daytime sleepiness, or an AHI of at least 15 events/hour, with a drop in the AHI of at least 50% and the AHI falling to under 5 events/hour when the patient changes from the supine to a non-supine position. Various methods for avoiding the supine position while sleeping have been utilized, and studied. Most devices involve some sort of physical barrier restricting the ability to lie supine, and there are many commercially available products some using foam wedges, while others use air-filled packages both of which are held in place with a belt. Many have even used tennis balls attached to the back of a night shirt to encourage avoidance of the supine position.

Data has demonstrated the efficacy of positional therapy devices. One study recruited patients with mild to moderate OSA and used either CPAP or a commercially available positional therapy device during a second night sleep study, switching to the other therapy for a third night sleep study. The authors found that the positional therapy device reduced the AHI to under 5 events/hour in 92% of the patients, and CPAP in 97% of the patients. The positional therapy device was not associated with reductions of total sleep time or sleep efficiency [27]. Oksenberg et al. identified patients with positional OSA and prescribed the tennis ball technique (TBT) for treatment. This involves use of a soft cloth belt wrapped around the chest so that a pouch in the belt holding a tennis ball is positioned in the middle of the back. After 6 months, a questionnaire was mailed to patients to assess their use of the TBT. Of the 50 respondents, 38% indicated that they had continued to use the belt; 24% reported initially using the belt, but stopping after learning to maintain the lateral position; and 38% said they had stopped using the belt, but did not maintain sleep in the lateral position. Patients continuing to use TBT reported an improvement in sleep quality, a decrease in snoring loudness, and an improvement in daytime alertness compared with the other groups. A PSG performed on 12 patients using the TBT demonstrated an improvement in AHI from 46.5 events/hour at baseline to 17.5 events/hour with use of the TBT; 58% of these patients had an AHI less than 10 events/hour and for 2 patients, the TBT did not work [24]. Another survey study with returned responses from 67 patients with positional OSA who had been prescribed the tennis ball technique (TBT) found that after a mean follow-up time of 2.5 yrs only 6% of respondents had continued using the TBT. Of those who were no longer using the TBT, 13.4% had taught themselves to avoid supine sleep. Of those who had discontinued TBT who had not taught themselves to avoid supine sleeping, 63% reported TBT was too uncomfortable, and 26% indicated it did not improve sleep quality or daytime alertness [3]. A more recent study recruited patients with mild to severe positional OSA and embedded an actigraph within a specialized positional device to assess hours of use of the device. Efficacy of the device was assessed using the change in AHI from baseline to 3 months, and demonstrated a drop in the AHI from 26.7 events/hour to 6.0

events/hour on the first night of use of the positional therapy device. The AHI remained stable at the 3-month assessment, and statistically significantly improved from baseline. The device was used about 73% of the nights for an average of 8 hours per night [12].

Newer devices which provide a vibrational stimulus to induce a positional change have hit the medical market. The devices are usually applied to the center of the chest, and held in place using soft straps that run around the patient's back. Use of a sleep position treatment (SPT) device has established efficacy. In a study of 101 patients with overall moderate positional OSA, use of a SPT device improved the AHI from 18.1 events/hour to 10.4 events/hour after 2 months, and the AHI supine from 35.3 events/hour to 17.5 events/hour. The changes in the AHIs were significant when compared to the control group [18].

A sleep position treatment device (SPT) was compared with autotitrating CPAP for the treatment of positional OSA. Patients used both a SPT device and the autotitrating CPAP device each for a 6-week period with the intent to demonstrate noninferiority in both AHI and adherence time. The baseline AHI was 21.5 events/hour; use of the SPT resulted in an AHI of 7.3 events/hour while use of CPAP led to an AHI of 3.7 events/hour. The difference between the treatment's AHIs was statistically significant, however was within the authors' noninferiority difference range. A greater number of patients in the autotitrating CPAP group compared to the SPT group achieved an AHI less than 5 events/hour. The group overall was not sleepy as reflected by an Epworth Sleepiness Scale less than 10, and although CPAP lowered the ESS to a greater degree than the SPT, the difference is unlikely to be clinically relevant. Average adherence to treatment, average nightly duration of use, and the percentage of nights with use at least 4 hours was significantly greater on SPT than on CPAP [2].

Surgery

Maxillomandibular Advancement (MMA)

A maxillomandibular advancement (MMA) is a multilevel skeletal procedure involving a LeFort I combined with bilateral sagittal split rami osteotomies. The procedures advance the soft palate, tongue base, and suprahyoid musculature leading to enlargement of the velo-orohypopharyngeal airway. In a meta-analysis of patients with severe OSA with an average AHI of 54 events/hour, MMA reduced the AHI by about 87% reaching values under 10 events/hour [5]. The analysis was based solely on multiple case series. Other outcome measures, such as sleepiness and cardiovascular metrics, were rarely reported. Although criteria for evaluating patients for MMA are not standardized, hypopharyngeal with or without velo-oropharyngeal narrowing are common, and usually associated clinically with retrognathia. The procedure can be associated with dental malocclusion and facial neurosensory deficits [5].

Uvulopalatopharyngoplasty (UPPP)

The uvulopalatopharyngoplasty is a soft palate procedure involving removal of tissue from the soft palate, the uvula, and the tonsils with the goal of reducing or restructuring the collapsible part of the soft palate. Meta-analysis of mostly male patients with a baseline AHI of 40.3 events/hour who underwent UPPP ended up with an AHI of 29.8 events/hour, an overall reduction of 33% [5]. Selection criteria were variable. The analysis was based mostly on observational studies; however, there were two small randomized controlled trials included. Reporting of side effects was inconsistent in the included trials; however, previous reviews reported difficulty swallowing, nasal regurgitation, taste disturbances, and voice changes [5, 8].

Laser-Assisted Uvuloplasty (LAUP)

This procedure uses laser to shorten the uvula and tighten the posterior soft palate. When the 2 RCTs were combined with the 6 case series, the overall reduction in AHI was 33%. Review of the RCTs however demonstrated minimal change in AHI, or an increase in the AHI after LAUP. The case series suggested a larger range of AHI improvement with 1 case series demonstrated a 73% reduction in AHI [5].

Radiofrequency Therapies

The use of thermal energy to different upper airway structures has been intended to reduce the size of collapsible structures. Targeted structures include the soft palate, the base of the tongue, and a multiple-level approach. The vast majority of the data in meta-analysis is from observational reports. In the single RCT, the post-surgical AHI was reduced by 21%. The observational reports demonstrated a combined AHI reduction from 23.4 events/hour to 14.2 events/hour [5].

Multilevel Surgery

The upper airway demonstrates complex airflow physiology and may have multiple levels of collapse. Many investigators have advocated a surgical approach to treatment that addresses multiple levels of the upper airway either simultaneously, or in a step-wise fashion. The vast majority of investigative reports regarding multilevel surgery consists solely of case series, but generally demonstrate improvement in AHI comparing the preoperative with postoperative measures. Simultaneous multilevel surgeries usually combine a UPPP with a tongue-specific procedure, such as radiofrequency treatment. A retrospective analysis was conducted [9] comparing a series of patients who underwent UPPP combined with radiofrequency treatment to the tongue base to a series of patients who underwent UPPP alone, and used the ESS and polysomnographic measures as outcome assessments. The pre-operative AHI in the UPPP-only group was 35.4 events/hour and in the UPPP + tongue base radiofrequency treatment was 43.9 events/hour (statistically significantly different). The postoperative AHI was 26.5 event/hour and 28.1 events/hour in the UPPP and UPPP + tongue base radiofrequency treatment group, respectively, both measures representing statistically significant improvements compared to preoperative values, but not when compared between groups. ESS was noted to improve from a preoperative level of 15 to a postoperative level of 8 in the UPPP + tongue base radiofrequency treatment group; similar data was not recorded in the UPPP-only group. A step-wise multilevel surgical series of 306 patients [31] underwent phase 1 surgery consisting of UPPP for palatal obstruction and genioglossus advancement with hyoid myotomy-suspension for obstruction at the level of the base of the tongue. Phase 2 surgery, consisting of maxillomandibular advancement, was offered to patients who failed phase 1 determined by a comparison between the residual RDI of patients after surgery and patients using nasal CPAP, and with baseline measures. The pre-operative RDI was 55.8 events/hour, the RDI on nasal CPAP was 7.2 events/hour, and the post-operative RDI was 9.2 events/hour. A similar trend was found with oxyhemoglobin saturation nadirs with the pre-operative value of 70.5%, nasal CPAP minimum saturation 86.7%, and post-operative saturation nadir of 86.6%.

A randomized assessment of multilevel surgery, consisting of a modified UPPP combined with radiofrequency tongue reduction, compared with ongoing medical management in patients with moderate to severe OSA demonstrated a statistically significantly greater improvement in AHI and sleepiness in patients who underwent surgical treatment. The resulting mean AHI in the surgery group was 20.8 events/hour (from a baseline of 47.9 events/hour), which is still in the moderate severity OSA category; however, it should be emphasized that this was associated with improvement in sleep-specific quality of life and general health status. The Epworth Sleepiness Scale in the surgery group decreased from 12.4 at baseline to 5.3 after surgery, where the ESS did not change medical management group (11.1 at baseline vs 10.5) [19].

Hypoglossal Nerve Stimulation (HNS)

The relationship between activation of the genioglossus and upper airway patency was the motivation for evaluating the use of stimulation of the hypoglossal nerve as a therapy for OSA. An impulse generator is implanted in the subcutaneous tissues of the upper chest, typically on the right side. The medial branch of the hypoglossal nerve typically on the right is exposed, and a stimulation lead is wrapped around it. A sensing lead is placed between the internal and external intercostal muscles at the fourth intercostal level. When a respiratory effort ensues, the stimulator is activated and provides an impulse to the hypoglossal nerve causing the tongue to move anteriorly. Patients with moderate-to-severe OSA who had either not tolerated PAP therapy, or who declined to use it were recruited to undergo implantation of the device. The patients had an AHI of 32 events/hour at baseline with a moderate amount of fatigue, and daytime sleepiness with an Epworth sleepiness scale of 11.6. Assessment after 12 months of treatment revealed a drop in the median AHI from 29.3 events/hour to 9.0 events/hour, and 66% of the participants had met the coprimary outcome of a drop in AHI by at least 50% and a reduction in AHI to 20 events/hour or less. Adverse events included tongue weakness, tongue soreness, abrasion on the underside of the tongue, and discomfort from the stimulation; however, none of these caused permanent issues [35]. HNS have now been implanted in over 10,000 patients worldwide. Five-year data are available from the initial trial and demonstrate persistent reductions in AHI, ESS, and QOL scores without the need for increased stimulation voltage [38].

Conclusion

OSA is a highly prevalent disorder that can be associated with considerable daytime impairment and significant cardiovascular consequences both of which provide a compelling indication for treatment. The rationale for the use of CPAP and the body of evidence that has accumulated provide a sound foundation supporting its use. The variety of options for administering CPAP therapy should allow for tailoring of treatment to an individual patient's needs; however, a significant minority of patients for whom CPAP is discussed and prescribed either do not tolerate the therapy, or refuse to use it. Therefore, alternatives to CPAP exist and should be offered when appropriate and in a judicious fashion.

References

1. Bartolucci ML, Bortolotti F, Corazza G, Incerti Parenti S, Paganelli C, Alessandri Bonetti G. Effectiveness of different mandibular advancement device designs in obstructive sleep apnoea therapy: a systematic review of randomised controlled trials with meta-analysis. J Oral Rehabil. 2021;48:469–86.
2. Berry RB, Uhles ML, Abaluck BK, Winslow DH, Schweitzer PK, Gaskins RA Jr, Doekel RC Jr, Emsellem HA. NightBalance sleep position treatment device versus auto-adjusting positive airway pressure for treatment of positional obstructive sleep apnea. J Clin Sleep Med. 2019;15:947–56.
3. Bignold JJ, Deans-Costi G, Goldsworthy MR, Robertson CA, Mcevoy D, Catcheside PG, Mercer JD. Poor long-term patient compliance with the tennis ball technique for treating positional obstructive sleep apnea. J Clin Sleep Med. 2009;5:428–30.
4. Block AJ, Faulkner JA, Hughes RL, Remmers JE, Thach B. Clinical conference in pulmonary disease. Factors influencing upper airway closure. Chest. 1984;86:114–22.
5. Caples SM, Rowley JA, Prinsell JR, Pallanch JF, Elamin MB, Katz SG, Harwick JD. Surgical modifications of the upper airway for obstructive sleep apnea in adults: a systematic review and meta-analysis. Sleep. 2010;33:1396–407.

6. Dellweg D, Kerl J, Hoehn E, Wenzel M, Koehler D. Randomized controlled trial of noninvasive positive pressure ventilation (NPPV) versus servoventilation in patients with CPAP-induced central sleep apnea (complex sleep apnea). Sleep. 2013;36:1163–71.
7. Ebben MR, Narizhnaya M, Segal AZ, Barone D, Krieger AC. A randomised controlled trial on the effect of mask choice on residual respiratory events with continuous positive airway pressure treatment. Sleep Med. 2014;15:619–24.
8. Franklin KA, Anttila H, Axelsson S, Gislason T, Maasilta P, Myhre KI, Rehnqvist N. Effects and side-effects of surgery for snoring and obstructive sleep apnea–a systematic review. Sleep. 2009;32:27–36.
9. Friedman M, Ibrahim H, Lee G, Joseph NJ. Combined uvulopalatopharyngoplasty and radiofrequency tongue base reduction for treatment of obstructive sleep apnea/hypopnea syndrome. Otolaryngol Head Neck Surg. 2003;129:611–21.
10. Gay P, Weaver T, Loube D, Iber C, Positive Airway Pressure Task, F., Standards of Practice, C. & American Academy of Sleep, M. Evaluation of positive airway pressure treatment for sleep related breathing disorders in adults. Sleep. 2006;29:381–401.
11. Gold AR, Schwartz AR. The pharyngeal critical pressure. The whys and hows of using nasal continuous positive airway pressure diagnostically. Chest. 1996;110:1077–88.
12. Heinzer RC, Pellaton C, Rey V, Rossetti AO, Lecciso G, Haba-Rubio J, Tafti M, Lavigne G. Positional therapy for obstructive sleep apnea: an objective measurement of patients' usage and efficacy at home. Sleep Med. 2012;13:425–8.
13. Holley AB, Lettieri CJ, Shah AA. Efficacy of an adjustable oral appliance and comparison with continuous positive airway pressure for the treatment of obstructive sleep apnea syndrome. Chest. 2011;140:1511–6.
14. Issa FG, Sullivan CE. Upper airway closing pressures in obstructive sleep apnea. J Appl Physiol Respir Environ Exerc Physiol. 1984;57:520–7.
15. Johal A, Haria P, Manek S, Joury E, Riha R. Ready-made versus custom-made mandibular repositioning devices in sleep apnea: a randomized clinical trial. J Clin Sleep Med. 2017;13:175–82.
16. Kuna ST, Bedi DG, Ryckman C. Effect of nasal airway positive pressure on upper airway size and configuration. Am Rev Respir Dis. 1988;138:969–75.
17. Kushida CA, Nichols DA, Holmes TH, Quan SF, Walsh JK, Gottlieb DJ, SIMON RD Jr, Guilleminault C, White DP, Goodwin JL, Schweitzer PK, Leary EB, Hyde PR, Hirshkowitz M, Green S, Mcevoy LK, Chan C, Gevins A, Kay GG, Bloch DA, Crabtree T, Dement WC. Effects of continuous positive airway pressure on neurocognitive function in obstructive sleep apnea patients: the Apnea Positive Pressure Long-term Efficacy Study (APPLES). Sleep. 2012;35:1593–602.
18. Laub RR, Tonnesen P, Jennum PJ. A sleep position trainer for positional sleep apnea: a randomized, controlled trial. J Sleep Res. 2017;26:641–50.
19. Mackay S, Carney AS, Catcheside PG, Chai-Coetzer CL, Chia M, Cistulli PA, Hodge JC, jones A, Kaambwa B, Lewis R, Ooi EH, Pinczel AJ, Mcardle N, Rees G, Singh B, Stow N, Weaver EM, Woodman RJ, Woods CM, Yeo A, Mcevoy RD. Effect of multilevel upper airway surgery vs medical management on the apnea-hypopnea index and patient-reported daytime sleepiness among patients with moderate or severe obstructive sleep apnea: the SAMS randomized clinical trial. JAMA. 2020;324:1168–79.
20. Madeiro F, Andrade RGS, Piccin VS, Pinheiro GDL, Moriya HT, Genta PR, Lorenzi-Filho G. Transmission of oral pressure compromises oronasal CPAP efficacy in the treatment of OSA. Chest. 2019;156:1187–94.
21. Masa JF, Corral J, Alonso ML, Ordax E, Troncoso MF, Gonzalez M, Lopez-Martinez S, Marin JM, Marti S, Diaz-Cambriles T, chiner E, Aizpuru F, Egea C, Spanish Sleep, N. Efficacy of different treatment alternatives for obesity hypoventilation syndrome. Pickwick study. Am J Respir Crit Care Med. 2015;192:86–95.
22. Masa JF, Mokhlesi B, Benitez I, Gomez De Terreros FJ, Sanchez-Quiroga MA, Romero A, Caballero-Eraso C, Teran-Santos J, Alonso-Alvarez ML, Troncoso MF, Gonzalez M, Lopez-Martin S, Marin JM, Marti S, Diaz-Cambriles T, Chiner E, Egea C, Barca J, Vazquez-Polo FJ,

Negrin MA, Martel-Escobar M, Barbe F, Corral J, Spanish Sleep N. Long-term clinical effectiveness of continuous positive airway pressure therapy versus non-invasive ventilation therapy in patients with obesity hypoventilation syndrome: a multicentre, open-label, randomised controlled trial. Lancet. 2019;393:1721–32.

23. Mazza S, Pepin JL, Naegele B, Rauch E, Deschaux C, Ficheux P, Levy P. Driving ability in sleep apnoea patients before and after CPAP treatment: evaluation on a road safety platform. Eur Respir J. 2006;28:1020–8.

24. Oksenberg A, Silverberg D, Offenbach D, Arons E. Positional therapy for obstructive sleep apnea patients: a 6-month follow-up study. Laryngoscope. 2006;116:1995–2000.

25. Patil SP, Ayappa IA, Caples SM, Kimoff RJ, Patel SR, Harrod CG. Treatment of adult obstructive sleep apnea with positive airway pressure: an American Academy of Sleep Medicine Clinical Practice Guideline. J Clin Sleep Med. 2019;15:335–43.

26. Penzel T, Moller M, Becker HF, Knaack L, Peter JH. Effect of sleep position and sleep stage on the collapsibility of the upper airways in patients with sleep apnea. Sleep. 2001;24:90–5.

27. Permut I, Diaz-Abad M, Chatila W, Crocetti J, Gaughan JP, D'alonzo GE, Krachman SL. Comparison of positional therapy to CPAP in patients with positional obstructive sleep apnea. J Clin Sleep Med. 2010;6:238–43.

28. Piper AJ, Wang D, Yee BJ, Barnes DJ, Grunstein RR. Randomised trial of CPAP vs bilevel support in the treatment of obesity hypoventilation syndrome without severe nocturnal desaturation. Thorax. 2008;63:395–401.

29. Ramar K, Dort LC, Katz SG, Lettieri CJ, Harrod CG, Thomas SM, Chervin RD. Clinical practice guideline for the treatment of obstructive sleep apnea and snoring with oral appliance therapy: an update for 2015. J Clin Sleep Med. 2015;11:773–827.

30. Remmers JE, Degroot WJ, Sauerland EK, Anch AM. Pathogenesis of upper airway occlusion during sleep. J Appl Physiol Respir Environ Exerc Physiol. 1978;44:931–8.

31. Riley RW, Powell NB, Guilleminault C. Obstructive sleep apnea syndrome: a review of 306 consecutively treated surgical patients. Otolaryngol Head Neck Surg. 1993;108:117–25.

32. Rowland S, Aiyappan V, Hennessy C, Catcheside P, Chai-Coetzer CL, Mcevoy RD, Antic NA. Comparing the efficacy, mask leak, patient adherence, and patient preference of three different CPAP interfaces to treat moderate-severe obstructive sleep apnea. J Clin Sleep Med. 2018;14:101–8.

33. Soghier I, Brozek JL, Afshar M, Tamae Kakazu M, Wilson KC, Masa JF, Mokhlesi B. Noninvasive ventilation versus CPAP as initial treatment of obesity hypoventilation syndrome. Ann Am Thorac Soc. 2019;16:1295–303.

34. Strohl KP, Redline S. Nasal CPAP therapy, upper airway muscle activation, and obstructive sleep apnea. Am Rev Respir Dis. 1986;134:555–8.

35. Strollo PJ Jr, Soose RJ, Maurer JT, De Vries N, Cornelius J, Froymovich O, Hanson RD, Padhya TA, Steward DL, Gillespie MB, Woodson BT, Van De Heyning PH, Goetting MG, Vanderveken OM, Feldman N, Knaack I, Strohl KP, Group, S. T. Upper-airway stimulation for obstructive sleep apnea. N Engl J Med. 2014;370:139–49.

36. Sullivan CE, Issa FG, Berthon-Jones M, Eves L. Reversal of obstructive sleep apnoea by continuous positive airway pressure applied through the nares. Lancet. 1981;1:862–5.

37. Vanderveken OM, Devolder A, Marklund M, Boudewyns AN, Braem MJ, Okkerse W, Verbraecken JA, Franklin KA, DE Backer WA, Van De Heyning PH. Comparison of a custom-made and a thermoplastic oral appliance for the treatment of mild sleep apnea. Am J Respir Crit Care Med. 2008;178:197–202.

38. Woodson BT, Strohl KP, Soose RJ, Gillespie MB, Maurer JT, De Vries N, Padhya TA, Badr MS, Lin HS, Vanderveken OM, Mickelson S, Strollo PJ Jr. Upper airway stimulation for obstructive sleep apnea: 5-year outcomes. Otolaryngol Head Neck Surg. 2018;159:194–202.

Chapter 8
Central Sleep Apnea: Pathophysiology and Clinical Management

M. Safwan Badr and Geoffrey Ginter

Keywords Central apnea · Hypoventilation · Hyperventilation · Hypocapnia · Cheyne–Stokes respiration · CPAP · Adaptive servo-ventilation

Central sleep apnea is a manifestation of breathing instability in a variety of clinical conditions and is often bundled under the rubric of obstructive sleep apnea. Central sleep apnea occurs because of a transient cessation of ventilatory motor output, under several physiologic or pathologic conditions. This chapter will address the pathogenesis, clinical features, and management of central sleep apnea.

Determinants of Central Apnea During NREM Sleep

Hypocapnia

The sleep state (specifically non-rapid eye movement or NREM sleep) removes the wakefulness "drive to breathe" and renders respiration critically dependent on chemical influences, especially partial pressure of carbon dioxide (PCO_2). Central apnea results if arterial PCO_2 is lowered below a highly sensitive "apneic threshold." [1, 2] Hypocapnia is a potent but not an omnipotent mechanism of reduced ventilatory motor output during NREM sleep. Several factors modulate and mitigate the effects of hypocapnia on ventilatory motor output and promote stability of respiration.

M. S. Badr (✉)
Division of Pulmonary, Critical Care and Sleep Medicine, Department of Internal Medicine, Harper University Hospital, Wayne State University School of Medicine, Detroit, MI, USA
e-mail: sbadr@med.wayne.edu

G. Ginter
Department of Internal Medicine, Harper University Hospital, Wayne State University School of Medicine, Detroit, MI, USA

Short-Term Potentiation

Actively induced hyperventilation (such as hypoxic hyperventilation) is associated with activation of an excitatory neural mechanism referred to as short-term potentiation (STP) [3–5], which results in a gradual return of ventilation toward the baseline upon cessation of the stimulus to breathe. STP has been demonstrated in humans as well as in animals, and is unaffected by the state of consciousness. STP may play a significant role in preserving rhythmic respiration by preventing abrupt drop in ventilation during transient hypocapnia such as following brief hypoxia or transient arousal. In fact, central apnea rarely occurs following termination of brief hypoxia, despite hypocapnia at or below the apneic threshold [3–5]. Similarly, although hypocapnia occurs during transient arousals from sleep, the activation of STP may mitigate the occurrence of central apnea under these conditions [6]. However, prolonged hypoxia may abolish STP, which may explain the development of periodic breathing after 20–25 min of hypoxia and the occurrence of central apnea upon termination of prolonged hypoxic exposure [5, 7].

Duration of Hyperpnea

The duration of hyperpnea is another important determinant of reduced ventilatory motor output following hyperventilation. Central apnea does not usually occur following brief arousal in sleeping humans [8] or dogs [9] possibly due to insufficient reduction in PCO_2 at the level of the central chemoreceptors.

In summary, the balance between hypocapnia and short-term potentiation determines the occurrence of post-hyperventilation apnea during stable sleep, while the duration of hyperventilation may determine whether the reduction in medullary PCO_2 is enough for the development of central apnea.

Role of Upper Airway Reflexes

While hypocapnia is the most common influence leading to central apnea, other mechanisms may also induce central apnea. For example, negative pressure–induced deformation of the isolated upper airway causes central apnea in dogs during both wakefulness and sleep [10]. Whether such reflexes contribute to the developments of central apnea in sleeping humans remains speculative. Conversely, central apnea occurs more frequently in the supine position [11–13] and may be reversed with nasal continuous positive airway pressure (CPAP) [14]. Likewise, there is evidence of supine dependency including that the lateral position amelioration of severity of central apnea and Cheyne–Stokes respiration [11–13].

Mechanisms Perpetuating Breathing Instability

Central apnea does not occur as a single event, but as cycles of apnea/hypopnea alternating with hyperpnea. Ventilatory control during sleep operates as a negative-feedback closed-loop cycle to maintain homeostasis of blood gas tensions within a physiologic range. Many authors have adopted the engineering concept of "loop gain" as a measure of ventilatory stability or susceptibility to central apnea and recurrent periodic breathing [15]. Loop gain represents the overall response of the plant (representing the lung and respiratory muscles); the controller (representing the ventilatory control centers and the chemoreceptors); and the delay, dilution, and diffusion inherent in transferring the signal between the plant and the controller. The formula for loop gain is as follows:

$$\text{Loop gain} = \text{Controller gain} \times \text{Plant gain}$$
$$= \frac{\Delta \text{Ventilation}}{\Delta PCO_2} \times \frac{\Delta PCO_2}{\Delta \text{Ventilation}}$$

The formula can be expanded to account for pulmonary blood flow (Q, equivalent to cardiac output) and carbon dioxide–carrying capacity of the blood (β); the derivation for this expanded equation can be found in the study by Ghazanshahi and Khoo [16]. These two factors comprise the rate of carbon dioxide delivery to the chemoreceptors and the lungs, which, when delayed, can increase loop gain by producing lag between the disturbance (initial change in ventilation or carbon dioxide) and the response. A greater loop gain represents increased reactivity of the ventilatory circuit to disturbances and, consequently, ventilatory instability [17]. Central sleep apnea is associated with increased loop gain, which can be observed in conditions such as congestive heart failure (CHF – increased controller gain and prolonged circulation time) or obesity and tetraplegia (increased plant gain resulting from decreased lung volumes) [17–19]. Conversely, a lower loop gain corresponds to greater ventilatory stability, as is observed during REM sleep [20]. A detailed discussion of the dynamics of ventilatory control is beyond the scope of this chapter; however, there are several excellent reviews that have discussed this aspect in detail [21–23].

The occurrence of central apnea is associated with several consequences that conspire to promote further breathing instability:

- Once ventilatory motor output ceases, rhythmic breathing does not resume at eupneic arterial PCO_2 ($PaCO_2$) due to inertia of the ventilatory control system; an increase in $PaCO_2$ by 4–6 mmHg above eupnea is required for resumption of respiratory effort [24].
- Central apnea is associated with narrowing or occlusion of the pharyngeal airway [25]. Thus, resumption of ventilation requires opening of a narrowed or occluded airway and overcoming tissue adhesion forces [26] and craniofacial gravitational forces.

Termination of central apnea is associated with variable changes in arterial blood gases (hypoxia and hypercapnia) and transient EEG arousal, resulting in ventilatory overshoot, subsequent hypocapnia, and a recurrence of apnea/hypopnea. This sequence explains why apnea rarely occurs as a single event (i.e., "apnea begets apnea") and why there is an overlap between central and obstructive apnea (upper airway obstruction often follows central apneas upon resumption of respiratory effort, i.e., mixed apnea).

Pathophysiologic Classification of Central Sleep Apnea

Central apnea syndrome may be present in a diverse group of conditions including heart failure and obstructive sleep apnea. The ICSD-3 lists several categories of central apnea: (1) Primary Central Sleep Apnea, (2) Central Sleep Apnea Due to Cheyne–Stokes Breathing Pattern, (3) Central Sleep Apnea Due to Medical Condition Not Cheyne–Stokes, (4) Central Sleep Apnea due to High Altitude Periodic Breathing, (5) Central Sleep Apnea Due to Drug or Substance Use, (6) Central Sleep Apnea of Infancy, (7) Central Sleep Apnea of Prematurity, and (8) Treatment-Emergent Central Sleep Apnea [27]. Central apneas are caused either by hyperventilation or hypoventilation. Primary central sleep apnea (CSA), Cheyne–Stokes respiration with central sleep apnea (CSA-CSR), and CSA at high altitude are examples of CSA-related to hyperventilation. Central sleep apnea due to drug or substance use is due to hypoventilation, whereas central apnea associated with other medical conditions may be due to either hyperventilation or hypoventilation. The underlying mechanisms influence the choice of therapy including optimization of medical therapy in central apnea associated with other conditions such as heart failure, hypothyroidism, or acromegaly.

The level of arterial PCO_2 during wakefulness is often used to classify central apnea as hypercapnic or non-hypercapnic. However, such classification does not capture the underlying pathogenesis as apnea represents hypoventilation or a consequence of hyperventilation.

Central Sleep Apnea Secondary to Hypoventilation

The sleep state is associated with reduced ventilatory motor output, increased upper airway resistance, and hypoventilation. This physiologic constellation carries pathologic consequences in patients with an underlying abnormality in ventilatory control or impaired pulmonary mechanics. Most afflicted patients suffer from a central nervous system disease (e.g., encephalitis), neuromuscular disease (e.g., post-polio syndrome), or severe abnormalities in pulmonary mechanics (e.g., kyphoscoliosis [28]). *Thus, the hallmark of this disease is alveolar hypoventilation representing nocturnal ventilatory failure or worsening of the underlying chronic disease.* Arousal from sleep restores alveolar ventilation to a variable degree; resumption of sleep reduces ventilation in a cyclical fashion.

Central apnea secondary to hypoventilation does not necessarily meet the strict definition of "apnea," since feeble ventilatory motor output may persist albeit below the thresholds required to preserve alveolar ventilation. Likewise, it may not meet the definition of "central" in patients with respiratory muscle disease or skeletal deformities. Consequently, the presenting clinical picture includes both features of the underlying ventilatory insufficiency (e.g., morning headache, cor pulmonale, peripheral edema, polycythemia, and abnormal pulmonary function tests) and features of the sleep apnea/hypopnea syndrome (e.g., poor nocturnal sleep, snoring, and daytime sleepiness).

A rare but interesting group of patients present with primary alveolar hypoventilation manifesting by daytime hypoventilation without an apparent identifiable cause and blunted chemo responsiveness [29, 30]. Congenital central hypoventilation syndrome (CCHS) results from a mutation in the gene that encodes the homeobox (PHOX) 2B gene.

The mechanism(s) responsible for hypercapnic central sleep apnea in a given patient influence(s) the management strategy, which aims to restore effective alveolar ventilation during sleep. Treatment of choice is assisted ventilation; nasal CPAP and supplemental oxygen are unlikely to alleviate the condition.

Central Apnea Secondary to Hyperventilation

Hypocapnia secondary to hyperventilation is the most common underlying mechanism of central apnea. A typical patient with non-hypercapnic central apnea has no evidence of a neuromuscular disorder, abnormal lung mechanics, or impaired responses to chemical stimuli. Accordingly, apnea is a result of a transient instability rather than a ventilatory control defect.

How does the first apnea begin? Several transient perturbations may trigger the initial event, including oscillation in sleep state [31], or transient hypoxia possibly due to retention of secretions or reduced lung volumes at sleep onset. Thus, hypoxia stimulates ventilation, subsequently leading to hypocapnia and apnea. The occurrence of apnea initiates the repetitive process of apnea–hyperpnea and leads to sustained breathing instability, manifested as periodic breathing (see above). In summary, non-hypercapnic central apnea is a heterogeneous entity that may be an idiopathic or a secondary condition. The pathogenesis may vary depending upon the clinical condition. However, hypocapnia secondary to hyperventilation is the common denominator in this group of disorders.

Central Apnea Risk Factors

Sleep State

Transient breathing instability and central apnea may occur during the transition from wakefulness to NREM sleep. As sleep state oscillates between wakefulness and light sleep [32–34], the level of $PaCO_2$ is at or below the hypocapnic level required to maintain rhythmic breathing during sleep (i.e., the "apneic threshold"), resulting in central apnea. Recovery from apnea is associated with transient wakefulness and hyperventilation. The subsequent hypocapnia elicits apnea upon resumption of sleep. Consolidation of sleep alleviates the oscillation in sleep and respiration and stabilizes $PaCO_2$ at a higher set point above the apneic threshold. Sleep onset is also associated with another type of central apnea, not preceded by hyperventilation. The transition from alpha to theta in normal subjects is associated with prolongation of breath duration [35].

Central apnea at sleep onset if often considered "physiologic," albeit not universal. Furthermore, events that occur during epochs scored as "wakefulness" are not captured. Whether sleep-onset central apnea is truly physiologic, or a reflection of increased loop gain is yet to be determined. The clinical implications and natural history of this "phenomenon" is unknown.

Central sleep apnea is uncommon during REM sleep as many studies suggest that breathing during REM sleep is impervious to chemical influences (REF), possibly due to increased ventilatory motor output during REM sleep [36, 37] relative to NREM sleep. In addition, there is evidence in animal studies that hypocapnia, per se, may decrease the amount of REM sleep [38]. The major barrier to answering this question in humans is the difficulty in conducting such experiments without disrupting REM sleep.

The loss of intercostal and accessory muscle activity during REM sleep leads to a reduction of alveolar ventilation. This may manifest as apparent central apnea or hypopnea in patients with compromised lung mechanics or neuromuscular disease. If severe diaphragm dysfunction is present, nadir tidal volume may be negligible and the event may appear as central apnea. Thus, central apnea during REM sleep represents transient hypoventilation rather than post-hyperventilation hypocapnia.

Age and Gender

Central sleep apnea is more prevalent in older adults relative to middle-aged individuals [39–41]. Physiologically, sleep state oscillations may precipitate central apnea in older adults [42]. Increased prevalence of comorbid conditions such as thyroid disease [43], congestive heart failure [44], atrial fibrillation [45], and cerebrovascular disease [46] may also contribute to increased susceptibility to develop central apnea in older adults.

Central sleep apnea is uncommon in premenopausal women [47]. There is evidence that women are less susceptible to the development of hypocapnic central apnea relative to men following mechanical ventilation. Physiologically, the hypocapnic apneic threshold is higher in men relative to women. Using nasal mechanical ventilation during stable NREM sleep, Zhou et al. [2] have shown that the apneic threshold was −3.5 versus −4.7 mmHg below room air level in men and women respectively. This difference was not due to progesterone. In fact, administration of testosterone to healthy premenopausal women for 12 days resulted in an elevation of the apneic threshold and a diminution in the magnitude of hypocapnic required for induction of central apnea during NREM sleep [48]. Conversely, suppression of testosterone with leuprolide acetate in healthy males decreases the hypocapnic apneic threshold and potentially stabilizing respiration [49]. Thus, male sex hormones are the most likely factor elevating the apneic threshold in men.

Medical Conditions

Sleep apnea is highly prevalent in patients with CHF [44, 50–52]. Javaheri et al. [51] demonstrated that 51% of male patients with CHF had sleep-disordered breathing, 40% had central sleep apnea, and 11% obstructive apnea. Risk factors for CSA in this group of patients include male gender, atrial fibrillation, age >60 years, and daytime hypocapnia (PCO_2 < 38 mmHg during wakefulness) [53]. Risk factors for OSA differed by gender; the only independent determinant in men was body mass index (BMI), whereas age over 60 was the only independent determinant in women.

Hyperventilation is a common breathing pattern in patients with CHF, who demonstrate daytime hypocapnia and minimal or no rise in P_{ET} CO_2 from wakefulness to sleep [54]. Chronic hyperventilation results in decreased plant gain [55, 56], which mitigates the magnitude of hypocapnia for a given increase in alveolar ventilation. In other words, steady-state hyperventilation and hypocapnia are potentially stabilizing rather than destabilizing as is commonly thought. Increased propensity to central apnea in patients with CHF is due to increased hypocapnic chemosensitivity (increased controller gain) and prolonged circulatory delay.

Sleep apnea is also common after a cerebrovascular accident (CVA) [46]; with central apnea being the predominant type in 40% of patients with sleep apnea after a CVA [57, 58]. Likewise, central apnea occurs in 30% of patients who are on stable methadone maintenance treatment [59]. Finally, several medical conditions predispose to the development of central apnea including hypothyroidism, acromegaly, and renal failure have an unexpectedly high prevalence of sleep apnea [60–62]. Nocturnal hemodialysis is associated with improvement in sleep apnea indices in patients with renal failure [62].

Cervical spinal cord injury (C-SCI) has also recently been identified as a risk factor for the development of central sleep apnea [63]. The mechanism underlying CSA in C-SCI is uncertain. Potential mechanisms include loss of intercostal muscle activity or decreased lung volume [64]. A reduction in lung volume results in increased plant gain, which causes an exaggerated change in PCO_2 in response to changes in ventilation [65]. SCI has also been shown to increase peripheral chemosensitivity, possibly due to potentiation of the neurocircuitry regulating the production of serotonin, which is implicated in plasticity of the respiratory circuit [66]. The combination of increased plant gain and increased peripheral chemosensitivity may promote instability via ventilatory overshoot in response to minor derangements in ventilation or PCO_2, leading to central apnea.

Some patients with central apnea have no apparent risk factor and are deemed to have "idiopathic central apnea." Typically, these patients demonstrate increased chemo-responsiveness and sleep state instability [67]. It is plausible that these patients will have occult cardiac or metabolic disease. For example, idiopathic central sleep apnea is more prevalent in patients with atrial fibrillation [45].

Central sleep apnea can also develop during treatment of obstructive sleep apnea. Treatment-emergent central sleep apnea (TECSA) is primarily associated with the initiation of CPAP therapy, but has been observed in other OSA therapies, including mandibular advancement devices and surgical intervention [68, 69]. TECSA may be either transient or persistent, often resolving spontaneously with persistent positive airway pressure (PAP) therapy [69]. Possible mechanisms underlying TECSA include increased elimination of CO_2 following relief of airway obstruction, hyperventilation due to PAP-related arousals, and over-titration causing activation of lung stretch receptors and subsequent inhibition of respiratory drive [68].

Clinical Features and Diagnosis

The clinical presentation includes features of the underlying disease and features of sleep apnea syndrome. Patients with central apnea secondary to hyperventilation may present with the usual symptoms of sleep apnea syndrome. Alternatively, they may present with *insomnia* and *poor nocturnal* addition. Frequent oscillation between wakefulness and stage 1 NREM sleep may promote *sleep fragmentation and poor nocturnal sleep* as the presenting symptoms.

Central sleep apnea may also be a found as an incidental polysomnographic finding in a patient with obstructive sleep apnea, either on the initial diagnostic study or after restoring upper airway patency with nasal CPAP. The latter is referred to as "complex sleep apnea," implying a distinct clinical entity. However, it is likely that this phenomenon represents unmasking of the underlying breathing instability in patients with obstructive sleep apnea and may resolve spontaneously [70, 71].

Nocturnal polysomnography is the standard diagnostic method including measurement of sleep and respiration, and also including detection of flow, measurement of oxyhemoglobin saturation, and detection of respiratory effort. Detection of respiratory effort is important to distinguish central from obstructive apnea. Most clinical sleep laboratories utilize surface recording of effort to detect displacement of the abdominal and thoracic compartments instead of esophageal pressure recording.

The presence of cardiogenic oscillations (pulse artifacts) on the flow signal has been used as an indirect index of central etiology. The underlying rationale is the pulse artifacts represent transmission of a pulse waveform from the thorax, and hence indicates a patent upper airway that allows the transmission of cardiogenic oscillation. Morrell et al. [72] used fiber optic nasopharyngoscopy to evaluate upper airway patency during central apnea; cardiogenic oscillations were present even when the airway is completely occluded. Thus, the presence of cardiogenic oscillations does not prove upper airway patency or central etiology.

Management

Central sleep apnea is a disorder with protean manifestations and underlying conditions. The presence of comorbid conditions and concomitant obstructive sleep apnea influence therapeutic approach significantly. Specific therapeutic options include positive pressure therapy, pharmacologic therapy, and supplemental oxygen.

Positive Pressure Therapy

CPAP therapy is the initial treatment of choice for central sleep apnea. Published practice parameters by the American Academy of Sleep Medicine recommends CPAP as a standard therapy, based on the preponderance of evidence supporting its use [73]. Most of this evidence comes from investigations on central apnea related to congestive heart failure (CHF), although other subtypes of central sleep apnea appear to respond to CPAP as well, especially if it occurs in combination with episodes of obstructive or mixed apnea. In fact, "pure" central apnea with no concomitant obstructive events is uncommon. If a comorbid clinical condition is present, such as heart failure, hypothyroidism, or acromegaly, optimization of medical therapy is also required and may ameliorate the severity of central apnea. Likewise, central sleep apnea in patients with obstructive sleep apnea may resolve with alleviation of upper airway obstruction with positive pressure therapy. Many patients with idiopathic central sleep apnea receive a trial of nasal CPAP, which has been shown to reverse central sleep apnea, even in the absence of obstructive respiratory events [14], especially supine-dependent central sleep apnea. The response may be due to preventing upper airway occlusion during central apnea and subsequent ventilatory overshoot [25]. Prevention of ventilatory overshoot may explain the reported combination of reduced apnea frequency and increased PCO_2 after CPAP [74]. Nasal CPAP is the initial option during a therapeutic titration study, despite the lack of systematic studies on nasal CPAP therapy in patients with idiopathic central apnea.

The exuberance regarding nasal CPAP therapy in patients with central apnea and CHF did not withstand the rigors of controlled clinical trials. The Canadian

Continuous Positive Airway Pressure trial, or Can PAP [75] tested the hypothesis that CPAP would improve the survival rate without heart transplantation in patients with heart failure and central sleep apnea. This type of central apnea corresponds to Central Sleep Apnea Due to Cheyne–Stokes Breathing Pattern, in the International Classification of Sleep Disorders – Third Edition (ICSD-3). Participants were randomly assigned to nasal CPAP or no CPAP. There was no difference in the overall event rates (death and heart transplantation) between the two groups after a 2-year follow-up, despite greater improvement in the CPAP group at 3 months in several intermediate outcomes including apnea–hypopnea index, ejection fraction, mean nocturnal oxyhemoglobin saturation, plasma norepinephrine levels, and the distance walked in 6 min at 3 months. Thus, nasal CPAP had no measured effect on survival, despite the effect on the "severity" of central apnea and several intermediate outcome variables. Therefore, current evidence supports the use of CPAP to alleviate the severity of central sleep apnea and improve daytime function and quality of life.

Noninvasive positive pressure ventilation (NIPPV) using pressure support mode (bi-level nasal positive pressure) is effective in restoring alveolar ventilation during sleep. Clinical indications include nocturnal ventilatory failure and central apnea secondary to hypoventilation. There is evidence that NIPPV exerts a salutary effect on survival in patients with ventilatory failure secondary to amyotrophic lateral sclerosis [76]. It is unclear whether NIPPV exerts a similar effect in other neuromuscular conditions associated with nocturnal ventilatory failure. However, the overall evidence supports the use of NIPPV in a pressure support mode to treat central sleep apnea secondary to hypoventilation, such as neuromuscular or chest wall–related nocturnal hypoventilation. If the ventilatory motor output is insufficient to "trigger" the mechanical inspiration, adding a backup rate ensure adequate ventilation.

Treatment of central apnea secondary to hyperventilation using nasal pressure support ventilation in the bi-level mode may result in worsening of central apnea and breathing instability owing to augmented ventilatory overshoot and hypocapnia [77]. The work of Meza et al. [78] provides empiric evidence that pressure-support ventilation results in periodic breathing and recurrent central apnea when the pressure gradient is above 7 cm H_2O. The addition of a backup rate would be required to maintain stable respiration, which would convert ventilatory support to controlled mechanical ventilation. In general, bi-level positive pressure therapy is unlikely to alleviate central apnea, without a backup rate. Nevertheless, bi-level PAP may ameliorate central apnea that accompanies severe obstructive apnea by preventing upper airway obstruction and ventilatory overshoot.

Recent technological advances allowed for variations in the mode of delivering positive pressure ventilation. One example is Adaptive Servo-Ventilation (ASV), which provides a small but varying amount of ventilatory support and a back-up rate, against a background of low level of CPAP. The device maintains ventilation at 90% of a running 3-min reference period; thus, changes in respiratory effort results in reciprocal changes in the magnitude of ventilatory support. There is evidence that ASV is more effective than CPAP, bi-level pressure support ventilation, or increased dead space in alleviating central sleep apnea [79, 80]. However, the Adaptive Servo-Ventilation for Central Sleep Apnea in Systolic Heart Failure (SERVE-HF) trial demonstrated a significant increase in both all-cause and cardiac mortality in individuals with CHF with a left ventricular ejection fraction (LVEF) <45%, leading the American Academy of Sleep Medicine to recommend against the use of ASV in this population [81, 82]. ASV is still permissible for patients with CSA with CHF with LVEF >45% [82]. In patients for whom there are no absolute contraindications to ASV, the decision to initiate ASV hinges on the efficacy of the treatment in normalizing AHI, patient preference, payers' preference, and the availability of the requisite support for adherence or troubleshooting.

Pharmacological Therapy

Pharmacologic therapy for central apnea remains elusive, and there are no controlled clinical trials demarcating the boundaries of effectiveness [83]. Several small clinical trials indicate that acetazolamide, theophylline, or zolpidem may be beneficial in the treatment of central apnea [84, 85]. Acetazolamide is a weak diuretic and a carbonic anhydrase inhibitor that causes mild metabolic acidosis. Acetazolamide ameliorates central sleep apnea when administered as a single dose of 250 mg before bedtime [18, 84]. Likewise, theophylline ameliorates the severity of Cheyne–Stokes respiration in patients with CHF [85], without adverse effect on sleep architecture. Zolpidem – a non-benzodiazepine sedative hypnotic – has been shown in one study to reduce the severity of central sleep apnea and improve sleep continuity [86]. However, there are no controlled studies demonstrating safety and efficacy; therefore, zolpidem cannot be recommended for the treatment of central apnea. Recently, serotonergic drugs have been investigated as possible therapies for central sleep apnea due to the modulatory role serotonin plays in the respiratory circuit. Buspirone, an anxiolytic and direct serotonin receptor agonist, has demonstrated some efficacy in treating central sleep apnea [87, 88]. Nevertheless, safety and efficacy of the pharmacologic agents await empiric proof. Pharmacologic therapy represents a major opportunity for future investigation.

Supplemental O_2 and CO_2

Several studies have demonstrated a salutary effect of supplemental O_2 in patients with idiopathic central sleep apnea and patients with Central Sleep Apnea Due to Cheyne–Stokes Breathing Pattern [89]. Several potential mechanisms may explain the stabilizing effect of supplemental oxygen on respiration. Oxygen dampens peripheral chemoreceptor responsiveness and minimizes the subsequent ventilatory overshoot. In addition, prolonged hyperoxia stimulates respiration, perhaps by elevating cerebral PCO_2 by the Haldane effect. Acute administration of oxygen is associated with diminished propensity to develop central apnea in normal subjects during sleep [90]. While long-term clinical trials are lacking, supplemental oxygen therapy is a promising adjunct for central apnea, especially in patients with CHF. Likewise, supplemental CO_2 abolishes central apnea in patients with pure central sleep apnea, by raising PCO_2 above the apneic threshold [91, 92]. However, this therapy is not practical given the need for a closed circuit to deliver supplemental CO_2.

Transvenous Phrenic Nerve Stimulation

A recent development in the treatment of CSA is the use of implantable device-based therapy to pace the diaphragm in response to cessation of respiratory drive. Transvenous phrenic nerve stimulation (TPNS) involves an implantable 2-lead system, including a sensory lead which detects pauses in respiration and a stimulatory lead affixed to the phrenic nerve, which initiates contraction of the corresponding hemidiaphragm via a pulse generator implanted in the pectoral region [93]. TPNS significantly reduces the frequency of central apnea, nocturnal oxyhemoglobin desaturations, and arousals while improving sleep architecture and subjective sleep quality [94]. Benefits of TPNS include portability, effective control of central sleep apnea symptoms, and avoidance of nonadherence. The most common adverse effect of TPNS is discomfort, occurring in up to one-third of patients, but less than 5% of patients receiving TPNS elect to discontinue therapy [95]. As a recent innovation, there are no long-term clinical trials following the safety and efficacy of TPNS; however, the implementation of implantable devices represents an area of significant potential utility in the treatment of central sleep apnea.

A Suggested Approach

The heterogeneity of central sleep apnea dictates individualized treatment approach, including optimal treatment of underlying medical conditions and attention to potential medication effects. A trial of nasal CPAP in the sleep laboratory is warranted to ascertain the magnitude of improvement with CPAP alone. The use of BPAP in a pressure support mode is likely to aggravate the severity of central apnea, unless accompanied by a backup rate. While contraindicated in patients with CHF and LVEF <45%, ASV may be beneficial in patients with CSR secondary to CHF with LVEF >45% who do not respond to nasal CPAP alone. Supplemental O_2 may be beneficial in patients with central apnea that persists on nasal CPAP, especially in patients with CHF-CSR.

Summary of Key Points
- Sleep-related withdrawal of the ventilatory drive to breathe is the common denominator among all cases of central apnea, whereas hypocapnia is the final common pathway leading to apnea in non-hypercapnic central apnea.
- The pathophysiologic heterogeneity may explain the protean clinical manifestations and the lack of a single effective therapy for all patients.
- Central sleep apnea is not a single clinical entity; instead, it is a manifestation of breathing instability in a variety of clinical conditions. Central apnea syndrome may be present in a diverse group of conditions including heart failure and obstructive sleep apnea.
- Central sleep apnea is caused either by hyperventilation or hypoventilation. Hypocapnia is the most potent and ubiquitous trigger of central sleep apnea. Central apnea rarely occurs as a single event; instead, it manifests by cycles of apnea/hypopnea alternating with hyperpnea.
- Central sleep apnea is classified into the following specific categories according to the ICSD-3: (1) Primary Central Sleep Apnea, (2) Central Sleep Apnea Due to Cheyne–Stokes Breathing Pattern, (3) Central Sleep Apnea Due to Medical Condition Not Cheyne–Stokes, (4) Central Sleep Apnea due to High Altitude Periodic Breathing, (5) Central Sleep Apnea Due to Drug or Substance Use, (6) Central Sleep Apnea of Infancy, (7) Central Sleep Apnea of Prematurity, and (8) Treatment-Emergent Central Sleep Apnea. The underlying mechanisms influence the choice of therapy including optimization of medical therapy in central apnea associated with other conditions such as heart failure, hypothyroidism, or acromegaly.
- Advanced age, male gender, and postmenopausal state in women are known determinants of central apnea. In contrast, central apnea is less common in REM sleep. Medical conditions which are associated with higher risk of central sleep apnea include CHF, CVA, chronic narcotics users, acromegaly, chronic renal failure, hypothyroidism, and spinal cord injury. Treatment-emergent central sleep apnea may also arise during treatment of obstructive sleep apnea.
- Clinical features are a combination of sleep apnea features and comorbid conditions. The diagnosis requires nocturnal polysomnography. Specific therapeutic options include positive pressure therapy, pharmacologic therapy, supplemental oxygen, and transvenous phrenic nerve stimulation. Nasal CPAP is the recommended initial treatment of choice.

References

1. Skatrud JB, Dempsey JA. Interaction of sleep state and chemical stimuli in sustaining rhythmic ventilation. J Appl Physiol Respir Environ Exerc Physiol. 1983;55(3):813–22.
2. Zhou XS, Shahabuddin S, Zahn BR, Babcock MA, Badr MS. Effect of gender on the development of hypocapnic apnea/hypopnea during NREM sleep. J Appl Physiol (1985). 2000;89(1):192–9.

3. Tawadrous FD, Eldridge FL. Posthyperventilation breathing patterns after active hyperventilation in man. J Appl Physiol. 1974;37(3):353–6.
4. Eldridge FL, Gill-Kumar P. Central neural respiratory drive and after discharge. Respir Physiol. 1980;40(1):49–63.
5. Badr MS, Skatrud JB, Dempsey JA. Determinants of poststimulus potentiation in humans during NREM sleep. J Appl Physiol (1985). 1992;73(5):1958–71.
6. Badr MS, Morgan BJ, Finn L, et al. Ventilatory response to induced auditory arousals during NREM sleep. Sleep. 1997;20(9):707–14.
7. Berssenbrugge A, Dempsey J, Iber C, Skatrud J, Wilson P. Mechanisms of hypoxia-induced periodic breathing during sleep in humans. J Physiol. 1983;343:507–24.
8. Badr MS, Kawak A. Post-hyperventilation hypopnea in humans during NREM sleep. Respir Physiol. 1996;103(2):137–45.
9. Chow CM, Xi L, Smith CA, Saupe KW, Dempsey JA. A volume-dependent apneic threshold during NREM sleep in the dog. J Appl Physiol (1985). 1994;76(6):2315–25.
10. Harms CA, Zeng YJ, Smith CA, Vidruk EH, Dempsey JA. Negative pressure-induced deformation of the upper airway causes central apnea in awake and sleeping dogs. J Appl Physiol (1985). 1996;80(5):1528–39.
11. Sahlin C, Svanborg E, Stenlund H, Franklin KA. Cheyne-Stokes respiration and supine dependency. Eur Respir J. 2005;25(5):829–33.
12. Oksenberg A, Arons E, Snir D, Radwan H, Soroker N. Cheyne-Stokes respiration during sleep: a possible effect of body position. Med Sci Monit. 2002;8(7):Cs61–5.
13. Szollosi I, Roebuck T, Thompson B, Naughton MT. Lateral sleeping position reduces severity of central sleep apnea / Cheyne-Stokes respiration. Sleep. 2006;29(8):1045–51.
14. Issa FG, Sullivan CE. Reversal of central sleep apnea using nasal CPAP. Chest. 1986;90(2):165–71.
15. Khoo MC, Kronauer RE, Strohl KP, Slutsky AS. Factors inducing periodic breathing in humans: a general model. J Appl Physiol Respir Environ Exerc Physiol. 1982;53(3):644–59.
16. Ghazanshahi SD, Khoo MC. Estimation of chemoreflex loop gain using pseudorandom binary CO2 stimulation. IEEE Trans Biomed Eng. 1997;44(5):357–66.
17. Sands SA, Mebrate Y, Edwards BA, et al. Resonance as the mechanism of daytime periodic breathing in patients with heart failure. Am J Respir Crit Care Med. 2017;195(2):237–46.
18. Ginter G, Sankari A, Eshraghi M, et al. Effect of acetazolamide on susceptibility to central sleep apnea in chronic spinal cord injury. J Appl Physiol (1985). 2020;128(4):960–6.
19. Bokov P, Essalhi M, Delclaux C. Loop gain in severely obese women with obstructive sleep apnoea. Respir Physiol Neurobiol. 2016;221:49–53.
20. Badr MS, Dingell JD, Javaheri S. Central sleep apnea: a brief review. Curr Pulmonol Rep. 2019;8(1):14–21.
21. Khoo MC. Determinants of ventilatory instability and variability. Respir Physiol. 2000;122(2–3):167–82.
22. Chapman KR, Bruce EN, Gothe B, Cherniack NS. Possible mechanisms of periodic breathing during sleep. J Appl Physiol (1985). 1988;64(3):1000–8.
23. Cherniack NS, Longobardo GS. Mathematical models of periodic breathing and their usefulness in understanding cardiovascular and respiratory disorders. Exp Physiol. 2006;91(2):295–305.
24. Leevers AM, Simon PM, Dempsey JA. Apnea after normocapnic mechanical ventilation during NREM sleep. J Appl Physiol (1985). 1994;77(5):2079–85.
25. Badr MS, Toiber F, Skatrud JB, Dempsey J. Pharyngeal narrowing/occlusion during central sleep apnea. J Appl Physiol (1985). 1995;78(5):1806–15.
26. Olson LG, Strohl KP. Airway secretions influence upper airway patency in the rabbit. Am Rev Respir Dis. 1988;137(6):1379–81.
27. Sateia MJ. International classification of sleep disorders-third edition: highlights and modifications. Chest. 2014;146(5):1387–94.
28. Mezon BL, West P, Israels J, Kryger M. Sleep breathing abnormalities in kyphoscoliosis. Am Rev Respir Dis. 1980;122(4):617–21.

29. Barlow PB, Bartlett D Jr, Hauri P, et al. Idiopathic hypoventilation syndrome: importance of preventing nocturnal hypoxemia and hypercapnia. Am Rev Respir Dis. 1980;121(1):141–5.
30. Weese-Mayer DE, Rand CM, Berry-Kravis EM, et al. Congenital central hypoventilation syndrome from past to future: model for translational and transitional autonomic medicine. Pediatr Pulmonol. 2009;44(6):521–35.
31. Pack AI, Cola MF, Goldszmidt A, Ogilvie MD, Gottschalk A. Correlation between oscillations in ventilation and frequency content of the electroencephalogram. J Appl Physiol (1985). 1992;72(3):985–92.
32. Trinder J, Whitworth F, Kay A, Wilkin P. Respiratory instability during sleep onset. J Appl Physiol (1985). 1992;73(6):2462–9.
33. Dunai J, Wilkinson M, Trinder J. Interaction of chemical and state effects on ventilation during sleep onset. J Appl Physiol (1985). 1996;81(5):2235–43.
34. Dunai J, Kleiman J, Trinder J. Ventilatory instability during sleep onset in individuals with high peripheral chemosensitivity. J Appl Physiol (1985). 1999;87(2):661–72.
35. Thomson S, Morrell MJ, Cordingley JJ, Semple SJ. Ventilation is unstable during drowsiness before sleep onset. J Appl Physiol (1985). 2005;99(5):2036–44.
36. Orem J. Neuronal mechanisms of respiration in REM sleep. Sleep. 1980;3(3–4):251–67.
37. Orem J, Lovering AT, Dunin-Barkowski W, Vidruk EH. Tonic activity in the respiratory system in wakefulness, NREM and REM sleep. Sleep. 2002;25(5):488–96.
38. Lovering AT, Fraigne JJ, Dunin-Barkowski WL, Vidruk EH, Orem JM. Hypocapnia decreases the amount of rapid eye movement sleep in cats. Sleep. 2003;26(8):961–7.
39. Phillips B, Cook Y, Schmitt F, Berry D. Sleep apnea: prevalence of risk factors in a general population. South Med J. 1989;82(9):1090–2.
40. Phillips BA, Berry DT, Schmitt FA, Magan LK, Gerhardstein DC, Cook YR. Sleep-disordered breathing in the healthy elderly. Clinically significant? Chest. 1992;101(2):345–9.
41. Ancoli-Israel S, Kripke DF, Klauber MR, Mason WJ, Fell R, Kaplan O. Sleep-disordered breathing in community-dwelling elderly. Sleep. 1991;14(6):486–95.
42. Pack AI, Silage DA, Millman RP, Knight H, Shore ET, Chung DC. Spectral analysis of ventilation in elderly subjects awake and asleep. J Appl Physiol (1985). 1988;64(3):1257–67.
43. Kapur VK, Koepsell TD, deMaine J, Hert R, Sandblom RE, Psaty BM. Association of hypothyroidism and obstructive sleep apnea. Am J Respir Crit Care Med. 1998;158(5 Pt 1):1379–83.
44. Bradley TD, Floras JS. Sleep apnea and heart failure: part II: central sleep apnea. Circulation. 2003;107(13):1822–6.
45. Leung RS, Huber MA, Rogge T, Maimon N, Chiu KL, Bradley TD. Association between atrial fibrillation and central sleep apnea. Sleep. 2005;28(12):1543–6.
46. Bassetti C, Aldrich MS. Sleep apnea in acute cerebrovascular diseases: final report on 128 patients. Sleep. 1999;22(2):217–23.
47. Bixler EO, Vgontzas AN, Lin HM, et al. Prevalence of sleep-disordered breathing in women: effects of gender. Am J Respir Crit Care Med. 2001;163(3 Pt 1):608–13.
48. Zhou XS, Rowley JA, Demirovic F, Diamond MP, Badr MS. Effect of testosterone on the apneic threshold in women during NREM sleep. J Appl Physiol (1985). 2003;94(1):101–7.
49. Mateika JH, Omran Q, Rowley JA, Zhou XS, Diamond MP, Badr MS. Treatment with leuprolide acetate decreases the threshold of the ventilatory response to carbon dioxide in healthy males. J Physiol. 2004;561(Pt 2):637–46.
50. Javaheri S, Parker TJ, Liming JD, et al. Sleep apnea in 81 ambulatory male patients with stable heart failure. Types and their prevalences, consequences, and presentations. Circulation. 1998;97(21):2154–9.
51. Javaheri S, Parker TJ, Wexler L, et al. Occult sleep-disordered breathing in stable congestive heart failure. Ann Intern Med. 1995;122(7):487–92.
52. Javaheri S. Central sleep apnea-hypopnea syndrome in heart failure: prevalence, impact, and treatment. Sleep. 1996;19(10 Suppl):S229–31.

53. Sin DD, Fitzgerald F, Parker JD, Newton G, Floras JS, Bradley TD. Risk factors for central and obstructive sleep apnea in 450 men and women with congestive heart failure. Am J Respir Crit Care Med. 1999;160(4):1101–6.
54. Xie A, Skatrud JB, Puleo DS, Rahko PS, Dempsey JA. Apnea-hypopnea threshold for CO_2 in patients with congestive heart failure. Am J Respir Crit Care Med. 2002;165(9):1245–50.
55. Dempsey JA, Sheel AW, Haverkamp HC, Babcock MA, Harms CA. [The John Sutton Lecture: CSEP, 2002]. Pulmonary system limitations to exercise in health. Can J Appl Physiol. 2003;28 Suppl:S2–24.
56. Dempsey JA, Smith CA, Przybylowski T, et al. The ventilatory responsiveness to CO(2) below eupnoea as a determinant of ventilatory stability in sleep. J Physiol. 2004;560(Pt 1):1–11.
57. Bassetti C, Aldrich MS, Chervin RD, Quint D. Sleep apnea in patients with transient ischemic attack and stroke: a prospective study of 59 patients. Neurology. 1996;47(5):1167–73.
58. Parra O, Arboix A, Bechich S, et al. Time course of sleep-related breathing disorders in first-ever stroke or transient ischemic attack. Am J Respir Crit Care Med. 2000;161(2 Pt 1):375–80.
59. Grunstein RR, Ho KY, Berthon-Jones M, Stewart D, Sullivan CE. Central sleep apnea is associated with increased ventilatory response to carbon dioxide and hypersecretion of growth hormone in patients with acromegaly. Am J Respir Crit Care Med. 1994;150(2):496–502.
60. Grunstein RR, Ho KY, Sullivan CE. Sleep apnea in acromegaly. Ann Intern Med. 1991;115(7):527–32.
61. Grunstein RR, Sullivan CE. Sleep apnea and hypothyroidism: mechanisms and management. Am J Med. 1988;85(6):775–9.
62. Hanly PJ, Pierratos A. Improvement of sleep apnea in patients with chronic renal failure who undergo nocturnal hemodialysis. N Engl J Med. 2001;344(2):102–7.
63. Sankari A, Bascom AT, Chowdhuri S, Badr MS. Tetraplegia is a risk factor for central sleep apnea. J Appl Physiol (1985). 2014;116(3):345–53.
64. Sankari A, Vaughan S, Bascom A, Martin JL, Badr MS. Sleep-disordered breathing and spinal cord injury: a state-of-the-art review. Chest. 2019;155(2):438–45.
65. Naughton MT. Loop gain in apnea. Am J Respir Crit Care Med. 2010;181(2):103–5.
66. Sankari A, Bascom AT, Riehani A, Badr MS. Tetraplegia is associated with enhanced peripheral chemoreflex sensitivity and ventilatory long-term facilitation. J Appl Physiol (1985). 2015;119(10):1183–93.
67. Xie A, Rutherford R, Rankin F, Wong B, Bradley TD. Hypocapnia and increased ventilatory responsiveness in patients with idiopathic central sleep apnea. Am J Respir Crit Care Med. 1995;152(6 Pt 1):1950–5.
68. Zhang J, Wang L, Guo H-J, Wang Y, Cao J, Chen B-Y. Treatment-emergent central sleep apnea: a unique sleep-disordered breathing. Chin Med J. 2020;133(22)
69. Zeineddine S, Badr MS. Treatment-emergent central apnea: physiologic mechanisms informing clinical practice. Chest. 2021;159(6):2449–57.
70. Dernaika T, Tawk M, Nazir S, Younis W, Kinasewitz GT. The significance and outcome of continuous positive airway pressure-related central sleep apnea during split-night sleep studies. Chest. 2007;132(1):81–7.
71. Wang D, Teichtahl H, Drummer O, et al. Central sleep apnea in stable methadone maintenance treatment patients. Chest. 2005;128(3):1348–56.
72. Morrell MJ, Badr MS, Harms CA, Dempsey JA. The assessment of upper airway patency during apnea using cardiogenic oscillations in the airflow signal. Sleep. 1995;18(8):651–8.
73. Aurora RN, Chowdhuri S, Ramar K, et al. The treatment of central sleep apnea syndromes in adults: practice parameters with an evidence-based literature review and meta-analyses. Sleep. 2012;35(1):17–40.
74. Naughton MT, Benard DC, Rutherford R, Bradley TD. Effect of continuous positive airway pressure on central sleep apnea and nocturnal PCO2 in heart failure. Am J Respir Crit Care Med. 1994;150(6 Pt 1):1598–604.
75. Bradley TD, Logan AG, Kimoff RJ, et al. Continuous positive airway pressure for central sleep apnea and heart failure. N Engl J Med. 2005;353(19):2025–33.

76. Aboussouan LS, Khan SU, Banerjee M, Arroliga AC, Mitsumoto H. Objective measures of the efficacy of noninvasive positive-pressure ventilation in amyotrophic lateral sclerosis. Muscle Nerve. 2001;24(3):403–9.
77. Johnson KG, Johnson DC. Bilevel positive airway pressure worsens central apneas during sleep. Chest. 2005;128(4):2141–50.
78. Meza S, Mendez M, Ostrowski M, Younes M. Susceptibility to periodic breathing with assisted ventilation during sleep in normal subjects. J Appl Physiol (1985). 1998;85(5):1929–40.
79. Teschler H, Döhring J, Wang YM, Berthon-Jones M. Adaptive pressure support servo-ventilation: a novel treatment for Cheyne-Stokes respiration in heart failure. Am J Respir Crit Care Med. 2001;164(4):614–9.
80. Morgenthaler TI, Gay PC, Gordon N, Brown LK. Adaptive servoventilation versus noninvasive positive pressure ventilation for central, mixed, and complex sleep apnea syndromes. Sleep. 2007;30(4):468–75.
81. Cowie MR, Woehrle H, Wegscheider K, et al. Adaptive servo-ventilation for central sleep apnea in systolic heart failure. N Engl J Med. 2015;373(12):1095–105.
82. Aurora RN, Bista SR, Casey KR, et al. Updated adaptive servo-ventilation recommendations for the 2012 AASM guideline: "The treatment of central sleep apnea syndromes in adults: practice parameters with an evidence-based literature review and meta-analyses". J Clin Sleep Med. 2016;12(5):757–61.
83. Hudgel DW, Thanakitcharu S. Pharmacologic treatment of sleep-disordered breathing. Am J Respir Crit Care Med. 1998;158(3):691–9.
84. DeBacker WA, Verbraecken J, Willemen M, Wittesaele W, DeCock W, Van deHeyning P. Central apnea index decreases after prolonged treatment with acetazolamide. Am J Respir Crit Care Med. 1995;151(1):87–91.
85. Javaheri S, Parker TJ, Wexler L, Liming JD, Lindower P, Roselle GA. Effect of theophylline on sleep-disordered breathing in heart failure. N Engl J Med. 1996;335(8):562–7.
86. Quadri S, Drake C, Hudgel DW. Improvement of idiopathic central sleep apnea with zolpidem. J Clin Sleep Med. 2009;5(2):122–9.
87. Maresh S, Prowting J, Vaughan S, et al. Buspirone decreases susceptibility to hypocapnic central sleep apnea in chronic SCI patients. J Appl Physiol (1985). 2020;129(4):675–82.
88. Giannoni A, Borrelli C, Mirizzi G, Richerson GB, Emdin M, Passino C. Benefit of buspirone on chemoreflex and central apnoeas in heart failure: a randomized controlled crossover trial. Eur J Heart Fail. 2021;23(2):312–20.
89. Javaheri S, Ahmed M, Parker TJ, Brown CR. Effects of nasal O2 on sleep-related disordered breathing in ambulatory patients with stable heart failure. Sleep. 1999;22(8):1101–6.
90. Chowdhuri S, Sinha P, Pranathiageswaran S, Badr MS. Sustained hyperoxia stabilizes breathing in healthy individuals during NREM sleep. J Appl Physiol (1985). 2010;109(5):1378–83.
91. Xie A, Rankin F, Rutherford R, Bradley TD. Effects of inhaled CO2 and added dead space on idiopathic central sleep apnea. J Appl Physiol (1985). 1997;82(3):918–26.
92. Badr MS, Grossman JE, Weber SA. Treatment of refractory sleep apnea with supplemental carbon dioxide. Am J Respir Crit Care Med. 1994;150(2):561–4.
93. Ding N, Zhang X. Transvenous phrenic nerve stimulation, a novel therapeutic approach for central sleep apnea. J Thorac Dis. 2018;10(3):2005–10.
94. Costanzo MR, Javaheri S, Ponikowski P, et al. Transvenous phrenic nerve stimulation for treatment of central sleep apnea: five-year safety and efficacy outcomes. Nat Sci Sleep. 2021;13:515–26.
95. Schwartz AR, Goldberg LR, McKane S, Morgenthaler TI. Transvenous phrenic nerve stimulation improves central sleep apnea, sleep quality, and quality of life regardless of prior positive airway pressure treatment. Sleep Breath. 2021;25(4):2053–63.

Chapter 9
Sleep and Hypoventilation

Amanda J. Piper

Keywords Sleep hypoventilation · hypercapnia · respiratory failure · obesity hypoventilation syndrome · neuromuscular disease · sleep disordered breathing

General Introduction

Sleep can present a significant challenge to respiration in people with respiratory or ventilatory control disorders. The normal physiological changes in breathing associated with sleep may be exaggerated in these populations, resulting in sleep disruption and hypoventilation. Sleep-related hypoventilation is most commonly seen in patients with morbid obesity, neuromuscular disorders (NMD) or severe chronic obstructive pulmonary disease (COPD). Failure to recognize and treat sleep hypoventilation leads to eventual daytime hypercapnia and premature mortality. However, signs and symptoms suggestive of sleep hypoventilation are often non-specific and vague, and so the condition may be overlooked or misdiagnosed preventing timely and appropriate intervention. In this chapter, the general mechanisms relevant to the development of sleep hypoventilation will be reviewed as well as issues specific to the major diagnostic groups likely to present with sleep hypoventilation.

A. J. Piper (✉)
Department of Respiratory and Sleep Medicine, Royal Prince Alfred Hospital, Camperdown, NSW, Australia

Faculty of Medicine and Health, University of Sydney, Camperdown, NSW, Australia
e-mail: amanda.piper@sydney.edu.au

© Springer Nature Switzerland AG 2022
M. S. Badr, J. L. Martin (eds.), *Essentials of Sleep Medicine*,
Respiratory Medicine, https://doi.org/10.1007/978-3-030-93739-3_9

Normal Sleep Breathing

When an individual goes from awake to sleep, a number of physiological changes occur within the respiratory system. These include a reduction in respiratory centre output to the upper airway and respiratory muscles, along with reduced chemoreceptor responsiveness to oxygen (O_2) and carbon dioxide (CO_2). As a consequence, upper airway resistance increases, lung volumes decrease and respiration can become more variable and shallower, resulting in a small fall in minute ventilation of around 10–15% along with rises in CO_2 of 2–7 mmHg [1, 2]. Oxygen saturation during sleep is also lower by around 2%. During rapid eye movement (REM) sleep, inhibition of postural muscles including the intercostal and accessory respiratory muscles leaves the diaphragm to maintain ventilation [1, 3]. Chemosensitivity to both O_2 and CO_2 is further reduced in this sleep stage [4]. These changes in ventilation and gas exchange are relatively minor and of little clinical consequence. However, when overlaid on pre-existing pulmonary or neuromuscular pathology, significant reductions in ventilation and abnormalities in gas exchange can occur [3]. These reductions are generally related to falls in tidal volume, and hence alveolar ventilation, and most marked in REM sleep [3] (Fig. 9.1). However, over time with ongoing attenuation of ventilatory responsiveness to chemostimulation, extension of hypoventilation into non-REM (NREM) and wakefulness eventually occurs. In addition, the reduction in lung volumes [5] and reduced activation of the upper airway muscles with the onset of sleep can produce flow limitation and upper airway collapse, resulting in an added challenge to breathing during sleep in some at risk populations.

Compensatory Mechanisms in Hypoventilation Syndromes

A number of defensive or compensatory mechanisms can be brought into play to minimize disturbance of gas exchange during sleep in those experiencing sleep hypoventilation. The most obvious of these is arousal from sleep in the face of significant changes in gas exchange. Through arousal, albeit brief, ventilation can be restored at least to some extent, limiting the degree of oxygen saturation fall and carbon dioxide accumulation. However, frequent arousal from sleep will impair sleep quality, producing daytime symptoms, and if persistent will contribute to attenuated chemosensitivity [6]. In addition, hypoxia impairs the arousal response to compromised ventilation [7]. In an ongoing cycle, longer periods of abnormal gas exchange occur before arousal produces some, although incomplete, restoration of ventilation with consequent higher levels of CO_2 and lower levels of oxygen. This further impairs ventilatory responsiveness to changes in gas exchange, eventually seeing the development of hypoventilation throughout the sleep period and eventually wakefulness [8].

In an attempt to improve sleep and breathing, patients may alter their sleeping position. Vital capacity (VC) is reduced from the upright to supine position in those

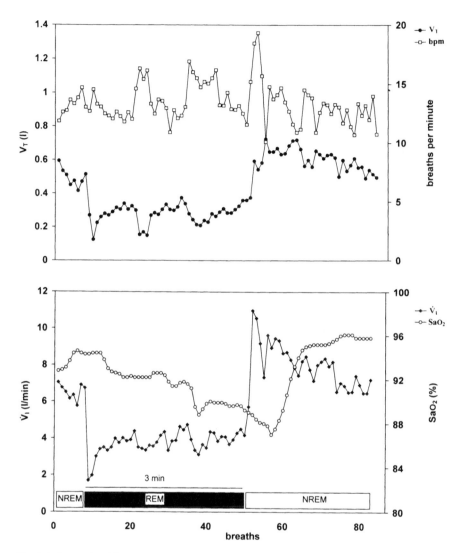

Fig. 9.1 In people with nocturnal hypoventilation, a significant fall in minute ventilation (Vi) during sleep occurs, most marked during REM sleep. As shown in the top panel, this fall in ventilation and oxygen saturation is primarily driven by a reduction in tidal volume (V_T) (bottom panel). (Reprinted with permission of the American Thoracic Society. Copyright © 2020 American Thoracic Society. All rights reserved. Becker et al. [3]. The American Journal of Respiratory and Critical Care Medicine is an official journal of the American Thoracic Society)

with diaphragmatic weakness or where diaphragmatic movement is restricted due to abdominal obesity. In order to minimize orthopnoea, the supine position may be avoided, or patients will use multiple pillows to assume a more upright position in bed. Some morbidly obese individuals have spent months or years in a chair at night in an attempt to both sleep and breathe.

Since the physiological changes occurring during sleep make breathing most vulnerable during the REM period, a reduction or absence of this sleep stage minimizes the likelihood of significant abnormalities in gas exchange occurring. However, this also produces sleep disruption and has been shown to be associated with poorer outcomes in some conditions [9].

Recruitment of accessory respiratory muscles such as the sternomastoid and scalene during inspiration and the abdominal muscle during expiration occurs in some patients with diaphragmatic dysfunction during wakefulness and NREM sleep. This is thought to be an adaptive mechanism to maintain ventilation particularly in NREM sleep in response to reduced neural drive [10]. With the normal loss of postural muscle tone during REM, accessory respiratory muscles are no longer able to contribute to maintaining ventilation, resulting in deterioration in gas exchange [11, 12]. In some patients however, persistence of extradiaphragmatic muscle activity during REM occurs [9, 13, 14]. In a group of patients with amyotrophic lateral sclerosis (ALS) and diaphragmatic dysfunction, those in whom sternomastoid activity continued in REM sleep not only maintained this sleep stage for longer but survival was also better compared to those individuals not exhibiting this behaviour [9]. More recently, persistence of neck muscle activity during sleep was evaluated in a group of severe COPD patients recovering from an exacerbation [14]. While no patient showed neck muscle activity while awake, 26 of the 29 studied demonstrated inspiratory neck muscle activity during sleep. In 17 patients, this occurred in Stage 3 sleep only while in 9, there was persistence of activity throughout sleep. Compared to those showing no or intermittent sleep neck muscle activity, patients where the neck muscles were activated throughout sleep experienced greater sleep disruption, more exacerbations in the year prior to the study and were more likely to be re-hospitalized over the next 6 months with an exacerbation. However, there was no difference between groups in awake $PaCO_2$ or nocturnal hypoventilation/ hypoxemia.

Irrespective of the primary underlying disorder, those with sleep hypoventilation exhibit a reduced responsiveness to CO_2. In response to abnormally low breathing during sleep, CO_2 rises transiently. If there is insufficient restorative ventilation between these abnormal breathing periods, CO_2 accumulates. In order to maintain pH levels, renal compensation with retention of bicarbonate occurs. However, these elevated blood bicarbonate levels blunt ventilatory responsiveness to CO_2 [15], contributing to further progression of respiratory failure. In obesity hypoventilation syndrome (OHS), patients with a lower ventilatory response to CO_2 spent a greater percentage of REM sleep in hypoventilation [16] (Fig. 9.2). Studies investigating how nocturnal non-invasive ventilation (NIV) achieves improved awake gas exchange in chronic hypoventilation found that an increase in ventilatory responsiveness to CO_2 was the main mechanism in patients with restrictive thoracic disorders [17], and played a significant role along with reduced gas trapping in those with chronic obstructive pulmonary disease (COPD) [18].

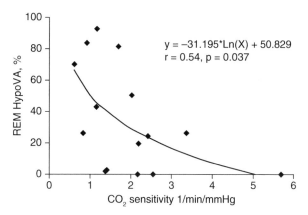

Fig. 9.2 In obesity, hypoventilation syndrome, a significant relationship between baseline CO_2 sensitivity and the amount of hypoventilation during REM sleep has been shown such that patients with lower CO_2 ventilatory responsiveness will spend more of REM sleep in hypoventilation. (From Chouri-Pontarollo et al. [16] with permission)

$$y = -31.195 * Ln(X) + 50.829$$
$$r = 0.54, p = 0.037$$

Identifying and Defining Sleep Hypoventilation

Traditionally, arterial blood gas measurements have been performed to detect raised CO_2, which is the hallmark of hypoventilation. However, repeated arterial punctures or the insertion of an arterial line to monitor CO_2 during sleep is not practical or appropriate to identify sleep hypoventilation. Furthermore, the development of awake hypercapnic respiratory failure is considered to be a late manifestation of sleep hypoventilation, particularly in those with neuromuscular or chest wall disorders. Consequently, clinicians have sought simpler, less invasive methods of identifying sleep hypoventilation before awake hypercapnia is present to prevent acute respiratory decompensation.

Daytime Measures to Identify Sleep Hypoventilation

Patients with sleep hypoventilation may complain of an array of symptoms, related to both sleep and daytime function (Table 9.1). However, symptoms alone are not a good guide in identifying possible sleep hypoventilation due to their vague and non-specific nature. Additionally, some individuals will not even be aware they are experiencing symptoms until effective therapy has been established. In other cases, reported symptoms may be erroneously attributed to the underlying disorder and further investigation of potential sleep breathing problems overlooked.

In neuromuscular disorders (NMD), a number of simple clinic tests have been used to identify those most at risk of sleep hypoventilation. The most widely used measure is VC, with a previous study in a mixed group of muscular dystrophies and myopathies finding a VC <40% of predicted identified those likely to have continuous hypoventilation while daytime respiratory failure was likely to been seen with a VC <25% of predicted [19]. Supine VC improves the predictive value of this measure

Table 9.1 Symptoms commonly associated with sleep hypoventilation

Daytime fatigue
Daytime sleepiness
Morning headaches
Sleep disruption
Orthopnoea
Dyspnoea
Confusion
Insomnia
Nightmares

[19], with a fall from the upright position >20% suggestive of diaphragm weakness [20] and therefore a higher suspicion of sleep hypoventilation. In ALS, VC is widely used as a predictor of survival and an indicator to commence nocturnal NIV [21], but has limited predictive power in identifying sleep hypoventilation. For instance, in a study of 250 patients with ALS, Boentert et al. [22] found that a third of those with an upright VC >75% of predicted showed sleep hypoventilation while, in contrast, almost half of those with a VC <in 50% predicted, no nocturnal hypoventilation was seen. Other simple measures of inspiratory muscle strength used in conjunction with VC measures are maximum inspiratory pressure (MIP) and sniff nasal inspiratory pressure (SNIP). This latter measurement is particularly useful in patients with facial muscle weakness who find it difficult to maintain a lip seal around a mouthpiece [23]. Nocturnal hypoventilation is unlikely to occur until MIP is <40 cmH_2O [19], but this test may give falsely low values in some patients due to leak around the mouthpiece or from an inability to sustain a maximal inspiratory effort [24]. In ALS patients, a SNIP <40 cmH_2O correlates well with nocturnal hypoxia [23]. Although there is a good correlation between MIP and SNIP in NMD, these tests are not interchangeable and whenever possible should be performed concurrently [25].

Measures of daytime pulmonary function have not been shown to be sufficiently sensitive to predict hypoventilation in OHS or COPD. In patients presenting with obesity and potential sleep disordered breathing, the goal is to identify those in whom an arterial blood gas should be taken in order to confirm a diagnosis of OHS. In this population, oxygen saturation by pulse oximetry (SpO_2) rather than spirometric measures is generally used as a screening tool to identify those at risk for awake hypercapnia. Chung et al. [26] showed an awake supine SpO_2 <91% had a 34.8% sensitivity and 96.6% specificity for detecting daytime hypercapnia in a group of super-obese individuals (body mass index [BMI] >50 kg/m^2) presenting to a sleep laboratory. In another study, a combination of clinic SpO_2 and FVC was found to be highly sensitive in detecting awake hypercapnia in obese individuals with an abnormal nocturnal oximetry, although specificity was low [27]. Only one study has sought to identify obesity-related sleep hypoventilation, a potential early stage of OHS [28, 29]. In a group of morbidly obese patients (BMI > 40 kg/m^2), an awake SpO_2 measured in the supine position of ≤93% was found to predict sleep hypoventilation with a sensitivity of 39% and specificity of 98% [30]. However, recent guidelines on evaluating and managing OHS suggest that SpO_2 during wakefulness should not be used to screen for OHS in obese patients with obstructive sleep apnoea (OSA) due to insufficient data [31]. Although patients with low awake PaO_2 or SpO_2 are more likely to desaturate at night [32], this is not necessarily related to hypoventilation alone, and overall daytime awake pulmonary function values do not correlate well with nocturnal desaturation [33].

Elevated levels of bicarbonate or base excess measured by venous or arterial bloods can be useful to suggest or screen out sleep hypoventilation. Base excess >3 mmol/L has been reported to be a significant predictor of sleep hypoventilation in ALS [22] and Duchenne muscular dystrophy (DMD) [34], although with only moderate sensitivity. In obese individuals with OSA, a serum bicarbonate <27 mmol/L makes the diagnosis of OHS very unlikely [31]. However, caution needs to be exercised when interpreting bicarbonate levels, as these can be influenced by factors other than a raised CO_2 [35].

Nocturnal Monitoring to Identify Sleep Hypoventilation

While awake testing in some populations can raise the suspicion of sleep hypoventilation, as discussed previously these measures remain limited in their ability to predict sleep hypoventilation and detect its severity. Consequently, more direct monitoring of gas exchange during sleep is needed to identify sleep hypoventilation at an earlier stage.

Nocturnal oximetry has been widely used as a potential surrogate for detecting sleep disordered breathing and hypoxemia. Although cyclical episodes of desaturation–resaturation may be suggestive of obstructive breathing, it does not reveal anything about CO_2 levels. Even if sustained hypoxemia is present, this cannot be used as evidence for hypoventilation, as this pattern can also occur with ventilation–perfusion mismatching. Furthermore, oximetry can miss sleep hypoventilation in around a third of individuals with NMD [22], and is not informative in those using supplemental oxygen. Adding a morning blood gas to nocturnal oximetry may still miss the presence of nocturnal hypoventilation in 20–30% of patients with neuromuscular disorders [22, 36]. Despite some technical limitations, transcutaneous carbon dioxide ($TcCO_2$) is now recommended to identify sleep hypoventilation across a range of respiratory disorders [37], with monitoring able to be performed both within sleep laboratories and in patient homes [38]. While advances in technology have significantly improved the relationship between $PaCO_2$ and $TcCO_2$ (Fig. 9.3), there may be an overestimation of CO_2 over time due to signal drift [40]. However, correction for this drift considerably improves the reliability of the measurement [39]. The addition of polygraphy and polysomnography to the assessment of patients with potential sleep hypoventilation provides additional information about the nature of the respiratory events, or in the case of polysomnography, sleep quality and duration. However, limited access, wait times,

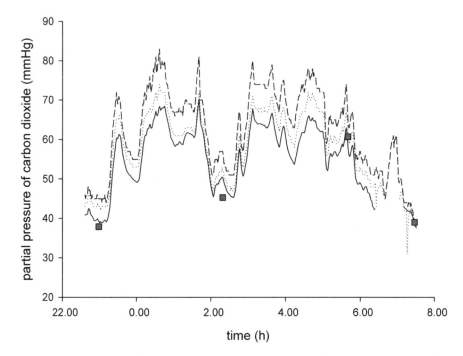

Fig. 9.3 Significant fluctuations in nocturnal CO_2 can occur which may be missed if a single blood gas measure is made. In this illustration, continuous monitoring by two transcutaneous carbon dioxide devices (the solid and broken lines) capture the variability in CO_2 levels that are occurring in this patient who is using nocturnal ventilatory support. Blood gases (represented by the grey boxes) can only capture CO_2 at a single point in time and can easily miss this variability. Improvements in technology in recent years have significantly improved the accuracy and reliability of transcutaneous CO_2 monitoring. (From Storre et al. [39] with permission)

cost and a lack of facilities to properly care for individuals with significant physical impediments in sleep laboratories often mean that more limited nocturnal monitoring is undertaken.

One of the difficulties in comparing studies of sleep hypoventilation has been the various definitions that have been employed to describe this phenomenon. Ogna and colleagues [41] compared the prevalence of hypoventilation in an unselected adult NMD population according to eight different definitions commonly found in the literature. Depending on the definition used, hypoventilation ranged from 10% to 61%, even when only definitions around $TcCO_2$ were used (Fig. 9.4). The most widely recognized definition at present is that proposed by the American Academy of Sleep Medicine [37] which suggests "an increase in the arterial $PaCO_2$ (or surrogate) to a value > 55 mmHg for $\geq$ 10 minutes, or a $\geq$ 10 mmHg increase in $PaCO_2$ (or surrogate) during sleep (in comparison to an awake supine value) to a value exceeding 50 mmHg for $\geq$ 10 minutes." However, these thresholds are based on expert consensus and may be less sensitive than other definitions in identifying patients with NMD and daytime normocapnia likely to require ventilatory support

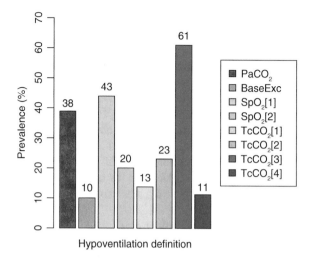

Fig. 9.4 Numerous definitions of sleep hypoventilation have appeared in the literature which will significantly impact on the prevalence of the disorder. This is illustrated by a study of 232 patients with neuromuscular disorders where the prevalence of sleep hypoventilation ranged from 10.3% to 61.2% depending on the definition used. Legend – $PaCO_2$: awake $PaCO_2$ >45 mmHg; BaseExc: awake base excess ≥4 mmol/L; SpO_2 [1]: nocturnal SpO_2 ≤88% for 5 consecutive minutes; SpO_2 [2]: mean nocturnal SpO_2 <90% or SpO_2 <90% during >10% of recording time; $TcCO_2$ [1]: $TcCO_2$ >55 mmHg; $TcCO_2$ [2]: increase in $TcCO_2$ ≥10 mmHg (in comparison to an awake supine value) to a value exceeding 50 mmHg for ≥10 min; $TcCO_2$ [3]: peak $TcCO_2$ >49 mmHg; $TcCO_2$ [4]: mean $TcCO_2$ >50 mmHg; $TcCO_2$: transcutaneous carbon dioxide. (From Ogna et al. [41] with permission)

within the next 24 months [42, 43]. There is also limited information around how these definitions relate to other clinical and patient reported outcomes [44].

Disease-Specific Issues in Sleep Hypoventilation

Obesity Hypoventilation Syndrome

Obesity hypoventilation syndrome (OHS) is diagnosed in obese individuals (BMI > 30 kg/m^2) who present with awake hypercapnia ($PaCO_2$ > 45 mmHg) when other known causes of hypoventilation such as lung or neuromuscular disease cannot be identified. Obstructive sleep apnoea is present in 90% of these individuals, with 70% showing an apnoea hypopnea index ≥30/hour [45]. In the remaining 10% hypoventilation alone is seen, particularly marked during REM sleep. The prevalence of OHS varies depending on the clinical setting these individuals are seen in and the BMI of the population. Current estimates put the prevalence of OHS in the general community at around 0.3%, [46] with the likelihood of OHS increasing with BMI. In obese patients referred to sleep clinics, 10–20% will have OHS [47, 48].

This disorder represents one of the most common causes of sleep hypoventilation seen in sleep laboratories and for some years has been a major indication for home NIV [49, 50].

Although upper airway obstruction is common in this condition, OHS is more than just severe OSA. This condition is associated with worse outcomes than eucapnic obesity with or without OSA, with patients presenting with more comorbidities including chronic heart failure and pulmonary hypertension [51, 52], worse social circumstances [53, 54], more healthcare resource use [54] and lower survival rates even after therapy is commenced [55, 56]. Unfortunately, appropriate treatment is often delayed with patients being misdiagnosed with obstructive pulmonary disease or congestive cardiac failure [58], or the diagnosis overlooked completely [59]. In some series, up to 70% of patients were diagnosed only after presenting with acute on chronic respiratory failure [55].

The mechanisms around the development of hypoventilation in some obese patients with or without OSA and not others are not fully understood, but involves a complex interplay between abnormal lung mechanics, respiratory drive, neurohormonal factors and sleep disordered breathing. The degree to which each of these factors contributes to hypoventilation in obesity likely varies between individuals and may influence clinical presentation and outcomes. Two distinct phenotypes of this disorder are currently recognized. Those with a high severity of OSA in conjunction with OHS appear to be younger, generally male, more obese and hypersomnolent with worse nocturnal and daytime gas exchange but with a lower cardiovascular and metabolic risk compared to the OHS without OSA phenotype [60].

In morbid obesity, deposition of adipose tissue around the abdomen and chest wall reduces lung volumes (particularly expiratory reserve volume) and thoracic compliance [61]. Breathing at these lower volumes increases airway resistance and promotes small airway closure, both of which place a further load on breathing [62]. This adds to an elevated work of breathing [63] and worsening ventilation perfusion distribution. In response to these changes in respiratory loads and lung mechanics, neural drive in morbid obesity is increased two to three times that seen in normal weight controls [62]. However OHS patients lack this augmented drive [64], and as a consequence minute ventilation is insufficient to maintain eucapnia, especially given CO_2 production is also increased due to obesity [65]. In addition, ventilatory responses to O_2 and CO_2 are diminished compared to eucapnic OSA [16, 66], as is the response to CO_2 loading during sleep compared to those with eucapnic obesity [67], further promoting CO_2 retention. A more blunted ventilatory responsiveness to CO_2 is associated with more severe hypoventilation during rapid eye movement (REM) sleep [16]. This reduced responsiveness appears to be secondary to sleep disordered breathing as improvements are seen after PAP use in many individuals even if BMI and lung function are unchanged [16, 66, 68].

The lower lung volumes associated with obesity increase the risk of upper airway obstruction during sleep. The majority of patients with OHS have significant OSA [45] which can be another contributor to CO_2 retention during sleep. Indeed, even awake upper airway resistance is significantly higher in OHS compared eucapnic obesity [69]. Following obstructed nocturnal breathing differences in the pattern of ventilation between eucapnic and hypercapnic patients with OSA have been observed [70]. The length of the ventilation recovery period between events compared to the event length is shortened [67, 71], while the magnitude by which ventilation increases post event is diminished in those with hypercapnic compared to their eucapnic counterparts [67]. This pattern permits an accumulation of CO_2 during the obstructed event with insufficient offloading of CO_2 in the post-arousal period. Over time, metabolic compensation by the kidneys to maintain pH produces an increase in bicarbonate levels, thereby further blunting ventilatory drive [72].

A common thread between sleep disordered breathing, altered respiratory mechanics and reduced respiratory drive in OHS may be some of the adipokines and hormones associated with obesity. Leptin is a protein designed to regulate appetite and energy expenditure which also acts as a powerful stimulant of ventilation. In both obesity and OSA, serum leptin levels are elevated, suggesting a compensatory response for the increased ventilatory load in order to maintain eucapnia [73]. Fasting serum leptin levels are higher again in OHS patients compared to eucapnic obese individuals [73]. Hyperleptinemia has been shown to be associated with a reduction in both respiratory drive and ventilatory responsiveness to CO_2 [74], and even when leptin levels are similar, the hypercapnic ventilatory response appears to be significantly lower in hypercapnic patients compared with those who were eucapnic [75]. It appears that the stimulatory effects of leptin are attenuated in OHS, likely from reduced leptin permeability across the blood-brain barrier [76]. Leptin also appears to be involved in maintaining neuromuscular drive to the upper airway muscles during sleep [77] and could account for the high frequency of OSA in many patients with OHS. In an interesting study in diet-induced obese mice, intra-nasal leptin used to bypass the blood–brain barrier significantly reduced obstructed breathing while also increasing minute ventilation during periods of non-flow limited breathing [78]. It remains unclear if similar benefits would be achieved in humans [79], but it does provide interesting insights into the potential of improving central concentrations of leptin in OHS.

Initial management of OHS involves commencing positive airway pressure (PAP) to stabilize breathing and gas exchange during sleep. There has been some debate around what form of PAP therapy is most appropriate both initially and as long-term treatment. Since upper airway obstruction is seen in the majority of patients, it is reasonable to start most OHS patients with concurrent OSA on continuous PAP (CPAP) therapy. This approach is supported by several RCTs [45, 80–82] and systematic reviews [83, 84] demonstrating that both medium (<3 months) [45, 80, 82] and long-term (>3 years) [81, 83] outcomes including resolution of awake $PaCO_2$ and symptoms, changes in pulmonary artery pressure, healthcare use and survival are similar whether CPAP or bilevel PAP therapy is used. Adherence to therapy appears to be a more important factor in PAP choice than the type of PAP [81, 85, 86]. Improvements with CPAP in terms of nocturnal gas exchange [82, 87], awake CO_2 [80, 81] and pulmonary hypertension [88] may be a little slower to emerge over the first weeks or months of therapy, but so long as patients are adherent to therapy, similar long-term outcomes including hospitalizations and survival are achieved with CPAP and bilevel therapy [81]. However, close monitoring during the early period of therapy is needed to identify non-responders. These include patients with more restrictive pulmonary mechanics, higher initial awake CO_2 levels [80] and lower baseline AHI [89, 90]. Bilevel therapy is recommended in the OHS-sleep hypoventilation only phenotype [91] and those presenting with acute on chronic hypercapnic respiratory failure [92]. Despite control of sleep disordered breathing and good adherence to PAP, at least 20% of patients with OHS will continue to experience some residual awake hypercapnia (generally 45–49 mmHg range) [85, 86] but with minimal clinical symptoms.

As weight is a central issue involved in the development of OHS, steps to address this should be undertaken. However, significant weight loss of around 25–35% is probably needed to resolve OHS, while losses <10% are unlikely to achieve clinically important outcomes [93]. Cardiovascular disease becomes the predominant cause of death following the use of PAP therapy, so early identification and follow up of cardiometabolic risk factors is needed [94].

A key aspect of defining OHS has been the presence of awake hypercapnia ($PaCO_2$ > 45 mmHg). Given the importance of identifying patients with OHS early, it has been suggested that the presence of diurnal hypercapnia already represents an advanced stage of OHS [28]. A recent European Respiratory Society task force divided hypoventilation into five stages [28]. Stage 0 represented eucapnic OSA. Stages I and II described obesity-related sleep hypoventilation (ORSH), with a bicarbonate level <27 mmol/L or ≥27 mmol/L, respectively. The taskforce saw daytime hypercapnia as being present only in the most advanced OHS stages of III and IV, with Stage IV having concurrent comorbidities. Similar to patients with neuromuscular and chest wall restriction, eucapnic obese individuals with nocturnal-only hypoventilation may eventually progress to these more advanced stages of OHS. Although longitudinal studies have not been performed to confirm this progression, in a cross-sectional study of obese individuals, those with a raised serum base excess (BE) ≥2 mmol/L were found to have ventilatory responses and sleep-breathing measures lying between those with normal awake $PaCO_2$ and BE and those with awake hypercapnia [29]. Whether isolated sleep hypoventilation is part of the OHS spectrum or whether it represents a distinct phenotype [30] has not been established. It is also unknown if early identification and intervention can prevent the development of full blown OHS with its attendant comorbidities and reduced survival.

Neuromuscular Disorders

Neuromuscular disorders (NMDs) cover a broad group of diseases where sleep hypoventilation occurs as a consequence of involvement of the respiratory motor neurons, peripheral nerves, the neuromuscular junction or the respiratory muscles themselves. These disorders can be inherited or acquired, rapidly or slowly progressive. Irrespective of the primary diagnosis, untreated many will develop respiratory complications and awake hypercapnia, with death from respiratory infection and respiratory failure common. Changes in respiratory muscle function and breathing control during sleep interact to produce hypoventilation, earliest and most marked in REM sleep, irrespective of the pathogenesis of the primary disorder.

The age of onset of sleep hypoventilation will vary considerably depending on the primary diagnosis. Sleep hypoventilation can be expected during early childhood in spinal muscular atrophy (SMA) type I and in some with SMA type 2, while in Duchenne muscular dystrophy (DMD) this usually occurs sometime during late adolescence or early adulthood. People with ALS commonly present in the fifth and sixth decades of life, with sleep hypoventilation generally occurring some 12 or so months after diagnosis [95, 96]. The stage at which diaphragm involvement occurs is central to the appearance of hypoventilation and this can vary considerably within and between disorders. Obesity and chest wall deformity will also influence the onset on sleep hypoventilation by further adding to respiratory muscle load/capacity imbalance.

Upper airway obstruction during sleep in neuromuscular disorders is not uncommon [22, 97]. These obstructive events may arise from the usual mechanical factors associated with OSA such as obesity, the supine position, enlarged tonsils or retrognathia. However, there are some aspects of NMD which may promote upper airway instability such as low lung volumes from respiratory muscle weakness, pharyngeal hypotonia and macroglossia [98]. A bimodal pattern of sleep disordered breathing has been reported in some disorders including DMD, acid maltase deficiency and ALS [22, 96, 99], with obstructive events more common initially, progressing to more "pseudocentral" events and hypoventilation with disease progression. This transition likely reflects increasing inspiratory muscle weakness, particularly that of the diaphragm, whereby insufficient inspiratory pressure is generated to create complete airway collapse [22, 98]. Obstructive events could also be related to obesity, an enlarged tongue with posterior displacement or reduced pharyngeal tone. In ALS, these obstructive events do not appear to be related to bulbar dysfunction [22], but have been associated with shorter survival [100, 101].

In some neuromuscular diseases, a primary abnormality in ventilatory control may be present in addition to peripheral muscle weakness. Myotonic dystrophy, the most common type of muscular dystrophy, has a high prevalence of both excessive daytime sleepiness and sleep disordered breathing [102]. However, there does not appear to be a direct relationship between sleepiness and abnormal nocturnal breathing, nor between pulmonary function and sleep disordered breathing [103, 104]. It is thought that neuronal loss in CNS structures regulating central respiratory drive might be an underlying contributor to sleep-breathing abnormalities in these patient [104, 105]. In ALS, periodic clustering of desaturation during sleep has been found in some patients despite normal respiratory function and neurophysiological phrenic nerve and diaphragm tests [106, 107]. These episodes occur despite normal respiratory movements, suggesting instability in central respiratory control. During NIV, upper airway obstruction with reduced respiratory drive has been shown to be a common reason for inadequate ventilatory support during NIV, with shorter survival even when these events are not associated with desaturation [100]. In investigating mechanisms for this, Sancho and colleagues [108] found those exhibiting upper airway obstruction with reduced respiratory drive during NIV had greater respiratory instability, with higher controller gain values and lower CO_2 reserves compare to ALS patients without these events. Moreover, these patients were more likely to have upper motor neuron predominant dysfunction at the bulbar level. Increasing EPAP or changing masks would have little effect on improving obstructive events if they are caused by hyperreflexia and adduction of the vocal folds [108].

In NMD, poor cough with secretion accumulation can also contribute to hypoventilation, with chest infection and pneumonia being major causes of respiratory morbidity and mortality [109]. Reduced inspiratory muscle strength limits the inspired volume able to be achieved pre-cough while impaired glottic control and weak expiratory muscles adversely impact the effectiveness of expiratory flow rates needed to expel secretions from the large airways. Cough augmentation and lung volume recruitment techniques form an essential part of the holistic management of these individuals, and may need to be introduced prior to the use of NIV.

COPD

Poor-quality sleep is common in COPD [110] and is predictive of exacerbations, emergency healthcare utilization and mortality [111, 112]. Although the source of this disruption may be caused by other factors such as medications, secretions, nicotine use and reflux, sleep disordered breathing is a common, frequently overlooked contributor.

Worsening respiratory mechanics and reduced inspiratory neural drive [10, 113] appear to underlie sleep hypoventilation in COPD. With the onset of sleep, neural drive decreases in parallel with reductions in ventilation [10]. In addition, diaphragm inefficiency brought on by hyperinflation is offset to some extent by recruitment of the accessory respiratory muscles in an attempt maintain ventilation. However, when this activity is lost during REM sleep, tidal volume is reduced with ensuing hypoventilation. Lung hyperinflation itself has been associated with increased arousal from sleep [114]. In some patients with COPD, increased upper airway resistance, even in the absence of frank obstruction may occur, contributing further to sleep hypoventilation [115].

Once awake hypercapnia develops, prognosis is poorer than in patients with hypoxemia alone [116]. However few studies have investigated isolated sleep-related hypoventilation and its consequences in COPD. Prevalence rates of sleep hypoventilation have varied considerably depending on how hypoventilation was defined and measured [14, 33, 117]. In studies of hypercapnic COPD patients using long-term oxygen therapy, prevalence rates of 21–43% have been reported [33, 117]. In a prospective, observational study of 100 stable COPD patients attending an inpatient rehabilitation program, Holmedahl et al. [118] identified sleep hypoventilation in 15 subjects, including 6 subjects with awake normocapnia. While BMI and AHI were similar between awake hypercapnic and normocapnic groups with sleep hypoventilation, FEV1 was significantly higher in the normocapnic group (1.45 vs 0.63L). In a small study of 21 selected patients with stable severe COPD without significant awake hypercapnia, Kitajima et al. [119] identified ten patients with episodic sleep hypoventilation, defined as an increase of ≥ 5 mmHg in $TcCO_2$ from baseline for

≥5 mins continuously accompanied by at least one episode of oxygen desaturation. Those demonstrating episodic sleep hypoventilation had higher markers of pulmonary hypertension and experienced more frequent admissions in the previous year than the group without these episodic events. Although early identification of sleep hypoventilation and intervention may reduce morbidity and mortality as seen in other hypoventilating disorders, this premise has not been tested in COPD. Currently non-invasive ventilatory support (NIV) is introduced in stable patients when awake or persistent hypercapnia is detected, usually when awake $PaCO_2$ values 50 mmHg or greater [120–123]. Recently published evidence-based guidelines support the use of NIV for COPD when the above conditions are present, with the suggestion that NIV settings need to target a significant reduction in CO_2 [124].

Generally, chronic hypoventilation is most likely seen in COPD with more severe airflow limitation. However, if upper airway obstruction occurs in those with only moderately altered respiratory mechanics, nocturnal and awake hypercapnia may be present at levels of lung function not normally associated with hypoventilation [125]. Obstructive sleep apnoea is not an uncommon finding in COPD, with prevalence rates ranging 3–65%, depending on the clinical population studied, severity of the underlying lung disease, BMI and age [126–128]. The occurrence of both disorders in the same patient is described as "overlap" and is of clinical relevance since these individuals usually have more severe hypoxemia and hypercapnia, as well as higher mortality rates compared to either disease alone [57, 126] (Fig. 9.5). Quality

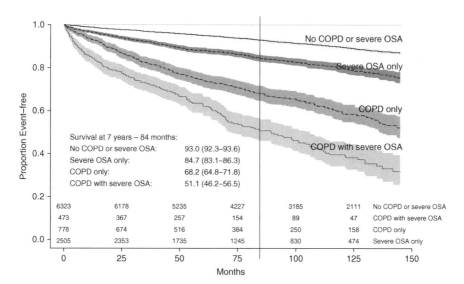

Fig. 9.5 Unadjusted Kaplan–Meier event-free survival curves showing the impact of severe obstructive sleep apnoea (OSA) (apnoea–hypopnea index >30) in people chronic obstructive pulmonary disease (COPD) compared to either disease alone. Outcome was defined as a composite of hospitalization due to myocardial infarction, stroke, congestive heart failure, cardiac revascularization procedures or death from any cause. (Reprinted with permission of the American Thoracic Society. Copyright © 2020 American Thoracic Society. All rights reserved. Kendzerska et al. [57]. Annals of the American Thoracic Society is an official journal of the American Thoracic Society)

of life among overlap patients is significantly worse than that of COPD-only patients, in addition to more cardiovascular morbidity, more frequent exacerbations and higher healthcare costs than either condition alone [127]. In contrast to COPD-only patients where sleep hypoventilation appears to be mainly a consequence of reduced neural respiratory drive [10], in overlap the fall in ventilation seen during sleep is largely due to an increase in upper airway resistance [129]. A small pilot study in overlap patients showed a high loop gain and low arousal threshold likely contributes to the development of OSA and its severity in these individuals [130].

When applying PAP therapy in overlap, the mode of therapy needs to balance reversal of abnormal respiratory mechanics against control of upper airway patency. Where upper airway obstruction predominates, CPAP therapy with or without supplemental oxygen can provide significant benefits including improved blood gases, reduced excerbations [131] and a lower mortality risk [126]. The survival benefit may be more marked in those with baseline hypercapnia [132] (Fig. 9.6). However, higher awake CO_2 levels and more time with SpO_2 <90% during sleep are independent factors predicting CPAP failure [133], when bilevel therapy would be the preferred management option. Close monitoring of hypercapnic overlap patients commencing CPAP is needed to ensure persistent sleep hypoventilation is not occurring.

Summary

Sleep hypoventilation is a frequent occurrence in patients with a wide range of disorders where diaphragmatic weakness, abnormal chest wall mechanics or altered respiratory drive are present. Hypoventilation during sleep can be present

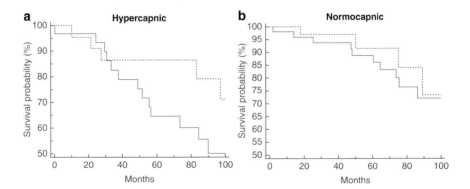

Fig. 9.6 Kaplan–Meier survival curves comparing continuous positive airway pressure (dotted line) to non-treated patients (continuous line) for (**a**) those who were hypercapnic at baseline and (**b**) normocapnic patients. In this study, CPAP treatment reduced the excess risk of death in the hypercapnic group (log rank test 4.16; $p = 0.04$) but not the normocapnic group (Log rank test 0.63; $p = 0.42$). (From Jaoude et al. [132] with permission)

months or years prior to the development of daytime hypercapnia. Recognition and early treatment is considered important since sleep hypoventilation can have a significant impact on quality of life, neurocognition function, health resource use and mortality. Although daytime measures of respiratory function can be helpful in identifying some individuals at risk of sleep hypoventilation, these have a limited ability to accurately detect nocturnal hypoventilation and its severity. Consequently, some measure of CO_2 during sleep is required to capture this disorder. Advancements in technology associated with transcutaneous carbon dioxide monitoring have seen this technique become more widely used to identify the presence and severity of sleep hypoventilation. However, more work is needed to better understand thresholds of CO_2 during sleep that are associated with poorer clinical outcomes.

References

1. Douglas NJ, White DP, Pickett CK, Weil JV, Zwillich CW. Respiration during sleep in normal man. Thorax. 1982;37:840–4.
2. Tabachnik E, Muller NL, Bryan AC, Levison H. Changes in ventilation and chest wall mechanics during sleep in normal adolescents. J Appl Physiol. 1981;51(3):557–64.
3. Becker HF, Piper AJ, Flynn WE, et al. Breathing during sleep in patients with nocturnal desaturation. Am J Respir Crit Care Med. 1999;159(1):112–8.
4. Douglas NJ, White DP, Weil JV, Pickett CK, Zwillich CW. Hypercapnic ventilatory response in sleeping adults. Am Rev Respir Dis. 1982;126(5):758–62.
5. Appelberg J, Nordahl G, Janson C. Lung volume and its correlation to nocturnal apnoea and desaturation. Respir Med. 2000;94(3):233–9.
6. White DP, Douglas NJ, Pickett CK, Zwillich CW, Weil JV. Sleep deprivation and the control of ventilation. Am Rev Respir Dis. 1983;128(6):984–6.
7. Hlavac MC, Catcheside PG, McDonald R, Eckert DJ, Windler S, McEvoy RD. Hypoxia impairs the arousal response to external resistive loading and airway occlusion during sleep. Sleep. 2006;29(5):624–31.
8. Piper A. Sleep abnormalities associated with neuromuscular disease: pathophysiology and evaluation. Semin Respir Crit Care Med. 2002;23(3):211–9.
9. Arnulf I, Similowski T, Salachas F, et al. Sleep disorders and diaphragmatic function in patients with amyotrophic lateral sclerosis. Am J Respir Crit Care Med. 2000;161(3):849–56.
10. Luo YM, He BT, Wu YX, et al. Neural respiratory drive and ventilation in patients with chronic obstructive pulmonary disease during sleep. Am J Respir Crit Care Med. 2014;190(2):227–9.
11. Bye PT, Ellis ER, Issa FG, Donnelly PM, Sullivan CE. Respiratory failure and sleep in neuromuscular disease. Thorax. 1990;45(4):241–7.
12. White JE, Drinnan MJ, Smithson AJ, Griffiths CJ, Gibson GJ. Respiratory muscle activity during rapid eye movement (REM) sleep in patients with chronic obstructive pulmonary disease. Thorax. 1995;50(4):376–82.
13. Bennett JR, Dunroy HM, Corfield DR, et al. Respiratory muscle activity during REM sleep in patients with diaphragm paralysis. Neurology. 2004;62(1):134–7.
14. Redolfi S, Grassion L, Rivals I, et al. Abnormal activity of neck inspiratory muscles during sleep as a prognostic indicator in chronic obstructive pulmonary disease. Am J Respir Crit Care Med. 2020;201(4):414–22.
15. Goldring RM, Turino GM, Heinemann HO. Respiratory-renal adjustments in chronic hypercapnia in man. Extracellular bicarbonate concentration and the regulation of ventilation. Am J Med. 1971;51(6):772–84.

16. Chouri-Pontarollo N, Borel JC, Tamisier R, Wuyam B, Levy P, Pepin JL. Impaired objective daytime vigilance in obesity-hypoventilation syndrome: impact of noninvasive ventilation. Chest. 2007;131(1):148–55.
17. Nickol AH, Hart N, Hopkinson NS, Moxham J, Simonds A, Polkey MI. Mechanisms of improvement of respiratory failure in patients with restrictive thoracic disease treated with non-invasive ventilation. Thorax. 2005;60(9):754–60.
18. Nickol A, Hart N, Hopkinson N, et al. Mechanisms of improvement of respiratory failure in patients with COPD treated with NIV. Int J Chron Obstruct Pulmon Dis. 2008;3(3):453–62.
19. Ragette R, Mellies U, Schwake C, Voit T, Teschler H. Patterns and predictors of sleep disordered breathing in primary myopathies. Thorax. 2002;57(8):724–8.
20. Fromageot C, Lofaso F, Annane D, et al. Supine fall in lung volumes in the assessment of diaphragmatic weakness in neuromuscular disorders. Arch Phys Med Rehabil. 2001;82(1):123–8.
21. Baumann F, Henderson RD, Morrison SC, et al. Use of respiratory function tests to predict survival in amyotrophic lateral sclerosis. Amyotroph Lateral Scler. 2010;11(1-2):194–202.
22. Boentert M, Glatz C, Helmle C, Okegwo A, Young P. Prevalence of sleep apnoea and capnographic detection of nocturnal hypoventilation in amyotrophic lateral sclerosis. J Neurol Neurosurg Psychiatry. 2018;89(4):418–24.
23. Morgan RK, McNally S, Alexander M, Conroy R, Hardiman O, Costello RW. Use of sniff nasal-inspiratory force to predict survival in amyotrophic lateral sclerosis. Am J Respir Crit Care Med. 2005;171(3):269–74.
24. Fitting JW. Sniff nasal inspiratory pressure: simple or too simple? Eur Respir J. 2006;27(5):881–3.
25. Oliveira MJP, Rodrigues F, Firmino-Machado J, et al. Assessment of respiratory muscle weakness in subjects with neuromuscular disease. Respir Care. 2018;63(10):1223–30.
26. Chung Y, Garden FL, Jee AS, et al. Supine awake oximetry as a screening tool for daytime hypercapnia in super-obese patients. Intern Med J. 2017;47(10):1136–41.
27. Mandal S, Suh ES, Boleat E, et al. A cohort study to identify simple clinical tests for chronic respiratory failure in obese patients with sleep-disordered breathing. BMJ Open Respir Res. 2014;1(1):e000022.
28. Randerath W, Verbraecken J, Andreas S, et al. Definition, discrimination, diagnosis and treatment of central breathing disturbances during sleep. Eur Respir J. 2017;49(1):1600959.
29. Manuel ARGM, Mbbs RG, Hart NP, Stradling JRMD. Is a raised bicarbonate, without hypercapnia, part of the physiologic spectrum of obesity-related hypoventilation? Chest. 2015;147(2):362–8.
30. Sivam S, Yee B, Wong K, Wang D, Grunstein R, Piper A. Obesity hypoventilation syndrome: early detection of nocturnal-only hypercapnia in an obese population. J Clin Sleep Med. 2018;14(9):1477–84.
31. Mokhlesi B, Masa JF, Brozek JL, et al. Evaluation and management of Obesity Hypoventilation Syndrome. An official American Thoracic Society clinical practice guideline. Am J Respir Crit Care Med. 2019;200(3):e6–e24.
32. Mulloy E, McNicholas WT. Ventilation and gas exchange during sleep and exercise in severe COPD. Chest. 1996;109(2):387–94.
33. Tarrega J, Anton A, Guell R, et al. Predicting nocturnal hypoventilation in hypercapnic chronic obstructive pulmonary disease patients undergoing long-term oxygen therapy. Respiration. 2011;82(1):4–9.
34. Hukins CA, Hillman DR. Daytime predictors of sleep hypoventilation in Duchenne muscular dystrophy. Am J Respir Crit Care Med. 2000;161(1):166–70.
35. Manthous CA, Mokhlesi B. Avoiding management errors in patients with obesity hypoventilation syndrome. Ann Am Thorac Soc. 2016;13(1):109–14.
36. Georges M, Nguyen-Baranoff D, Griffon L, et al. Usefulness of transcutaneous PCO2 to assess nocturnal hypoventilation in restrictive lung disorders. Respirology. 2016;21(7):1300–6.
37. Berry RB, Budhiraja R, Gottlieb DJ, et al. Rules for scoring respiratory events in sleep: update of the 2007 AASM Manual for the Scoring of Sleep and Associated Events. Deliberations of

the Sleep Apnea Definitions Task Force of the American Academy of Sleep Medicine. J Clin Sleep Med. 2012;8(5):597–619.

38. Duiverman ML, Vonk JM, Bladder G, et al. Home initiation of chronic non-invasive ventilation in COPD patients with chronic hypercapnic respiratory failure: a randomised controlled trial. Thorax. 2020;75(3):244–52.

39. Storre JH, Magnet FS, Dreher M, Windisch W. Transcutaneous monitoring as a replacement for arterial PCO(2) monitoring during nocturnal non-invasive ventilation. Respir Med. 2011;105(1):143–50.

40. Berlowitz DJ, Spong J, O'Donoghue FJ, et al. Transcutaneous measurement of carbon dioxide tension during extended monitoring: evaluation of accuracy and stability, and an algorithm for correcting calibration drift. Respir Care. 2011;56(4):442–8.

41. Ogna A, Quera Salva MA, Prigent H, et al. Nocturnal hypoventilation in neuromuscular disease: prevalence according to different definitions issued from the literature. Sleep Breath. 2016;20(2):575–81.

42. Orlikowski D, Prigent H, Quera Salva MA, et al. Prognostic value of nocturnal hypoventilation in neuromuscular patients. Neuromuscul Disord. 2017;27(4):326–30.

43. Ward S, Chatwin M, Heather S, Simonds AK. Randomised controlled trial of non-invasive ventilation (NIV) for nocturnal hypoventilation in neuromuscular and chest wall disease patients with daytime normocapnia. Thorax. 2005;60(12):1019–24.

44. Ogna A, Nardi J, Prigent H, et al. Prognostic value of initial assessment of residual hypoventilation using nocturnal capnography in mechanically ventilated neuromuscular patients: a 5-year follow-up study. Front Med. 2016;3:40.

45. Masa JF, Corral J, Alonso ML, et al. Efficacy of different treatment alternatives for obesity hypoventilation syndrome. Pickwick study. Am J Respir Crit Care Med. 2015;192(1):86–95.

46. Littleton SW, Mokhlesi B. The Pickwickian syndrome—obesity hypoventilation syndrome. Clin Chest Med. 2009;30(3):467–78.

47. BaHammam AS. Prevalence, clinical characteristics, and predictors of obesity hypoventilation syndrome in a large sample of Saudi patients with obstructive sleep apnea. Saudi Med J. 2015;36(2):181–9.

48. Balachandran JS, Masa JF, Mokhlesi B. Obesity hypoventilation syndrome: epidemiology and diagnosis. Sleep Med Clin. 2014;9(3):341–7.

49. Garner DJ, Berlowitz DJ, Douglas J, et al. Home mechanical ventilation in Australia and New Zealand. Eur Respir J. 2013;41(1):39–45.

50. Melloni B, Mounier L, Laaban JP, Chambellan A, Foret D, Muir JF. Home-based care evolution in chronic respiratory failure between 2001 and 2015 (Antadir Federation Observatory). Respiration. 2018:1–9.

51. Alawami M, Mustafa A, Whyte K, Alkhater M, Bhikoo Z, Pemberton J. Echocardiographic and electrocardiographic findings in patients with obesity hypoventilation syndrome. Intern Med J. 2015;45(1):68–73.

52. Kessler R, Chaouat A, Schinkewitch P, et al. The obesity-hypoventilation syndrome revisited: a prospective study of 34 consecutive cases. Chest. 2001;120(2):369–76.

53. Jennum P, Ibsen R, Kjellberg J. Social consequences of sleep disordered breathing on patients and their partners. A controlled national study. Eur Respir J. 2014;43(1):134–44.

54. Jennum P, Kjellberg J. Health, social and economical consequences of sleep-disordered breathing: a controlled national study. Thorax. 2011;66(7):560–6.

55. Castro-Añón O, Pérez de Llano LA, De la Fuente SS, et al. Obesity-hypoventilation syndrome: increased risk of death over sleep apnea syndrome. PLoS One. 2015;10(2):e0117808.

56. Kreivi HR, Italuoma T, Bachour A. Effect of ventilation therapy on mortality rate among obesity hypoventilation syndrome and obstructive sleep apnoea patients. ERJ Open Res. 2020;6(2)

57. Kendzerska T, Leung RS, Aaron SD, Ayas N, Sandoz JS, Gershon AS. Cardiovascular outcomes and all-cause mortality in patients with obstructive sleep apnea and chronic obstructive pulmonary disease (overlap syndrome). Ann Am Thorac Soc. 2019;16(1):71–81.

58. Marik PE, Desai H. Characteristics of patients with the "malignant obesity hypoventilation syndrome" admitted to an ICU. J Intensive Care Med. 2013;28(2):124–30.
59. Quint JK, Ward L, Davison AG. Previously undiagnosed obesity hypoventilation syndrome. Thorax. 2007;62(5):462–3.
60. Masa JF, Corral J, Romero A, et al. Protective cardiovascular effect of sleep apnea severity in obesity hypoventilation syndrome. Chest. 2016;150(1):68–79.
61. Pelosi P, Croci M, Ravagnan I, Vicardi P, Gattinoni L. Total respiratory system, lung, and chest wall mechanics in sedated-paralyzed postoperative morbidly obese patients. Chest. 1996;109(1):144–51.
62. Steier J, Jolley CJ, Seymour J, Roughton M, Polkey MI, Moxham J. Neural respiratory drive in obesity. Thorax. 2009;64(8):719–25.
63. Lee MY, Lin CC, Shen SY, Chiu CH, Liaw SF. Work of breathing in eucapnic and hypercapnic sleep apnea syndrome. Respiration. 2009;77(2):146–53.
64. Lopata M, Onal E. Mass loading, sleep apnea, and the pathogenesis of obesity hypoventilation. Am Rev Respir Dis. 1982;126(4):640–5.
65. Javaheri S, Simbartl LA. Respiratory determinants of diurnal hypercapnia in obesity hypoventilation syndrome. What does weight have to do with it? Ann Am Thorac Soc. 2014;11(6):945–50.
66. Fernandez Alvarez R, Rubinos Cuadrado G, Ruiz Alvarez I, et al. Hypercapnia response in patients with obesity-hypoventilation syndrome treated with non-invasive ventilation at home. Arch Bronconeumol (Engl Ed). 2018;54(9):455–9.
67. Berger KI, Ayappa I, Sorkin IB, Norman RG, Rapoport DM, Goldring RM. Postevent ventilation as a function of CO_2 load during respiratory events in obstructive sleep apnea. J Appl Physiol. 2002;93(3):917–24.
68. Redolfi S, Corda L, La Piana G, Spandrio S, Prometti P, Tantucci C. Long-term non-invasive ventilation increases chemosensitivity and leptin in obesity-hypoventilation syndrome. Respir Med. 2007;101(6):1191–5.
69. Lin CC, Wu KM, Chou CS, Liaw SF. Oral airway resistance during wakefulness in eucapnic and hypercapnic sleep apnea syndrome. Respir Physiol Neurobiol. 2004;139(2):215–24.
70. Berger KI, Ayappa I, Sorkin IB, Norman RG, Rapoport DM, Goldring RM. CO(2) homeostasis during periodic breathing in obstructive sleep apnea. J Appl Physiol. 2000;88(1):257–64.
71. Ayappa I, Berger KI, Norman RG, Oppenheimer BW, Rapoport DM, Goldring RM. Hypercapnia and ventilatory periodicity in obstructive sleep apnea syndrome. Am J Respir Crit Care Med. 2002;166(8):1112–5.
72. Berger KI, Goldring RM, Rapoport DM. Obesity hypoventilation syndrome. Semin Respir Crit Care Med. 2009;30:253–61.
73. Phipps PR, Starritt E, Caterson I, Grunstein RR. Association of serum leptin with hypoventilation in human obesity. Thorax. 2002;57(1):75–6.
74. Campo A, Fruhbeck G, Zulueta JJ, et al. Hyperleptinemia, respiratory drive and hypercapnic response in obese patients. Eur Respir J. 2007;30:223–31.
75. Makinodan K, Yoshikawa M, Fukuoka A, et al. Effect of serum leptin levels on hypercapnic ventilatory response in obstructive sleep apnea. Respiration. 2008;75(3):257–64.
76. Schwartz MW, Peskind E, Raskind M, Boyko EJ, Porte D Jr. Cerebrospinal fluid leptin levels: relationship to plasma levels and to adiposity in humans. Nat Med. 1996;2(5):589–93.
77. Polotsky M, Elsayed-Ahmed AS, Pichard L, et al. Effects of leptin and obesity on the upper airway function. J Appl Physiol. 2012;112(10):1637–43.
78. Berger S, Pho H, Fleury-Curado T, et al. Intranasal leptin relieves sleep disordered breathing in mice with diet induced obesity. Am J Respir Crit Care Med. 2019;199(6):773–83.
79. Ip MSM, Mokhlesi B. Activating leptin receptors in the central nervous system using intranasal leptin. A novel therapeutic target for sleep-disordered breathing. Am J Respir Crit Care Med. 2019;199(6):689–91.
80. Howard ME, Piper AJ, Stevens B, et al. A randomised controlled trial of CPAP versus non-invasive ventilation for initial treatment of obesity hypoventilation syndrome. Thorax. 2017;72(5):437–44.

81. Masa JF, Mokhlesi B, Benitez I, et al. Long-term clinical effectiveness of continuous positive airway pressure therapy versus non-invasive ventilation therapy in patients with obesity hypoventilation syndrome: a multicentre, open-label, randomised controlled trial. Lancet. 2019;393(10182):1721–32.
82. Piper AJ, Wang D, Yee BJ, Barnes DJ, Grunstein RR. Randomised trial of CPAP vs bilevel support in the treatment of obesity hypoventilation syndrome without severe nocturnal desaturation. Thorax. 2008;63(5):395–401.
83. Royer CP, Schweiger C, Manica D, Rabaioli L, Guerra V, Sbruzzi G. Efficacy of bilevel ventilatory support in the treatment of stable patients with obesity hypoventilation syndrome: systematic review and meta-analysis. Sleep Med. 2018;53:153–64.
84. Soghier I, Brozek JL, Afshar M, et al. Noninvasive ventilation versus CPAP as initial treatment of obesity hypoventilation syndrome. Ann Am Thorac Soc. 2019;16(10):1295–303.
85. Bouloukaki I, Mermigkis C, Michelakis S, et al. The association between adherence to positive airway pressure therapy and long-term outcomes in patients with obesity hypoventilation syndrome: a prospective observational study. J Clin Sleep Med. 2018;14(9):1539–50.
86. Mokhlesi B, Tulaimat A, Evans AT, et al. Impact of adherence with positive airway pressure therapy on hypercapnia in obstructive sleep apnea. J Clin Sleep Med. 2006;2(1):57–62.
87. Salord N, Mayos M, Miralda RM, et al. Continuous positive airway pressure in clinically stable patients with mild-to-moderate obesity hypoventilation syndrome and obstructive sleep apnoea. Respirology. 2013;18(7):1135–42.
88. Masa JF, Mokhlesi B, Benítez I, et al. Echocardiographic changes with positive airway pressure therapy in obesity hypoventilation syndrome. Long-term Pickwick randomized controlled clinical trial. Am J Respir Crit Care Med. 2020;201(5):586–97.
89. Banerjee D, Yee BJ, Piper AJ, Zwillich CW, Grunstein RR. Obesity hypoventilation syndrome: hypoxemia during continuous positive airway pressure. Chest. 2007;131(6):1678–84.
90. Perez de Llano LA, Golpe R, Ortiz Piquer M, et al. Clinical heterogeneity among patients with obesity hypoventilation syndrome: therapeutic implications. Respiration. 2008;75(1):34–9.
91. Masa JF, Benítez I, Sánchez-Quiroga M, et al. Long-term noninvasive ventilation in obesity hypoventilation syndrome without severe OSA: the Pickwick randomized controlled trial. Chest. 2020:S0012-3692(20)30711-X.; https://doi.org/10.1016/j.chest.2020.03.068.
92. Carrillo A, Ferrer M, Gonzalez-Diaz G, et al. Noninvasive ventilation in acute hypercapnic respiratory failure caused by obesity hypoventilation syndrome and chronic obstructive pulmonary disease. Am J Respir Crit Care Med. 2012;186(12):1279–85.
93. Kakazu MT, Soghier I, Afshar M, et al. Weight loss interventions as treatment of obesity hypoventilation syndrome. A systematic review. Ann Am Thorac Soc. 2020;17(4):492–502.
94. Borel J-C, Burel B, Tamisier R, et al. Comorbidities and mortality in hypercapnic obese under domiciliary noninvasive ventilation. PLoS One. 2013;8(1):e52006.
95. Lo Coco D, Marchese S, Corrao S, et al. Development of chronic hypoventilation in amyotrophic lateral sclerosis patients. Respir Med. 2006;100(6):1028–36.
96. Prell T, Ringer TM, Wullenkord K, et al. Assessment of pulmonary function in amyotrophic lateral sclerosis: when can polygraphy help evaluate the need for non-invasive ventilation? J Neurol Neurosurg Psychiatry. 2016;87(9):1022–6.
97. Reyhani A, Benbir Senel G, Karadeniz D. Effects of sleep-related disorders on the prognosis of amyotrophic lateral sclerosis. Neurodegener Dis. 2019;19(3-4):148–54.
98. Aboussouan LS. Sleep-disordered breathing in neuromuscular disease. Am J Respir Crit Care Med. 2015;191(9):979–89.
99. Suresh S, Wales P, Dakin C, Harris MA, Cooper DG. Sleep-related breathing disorder in Duchenne muscular dystrophy: disease spectrum in the paediatric population. J Paediatr Child Health. 2005;41(9-10):500–3.
100. Georges M, Attali V, Golmard JL, et al. Reduced survival in patients with ALS with upper airway obstructive events on non-invasive ventilation. J Neurol Neurosurg Psychiatry. 2016;87(10):1045–50.

101. Quaranta VN, Carratù P, Damiani MF, et al. The prognostic role of obstructive sleep apnea at the onset of amyotrophic lateral sclerosis. Neurodegener Dis. 2017;17(1):14–21.
102. Bianchi ML, Losurdo A, Di Blasi C, et al. Prevalence and clinical correlates of sleep disordered breathing in myotonic dystrophy types 1 and 2. Sleep Breath. 2014;18(3):579–89.
103. Laberge L, Dauvilliers Y, Bégin P, Richer L, Jean S, Mathieu J. Fatigue and daytime sleepiness in patients with myotonic dystrophy type 1: to lump or split? Neuromuscul Disord. 2009;19(6):397–402.
104. van der Meche FG, Bogaard JM, van der Sluys JC, Schimsheimer RJ, Ververs CC, Busch HF. Daytime sleep in myotonic dystrophy is not caused by sleep apnoea. J Neurol Neurosurg Psychiatry. 1994;57(5):626–8.
105. Ono S, Takahashi K, Jinnai K, et al. Loss of catecholaminergic neurons in the medullary reticular formation in myotonic dystrophy. Neurology. 1998;51(4):1121–4.
106. Atalaia A, De Carvalho M, Evangelista T, Pinto A. Sleep characteristics of amyotrophic lateral sclerosis in patients with preserved diaphragmatic function. Amyotroph Lateral Scler. 2007;8(2):101–5.
107. de Carvalho M, Costa J, Pinto S, Pinto A. Percutaneous nocturnal oximetry in amyotrophic lateral sclerosis: periodic desaturation. Amyotroph Lateral Scler. 2009;10(3):154–61.
108. Sancho J, Burés E, Ferrer S, Ferrando A, Bañuls P, Servera E. Unstable control of breathing can lead to ineffective noninvasive ventilation in amyotrophic lateral sclerosis. ERJ Open Res. 2019;5(3):00099-2019.
109. Benditt JO. Respiratory care of patients with neuromuscular disease. Respir Care. 2019;64(6):679–88.
110. McSharry DG, Ryan S, Calverley P, Edwards JC, McNicholas WT. Sleep quality in chronic obstructive pulmonary disease. Respirology. 2012;17(7):1119–24.
111. Omachi TA, Blanc PD, Claman DM, et al. Disturbed sleep among COPD patients is longitudinally associated with mortality and adverse COPD outcomes. Sleep Med. 2012;13(5):476–83.
112. Shorofsky M, Bourbeau J, Kimoff J, et al. Impaired sleep quality in COPD is associated with exacerbations: the CanCOLD cohort study. Chest. 2019;156(5):852–63.
113. Jolley CJ, Luo YM, Steier J, et al. Neural respiratory drive in healthy subjects and in COPD. Eur Respir J. 2009;33(2):289–97.
114. Kwon JS, Wolfe LF, Lu BS, Kalhan R. Hyperinflation is associated with lower sleep efficiency in COPD with co-existent obstructive sleep apnea. COPD. 2009;6(6):441–5.
115. O'Donoghue FJ, Catcheside PG, Eckert DJ, McEvoy RD. Changes in respiration in NREM sleep in hypercapnic chronic obstructive pulmonary disease. J Physiol. 2004;559(2):663–73.
116. Costello R, Deegan P, Fitzpatrick M, McNicholas WT. Reversible hypercapnia in chronic obstructive pulmonary disease: a distinct pattern of respiratory failure with a favorable prognosis. Am J Med. 1997;102(3):239–44.
117. O'Donoghue FJ, Catcheside PG, Ellis EE, et al. Sleep hypoventilation in hypercapnic chronic obstructive pulmonary disease: prevalence and associated factors. Eur Respir J. 2003;21(6):977–84.
118. Holmedahl NH, Overland B, Fondenes O, Ellingsen I, Hardie JA. Sleep hypoventilation and daytime hypercapnia in stable chronic obstructive pulmonary disease. Int J Chron Obstruct Pulmon Dis. 2014;9:265–75.
119. Kitajima T, Marumo S, Shima H, et al. Clinical impact of episodic nocturnal hypercapnia and its treatment with noninvasive positive pressure ventilation in patients with stable advanced COPD. Int J Chron Obstruct Pulmon Dis. 2018;13:843–53.
120. Kohnlein T, Windisch W, Kohler D, et al. Non-invasive positive pressure ventilation for the treatment of severe stable chronic obstructive pulmonary disease: a prospective, multicentre, randomised, controlled clinical trial. Lancet Respir Med. 2014;2(9):698–705.
121. Murphy PB, Rehal S, Arbane G, et al. Effect of home noninvasive ventilation with oxygen therapy vs oxygen therapy alone on hospital readmission or death after an acute COPD exacerbation: a randomized clinical trial. JAMA. 2017;317(21):2177–86.

122. Struik FM, Lacasse Y, Goldstein RS, Kerstjens HAM, Wijkstra PJ. Nocturnal noninvasive positive pressure ventilation in stable COPD: a systematic review and individual patient data meta-analysis. Respir Med. 2014;108(2):329–37.
123. Windisch W, Geiseler J, Simon K, Walterspacher S, Dreher M. German national guideline for treating chronic respiratory failure with invasive and non-invasive ventilation - revised edition 2017: part 2. Respiration. 2018;96(2):171–203.
124. Ergan B, Oczkowski S, Rochwerg B, et al. European Respiratory Society guidelines on long-term home non-invasive ventilation for management of COPD. Eur Respir J. 2019;54(3):1901003.
125. Crummy F, Piper AJ, Naughton MT. Obesity and the lung: 2. Obesity and sleep-disordered breathing. Thorax. 2008;63(8):738–46.
126. Marin JM, Soriano JB, Carrizo SJ, Boldova A, Celli BR. Outcomes in patients with chronic obstructive pulmonary disease and obstructive sleep apnea. The overlap syndrome. Am J Respir Crit Care Med. 2010;182(3):325–31.
127. Shawon MS, Perret JL, Senaratna CV, Lodge C, Hamilton GS, Dharmage SC. Current evidence on prevalence and clinical outcomes of co-morbid obstructive sleep apnea and chronic obstructive pulmonary disease: a systematic review. Sleep Med Rev. 2017;32:58–68.
128. Soler X, Gaio E. High prevalence of obstructive sleep apnea in patients with moderate to severe chronic obstructive pulmonary disease. Ann Am Thorac Soc. 2015;12(8):1219–25.
129. He BT, Lu G, Xiao SC, et al. Coexistence of OSA may compensate for sleep related reduction in neural respiratory drive in patients with COPD. Thorax. 2017;72(3):256–62.
130. Messineo L, Lonni S, Magri R, et al. Lung air trapping lowers respiratory arousal threshold and contributes to sleep apnea pathogenesis in COPD patients with overlap syndrome. Respir Physiol Neurobiol. 2020;271:103315.
131. Konikkara J, Tavella R, Willes L, Kavuru M, Sharma S. Early recognition of obstructive sleep apnea in patients hospitalized with COPD exacerbation is associated with reduced readmission. Hosp Pract (1995). 2016;44(1):41–7.
132. Jaoude P, Kufel T, El-Solh A. Survival benefit of CPAP favors hypercapnic patients with the overlap syndrome. Lung. 2014;192(2):251–8.
133. Kuklisova Z, Tkacova R, Joppa P, Wouters E, Sastry M. Severity of nocturnal hypoxia and daytime hypercapnia predicts CPAP failure in patients with COPD and obstructive sleep apnea overlap syndrome. Sleep Med. 2017;30:139–45.

Chapter 10
Perioperative Care of Patients with Obstructive Sleep Apnea Syndrome

Kara L. Dupuy-McCauley, Haven R. Malish, and Peter C. Gay

Keywords Perioperative complications · Postoperative monitoring · Obstructive sleep apnea · Questionnaires · Perioperative guidelines · Sleep apnea guidelines · Postoperative CPAP · Hospital sleep apnea

Introduction

Obstructive sleep apnea (OSA) is a prevalent chronic condition, which is characterized by repeated episodes of collapse of the upper airway during sleep, leading to episodic hypoxemia, sympathetic nervous system activation, and arousal from sleep [1, 2]. Patients with obstructive sleep apnea have anatomical narrowing of the upper airway (UA) leading to increased resistance, such that the force of the UA dilator muscles is insufficient to prevent collapse [1]. As anesthesia, sedation, and analgesia can approximate certain aspects of the sleep state, patients with OSA are at risk for worsening of disordered breathing events in the postoperative period and increased postoperative cardiopulmonary complications.

Several anesthesia and sleep societies have proposed guidelines for the postoperative management of this patient population, aimed at reducing the risk of postoperative cardiopulmonary complications [3–8], although there are limited data regarding the impact of implantation of these guidelines. This chapter will review the most recent evidence regarding postoperative risks to the patient with OSA and

K. L. Dupuy-McCauley
Center for Sleep Medicine, Mayo Clinic, Rochester, MN, USA

H. R. Malish
Sleep Medicine, Mayo Clinic, Rochester, MN, USA

P. C. Gay (✉)
Department of Medicine, Mayo Clinic, Rochester, MN, USA
e-mail: gay.peter@mayo.edu

© Springer Nature Switzerland AG 2022
M. S. Badr, J. L. Martin (eds.), *Essentials of Sleep Medicine*,
Respiratory Medicine, https://doi.org/10.1007/978-3-030-93739-3_10

the current recommendations regarding the care of patients with OSA during the perioperative period.

Epidemiology and Risk Factors for OSA

The prevalence of OSA is thought to be 15–30% in males and 10–15% in females in the general population of North America, but prevalence is increasing [9, 10] and may vary based on population characteristics. For instance, OSA is more common in older age, increased body mass index (BMI), and male gender [11]. Craniofacial structure may also influence the presence of OSA [12], as well as ethnicity with OSA being more common in those of East Asian and African American descent [13, 14].

The association between obesity and OSA warrants special consideration owing to the alarming increase in the prevalence of obesity in the United States. Obesity is associated with increased risk of OSA [10, 15], and may account for 58% of cases of OSA with an AHI $\geq$ 15 [16]. In 2015–2016, the prevalence of obesity was 37.9% in men and 41.1% in women [17]. The prevalence of severe obesity (BMI $\geq$ 40 kg/m^2) has increased from 5.7% to 7.7% from 2007 to 2016. Projections from this data suggest that by 2030, almost half of United States adults will be obese and almost one-fourth will be severely obese [17], and with this increase in weight, we will certainly see an increase in prevalence of OSA.

In a population of patients presenting for bariatric surgery, prevalence of OSA was very high and increased as BMI increased: For BMI 35–39.9 kg/m^2 – 71%, BMI 40–49.9 kg/m^2 – 74%, and BMI > 60 kg/m^2 – 95% [18].

Postoperative Risks Associated with OSA

OSA is a well-established risk factor for increased complications after surgery [19–35]. The most common of these would be respiratory-related adverse outcomes including worsening of OSA, acute respiratory failure requiring non-invasive ventilation or tracheal intubation with mechanical ventilation, pulmonary edema, acute respiratory distress syndrome (ARDS), and oxyhemoglobin desaturation [20, 24–26, 36–39]. Patients also may be at risk for cardiovascular complications including atrial fibrillation, myocardial infarction, cardiac arrest, congestive heart failure (CHF), cerebrovascular accident (CVA), venous thromboembolism (VTE), and shock [19, 20, 22, 24, 26, 39–41]. Several studies have shown increased risk of mortality, and other miscellaneous complications such as acute renal failure, wound hematomas or seromas, ICU transfer, and prolonged length of stay in hospital [24, 31].

Patients who have OSA overlapping with either obesity hypoventilation syndrome (OHS) or chronic obstructive pulmonary disease (COPD) have higher risk of pulmonary and cardiac complications, ICU transfer, and increased length of stay compared with OSA alone [23, 29].

It is important to note that these studies are heterogeneous as far as surgical procedures performed, methods and statistical analysis, and the evidence is of varying quality. In a more recent meta-analysis of the existing literature, OSA remained associated with myocardial infarction, atrial fibrillation, pneumonia, respiratory failure, oxygen desaturation, postoperative delirium, acute kidney injury, venous thromboembolism, length of hospital stay, 30-day mortality, unplanned ICU admission, and increased hospital admission costs, but was not found to be associated with CHF, CVA, risk of reintubation, in-hospital mortality, surgical site infection, or postoperative bleeding [42]. As an example of variance between postoperative risk and procedure performed, a meta-analysis examining outcomes after cardiac surgery specifically determined OSA was associated with increased risk of pooled major adverse cardiovascular and cerebrovascular events up to 30 days after surgery (all-cause mortality, myocardial infarction, myocardial injury, nonfatal cardiac arrest, revascularization process, pulmonary embolism, deep venous thrombosis, newly documented atrial fibrillation, CVA, and CHF), new-onset atrial fibrillation, postoperative tracheal intubation and mechanical ventilation, but not with ICU or hospital length-of-stay, infection, sepsis, or ICU readmission [43].

It is also important to acknowledge that some of these studies separate out mild, moderate, and severe OSA, whereas others do not. This is an important consideration because mild OSA may not portend the same postoperative consequences as moderate or severe disease. For instance, Chan and colleagues found in a post hoc analysis of their study on OSA and postoperative cardiovascular complications that severe OSA was associated with a higher risk of postoperative cardiac death, myocardial injury, CHF, new-onset atrial fibrillation, unplanned admission or readmission to the ICU, and unplanned tracheal intubation or lung ventilation, while moderate OSA was associated with postoperative cardiac death, unplanned ICU readmission, unplanned tracheal intubation, and infections, and mild OSA was only associated with unplanned ICU admission or readmission to the ICU, unplanned tracheal intubation or lung ventilation, and pneumonia [22].

Despite limitations in ability to determine precisely how severity of OSA, and type of surgery being performed might influence the risk of specific postoperative outcomes, it is clear that OSA does lead to a general increased postoperative risk and therefore it would follow that there may be a benefit to identifying people with OSA prior to surgery.

Preoperative Evaluation

Preoperative Risk Assessment and OSA Screening Protocols

Despite the increasing prevalence of OSA, many patients presenting for outpatient surgery (67%) remain undiagnosed [22]. In the case of elective, outpatient surgery, it may be possible to capture this population of patients through routine screening during preoperative evaluation and refer for evaluation of sleep-disordered breathing in advance of a planned surgical procedure if screening is positive. The American Society of Anesthesiologists (ASA) recommends that screening for OSA, which is now encouraged in most US hospitals, should begin with a thorough history and physical exam [3]. The history should focus on eliciting any risk factors for OSA that the patient may have including age, gender, ethnicity, presence of obesity, and common comorbid associated conditions including hypertension, history of stroke, history of myocardial infarction, diabetes mellitus, or abnormal cephalometric measurements. This would also include assessment of any congenital conditions and disease states that may be associated with OSA including Down's syndrome, acromegaly, neuromuscular disease, and cerebral palsy. Questions regarding the symptoms of OSA may include considering the presence of snoring, witnessed apneic episodes, frequent arousals during sleep, morning headaches, and daytime somnolence. Other important aspects of the history may include difficulty with previous anesthetic administration or history of difficult intubation. The physical exam should include assessment of the craniofacial structure, nasal passages, features of the posterior oropharynx (including tonsils and tongue size), and neck circumference. A neck circumference of >17 inches (43 cm) in men, and > 16 inches (40 cm) in women is a positive predictor for the presence of OSA [3, 7].

After preoperative evaluation, the decision may be made to manage the patient expectantly despite suspected OSA, or to delay surgery and have the patient pursue a more urgent evaluation and treatment for sleep disordered breathing.

Preoperative Screening for Suspected OSA

Several questionnaires have been developed for the purpose of screening for OSA and most have been assessed for use in the preoperative population and compared via meta-analysis [44, 45]. The ASA, Society of Anesthesia and Sleep Medicine (SASM), and the American Academy of Sleep Medicine (AASM) recommend routine preoperative screening for OSA to identify patients at increased risk of perioperative complications [46–48]. While there is consensus that risk of OSA should be evaluated and documented, this does not necessarily mean that the plan for surgery must be altered. The SASM guidelines state that there is insufficient evidence to advocate cancelling or delaying surgery with the intent of pursuing a sleep evaluation in patients with suspected OSA unless there is significant evidence of serious uncontrolled comorbid disease or gas exchange abnormality [5].

The Berlin Questionnaire

The Berlin Questionnaire was designed for use in an outpatient primary care setting and assesses five questions on snoring, three on excessive daytime sleepiness, one on sleepiness while driving, and one on history of hypertension [49]. Age, gender, weight, height, and neck circumference are also recorded. The Berlin Questionnaire's predictive performance is population dependent: In a primary care setting of 744 patients, it carried a sensitivity of 0.89, and specificity of 0.71. Half of high-risk patients it identifies are subsequently found to have at least moderate OSA (at AHI > 15) by polysomnography. In the preoperative setting, one study found the Berlin Questionnaire classified 24% of patients presenting for elective surgery as high risk [50]. Another study of preoperative use of the Berlin Questionnaire determined it had a sensitivity and specificity of 69% and 56% respectively in detecting OSA with AHI > 5, 79% and 51% respectively in detecting OSA with AHI > 15, and 87% and 46% respectively in detecting OSA with AHI > 30 [51]. Despite its varied performance in different patient populations, this data regarding use in the presurgical population suggests a moderately high sensitivity especially in moderate-to-severe OSA, and therefore supports the Berlin Questionnaire as a reasonable tool to rule out OSA in the preoperative setting [51].

The American Society of Anesthesiologists' Checklist

In the 2006 edition of the guidelines for the perioperative management of patients with OSA, the ASA taskforce on OSA developed a 14-item, provider-administered checklist to assist anesthesiologists in identifying OSA [52]. Patients endorsing symptoms or signs in two or more of the three categories (physical characteristics, history of airway obstruction during sleep, and complaints of somnolence) are considered high risk of having OSA. Like the Berlin Questionnaire and the STOP-Bang Questionnaire, the ASA checklist exhibits a relatively good sensitivity in detective OSA with an AHI of >5, >15, and > 30; 72%, 79%, and 87%, respectively. The specificity remains rather low at 38%, 37%, and 36%, respectively, making is another reasonable screening tool to rule *out* OSA [51].

The STOP Questionnaire

A condensed modification of the questions in the Berlin Questionnaire, the STOP Questionnaire was developed and validated to facilitate widespread OSA screening in surgical patients (S: Snore loudly, T: daytime Tiredness, O: Observed to stop breathing during sleep, P: high blood Pressure). In the presurgical population, the sensitivity of the STOP questionnaire at an AHI of >5, >15, and > 30 events/h cutoff levels was found to be 66%, 74%, and 80%, respectively, with a specificity of 60%, 53% and 49%, respectively [46].

The STOP-Bang Model

The STOP-Bang Questionnaire adds demographic and physical features (B: BMI >35 kg/m^2, A: Age > 50 years, N: Neck circumference > 40 cm, G: male Gender) to the STOP Questionnaire, and has the highest sensitivity in ruling OSA, especially in moderate-to-severe disease.

A meta-analysis of the use of the STOP-Bang Questionnaire in the presurgical population found a pooled prevalence of 68.4%, 39.2%, and 18.7% for any OSA, moderate-to-severe OSA, and severe OSA respectively, with corresponding sensitivities of 84%, 91%, and 96% respectively and specificity of 43%, 32%, and 29%, respectively [53]. A recent prospective cohort study of preoperative patients found that a STOP-Bang score of 5–8 may be significantly more suggestive of moderate-to-severe OSA than scores of 3–4: 78% prevalence versus 53% respective prevalence of moderate-to-severe OSA [54]. A study of an ethnically diverse population of bariatric patients found that the STOP-Bang previously validated cutoff of ≥4 achieved a sensitivity of >80% and specificity of 50–60%, which is similar to other populations [55]. The STOP-Bang has also been assessed in a variety of ethnic groups (Chinese, Indian, Malay, Caucasian) and there are recommendations in those groups for alternative BMI thresholds and STOP-Bang score cutoffs for optimal sensitivity and specificity in these patient populations [56]. Taken together, these data suggest that the STOP-Bang may be an appropriate assessment tool for a wide variety of patient populations but with alternative cutoffs for certain groups.

Sleep Apnea Clinical Score

The Sleep Apnea Clinical Score (SACS) was validated in the outpatient sleep laboratory environment and shown to have a high positive predictive value for OSA [57]. The SACS score was initially validated in postsurgical patients to identify patients who desaturated in the postoperative hospital ward area [58]. A large prospective study enrolled nearly 700 patients using the SACS and showed a higher risk of OSA (32% of all patients) was associated with a much higher likelihood of a postoperative 4% oxygen desaturation index (ODI) >10 events/h and recurrent post anesthesia care unit (PACU) respiratory events [59]. Subsequent postoperative hospital ward episodes of respiratory complications were also associated with a high SACS (odds ratio 3.5, $P < 0.001$), especially if they also had recurrent respiratory events in the PACU during 90 min of observation, whereby the likelihood of a postoperative respiratory event was profoundly increased (odds ratio 21.0, $P < 0.001$). There was no significant benefit with the SACS questionnaire in predicting cardiac complications or prolonged hospital stay.

Preoperative Screening in Suspected OSA

The use of one screening tool over another is not mandatory, and most guidelines leave this decision of which tool to use up to the provider who is performing the preoperative assessment. Optimal preoperative evaluation must also include consideration of the risk inherent to the particular type of surgery being performed, risk of other patient comorbidities, and past difficulties with anesthesia or intubation in addition to screening for OSA [60].

The left side of Fig. 10.1 summarizes one possible preoperative approach in the suspected OSA patient. Those with ≥2 on the STOP, or ≥ 3 on the STOP-Bang Questionnaire are considered high risk of having undiagnosed OSA.

In certain situations, preoperative assessment by a sleep physician may be warranted for consideration of polysomnography or home sleep testing if time and resources permit. An early consult would typically allow the sleep physician adequate time to prepare a perioperative management plan, which may include a period of at-home positive airway pressure (PAP) treatment prior to surgery for the

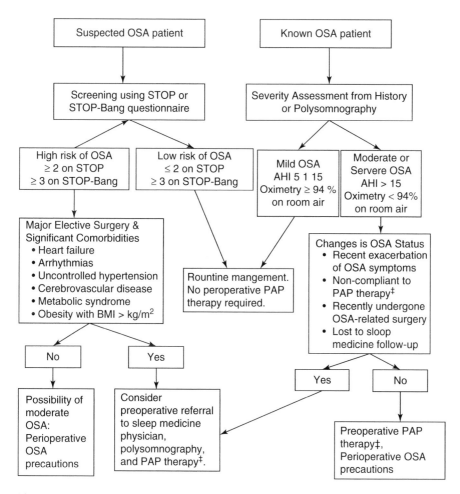

Fig. 10.1 An approach to those with suspected or known obstructive sleep apnea (OSA) prior to surgery in the ambulatory setting. ‡ Positive airway pressure (PAP) therapy may include continuous, bi-level, or auto-titrating PAP. (Adapted with kind permission from Springer Science + Business Media [60])

purpose of acclimatization. Ultimately, the decision for further preoperative sleep study testing would depend on the clinical judgment and expertise of the team of physicians providing perioperative care after careful screening and assessment. Patients determined to be at low risk for presence of OSA may be managed expectantly with no further diagnostic testing prior to surgery. For those deemed at high risk for OSA, there are a variety of possible courses of action. In some cases, major elective surgery may be deferred in patients with a high clinical suspicion of complicated, severe OSA. In other cases, there may be patients who are deemed high risk according to an OSA screening questionnaire, but who otherwise are without significant comorbidities or are scheduled to undergo a low risk procedure, and in that case, the physician team may elect to proceed to surgery without delay [61]. And there may be other situations where the risk of delaying the surgery outweighs the benefits of identifying and treating OSA preoperatively and so the patient is taken to surgery even in the setting of clinical suspicion of severe or complicated OSA. The literature is vague and lacking in the scientific evidence to support definitive guidelines regarding risks and benefits of cancelling most types of procedures.

Preoperative Screening in Known OSA

A potential preoperative evaluation approach for patients with known OSA is illustrated on the right side of Fig. 10.1. Although the original severity of the sleep-disordered breathing must be known or estimated in this case, the treatment status would be an important factor in preoperative risk assessment. The use of PAP devices (CPAP, bi-level PAP [BPAP], auto-titrating CPAP [APAP]), and the compliance should be assessed for those who have been prescribed PAP therapy. Patients who have been lost to sleep medicine follow-up and/or those who are noncompliant with therapy, those who have had recent exacerbation of OSA symptoms, and those who have undergone OSA-related airway surgery may benefit from preoperative referral for additional evaluation with a sleep medicine physician. Long-standing OSA, especially in the case of suboptimal treatment or lack of treatment, may have systemic complications, including hypoxemia, hypercarbia, polycythemia, and cor pulmonale. Pulse oximetry may be a simple screening tool in the preoperative clinic. Some advocate that an oxygen saturation value of <94% on room air in the absence of other causes should be a red flag for possible severe long-standing OSA [60], which may be another reason to refer to sleep preoperatively.

Preoperative OSA Treatment

The ASA, SASM, and AASM agree that patients with OSA who have been on PAP therapy should continue PAP therapy in the preoperative period [3, 5, 7]. The ASA recommends that initiation of PAP should be considered, particularly in patients with severe OSA, but that the preoperative use of an oral appliance, or weight loss, may also be acceptable considerations [3]. Initiation of PAP therapy for those with untreated OSA or re-initiation of preoperative PAP in the non-PAP-adherent OSA patient should be considered, although the benefit of using PAP in the time period leading up to surgery as a means to reduce postoperative cardiopulmonary risk in patients with OSA is uncertain [62].

Intraoperative OSA Management

Tracheal Intubation

The surgical and anesthesia team should be aware of a patient's previous diagnosis of OSA, or that the patient is "high risk" for OSA but has not undergone a formal sleep evaluation. The ASA guidelines state that patients with OSA should be presumed to have a "difficult airway," meaning there would potentially be difficulty with tracheal intubation, facemask ventilation, or both [3], and the patient should be managed in accordance with the ASA practice guidelines for management of the difficult airway [63]. The SASM advocates that patients at high risk for OSA should proceed to surgery in the same manner as those who have confirmed OSA, but that known or suspected OSA should be considered an independent risk factor for difficult intubation, difficult mask ventilation, or a combination of both [5, 6]. The AASM recommends that the patient be considered a "high-risk intubation," and advocates against the use of unsupervised preoperative sedation [7].

These recommendations are based upon literature suggesting OSA is associated with difficult intubation [36, 37, 64–68]. The reverse association is true as well, patients with a history of difficult intubation have a high prevalence of OSA. This was discovered retrospectively by Hiremath and colleagues [36], and subsequently confirmed with a prospective study done by Chung and colleagues [69]. A variety of other studies examining this association exist as well. A retrospective case-controlled study of 253 patients was conducted to determine the occurrence of difficult intubation in OSA patients. The OSA patients were matched with controls of the same age, gender, and type of surgery. Difficult intubation was assessed by laryngoscopy using the Cormack and Lehane classification [70], and was found to occur eight times as often in OSA patients versus controls (22% vs. 3%, $P < 0.05$) [37]. In OSA patients undergoing ear, nose, and throat surgery, a 44% prevalence of difficult intubation has similarly been reported [71]. Furthermore, patients with severe OSA (AHI >40) were found to have a much higher prevalence of difficult intubation [72]. Increased prevalence of obesity in the OSA population is not the only factor that explains this association. A study of more than 1500 nonobese and obese patients concluded that increased age, male gender, pharyngo-oral pathology, and the presence of OSA are all associated with a more frequent occurrence of difficult intubation [73]. This suggests that patients who are found to have a difficult airway in the absence of any documented OSA should be referred for evaluation by a sleep medicine provider.

Choice of Anesthetics/Anesthetic Technique

One aspect of planning and preparation for surgical procedures in patients with OSA is the choice of anesthesia strategy, which may present an opportunity to reduce risk in patients with OSA. Sedative, anesthetic, and analgesic medications mimic the sleep state by increasing collapsibility of the upper airway, reducing hypoxic and hypercapnic respiratory drives, decreasing activity of the respiratory muscles, increasing dependence upon the diaphragm, decreasing respiratory stimulation, and decreasing lung volumes, which may be especially detrimental to patients with OSA [74–81]. The ASA recommends general anesthesia with tracheal intubation as opposed to deep sedation without a secure airway [3]. The ASA also recommends that CPAP or a mandibular advancement device may be used during sedation to facilitate the airway remaining open.

Patients with OSA are felt to be at higher risk for adverse respiratory events from the use of propofol and neuromuscular blockade, but there is insufficient data to assess the risk associated with inhalational anesthetic agents, alpha-2-agonists (such as dexmedetomidine and clonidine), and ketamine [6]. However, data from studies of obese patients suggest that desflurane and sevoflurane may facilitate or more rapid and consistent postoperative recovery, which may be relevant to many patients with OSA, given the high association between OSA and obesity [82]. A strategy of regional anesthesia is preferred over general anesthesia in patients with OSA due to findings from several population-based studies showing decreased odds for mechanical ventilation, critical care admission, and prolonged hospital length of stay [3, 6, 52, 83–86].

Use of intravenous benzodiazepines may put patients with OSA at increased risk for upper airway collapse and subsequent respiratory complications. Much of this literature comes from the use of intravenous benzodiazepines during drug-induced sleep endoscopy (DISE), where IV benzodiazepines are used to induce collapse of the upper airway [87]. There are additional retrospective studies to suggest that patients with OSA are more prone to hypoxia and airway collapse when subjected to IV midazolam than those with primary snoring and no OSA diagnosis [88].

There are no prospective, randomized, controlled trials comparing the safety, efficacy, and impact on respiratory status of different anesthetic, analgesic, and sedative strategies in patients with OSA. However, a promising technique of opioid-free analgesia is emerging and may be a safer approach to anesthesia in the OSA population. This opioid-free strategy is based in the principle of multimodal anesthesia and would typically consist of using multiple anesthetic and analgesic agents in subtherapeutic doses simultaneous. For example, a continuous infusion of lidocaine and dexmedetomidine might be supplemented with a low dose of a volatile anesthetic agent and intermittent dosing of acetaminophen, ketamine, ibuprofen, and ketorolac. This innovative technique may provide adequate anesthesia and analgesia without exposing patients to the unwanted respiratory side-effects and possible addictive properties of opioids [89].

Extubation

The ASA and AASM recommend that patients with OSA be extubated awake and in the non-supine position unless contraindicated [3, 7], and the ASA adds that neuromuscular blockade should be fully reversed prior to extubation [3].

Postoperative OSA Management

Postoperative Pain Control

Postoperative analgesia can adversely influence respiration in surgical patients with OSA. In the acute setting, analgesia is commonly achieved with opioids, which may affect the central nervous system and whose effects may be potentiated by other sedative and anesthetic agents. Opioids depress the central respiratory drive, decrease consciousness, and decrease supraglottic muscle tone, leading to increased risk of upper airway obstruction [90]. In a retrospective study of 1600 patients who had received postoperative patient-controlled analgesia with IV opioids, eight cases of serious respiratory depression were reported [91]. Contributing factors were the concurrent use of a background infusion of opioids, advanced age, concomitant administration of sedative or hypnotic medications, and a preexisting history of sleep apnea. A review conducted to identify the risk factors for respiratory depression subsequent to patient-controlled analgesia concluded that there is no single indicator for respiratory depression but that OSA, whether suspected or verified by patient history, is a risk factor [92].

A recent review of critical perioperative complications (including death) in patients with OSA identified morbid obesity, male sex, undiagnosed/untreated OSA, suboptimal use of postoperative CPAP, need for opioid analgesia, and lack of appropriate postoperative monitoring as risk factors [28]. The majority of patients who had adverse outcomes in this study had consumed a typical, or even a less-than-typical amount of opioids, which may suggest increased sensitivity to opioids in this population as an explanation [93].

Because of the myriad effects of opioids on the CNS and respiratory systems, and the complex interaction between sleep disordered breathing, obesity, and sleep architecture, it is difficult to predict the respiratory consequences of opioid administration in the OSA population. Opioids can cause increased severity of obstructive events, elicitation of centrally mediated apneic events (central sleep apnea [CSA] or ataxic breathing), and hypoventilation. For instance, a randomized study of remifentanil use in patients with moderate OSA actually showed a decrease in the number of obstructive events with an increase in central apneas [94]. This decrease in obstructive events may be attributed to the decrease in REM sleep that typically occurs on the first night after surgery, but this report highlights the complex interaction between multiple factors postoperatively. And the literature on this subject must be interpreted with caution as there may be varying measures of respiratory changes.

The ASA guidelines recommend avoidance of opioids when possible in patients with OSA, especially in the form of continuous infusion, and they recommend caution with other known respiratory depressants such as benzodiazepines and barbiturates [3]. The AASM and SASM recommend caution with the use of sedatives, hypnotics, and anxiolytics in the postoperative period [6, 7]. Bearing in mind these guidelines, one might consider strategies to minimize opioid exposure in this population. One such strategy might involve careful titration of opioids so as to provide the minimum amount required to achieve adequate pain control [7]. Another potential strategy would be a multimodal approach using combinations of analgesics from different classes and different sites of analgesic administration for perioperative pain management [95–97]. Such an approach may include peripheral nerve block catheters or neuro-axial catheters dispensing local anesthetic agents (without opioids) and opioid-sparing analgesic agents, such as nonsteroidal anti-inflammatory drugs, COX-2 inhibitors, acetaminophen, pregabalin, tramadol, and dexamethasone [98]. But caution should still be exercised even despite opioid-sparing techniques. A large retrospective study of patients who had undergone laparoscopic surgery found an association between use of gabapentin and respiratory depression. This association tended to be present in patients who were older, had received midazolam, and had a slightly higher intraoperative dose of opioids [99]. This might suggest that even in the absence of postoperative opioid use, there may still be consequences to polypharmacy, and an effective postoperative monitoring strategy to identify those at risk for respiratory complications is important.

Postoperative Monitoring

The preservation of arousal mechanisms is vital when it comes to self-protection from airway obstruction and hypoventilation. When arousal responses are suppressed by sedative, anesthetic, and analgesic medications, the patient can have increased risk of asphyxia, cardiopulmonary arrest, and death [100]. Proper monitoring for return of these arousal mechanisms is key in ensuring patient safety in the postoperative setting. In patients with OSA, most respiratory complications occur on the general hospital ward in the first 24 hours post-surgery [28, 35, 101]. A closed claims analysis of postoperative opioid-induced respiratory depression revealed that 25% of claims were related to OSA [101], highlighting the importance of proper postoperative monitoring, especially for those patients who are within the 24-hour postoperative window, who have a diagnosis or are at high risk for OSA, and who are receiving opioid analgesia. A recent review of postoperative critical events associated with OSA by Bolden and colleagues found events were most likely to occur in the first 24 hours after surgery and that death or brain damage was less common in patients receiving supplemental oxygen and in patients with respiratory monitoring in place at the time of the event. Death or brain damage was more common in patients receiving sedatives in addition to opioids, and in patients who were not being closely observed [102]. This would seem to advise use of supplemental oxygen when appropriate, close observation, and avoidance of polypharmacy with multiple CNS depressants if feasible.

Oximetry

While there is no general consensus on an appropriate postoperative monitoring strategy for patients with OSA, the ASA and AASM both recommend continuous pulse oximetry postoperatively for this patient population [3, 7], although no mention is made of the setting in which this monitoring should occur (e.g., PACU vs. general medical ward), and the ASA acknowledges that the optimal duration for postoperative monitoring has not been established [3].

Gali and colleagues found that patients at risk for OSA who had recurrent respiratory events (bradypnea, apnea, oxygen desaturation, and pain–sedation mismatch) in the immediate postoperative period had the highest oxygen desaturation index on continuous pulse oximetry and were at the highest risk of postoperative respiratory complications. In this study, patients were assessed at 30, 60, and 90 minutes postoperatively, which may be an acceptable strategy to identify patients who may benefit from a higher level of care or more intensive monitoring [58].

Chan and colleagues also looked at postoperative patients at high risk for OSA and found that prolonged oxygen desaturations <80% during the first three postoperative nights portended a higher risk of postoperative cardiovascular events [103], again suggesting that oximetry may provide a clue as to which patients may benefit from closer monitoring.

These two studies would suggest that continuous pulse oximetry might be an important tool for risk stratification; however, other studies have failed to show a significant impact on clinical outcomes as a results of continuous pulse oximetry in the postoperative setting. A systematic review and meta-analysis of continuous pulse oximetry and capnography monitoring found that continuous remote pulse oximetry improved detection of oxygen desaturation and was associated with a trend toward decreased ICU transfer when compared to intermittent oxygen assessment, but did not significantly reduce mortality [104]. In the previously mentioned closed claims analysis by Lee and colleagues, it should be noted that one-third of the patients who experienced complications from postoperative opioid-induced respiratory depression were being monitored with oximetry [101], which reinforces concerns that while continuous pulse oximetry may bring attention to oxygen desaturation, we are not currently able to translate that into definitively improved patient outcomes.

Capnography

One conjecture as to why continuous oximetry does not necessarily translate into improved postoperative outcomes is that oxygen desaturation is a late sign of hypoventilation particularly for patients receiving supplemental oxygen, and perhaps continuous capnography monitoring might more effectively predict respiratory failure. In the assessment of capnography, a systematic review found that capnography derangements preceded changes in oxygen saturation in the setting of supplemental oxygen administration [104].

But capnography may not be accurate in the setting of PAP use. End-tidal carbon dioxide tension (ET-CO_2) and transcutaneous carbon dioxide monitoring (tc-CO_2) accuracy have been compared in a sleep laboratory with $PaCO_2$ levels in patients wearing a nasal cannula or using nocturnal positive-pressure ventilatory assistance [105]. ET-CO_2 tension and tc-CO_2 during diagnostic and therapeutic sleep studies did not accurately reflect the simultaneous $PaCO_2$ levels when PAP therapy was applied. It may be that ET-CO_2 and tc-CO_2 could be used to identify trends in CO_2 levels in patients on PAP rather than serving as a surrogate for arterial $PaCO_2$ levels, but more research is needed to define the clinical utility of such a strategy.

Capnography is not used on a routine basis in a clinical setting and there is no prospective data on whether capnography may improve outcomes or reduce postoperative complications. But although there are no current guideline recommendations advocating its use in postoperative patients, emerging research suggests that capnography may soon become more widely adopted as a tool for early detection of respiratory failure. A prospective, blinded, multicenter, observational trial found that adding capnography and the Integrated Pulmonary Index algorithm, an algorithm-derived value based on SpO_2, $EtCO_2$, pulse, and respiratory rate, to traditional pulse oximetry afforded an average additional 8–11 minutes lead time prior to an adverse respiratory event when compared to standard postoperative monitoring with pulse oximetry alone [106]. This suggests that capnography may soon become an important tool to facilitate early detection of postoperative respiratory compromise, hopefully leading to early intervention and decreased respiratory risk.

Management Algorithms

PACU

While the literature is insufficient to provide evidence-based guidance regarding specific postoperative monitoring strategies, one might consider the surgery type and risk, patient characteristics, as well as anesthesia and analgesia-specific factors when planning for the postoperative period. The 2006 ASA guidelines, directed by expert consensus in the absence of good clinical evidence at the time, urged guidance of OSA patient disposition by a weighted scoring system and patient risk factors [52]. Perioperative risk was broadly divided into severity and treatment of OSA, invasiveness of the surgery, anesthesia used, and postoperative opioid requirements. The scoring system was somewhat involved and did not recognize the importance of recurrent PACU events in predicting more episodes of oxygen desaturation and increased postoperative respiratory complications [59].

Taking into account 2006 ASA guidelines and recent evidence for identifying patients most at risk for postoperative respiratory complications, Seet and Chung [60] proposed an algorithm using recurrent PACU events as a predictive indicator to guide postoperative disposition of the known or suspected OSA patient (Fig. 10.2). A PACU event occurs if in one 30-min time block, the patient has any of the following: (1) apnea for ≥10 s (only one episode needed for yes), (2) bradypnea of ≤8 bpm (three episodes needed for yes), (3) desaturations to <90% (three episodes needed for yes), or (4) pain-sedation mismatch, as characterized by high pain scores and high sedation levels observed simultaneously.

A recurrent PACU event occurs when any one of the PACU respiratory events occur in two separate 30-min time blocks (not necessarily the same event or consecutive blocks). Patients who are at high risk of OSA on the screening questionnaires and have recurrent PACU respiratory events are more likely to have postoperative respiratory complications. It may be prudent to monitor these patients postoperatively with continuous oximetry in an area where early medical intervention can occur. The monitoring can occur in the step-down unit, on the surgical ward near the nursing station, or with remote pulse oximetry with telemetry (Fig. 10.2).

Close postoperative monitoring would certainly be called for in patients with known OSA with recurrent PACU events, but also in the absence of recurrent events if the patient's OSA is severe or if they are not using PAP (left side of Fig. 10.2). In the absence of severe OSA, nonadherence, and recurrent PACU events, patients with at least moderate OSA, or parenteral/higher dose oral opioids (codeine 60 mg every 4 h or equivalent) may be managed postoperatively on the surgical ward with periodic oximetry monitoring. The ASA also recommends that all patients be provided supplemental oxygen on a continuous basis until they are able to maintain their baseline oxygen saturation while on room air [3].

For those with previously undiagnosed but suspected OSA in the postoperative or medical inpatient setting, our institution has developed an obstructive apnea systematic intervention strategy (OASIS) protocol, as outlined in the top half of Fig. 10.3. PACU utilization, overnight oximetry, ABG, inpatient events, and discussion with the primary team are often enough to guide initial decision-making. Appropriate setting (outpatient vs. inpatient) and timing (before or after discharge) of a comprehensive sleep medicine assessment may be determined based on local resources and testing availability.

Postoperative Use of Positive Airway Pressure

When possible, patients with known OSA who are already on PAP therapy should bring their own equipment to the hospital and PAP should be used liberally perioperatively unless a contraindication exists [3]. Contraindications to PAP therapy

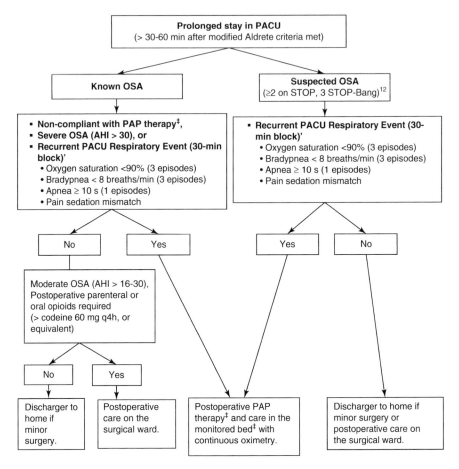

Fig. 10.2 Postoperative management of the known or suspected OSA patient after general anesthesia Number of occurrences of more than one set of events in each 30-min evaluation period while in the post-anesthesia care unit (PACU), including repeat occurrence of the same event set. ‡PAP therapy may include continuous, bi-level or auto-titrating PAP. †Monitored bed – inpatient area that would lend itself to early nursing intervention and includes continuous oximetry monitoring (e.g., intensive care unit, step-down unit, or remote pulse oximetry with telemetry in surgical ward). (Adapted with kind permission from Springer Science+Business Media [60])

include cardiac or respiratory arrest, severe encephalopathy, severe upper gastrointestinal bleeding, hemodynamic instability, cardiac arrhythmia, upper airway obstruction, high risk for aspiration, copious secretions, recent facial trauma, inability to clear secretions, and lack of cooperation from the patient [108]. Patients without a formal diagnosis of OSA, or who have OSA but are not on PAP therapy in the outpatient setting may warrant consideration of initiation of PAP postoperatively while hospitalized. CPAP and APAP are equally effective in the perioperative management of OSA as demonstrated by decrease in AHI, improvement in oxygenation, and shortened length of stay [109]. If the patient has a home machine, it is reasonable to start at the home pressure setting, but with the acknowledgement that the

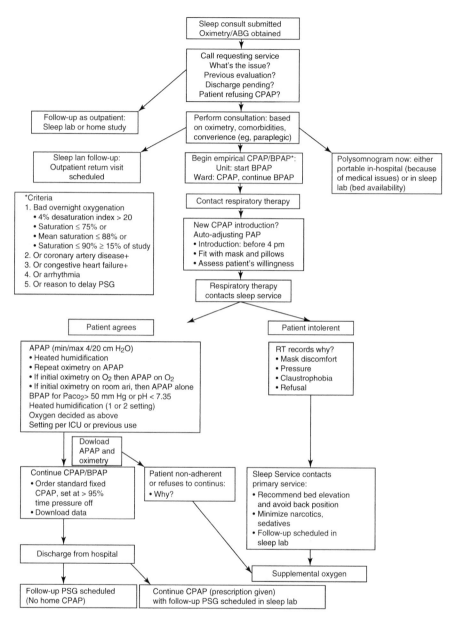

Fig. 10.3 Obstructive apnea systematic intervention strategy (OASIS) for assessing postoperative or medical patients for sleep-disordered breathing, with follow-through management algorithm based on patients' PAP willingness. ABG Arterial blood gas, CPAP continuous PAP, BPAP bi-level PAP, PSG polysomnography, APAP auto-adjusting PAP, PSG polysomnography, RT respiratory therapy. (Adapted from [107])

pressure need may need to be titrated to meet the fluctuating needs of the postoperative patient and to accommodate for increased time in the supine position, thoracic pain, postoperative distortions in sleep architecture, and CNS depressant medications. Sleep-related breathing disturbances are typically the highest on the third night postoperatively, likely due to "REM rebound," or increased proportion of REM sleep after the distortion in sleep architecture, (with decreased sleep efficiency, slow wave sleep and REM sleep) which typically accompanies postoperative night one [110]. This fluctuating severity of sleep disordered breathing in the postoperative period reinforces the concept that PAP needs may also vary and patients should be continuously monitored, and PAP adjusted appropriately. For patients who do not have a prior pressure setting, use of APAP or manual bedside titration may be more appropriate [111].

In those for which inpatient PAP initiation is desired, early assessment (prior to 4 p.m.) by the respiratory therapist mask fit and patient willingness is recommended. Once PAP is initiated, close follow-up is needed to assess patient tolerance. In the case of intolerance, troubleshooting may be attempted, including mask fit, pressure setting, addressing claustrophobia, and assessing if the treatment aligns with the patient's wishes and values. Upon discharge, the patient may need a formal sleep evaluation in the outpatient setting if continuation of PAP therapy is desired. In certain institutions, the patient may be qualified for PAP therapy in the inpatient setting and discharged with a prescription and routine sleep medicine follow up. The recommended follow through of inpatient PAP initiation is outlined in the bottom half of Fig. 10.3.

As there are no universal guidelines for discharge into an unmonitored setting, patients with known or suspected OSA should be discharged at the discretion of the inpatient care team when they are able to maintain oxygen saturation on room air [3], taking into account severity of OSA, type of surgery performed, and postoperative course (Fig. 10.2). Ambulatory surgical centers managing OSA patients should have transfer agreements to inpatient facilities and should be equipped to manage contingencies associated with OSA.

Positive Airway Pressure and Postoperative Risk Reduction

No consensus has emerged regarding the ability of PAP to reduce cardiopulmonary complications in patients with OSA. It is difficult to assess this body of literature as a whole due to its heterogeneous characteristics when it comes to the timing of PAP initiation (i.e., was PAP used in the preoperative period leading up to surgery vs. implementation during hospital admission), and low PAP compliance. Low PAP compliance has been a consistent hinderance to assessing OSA outcomes associated with PAP use in general, and PAP use tends to be even lower in the perioperative period [112]. Nagappa and colleagues performed a systematic review and meta-analysis of the existing studies on outcomes in OSA patients undergoing surgery. They examined six studies of 904 patients and found that use of perioperative CPAP did not decrease postoperative complications but it did lower the AHI and provided a trend toward decrease length of hospital stay [62]. A large cohort study by Mutter et al. deduced that CPAP decreased cardiovascular complications by demonstrating increased risk in patients who had undiagnosed OSA (versus diagnosed OSA), and patients who had a preoperative diagnosis of OSA and a CPAP prescription [40]. A smaller retrospective case–control study suggested that despite CPAP use being low in general, those who had been using CPAP prior to admission were at less risk of serious postoperative complications, total ICU length-of-stay, unplanned ICU admission, and length of hospital stay [35].

More recently, a large retrospective database study of over 28,000 patients was performed to assess differences in postoperative outcomes between those with previously diagnosed OSA and preoperatively suspected OSA. The rate of adverse perioperative outcomes (reintubation, mechanical ventilation, direct ICU admission after surgery, prolonged hospital length-of-stay, and all-cause 30-day mortality) was higher in those with suspected OSA after adjusting for potential confounders. But a subgroup analysis did not find any link between those who were diagnosed with OSA and compliant with CPAP versus those who were diagnosed and who were not compliant with CPAP, suggesting that PAP may not influence postoperative outcomes. However, this was based on self-reported PAP compliance, which can be inaccurate [113].

A review of perioperative CPAP use by Chung and colleagues highlighted several studies examining the perioperative benefits of CPAP and while some of the case series and cohort studies showed benefits from CPAP including decreased postoperative complications, and decreased length of hospital admission and ICU stay, the two RCTs did not show the same benefit [114].

The bariatric population offers an exceptional opportunity to study CPAP-related postoperative outcomes due to the high prevalence of OSA. A retrospective study of 53 patients undergoing bariatric surgery found no differences in postoperative complications, or hospital length of stay; however, similar to other literature on the subject, there were significant limitations including retrospective nature of the study, small sample size, use of oxygen desaturation index from pulse oximetry to define OSA presence and severity, and lack of CPAP adherence data [115]. Additionally, all patients with moderate-to-severe OSA were treated with CPAP, which may be a major confounder, being that other studies have shown varying postoperative risk based upon severity of OSA [22].

Although many of the studies suggesting benefit from perioperative CPAP use have significant limitations, they appear to be building the foundation of a body of evidence that may eventually show definitive reduction in postoperative complications as a result of PAP use.

And looking beyond the OSA population, there are compelling RCTs in patients without OSA that show a more conclusive postoperative PAP benefit. A meta-analysis of 9 RCTs of abdominal surgery patients without OSA found that CPAP reduced postoperative pulmonary complications when used perioperatively [116]. Similar benefits have been shown when prophylactic CPAP is used after cardiothoracic surgery [117, 118].

Although the data surrounding risk reduction afforded by CPAP in OSA patients is inconclusive, it's important to acknowledge the lack of large, prospective data, and also to consider some of the roadblocks such as poor adherence that have limited this type of investigation. Therefore, it's reasonable to consider the possibility that we simply do not have all the information at this point in time to make a fair assessment and it therefore may be reasonable to advocate for perioperative PAP use in patients with OSA when possible.

Conclusion

While it is clear that patients with OSA are at increased risk of postoperative cardiopulmonary complications, there is less certainty when it comes to what perioperative interventions might mitigate these risks. Emphasis has been placed on preoperative screening for suspect OSA and minimizing risk for known and suspected OSA patients by optimizing management of comorbidities and initiating OSA treatment preoperatively. The better question to ask is not who has OSA but who has an OSA phenotype that will result in postoperative complications. Our institution his implemented in-hospital sleep consultative services in combination with OASIS with a close follow-through protocol to aid workup and initial management of perioperative inpatients with suspected OSA. Many hospitals throughout the country have adopted their own approaches in screening and monitoring suspected and known OSA patients perioperatively, and have developed in-hospital sleep consultative services. But more evidence-based guidelines will need to be established before there can be a single algorithm to manage patients within the OSA population presenting for surgery.

OSA is a common entity and will likely continue to increase in prevalence in the coming years. We must strive to develop best practices to manage and monitor patients with OSA from the preoperative period to their discharge home from the hospital with the aim of reducing unnecessary postoperative risk. By combining preoperative screening, perioperative optimization of comorbidities, and identification of recurrent postoperative and PACU events, optimal risk identification, prevention, and intervention strategies will hopefully be achieved as we pursue more robust prospective outcomes data.

Summary of Key Points
- OSA is a common, chronic health condition associated with increased risk of cardiopulmonary complications in the post-surgical period.
- Several organizations have developed recommendations for management of patients with OSA presenting for surgery.
- Questionnaires have been validated for use in the preoperative setting to assess for risk of OSA and provide an opportunity for sleep medicine referral if deemed necessary.

- When additional factors were included, the STOP-Bang Questionnaire had the highest sensitivity in detecting those at risk for OSA, especially moderate-to-severe disease.
- Algorithms developed to minimize perioperative risk in those with known or suspected OSA consider the patients' risk of suspected OSA, severity of known OSA, type of surgery, comorbidities, and changes in OSA status.
- Early identification of patients with OSA may forewarn the clinician of potential difficulty with airway maintenance intra- and postoperatively, perhaps influencing choice of anesthetic/sedation/analgesia technique and postoperative monitoring environment.
- We advocate an algorithm using recurrent PACU events as a predictive indicator to guide postoperative disposition of the known or suspected OSA patient.
- For those with previously undiagnosed but suspected OSA in the postoperative or medical inpatients setting, our institution has developed an OASIS protocol.
- More prospective data is needed to guide recommendations for perioperative strategies to reduce postoperative risk in this patient population

References

1. Patil SP, Schneider H, Schwartz AR, Smith PL. Adult obstructive sleep apnea: pathophysiology and diagnosis. Chest. 2007;132:325–37.
2. Somers VK, Dyken ME, Clary MP, Abboud FM. Sympathetic neural mechanisms in obstructive sleep apnea. J Clin Invest. 1995;96:1897–904.
3. American Society of Anesthesiologists Task Force on Perioperative Management of patients with obstructive sleep a. Practice guidelines for the perioperative management of patients with obstructive sleep apnea: an updated report by the American Society of Anesthesiologists Task Force on Perioperative Management of patients with obstructive sleep apnea. Anesthesiology. 2014;120:268–86.
4. Ayas NT, Laratta CR, Coleman JM, Doufas AG, Eikermann M, Gay PC, Gottlieb DJ, Gurubhagavatula I, Hillman DR, Kaw R, Malhotra A, Mokhlesi B, Morgenthaler TI, Parthasarathy S, Ramachandran SK, Strohl KP, Strollo PJ, Twery MJ, Zee PC, Chung FF, Sleep ATSAo, Respiratory N. Knowledge gaps in the perioperative management of adults with obstructive sleep apnea and obesity hypoventilation syndrome. An official American Thoracic Society workshop report. Ann Am Thorac Soc. 2018;15:117–26.
5. Chung F, Memtsoudis SG, Ramachandran SK, Nagappa M, Opperer M, Cozowicz C, Patrawala S, Lam D, Kumar A, Joshi GP, Fleetham J, Ayas N, Collop N, Doufas AG, Eikermann M, Englesakis M, Gali B, Gay P, Hernandez AV, Kaw R, Kezirian EJ, Malhotra A, Mokhlesi B, Parthasarathy S, Stierer T, Wappler F, Hillman DR, Auckley D. Society of Anesthesia and Sleep Medicine Guidelines on preoperative screening and assessment of adult patients with obstructive sleep apnea. Anesth Analg. 2016;123:452–73.
6. Memtsoudis SG, Cozowicz C, Nagappa M, Wong J, Joshi GP, Wong DT, Doufas AG, Yilmaz M, Stein MH, Krajewski ML, Singh M, Pichler L, Ramachandran SK, Chung F. Society of Anesthesia and Sleep Medicine Guideline on intraoperative management of adult patients with obstructive sleep apnea. Anesth Analg. 2018;127:967–87.

7. Meoli AL, Rosen CL, Kristo D, Kohrman M, Gooneratne N, Aguillard RN, Fayle R, Troell R, Kramer R, Casey KR, Coleman J Jr, Clinical Practice Review C, American Academy of Sleep M. Upper airway management of the adult patient with obstructive sleep apnea in the perioperative period–avoiding complications. Sleep. 2003;26:1060–5.

8. Adesanya AO, Lee W, Greilich NB, Joshi GP. Perioperative management of obstructive sleep apnea. Chest. 2010;138:1489–98.

9. Young T, Palta M, Dempsey J, Peppard PE, Nieto FJ, Hla KM. Burden of sleep apnea: rationale, design, and major findings of the Wisconsin Sleep Cohort study. WMJ. 2009;108:246–9.

10. Peppard PE, Young T, Barnet JH, Palta M, Hagen EW, Hla KM. Increased prevalence of sleep-disordered breathing in adults. Am J Epidemiol. 2013;177:1006–14.

11. Young T, Palta M, Dempsey J, Skatrud J, Weber S, Badr S. The occurrence of sleep-disordered breathing among middle-aged adults. N Engl J Med. 1993;328:1230–5.

12. Dempsey JA, Skatrud JB, Jacques AJ, Ewanowski SJ, Woodson BT, Hanson PR, Goodman B. Anatomic determinants of sleep-disordered breathing across the spectrum of clinical and nonclinical male subjects. Chest. 2002;122:840–51.

13. Li KK, Kushida C, Powell NB, Riley RW, Guilleminault C. Obstructive sleep apnea syndrome: a comparison between Far-East Asian and white men. Laryngoscope. 2000;110:1689–93.

14. Pranathiageswaran S, Badr MS, Severson R, Rowley JA. The influence of race on the severity of sleep disordered breathing. J Clin Sleep Med. 2013;9:303–9.

15. Young T, Skatrud J, Peppard PE. Risk factors for obstructive sleep apnea in adults. JAMA. 2004;291:2013–6.

16. Young T, Peppard PE, Taheri S. Excess weight and sleep-disordered breathing. J Appl Physiol (1985). 2005;99:1592–9.

17. Hales CM, Fryar CD, Carroll MD, Freedman DS, Ogden CL. Trends in obesity and severe obesity prevalence in US youth and adults by sex and age, 2007-2008 to 2015-2016. JAMA. 2018;319:1723–5.

18. Lopez PP, Stefan B, Schulman CI, Byers PM. Prevalence of sleep apnea in morbidly obese patients who presented for weight loss surgery evaluation: more evidence for routine screening for obstructive sleep apnea before weight loss surgery. Am Surg. 2008;74:834–8.

19. Abdelsattar ZM, Hendren S, Wong SL, Campbell DA Jr, Ramachandran SK. The impact of untreated obstructive sleep apnea on cardiopulmonary complications in general and vascular surgery: a cohort study. Sleep. 2015;38:1205–10.

20. Mokhlesi B, Hovda MD, Vekhter B, Arora VM, Chung F, Meltzer DO. Sleep-disordered breathing and postoperative outcomes after bariatric surgery: analysis of the nationwide inpatient sample. Obes Surg. 2013;23:1842–51.

21. Memtsoudis SG, Stundner O, Rasul R, Chiu YL, Sun X, Ramachandran SK, Kaw R, Fleischut P, Mazumdar M. The impact of sleep apnea on postoperative utilization of resources and adverse outcomes. Anesth Analg. 2014;118:407–18.

22. Chan MTV, Wang CY, Seet E, Tam S, Lai HY, Chew EFF, Wu WKK, Cheng BCP, Lam CKM, Short TG, Hui DSC, Chung F. Postoperative vascular complications in unrecognized obstructive sleep apnea study I. Association of unrecognized obstructive sleep apnea with postoperative cardiovascular events in patients undergoing major noncardiac surgery. JAMA. 2019;321:1788–98.

23. Raveendran R, Wong J, Singh M, Wong DT, Chung F. Obesity hypoventilation syndrome, sleep apnea, overlap syndrome: perioperative management to prevent complications. Curr Opin Anaesthesiol. 2017;30:146–55.

24. Kaw R, Chung F, Pasupuleti V, Mehta J, Gay PC, Hernandez AV. Meta-analysis of the association between obstructive sleep apnoea and postoperative outcome. Br J Anaesth. 2012;109:897–906.

25. Memtsoudis S, Liu SS, Ma Y, Chiu YL, Walz JM, Gaber-Baylis LK, Mazumdar M. Perioperative pulmonary outcomes in patients with sleep apnea after noncardiac surgery. Anesth Analg. 2011;112:113–21.

26. Opperer M, Cozowicz C, Bugada D, Mokhlesi B, Kaw R, Auckley D, Chung F, Memtsoudis SG. Does obstructive sleep apnea influence perioperative outcome? A qualitative systematic review for the Society of Anesthesia and Sleep Medicine Task Force on preoperative preparation of patients with sleep-disordered breathing. Anesth Analg. 2016;122:1321–34.

27. Lindenauer PK, Stefan MS, Johnson KG, Priya A, Pekow PS, Rothberg MB. Prevalence, treatment, and outcomes associated with OSA among patients hospitalized with pneumonia. Chest. 2014;145:1032–8.

28. Subramani Y, Nagappa M, Wong J, Patra J, Chung F. Death or near-death in patients with obstructive sleep apnoea: a compendium of case reports of critical complications. Br J Anaesth. 2017;119:885–99.

29. Kaw R, Bhateja P, Paz YMH, Hernandez AV, Ramaswamy A, Deshpande A, Aboussouan LS. Postoperative complications in patients with unrecognized obesity hypoventilation syndrome undergoing elective noncardiac surgery. Chest. 2016;149:84–91.

30. Hai F, Porhomayon J, Vermont L, Frydrych L, Jaoude P, El-Solh AA. Postoperative complications in patients with obstructive sleep apnea: a meta-analysis. J Clin Anesth. 2014;26:591–600.

31. D'Apuzzo MR, Browne JA. Obstructive sleep apnea as a risk factor for postoperative complications after revision joint arthroplasty. J Arthroplast. 2012;27:95–8.

32. Masaraccchia MM, Sites BD, Herrick MD, Liu H, Davis M. Association between sleep apnea and perioperative outcomes among patients undergoing shoulder arthroscopy. Can J Anaesth. 2018;65:1314–23.

33. Fiorentino M, Hwang F, Pentakota SR, Livingston DH, Mosenthal AC. Pulmonary complications in trauma patients with obstructive sleep apnea undergoing pelvic or lower limb operation. Trauma Surg Acute Care Open. 2020;5:e000529.

34. Golaz R, Tangel VE, Lui B, Albrecht E, Pryor KO, White RS. Post-operative outcomes and anesthesia type in total hip arthroplasty in patients with obstructive sleep apnea: a retrospective analysis of the State Inpatient Databases. J Clin Anesth. 2021;69:110159.

35. Gupta RM, Parvizi J, Hanssen AD, Gay PC. Postoperative complications in patients with obstructive sleep apnea syndrome undergoing hip or knee replacement: a case-control study. Mayo Clin Proc. 2001;76:897–905.

36. Hiremath AS, Hillman DR, James AL, Noffsinger WJ, Platt PR, Singer SL. Relationship between difficult tracheal intubation and obstructive sleep apnoea. Br J Anaesth. 1998;80:606–11.

37. Siyam MA, Benhamou D. Difficult endotracheal intubation in patients with sleep apnea syndrome. Anesth Analg. 2002;95:1098–102, table of contents.

38. Rennotte MT, Baele P, Aubert G, Rodenstein DO. Nasal continuous positive airway pressure in the perioperative management of patients with obstructive sleep apnea submitted to surgery. Chest. 1995;107:367–74.

39. Mokhlesi B, Hovda MD, Vekhter B, Arora VM, Chung F, Meltzer DO. Sleep-disordered breathing and postoperative outcomes after elective surgery: analysis of the nationwide inpatient sample. Chest. 2013;144:903–14.

40. Mutter TC, Chateau D, Moffatt M, Ramsey C, Roos LL, Kryger M. A matched cohort study of postoperative outcomes in obstructive sleep apnea: could preoperative diagnosis and treatment prevent complications? Anesthesiology. 2014;121:707–18.

41. Karimi N, Kelava M, Kothari P, Zimmerman NM, Gillinov AM, Duncan AE. Patients at high risk for obstructive sleep apnea are at increased risk for atrial fibrillation after cardiac surgery: a cohort analysis. Anesth Analg. 2018;126:2025–31.

42. Ng KT, Lee ZX, Ang E, Teoh WY, Wang CY. Association of obstructive sleep apnea and postoperative cardiac complications: a systematic review and meta-analysis with trial sequential analysis. J Clin Anesth. 2020;62:109731.

43. Nagappa M, Ho G, Patra J, Wong J, Singh M, Kaw R, Cheng D, Chung F. Postoperative outcomes in obstructive sleep apnea patients undergoing cardiac surgery: a systematic review and meta-analysis of comparative studies. Anesth Analg. 2017;125:2030–7.

44. Abrishami A, Khajehdehi A, Chung F. A systematic review of screening questionnaires for obstructive sleep apnea. Can J Anaesth. 2010;57:423–38.
45. Ramachandran SK, Josephs LA. A meta-analysis of clinical screening tests for obstructive sleep apnea. Anesthesiology. 2009;110:928–39.
46. Chung F, Yegneswaran B, Liao P, Chung SA, Vairavanathan S, Islam S, Khajehdehi A, Shapiro CM. STOP questionnaire: a tool to screen patients for obstructive sleep apnea. Anesthesiology. 2008;108:812–21.
47. Seet E, Chua M, Liaw CM. High STOP-BANG questionnaire scores predict intraoperative and early postoperative adverse events. Singap Med J. 2015;56:212–6.
48. Proczko MA, Stepaniak PS, de Quelerij M, van der Lely FH, Smulders JF, Kaska L, Soliman Hamad MA. STOP-Bang and the effect on patient outcome and length of hospital stay when patients are not using continuous positive airway pressure. J Anesth. 2014;28:891–7.
49. Netzer NC, Stoohs RA, Netzer CM, Clark K, Strohl KP. Using the Berlin questionnaire to identify patients at risk for the sleep apnea syndrome. Ann Intern Med. 1999;131:485–91.
50. Chung F, Ward B, Ho J, Yuan H, Kayumov L, Shapiro C. Preoperative identification of sleep apnea risk in elective surgical patients, using the Berlin questionnaire. J Clin Anesth. 2007;19:130–4.
51. Chung F, Yegneswaran B, Liao P, Chung SA, Vairavanathan S, Islam S, Khajehdehi A, Shapiro CM. Validation of the Berlin questionnaire and American Society of Anesthesiologists checklist as screening tools for obstructive sleep apnea in surgical patients. Anesthesiology. 2008;108:822–30.
52. Gross JB, Bachenberg KL, Benumof JL, Caplan RA, Connis RT, Cote CJ, Nickinovich DG, Prachand V, Ward DS, Weaver EM, Ydens L, Yu S, American Society of Anesthesiologists Task Force on Perioperative M. Practice guidelines for the perioperative management of patients with obstructive sleep apnea: a report by the American Society of Anesthesiologists Task Force on Perioperative Management of patients with obstructive sleep apnea. Anesthesiology. 2006;104:1081–93; quiz 1117-1088
53. Nagappa M, Liao P, Wong J, Auckley D, Ramachandran SK, Memtsoudis S, Mokhlesi B, Chung F. Validation of the STOP-Bang questionnaire as a screening tool for obstructive sleep apnea among different populations: a systematic review and meta-analysis. PLoS One. 2015;10:e0143697.
54. Seguin L, Tamisier R, Deletombe B, Lopez M, Pepin JL, Payen JF. Preoperative screening for obstructive sleep apnea using alternative scoring models of the sleep tiredness observed pressure-body mass index age neck circumference gender questionnaire: an external validation. Anesth Analg. 2020;131:1025–31.
55. Kreitinger KY, Lui MMS, Owens RL, Schmickl CN, Grunvald E, Horgan S, Raphelson JR, Malhotra A. Screening for obstructive sleep apnea in a diverse bariatric surgery population. Obesity (Silver Spring). 2020;28:2028–34.
56. Waseem R, Chan MTV, Wang CY, Seet E, Tam S, Loo SY, CKM L, Hui DS, Chung F. Diagnostic performance of the STOP-Bang questionnaire as a screening tool for obstructive sleep apnea in different ethnic groups. J Clin Sleep Med. 2020;17:521.
57. Flemons WW, Whitelaw WA, Brant R, Remmers JE. Likelihood ratios for a sleep apnea clinical prediction rule. Am J Respir Crit Care Med. 1994;150:1279–85.
58. Gali B, Whalen FX Jr, Gay PC, Olson EJ, Schroeder DR, Plevak DJ, Morgenthaler TI. Management plan to reduce risks in perioperative care of patients with presumed obstructive sleep apnea syndrome. J Clin Sleep Med. 2007;3:582–8.
59. Gali B, Whalen FX, Schroeder DR, Gay PC, Plevak DJ. Identification of patients at risk for postoperative respiratory complications using a preoperative obstructive sleep apnea screening tool and postanesthesia care assessment. Anesthesiology. 2009;110:869–77.
60. Seet E, Chung F. Management of sleep apnea in adults – functional algorithms for the perioperative period: continuing professional development. Can J Anaesth. 2010;57:849–64.
61. Stierer TL, Wright C, George A, Thompson RE, Wu CL, Collop N. Risk assessment of obstructive sleep apnea in a population of patients undergoing ambulatory surgery. J Clin Sleep Med. 2010;6:467–72.

62. Nagappa M, Mokhlesi B, Wong J, Wong DT, Kaw R, Chung F. The effects of continuous positive airway pressure on postoperative outcomes in obstructive sleep apnea patients undergoing surgery: a systematic review and meta-analysis. Anesth Analg. 2015;120:1013–23.
63. Apfelbaum JL, Hagberg CA, Caplan RA, Blitt CD, Connis RT, Nickinovich DG, Hagberg CA, Caplan RA, Benumof JL, Berry FA, Blitt CD, Bode RH, Cheney FW, Connis RT, Guidry OF, Nickinovich DG, Ovassapian A, American Society of Anesthesiologists Task Force on Management of the Difficult A. Practice guidelines for management of the difficult airway: an updated report by the American Society of Anesthesiologists Task Force on Management of the Difficult Airway. Anesthesiology. 2013;118:251–70.
64. Acar HV, Yarkan Uysal H, Kaya A, Ceyhan A, Dikmen B. Does the STOP-Bang, an obstructive sleep apnea screening tool, predict difficult intubation? Eur Rev Med Pharmacol Sci. 2014;18:1869–74.
65. Corso RM, Petrini F, Buccioli M, Nanni O, Carretta E, Trolio A, De Nuzzo D, Pigna A, Di Giacinto I, Agnoletti V, Gambale G. Clinical utility of preoperative screening with STOP-Bang questionnaire in elective surgery. Minerva Anestesiol. 2014;80:877–84.
66. Gokay P, Tastan S, Orhan ME. Is there a difference between the STOP-BANG and the Berlin Obstructive Sleep Apnoea Syndrome questionnaires for determining respiratory complications during the perioperative period? J Clin Nurs. 2016;25:1238–52.
67. Kheterpal S, Han R, Tremper KK, Shanks A, Tait AR, O'Reilly M, Ludwig TA. Incidence and predictors of difficult and impossible mask ventilation. Anesthesiology. 2006;105:885–91.
68. Nagappa M, Wong DT, Cozowicz C, Ramachandran SK, Memtsoudis SG, Chung F. Is obstructive sleep apnea associated with difficult airway? Evidence from a systematic review and meta-analysis of prospective and retrospective cohort studies. PLoS One. 2018;13:e0204904.
69. Chung F, Yegneswaran B, Herrera F, Shenderey A, Shapiro CM. Patients with difficult intubation may need referral to sleep clinics. Anesth Analg. 2008;107:915–20.
70. Cormack RS, Lehane J. Difficult tracheal intubation in obstetrics. Anaesthesia. 1984;39:1105–11.
71. Gentil B, de Larminat JM, Boucherez C, Lienhart A. Difficult intubation and obstructive sleep apnoea syndrome. Br J Anaesth. 1994;72:368.
72. Kim JA, Lee JJ. Preoperative predictors of difficult intubation in patients with obstructive sleep apnea syndrome. Can J Anaesth. 2006;53:393–7.
73. Ezri T, Medalion B, Weisenberg M, Szmuk P, Warters RD, Charuzi I. Increased body mass index per se is not a predictor of difficult laryngoscopy. Can J Anaesth. 2003;50:179–83.
74. Mezzanotte WS, Tangel DJ, White DP. Waking genioglossal electromyogram in sleep apnea patients versus normal controls (a neuromuscular compensatory mechanism). J Clin Invest. 1992;89:1571–9.
75. Eastwood PR, Platt PR, Shepherd K, Maddison K, Hillman DR. Collapsibility of the upper airway at different concentrations of propofol anesthesia. Anesthesiology. 2005;103:470–7.
76. Eastwood PR, Szollosi I, Platt PR, Hillman DR. Comparison of upper airway collapse during general anaesthesia and sleep. Lancet. 2002;359:1207–9.
77. Hillman DR, Chung F. Anaesthetic management of sleep-disordered breathing in adults. Respirology. 2017;22:230–9.
78. Dahan A, Teppema LJ. Influence of anaesthesia and analgesia on the control of breathing. Br J Anaesth. 2003;91:40–9.
79. Douglas NJ, White DP, Weil JV, Pickett CK, Zwillich CW. Hypercapnic ventilatory response in sleeping adults. Am Rev Respir Dis. 1982;126:758–62.
80. Horner RL, Hughes SW, Malhotra A. State-dependent and reflex drives to the upper airway: basic physiology with clinical implications. J Appl Physiol (1985). 2014;116:325–36.
81. Rehder K, Sessler AD, Marsh HM. General anesthesia and the lung. Am Rev Respir Dis. 1975;112:541–63.
82. Ogunnaike BO, Jones SB, Jones DB, Provost D, Whitten CW. Anesthetic considerations for bariatric surgery. Anesth Analg. 2002;95:1793–805.
83. Memtsoudis SG, Stundner O, Rasul R, Sun X, Chiu YL, Fleischut P, Danninger T, Mazumdar M. Sleep apnea and total joint arthroplasty under various types of anesthesia: a population-based study of perioperative outcomes. Reg Anesth Pain Med. 2013;38:274–81.

84. Ambrosii T, Sandru S, Belii A. The prevalence of perioperative complications in patients with and without obstructive sleep apnoea: a prospective cohort study. Rom J Anaesth Intens Care. 2016;23:103–10.
85. Liu SS, Chisholm MF, Ngeow J, John RS, Shaw P, Ma Y, Memtsoudis SG. Postoperative hypoxemia in orthopedic patients with obstructive sleep apnea. HSS J. 2011;7:2–8.
86. Naqvi SY, Rabiei AH, Maltenfort MG, Restrepo C, Viscusi ER, Parvizi J, Rasouli MR. Perioperative complications in patients with sleep apnea undergoing total joint arthroplasty. J Arthroplast. 2017;32:2680–3.
87. Vroegop AV, Vanderveken OM, Boudewyns AN, Scholman J, Saldien V, Wouters K, Braem MJ, Van de Heyning PH, Hamans E. Drug-induced sleep endoscopy in sleep-disordered breathing: report on 1,249 cases. Laryngoscope. 2014;124:797–802.
88. Lee CH, Mo JH, Kim BJ, Kong IG, Yoon IY, Chung S, Kim JH, Kim JW. Evaluation of soft palate changes using sleep videofluoroscopy in patients with obstructive sleep apnea. Arch Otolaryngol Head Neck Surg. 2009;135:168–72.
89. Boysen PG 2nd, Pappas MM, Evans B. An evidence-based opioid-free anesthetic technique to manage perioperative and periprocedural pain. Ochsner J. 2018;18:121–5.
90. Macintyre PE, Loadsman JA, Scott DA. Opioids, ventilation and acute pain management. Anaesth Intensive Care. 2011;39:545–58.
91. Etches RC. Respiratory depression associated with patient-controlled analgesia: a review of eight cases. Can J Anaesth. 1994;41:125–32.
92. Hagle ME, Lehr VT, Brubakken K, Shippee A. Respiratory depression in adult patients with intravenous patient-controlled analgesia. Orthop Nurs. 2004;23:18–27; quiz 28-19
93. Lam KK, Kunder S, Wong J, Doufas AG, Chung F. Obstructive sleep apnea, pain, and opioids: is the riddle solved? Curr Opin Anaesthesiol. 2016;29:134–40.
94. Bernards CM, Knowlton SL, Schmidt DF, DePaso WJ, Lee MK, McDonald SB, Bains OS. Respiratory and sleep effects of remifentanil in volunteers with moderate obstructive sleep apnea. Anesthesiology. 2009;110:41–9.
95. Pyati S, Gan TJ. Perioperative pain management. CNS Drugs. 2007;21:185–211.
96. White PF. The changing role of non-opioid analgesic techniques in the management of postoperative pain. Anesth Analg. 2005;101:S5–22.
97. Joshi GP. Multimodal analgesia techniques for ambulatory surgery. Int Anesthesiol Clin. 2005;43:197–204.
98. Raghavendran S, Bagry H, Detheux G, Zhang X, Brouillette RT, Brown KA. An anesthetic management protocol to decrease respiratory complications after adenotonsillectomy in children with severe sleep apnea. Anesth Analg. 2010;110:1093–101.
99. Cavalcante AN, Sprung J, Schroeder DR, Weingarten TN. Multimodal analgesic therapy with gabapentin and its association with postoperative respiratory depression. Anesth Analg. 2017;125:141–6.
100. Lynn LA, Curry JP. Patterns of unexpected in-hospital deaths: a root cause analysis. Patient Saf Surg. 2011;5:3.
101. Lee LA, Caplan RA, Stephens LS, Posner KL, Terman GW, Voepel-Lewis T, Domino KB. Postoperative opioid-induced respiratory depression: a closed claims analysis. Anesthesiology. 2015;122:659–65.
102. Bolden N, Posner KL, Domino KB, Auckley D, Benumof JL, Herway ST, Hillman D, Mincer SL, Overdyk F, Samuels DJ, Warner LL, Weingarten TN, Chung F. Postoperative critical events associated with obstructive sleep apnea: results from the Society of Anesthesia and Sleep Medicine Obstructive Sleep Apnea Registry. Anesth Analg. 2020;131:1032–41.
103. Chan MT, Wang CY, Seet E, Tam S, Lai HY, Walker S, Short TG, Halliwell R, Chung F, Investigators P. Postoperative vascular complications in unrecognised Obstructive Sleep apnoea (POSA) study protocol: an observational cohort study in moderate-to-high risk patients undergoing non-cardiac surgery. BMJ Open. 2014;4:e004097.

104. Lam T, Nagappa M, Wong J, Singh M, Wong D, Chung F. Continuous pulse oximetry and capnography monitoring for postoperative respiratory depression and adverse events: a systematic review and meta-analysis. Anesth Analg. 2017;125:2019–29.

105. Sanders MH, Kern NB, Costantino JP, Stiller RA, Strollo PJ Jr, Studnicki KA, Coates JA, Richards TJ. Accuracy of end-tidal and transcutaneous PCO2 monitoring during sleep. Chest. 1994;106:472–83.

106. Chung F, Wong J, Mestek ML, Niebel KH, Lichtenthal P. Characterization of respiratory compromise and the potential clinical utility of capnography in the post-anesthesia care unit: a blinded observational trial. J Clin Monit Comput. 2020;34:541–51.

107. Gay PC. Sleep and sleep-disordered breathing in the hospitalized patient. Respir Care. 2010;55:1240–54.

108. Organized jointly by the American Thoracic Society tERStESoICM, the Societe de Reanimation de Langue F, approved by Ats Board of Directors D. International Consensus Conferences in Intensive Care Medicine: noninvasive positive pressure ventilation in acute respiratory failure. Am J Respir Crit Care Med. 2001;163:283–91.

109. Liao P, Luo Q, Elsaid H, Kang W, Shapiro CM, Chung F. Perioperative auto-titrated continuous positive airway pressure treatment in surgical patients with obstructive sleep apnea: a randomized controlled trial. Anesthesiology. 2013;119:837–47.

110. Chung F, Liao P, Yegneswaran B, Shapiro CM, Kang W. Postoperative changes in sleep-disordered breathing and sleep architecture in patients with obstructive sleep apnea. Anesthesiology. 2014;120:287–98.

111. Hillman DR, Jungquist CR, Auckley D. Perioperative implementation of noninvasive positive airway pressure therapies. Respir Care. 2018;63:479–87.

112. Guralnick AS, Pant M, Minhaj M, Sweitzer BJ, Mokhlesi B. CPAP adherence in patients with newly diagnosed obstructive sleep apnea prior to elective surgery. J Clin Sleep Med. 2012;8:501–6.

113. Fernandez-Bustamante A, Bartels K, Clavijo C, Scott BK, Kacmar R, Bullard K, Moss AFD, Henderson W, Juarez-Colunga E, Jameson L. Preoperatively screened obstructive sleep apnea is associated with worse postoperative outcomes than previously diagnosed obstructive sleep apnea. Anesth Analg. 2017;125:593–602.

114. Chung F, Nagappa M, Singh M, Mokhlesi B. CPAP in the perioperative setting: evidence of support. Chest. 2016;149:586–97.

115. Meurgey JH, Brown R, Woroszyl-Chrusciel A, Steier J. Peri-operative treatment of sleep-disordered breathing and outcomes in bariatric patients. J Thorac Dis. 2018;10:S144–52.

116. Ferreyra GP, Baussano I, Squadrone V, Richiardi L, Marchiaro G, Del Sorbo L, Mascia L, Merletti F, Ranieri VM. Continuous positive airway pressure for treatment of respiratory complications after abdominal surgery: a systematic review and meta-analysis. Ann Surg. 2008;247:617–26.

117. Zarbock A, Mueller E, Netzer S, Gabriel A, Feindt P, Kindgen-Milles D. Prophylactic nasal continuous positive airway pressure following cardiac surgery protects from postoperative pulmonary complications: a prospective, randomized, controlled trial in 500 patients. Chest. 2009;135:1252–9.

118. Squadrone V, Coha M, Cerutti E, Schellino MM, Biolino P, Occella P, Belloni G, Vilianis G, Fiore G, Cavallo F, Ranieri VM, Piedmont Intensive Care Units N. Continuous positive airway pressure for treatment of postoperative hypoxemia: a randomized controlled trial. JAMA. 2005;293:589–95.

Chapter 11
Sleep-Disordered Breathing (SDB) in Pediatric Populations

Carol L. Rosen

Keywords Pediatrics · Infant · Child · Adolescent · Polysomnography · Sleep apnea syndromes · Sleep-disordered breathing · Obstructive sleep apnea · Central sleep apnea · Central hypoventilation · Control of breathing · Hypoventilation · Apnea of prematurity · Airway obstruction · Achondroplasia · Cleft lip and palate · Chiari malformation · Congenital central hypoventilation syndrome · Craniofacial abnormalities · Craniosynostosis · Down's syndrome · Joubert syndrome · Muscular dystrophy · Neuromuscular weakness · *PHOX2B* · Pierre Robin syndrome · Prader · Willi syndrome · Rett syndrome · ROHHAD · Sickle cell disease · Spina bifida · Spinal muscular atrophy

Introduction

When evaluating sleep-disordered breathing (SDB) in children, the sleep medicine specialist will see a broad range of respiratory problems beyond collapse of the upper airway. In addition to obstructive sleep apnea (OSA), the specialist should be prepared to evaluate control of breathing disorders, hypoventilation due to neuro-muscular or thoracic cage disorders, and worsening sleep-related gas-exchange associated with chronic pulmonary conditions. The age spectrum will include infants to young adults with intellectual and other disabilities. Many referred children will have other comorbidities associated with increased risk of SDB such as obesity, genetic or craniofacial disorders, central nervous system (CNS) disorders,

C. L. Rosen (✉)
Department of Pediatrics, Case Western Reserve University School of Medicine, Cleveland, OH, USA
e-mail: carol.rosen@case.edu

© Springer Nature Switzerland AG 2022
M. S. Badr, J. L. Martin (eds.), *Essentials of Sleep Medicine*, Respiratory Medicine, https://doi.org/10.1007/978-3-030-93739-3_11

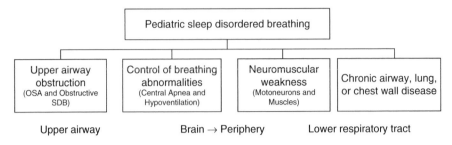

Fig. 11.1 Overview of pediatric sleep-disordered breathing

or neuromuscular disorders. Figure 11.1 presents a useful framework for thinking about the SDB in children in terms of understanding symptoms, signs, comorbidities, Polysomnography (PSG) findings, and planning a diagnosis and/or management approach.

This chapter provides summaries of the differences between pediatric and adult presentation of OSA, obstructive SDB in children, distinctive patient groups who are at high risk for SDB and respiratory-related hypoventilation and commonly referred for SDB evaluation, unique features of SDB in the first year of life, control of breathing disorders (central hypoventilation and central sleep apnea), and the basics of accommodating and evaluating children in sleep laboratory. More comprehensive references are listed for many topics.

Obstructive Sleep Apnea and Obstructive SDB in Children and Teens [1–4]

OSA is characterized by repeated episodes of partial upper airway obstruction and/or intermittent complete obstruction associated with disruption of gas exchange and sleep patterns. Anatomic and neuromotor problems contribute to its pathophysiology. The prevalence of OSA in healthy children is 1–5% but can exceed 50% in children with certain medical conditions (e.g., Down's syndrome, neuromuscular diseases, and craniofacial disorders). OSA has two age peaks in childhood. The first peak is in early childhood from ages 2–6 years, coinciding with normal lymphoid hyperplasia of tonsils and adenoids that surround the upper airway. The second peak appears after puberty, coinciding with weight gain and/or obesity. Table 11.1 summarizes risk factors for OSA in children.

Habitual snoring, prevalence 10%, is often the key presenting symptom, but not all snoring children have OSA. Table 11.2 lists symptoms and signs typically seen in children with OSA [1].

Clinical assessment does not reliably predict the presence or severity of OSA in children, but history and physical examination aids in risk assessment for OSA. In a large randomized controlled study of adenotonsillectomy in school-aged children

Table 11.1 Risk factors for obstructive OSA

Adenotonsillar hypertrophy
Comorbid conditions (obesity, craniofacial, neuromuscular, genetic)
Airway inflammation (nasal allergies, asthma)
Positive family history (two- to four-fold ↑ risk)
African American heritage (two- to four-fold ↑ risk)
Perinatal influences (prematurity, three-fold ↑ risk)
Prior adenotonsillectomy (unmasks anatomic and functional influences)
Socio-demographic (environmental tobacco smoke, neighborhood disadvantage, sleep deprivation)

Table 11.2 Symptoms and signs of OSA in children

History	Physical exam
Frequent snoring (≥3 nights/week)	Underweight or overweight
Labored breathing during sleep	Tonsillar hypertrophy
Gasping or snorting	Adenoidal facies or open mouth posture
Sleep enuresis (especially secondary)	Micro- or retrognathia
Sleeps sitting up or with neck hyperextended	High-arched palate
Cyanosis during sleep	Pectus deformity
Morning headaches	Hypertension
Daytime sleepiness	
Attention, behavior, or learning problems	

in which all participants had snoring, adenotonsillar hypertrophy, a standardized clinical history, and physical examination by pediatric ENT specialists, clinical parameters explained only 3% of the variance in the AHI [5, 6].

Laboratory-based PSG plays an important role in the diagnosis of OSA in children [1, 2, 7–12]. Although home-based sleep apnea testing (HSAT) is widely used in adults to diagnosis OSA in adult patients with high pretest probability of OSA, its use in children has been much more limited, reflecting concerns about safety feasibility, and reliability of collecting multiple respiratory signals in this population. Home sleep apnea testing (HSAT) devices are currently not recommended for use in children, but further research is needed to validate these approaches in children. More references on this topic are supplied later in the chapter.

Untreated OSA is associated with adverse consequences (attentional, behavioral, or learning problems; reduced quality of life, impaired growth, hypertension/cardiovascular stress, metabolic alterations and systemic inflammation, increased healthcare costs). In healthy children, adenotonsillar hypertrophy is the commonest cause of OSA and adenotonsillectomy is the first line of treatment, but success rates decrease significantly in children with underlying comorbidities. In a large randomized controlled trial of adenotonsillectomy in school-aged children with adenotonsillar hypertrophy and mild to moderate OSA, surgical treatment improved OSA symptoms, quality of life, PSG findings, behavior, and sleepiness [5, 13–15].

Patients should be reevaluated postoperatively for residual signs and symptoms to determine whether further treatment is required [9]. In otherwise healthy children, risk factors for persistence of OSA post-surgery includes obesity, African-American race/ethnicity, and higher obstructive apnea hypopnea indices [5]. In children with complex chronic conditions, residual SDB is common (30–60%) and anatomic and neuromotor problems are major contributors, so other surgical procedures and nonsurgical management may be needed [16].

Most children who do not respond to adenotonsillectomy or who are not candidates for adenotonsillectomy can be managed with PAP therapy [17, 18], but like adults, adherence is a challenge. Intranasal corticosteroids are an option for children with mild postoperative OSA or those who have not undergone adenotonsillectomy. Watchful waiting with supportive care may be appropriate for mild-moderate OSA [5]. Weight management and other lifestyle changes (exercise, sufficient and regular sleep) are recommended for patients who are overweight or obese. Novel dental or orthodontic treatments (e.g., rapid maxillary expansion, oral appliance to advance the mandible) may have a role in selected patients but more studies are needed to develop guidelines for this treatment of pediatric OSA. Positioning therapy may have a role in some selected patients.

Differences Between OSA Presentation Between Children and Adults

The clinical presentation and management of OSA differs between children and adults, but preteens and teens often present with a more adult-like picture (Table 11.3).

In children, adenotonsillar hypertrophy is the biggest risk factor for OSA, while obesity begins to play a stronger role in adolescence. There is no gender

Table 11.3 Comparison of OSA presentation in a child, adult, or obese child/teen

	Child	Adult	Obese child/teen
Gender	M = F	M>> > F	M> > F
Peak age	2–8 years	Mid-life	Preteen/Teen
Obesity	+	++++	++++
Craniofacial, genetic, or neuromuscular disorders	+++	+	++
Chief complaint for seeking medical attention	Snore Behavior/learning	Sleepiness	Snore, sleepiness Behavior/learning
Arousal	±	++++	+ to ++++
Respiratory pattern	Obstructive hypopneas ± hypoventilation	OSA	Obstructive hypoventilation to frank OSA
Treatment role for adenotonsillectomy	Common	Rare	Yes, but ↑ likelihood of residual OSA after surgery

Table 11.4 Comparison of OSA severity by obstructive AHI in pediatric and adult patients

	Pediatric	Adult
Mild	1–4.99	5–14.99
Moderate	5–9.99	15–29.99
Severe	≥10	≥30

predisposition in prepubertal children, but a male predominance appears in puberty. Overall children are much better defenders against upper airway collapse than adults, so their obstructive apnea hypopnea indices (AHI) are lower and OSA severity is scaled differently (Table 11.4) [19].

Association with Obesity

The prevalence of obesity across all age groups has more than doubled in school-aged children and tripled in teens, up to 18% in both age group. Obesity and OSA are independently associated with longer-term adverse cardiovascular, metabolic, and neuropsychological consequences. OSA occurs more often and may be more severe in children and adolescents who are overweight or obese compared with lean children. In a large randomized controlled trial of adenotonsillectomy in school-aged children with adenotonsillar hypertrophy and mild-to-moderate OSA, surgery normalized weight in children who had failure to thrive, but increased in risk for obesity in overweight children [20]. While treatment options for obesity-related OSA includes adenotonsillectomy, "cure" is less likely [5, 21]. Obese teens with OSA have enlarged tonsils and smaller airways compared to lean controls or obese controls without OSA [22]. PAP therapy is generally successful in relieving OSA but limited by generally poor compliance. There is increasing experience with bariatric surgery in youth with extreme obesity which may be a future OSA treatment option to this special population.

Special Populations at Higher Risk for OSA and Obstructive SDB [23–30]

Table 11.5 lists patient groups with genetic, craniofacial, CNS, or neuromuscular disorders who have higher risk of OSA/obstructive SDB due to a combination of factors (craniofacial anatomy, muscular weakness, hypotonia, control of breathing abnormalities, association with obesity).

In some patient groups, PSG is needed to evaluate SDB status before and after prescribing advanced ventilatory support or applying newer medical, surgical, or gene therapies, so key features of these unique patient groups are reviewed.

Table 11.5 Conditions associated with obstructive SDB

Down's syndrome (trisomy 21)
Prader–Willi syndrome
Craniofacial (Pierre Robin sequence, craniosynostoses, Treacher Collins syndrome, cleft lip/palate)
Skeletal dysplasias or connective tissue disorders (achondroplasia, Marfan syndrome)
Sickle cell disease
Neuromuscular disorders (spinal muscular atrophy, Duchenne muscular dystrophy, myotonic muscular dystrophy)
Storage diseases (mucopolysaccharidoses, glycogen storage diseases)
Epilepsy and vagal nerve stimulator

Down's Syndrome [31–34]

Down's Syndrome (also known as trisomy 21) is a common (prevalence 1/800 live births) genetic disorder and the most frequent genetic form of intellectual disability. Hallmarks of the syndrome include intellectual disability, hypotonia, craniofacial abnormalities, short stature, increased incidence of hypothyroidism, and congenital cardiac defects (50% of individuals). Life expectancy is now 60 years. OSA is highly prevalent in children with Down's syndrome (estimates are 30–60% depending on selection criteria) and 90% in adults (almost 70% in the severe range). Worsening of OSA over time is related to increasing age, obesity, and associated hypothyroidism. Predisposing factors for OSA include midfacial hypoplasia, mandibular hypoplasia, small crowded airways, hypotonia, and development of obesity. Symptoms and signs of OSA are underreported by caregivers and managing clinicians. Because sleep disturbances are either unrecognized or thought to be normal in children with Down's syndrome, the American Academy of Pediatrics guidelines for health care supervision in this group recommends referral to a sleep laboratory for polysomnography before 4 years of age [35]. Adenotonsillectomy is the first line of treatment in many cases, but often does not "cure" OSA. PAP therapy is highly effective, can be challenging to implement in this patient group, but often successful with behavioral support. Recognition and treatment of other comorbidities, such as gastroesophageal reflux (GER) in infants, weight management, rhinitis, asthma, or hypothyroidism (seen in up to one-third of children) is essential. Hypoglossal nerve stimulation in another therapy currently under investigation for this patient group. Some specialists have suggested that the increased prevalence of Alzheimer's disease in adults with Down's syndrome may be related in part to hypoxemia and sleep fragmentation from untreated OSA.

Prader–Willi Syndrome [36–42]

Prader–Willi syndrome is a rare (1 in 10,000–25,000 live births) autosomal dominant disorder resulting from the partial deletion or lack of expression of a region of genes on the paternal chromosome 15 or maternal uniparental disomy 15. Clinical features in infancy include diminished fetal activity, infantile hypotonia, and failure to thrive. In early childhood, progressive significant weight gain due to ravenous appetite appears to result in risk for morbid obesity. Other features include short stature, small hands and feet, hypogonadotropic hypogonadism, and intellectual disability. Several features predispose these patients to ventilatory problems: generalized hypotonia, abnormal arousal and ventilatory responses to hypoxia and hypercapnia, scoliosis, and developing obesity. Elevated central apnea indices can be seen in infancy, sometimes with sleep-related desaturation. In childhood and adulthood, obstructive SDB is common. A combination of factors (hypotonia, craniofacial dysmorphism, and viscous secretions) lead to OSA along with adenotonsillar hypertrophy and obesity. Finally, excessive daytime sleepiness (out of proportion to SDB and related to hypothalamic dysfunction) can appear in childhood and affects up to 50% of adults with a narcolepsy-like phenotype. Sleep architecture is also unusual with shorter REM latencies and increased REM cycles. Sleep apnea or sleep disturbance is a minor diagnostic criterion. GH is now routinely prescribed to improve development, growth, and body composition (increased muscle mass and decreased fat mass). Some studies report improvement in resting ventilation and inspiratory drive with this therapy. PSG is often performed prior to GH therapy. Untreated respiratory disorders can contribute to morbidity and premature death in PWS.

Craniofacial Abnormalities [24, 26]

Children with craniofacial syndromes are at high risk for obstructive SDB and OSA. OSA can develop because of both anatomic features that reduce the size of the airway and neuromotor deficits that impair the airway patency during sleep. Midface hypoplasia in children with craniosynostosis and glossoptosis and/or micrognathia in children with Pierre Robin sequence are well-recognized OSA risk factors but the etiology is multifactorial with multilevel airway obstruction. Screening questionnaires for OSA are not validated in this patient population and should not be a surrogate for objective diagnostic testing, so the threshold PSG is low. Some treatments are like those used in healthy children such as adenotonsillectomy, positive airway pressure, positive pressure ventilation, and in refractory cases, tracheostomy. However, distinct treatments include positioning, nasopharyngeal airways, tongue lip adhesion, and mandibular distraction osteogenesis in children with Pierre Robin sequence and midface advancement in children with craniosynostoses.

Pierre Robin Sequence

Pierre Robin sequence (prevalence 1 in 8500–14,000 individuals) is a triad of micrognathia, glossoptosis, and airway obstruction. Infants with this condition are at increased risk of oropharyngeal obstruction and feeding difficulties. About 20–40% of cases of Pierre Robin sequence occur in isolation (by itself) but the rest of cases occur as part of a syndrome that affects other organs and tissues in the body (e.g., Stickler syndrome, Treacher Collins syndrome). Pierre Robin sequence is the most common cause of syndromic micrognathia. Hypoplasia of the mandible leads to OSA due to obstruction at the base of the tongue from glossoptosis and reduced oropharyngeal size.

Cleft Lip/Palate [43]

Cleft lip/palate (1 per 1600 births) is an isolated condition in 70% of cases and part of a syndrome with other anomalies in the rest. Upper airway obstruction is more common in infants who have a cleft palate as part of the Pierre Robin sequence but breathing abnormalities during sleep are seen across the cleft lip/palate spectrum. Most children with cleft palate undergo primary palatoplasty between 9 and 12 months of age, but some children are left with velopharyngeal insufficiency needing further corrective surgery. OSA occurring after surgical correction of velopharyngeal insufficiency is well documented in children with cleft palate.

Craniosynostosis

Craniosynostosis, affecting 1 in 2500 births, occurs as part of a syndrome in 40% of cases. Apert, Crouzon, and Pfeiffer are well-known syndromes with craniosynostosis and are associated with mutations in the fibroblast growth receptor gene. Between 40% and 70% of children with syndromic craniosynostosis will have OSA. Although midface hypoplasia is the predominant causal factor for OSA in these children, multiple other factors such as adenotonsillar hypertrophy and choanal atresia contribute. Central apneas are also reported in some children with craniosynostosis and may be explained by pressure on the respiratory centers due to an underlying Chiari malformation or narrowing of the craniocervical junction.

Treacher Collins Syndrome

Treacher Collins syndrome is a rare (1 in 50,000 live births) autosomal dominant disorder associated with severe OSA. Family history is negative in about 50% of patients. Patients with this syndrome carry mutations in the *TCOF1* gene that encodes instructions for a protein involved in forming bones and other tissues of the face. Classic features include micrognathia, zygomatico-temporo-maxillary dysostosis, mandibular hypoplasia, choanal atresia, underdevelopment of the auricles, down slant of the eyelids, coloboma of the eyelids, and hypoplasia of the zygomatic bone and lateral orbital wall. Abnormalities in these structures explain the high frequency of OSA, 54% in children to 41% in adults. Surgical relief of upper airway obstruction is complicated due to multiple sites of obstruction. Skillful determination of the most useful site(s) for reconstructive surgery is key to a successful outcome.

Skeletal Dysplasias [44–46]

Skeletal dysplasias are rare genetic disorders that affect bones and joints leading to impaired growth and development, leaving affected children with short and/or deformed limbs. *Achondroplasia* is the most common (incidence 1 in 15–40,000 live births) form of disproportionate short stature. Over 80% of individuals with achondroplasia have parents with normal stature and are born with a de novo gene mutation. Two specific gain of function mutations in the fibroblast growth receptor 3 gene cause more than 95% of cases. Clinical features include short stature, shortened limbs, macrocephaly, frontal bossing, and midface hypoplasia. Although life expectancy is near normal, mortality rates are increased at all ages. One-third or more patients may have significant obstructive SDB. Patients with achondroplasia are at higher risk for OSA because of craniofacial dysmorphism, but also at greater risk for central sleep apnea because of cervicomedullary compression. They are also at higher risk for nocturnal sleep–related hypoxemia with or without hypoventilation because of thoracolumbar kyphosis, a small thorax, hypotonia, and tendency for obesity. PSG results are often abnormal and include a range of findings: central apnea, obstructive apneas, hypopneas, gas exchange abnormalities. The American Academy of Pediatrics recommends increased monitoring and evaluation for neurologic signs, especially in the first years of life [47]. Medical and surgical therapies that can improve OSA include adenotonsillectomy, targeted craniofacial surgeries, PAP therapy, and weight management. Other neurosurgeries may be needed for signs of brainstem compression. Evidence-based best practices are not established.

Sickle Cell Disease [48, 49]

Sickle cell disease (SCD), the most common inherited blood disorder in the US, affects 1 in 500 African Americans. It is characterized by chronic hemolytic anemia and complications related to recurrent vaso-occlusion. One of the strongest triggers for vaso-occlusion is oxyhemoglobin desaturation which has been linked to several complications of SCD, such as increased pain, greater risk of CNS events, cognitive dysfunction, history of acute chest syndrome. The prevalence of OSA in children with SCD is higher than in the general pediatric population. Habitual snoring and lower waking SpO_2 values were the strongest OSA risk factors in a cohort study of children with sickle cell anemia, unselected for OSA symptoms or asthma [50]. Because OSA is a treatable condition with adverse health outcomes, greater efforts are needed to screen, diagnose, and treat OSA in the high-risk vulnerable population. Of note, in patient with sickle cell disease, lower than normal SpO_2 values during sleep may not always be true hypoxemia because the oxyhemoglobin dissociation curve for Hb S is shifted to the right, compared to Hb A.

Neuromuscular Diseases

The term neuromuscular disease (NMD) encompasses a large variety of disorders that result in abnormal muscle function. Advances in understanding these diseases, their natural history, and increasing availability of mechanical ventilation for these patients have improved survival. [51, 52] Both spinal muscular atrophy (SMA) and Duchenne muscular dystrophy (DMD) are fatal monogenic neuromuscular disorders caused by loss-of-function mutations. The availability of advanced home-based options for ventilatory support and development of novel genetic and molecular therapies [53–56] provides an opportunity to use SDB as an outcome measure while also allowing the use of polysomnography as a validation tool in the assessments of effectiveness of therapies.

Spinal Muscular Atrophy [55, 57–59]

Spinal muscular atrophy (SMA), prevalence 1 in 7000–10,000 live births, is a diverse group of hereditary motor neuron disorders. Most cases are caused by a progressive loss of motor neurons due to the absence of the survival motor neuron (SMN1) protein. Historically five types have been described. Type 1 patients have a fatal course before age 2 years. Type 2 patients live into adulthood, and types 3 and 4 have a normal life span. Especially in type 1 patients, clinical features include progressive proximal weakness with intercostal muscles affected more than the diaphragm resulting in thoracoabdominal asynchrony (paradox) and a bell-shaped chest. Cardiac muscle is not affected. SDB is characterized by hypoventilation related to neuromuscular weakness. However, bulbar dysfunction and acquired maxillary hypoplasia can lead to upper airway obstruction while aspiration, impaired cough, and scoliosis lead to hypoxemia from to lower airway, parenchymal, and chest wall problems. Two novel genetic therapies, an RNA transcript modifier and a gene replacement are changing the natural history of this disease. Infants who historically would have succumbed by age 2 years are now sitting and standing, and some are walking. Children with more advanced disease are either experiencing disease stabilization or a return of recently lost abilities.

Duchenne Muscular Dystrophy [55, 58, 60–63]

Duchenne muscular dystrophy (DMD), affecting 20 per 100,000 live male births, is an X-linked, recessive disorder of the dystrophin gene which supplies structure and function to skeletal and cardiac muscle. Progressive weakness appears around 3 to 6 years of age, wheelchair is needed for mobility by 12 years of age, and scoliosis appears when the patient becomes nonambulatory. Chronic respiratory insufficiency and cardiomyopathy leading to premature death appears in the second decade of life. OSA is the predominant phenotypic of SDB at younger ages, sleep-related hypoventilation at older ages, with significant overlap given the propensity for obesity and variable progression of muscle weakness. Twenty-five percent of unexpected deaths occur at night. There is poor correlation between patient-reported symptoms and the presence of SDB, so the threshold for PSG should be low. PSG is the gold standard evaluation for SDB in children with DMD. Overnight oximetry can show sleep-related hypoxemia, but hypoventilation will be missed by oximetry alone, so PSG must include CO_2 monitoring. Central sleep apnea has been described in this patient groups, but it is unclear whether these "central" events are truly central or are classified as central on PSG due to poor signaling in the setting of decreased muscle strength. Noninvasive ventilatory support has changed the natural history, but novel gene therapies are in clinical trials may further improve outcomes.

Myotonic Muscular Dystrophy

Myotonic muscular dystrophy (prevalence 1 in 8000) is an autosomal dominant neuromuscular disease linked to cardiotocography (CTG) repeat expansions of two different genes with variable severity affecting all ages. Features of the adult-onset form of this multisystem disorder include progressive muscle weakness, excessive daytime sleepiness, fatigue, cataracts, endocrine dysfunction, and cardiac arrhythmias [64, 65]. Sleep apnea is highly prevalent. In the rare congenital form, inherited maternally in 90% of cases, infants present with severe skeletal, neuromuscular, and cognitive abnormalities [66]. The mortality rate is high related to need for ventilatory support. The childhood form is later onset and less severe.

Storage Diseases

Mucopolysaccharidosis refers to a heterogeneous group of rare (0.6–5:100,000 live births) genetic lysosomal storage diseases inherited disorders in which the body is unable to properly breakdown mucopolysaccharides with life expectancies of 20 years. Hunter and Hurler syndromes are examples of older names for these conditions. The cardinal abnormalities are musculoskeletal and cardiovascular. Upper airway obstruction is common in all forms of these disorders due to adenotonsillar enlargement, large and protruded tongue, reduced retropalatal and retroglossal space, narrow trachea, narrow airway, short neck, and small thoracic cage. Early recognition of OSA and proper treatment may reduce the high cardiovascular mortality and improve quality of life. There is no cure, but treatments such as bone marrow transplantation and enzyme replacement therapy may help with management of one subtype.

Glycogen storage diseases are caused by defective enzymes involved in the breakdown or synthesis of glycogen. The build-up of glycogen causes progressive muscle weakness and affects the function of the heart, skeletal muscles, liver, and nervous system. Of those, type 2, also known as Pompe disease (1: 40,000 live births) significantly affects respiratory muscles and is associated with SDB. There are three phenotypes based on the amount of residual enzyme activity that present in infancy, childhood, or adulthood. Skeletal muscle weakness and respiratory dysfunction are the hallmarks of the phenotype in adults, and respiratory failure is progressive in all forms. In the infantile form, clinical features of hypotonia, cardiomyopathy, and weakness are present within the first days to months of life.

Enzyme replacement therapy become the standard of care for the treatment of Pompe disease and has been available for more than a decade. The majority of patients with adult onset phenotype show improved ambulatory function and muscle strength, stabilization of pulmonary function, and increased survival that seems to peak at 3–5 years of treatment and is followed by a plateau or secondary decline with considerable individual variation after 10 years [67]. In infants and children with infantile or late onset forms, OSA and hypoventilation are common PSG findings, even in the absence of symptoms, with stabilization and improvements in PSG findings after 3 years of enzyme replacement therapy [68, 69]. They also have improved outcomes in terms of survival, remaining ventilator-free, and cardiac, skeletal muscle, and pulmonary function [70–74].

Epilepsy and Vagal Nerve Stimulators

All types of seizures can occur during sleep and some seizures occur only in sleep. Seizures during sleep can be associated with cardiopulmonary events: ictal and post-ictal apnea, tachypnea, tachycardia, bradycardia, and hypoxemia. Central or obstructive apneas may precede the seizure, occur during the seizure, or be the only clinical manifestation of the seizures. Ictal apnea can potentially contribute to sudden unexpected death in epilepsy which occurs more often during sleep.

Patients with vagal nerve stimulators (VNS) for intractable epilepsy should be screened for SDB. [75] About one-third will develop mild OSA and a small number will develop severe OSA. Apneas, hypopneas, desaturations, and tachypnea have been reported to occur exclusively during VNS activation, but not when the VNS is inactive. VNS may affect breathing either by its effect on the upper airway musculature or by its effect on central control of breathing. Vagal efferent nerves alter neuromuscular signal to the upper airway musculature of the pharynx and larynx, resulting in airway narrowing and obstruction. Vagal projection to the brainstem can also affect the rate and depth of respiration. Severity of the airway obstruction is related to the frequency of the VNS. Treatment needs to be individualized, but options include PAP therapy, changing the VNS settings, or stopping therapy.

Disorders Associated with Central Control of Breathing Abnormalities [76–78]

Central control of breathing abnormalities are a unique part of SDB in childhood. Table 11.6 list conditions associated with central apnea respiratory patterns with or without hypoventilation.

Table 11.6 Conditions associated with central apnea respiratory patterns with or without hypoventilation

Immature control of breathing
High altitude–induced periodic breathing

State-related changes in control of breathing
  Transition to sleep
  Low apnea hypocapnia threshold
  High loop gain
  High ventilatory response to arousal

Treatment emergent central apnea
Obesity hypoventilation syndrome (usually with another syndrome, e.g., Prader–Willi)
Cardiomyopathy and Cheyne–stokes respiration with congestive heart failure
Medication effect (e.g., narcotic-induced, baclofen, valproic acid)

Impaired central control of breathing/autonomic dysfunction
  CCHS
  ROHHAD
  Familial dysautonomia
  Rett syndrome

Genetic syndromes (e.g., Prader–Willi syndrome, Joubert syndrome)

CNS malformations or CNS tumors
  Hindbrain malformations (Chiari I, Chiari II with myelomeningocele)
  Foramen magnum stenosis or cervical medullary compression

Mitochondrial disorders

Central Sleep Apnea

Central sleep apnea in early infancy is usually part of immaturity of respiratory control. Although the mean central sleep apnea index during sleep is usually under 1/h, some normal children have values up to 4–5 events/h.

Elevated central apnea indices in children are reported in the setting of high altitude [79–82], state-related changes in control of breathing [83], certain genetic or metabolic disorders [84–88], CNS malformation or tumors [89–92], cardiac dysfunction [93], and as a medication effect [94–96]. One group has reported on "idiopathic" central apnea in pediatric patients, but potentially explanatory medical conditions were present [97]. Frequent prolonged (>20–25 s) central apneas, bradypnea with slow respiratory rates for age (rates less than 12/h), extreme elevation of periodic breathing indices or Biot's breathing suggest a problem requiring CNS imaging.

Central Hypoventilation Syndromes [98]

Hypoventilation refers to an increased arterial concentration of carbon dioxide due to inadequate gas exchange. Central hypoventilation means a deficiency in the central nervous system, rather than the respiratory system, is the root of the problem. Central hypoventilation is uncommon and may be due to a variety of conditions which are either congenital or acquired (Table 11.6). Current therapy for central hypoventilation focuses on achieving normal gas exchange, primarily through mechanical ventilatory support. Early identification of central hypoventilation and initiation of ventilatory support can improve adverse outcomes associated with chronic hypoxemia.

CCHS [99–101]

Congenital central hypoventilation syndrome (CCHS) is a rare, lifelong genetic disorder that causes central alveolar hypoventilation. Paired-like homeobox 2B (*PHOX2B*) mutations are found in almost all patients with CCHS. This gene encodes a key transcription factor that regulates neural crest cell migration and development of the autonomic nervous system. Deficiencies in central integration of chemoreceptor inputs cause autonomic dysfunction and loss of respiratory drive in CCHS. In addition, many patients have other symptoms of autonomic dysfunction (e.g., Hirschsprung disease and neural crest tumors) in addition to hypoventilation. Most patients present during the neonatal period, but late onset CCHS may present in later infancy, childhood, or even adulthood under various circumstances (e.g., respiratory infection, anesthesia). Since its original description in 1970 [102], this condition has evolved from a life-threatening neonatal onset disorder to include broader and milder clinical presentations, affecting children, adults, and families. Genes other than *PHOX2B* have been found to cause CCHS in rare cases.

In CCHS, the hypoventilation is worse in sleep compared to wakefulness. CCHS is unique in that it is the only respiratory disorder in which SDB is worse in NREM compared to REM sleep. Hypercapnia is greatest in NREM sleep because intact central chemoreception is essential to support normal ventilation in that state. Hypercapnia is milder in REM sleep and minimal to absent in wakefulness because central chemoreception is less important to ventilatory control in those states. The hypoventilation is caused by a shallow, low tidal volume (2 cc/kg) pattern of breathing rather than recurrent prolonged central apneas or slow respiratory rate. Patients with CCHS have absent or negligible ventilatory and reduced arousal sensitivity to hypercapnia and hypoxemia, so they do not show signs of respiratory distress when challenged with hypercarbia or hypoxia. Residual peripheral chemoreceptor function may allow for adequate ventilation during wakefulness.

Most *PHOX2B* mutations occur de novo, but 5–10% of cases are inherited in an autosomal dominant pattern with variable penetrance depending on the genotype. Most patients (90%) with CCHS will be heterozygous for extra polyalanine repeats in a specific region of the *PHOX2B* gene. The normal genotype is referred to as 20/20, while the mutated proteins produce extra repeats described as 20/24 to 20/33. The length of the polyalanine repeat expansion correlates with disease severity. A larger repeat region is associated with a more severe clinical phenotype more likely to present in the newborn period. In contrast, late-onset CCHS is more likely to be associated with a smaller repeat region and a milder clinical phenotype. The remaining 10% of patients, typically those with the most severe CCHS phenotypes, will be heterozygous for a non-polyalanine repeat-type mutations causing missense, nonsense, or frameshifts in the *PHOX2B* gene. Testing for a *PHOX2B* gene mutation is needed to confirm the diagnosis. Between 5% and 10% of cases are inherited in an autosomal dominant pattern from an affected and/or asymptomatic parent with somatic mosaicism for the expansion mutation. Parents and siblings should also be screened the mutation since there will be a 50% chance of recurrence with each future pregnancy. Genotype–phenotype associations allow for anticipatory guidance and improved clinical care. At present, management relies on lifelong ventilatory support (invasive and noninvasive ventilation and diaphragmatic pacing) and close follow up of dysautonomic progression. Infants with CCHS often require mechanical ventilation 24 h per day until wake–sleep periods are more stable and predictable, so they undergo tracheostomy.

ROHHAD [103–106]

ROHHAD (rapid onset obesity with hypothalamic dysfunction, hypoventilation, and autonomic dysregulation) is a rare disorder that presents between 3 and 10 years of age. Rapid onset weight gain usually occurs first; but hypoventilation, hypothalamic dysfunction, or tumors may bring the patient to medical attention. The hypothalamic dysfunction either precedes or follows weight gain and includes central hypothyroidism, growth hormone deficiency, diabetes insipidus, hyperprolactinemia, precocious/delayed puberty, thermal dysregulation, or corticotrophin deficiency. Once severe hypoventilation develops, ventilatory support is needed. Children are at high risk for respiratory arrest and mortality is high. Children with ROHHAD are also at risk for developing neural crest tumors. Developmental delay, regression, and behavioral problems are common. *PHOX2B* mutations are not seen and no candidate genes have been found. The cause is unknown but may be related to autoimmune inflammation of the CNS. ROHHAD can be diagnosed in children older than 18 months based on the development of rapid weight gain, endocrine defects, and central hypoventilation with other features of hypothalamic dysfunction. Repeated evaluations are needed in children as the syndrome evolves. Treatment is supportive and includes ventilatory support at night, as needed. Unrecognized or inadequately treated hypoventilation may have devastating consequences including death.

Familial Dysautonomia [107–109]

Familial dysautonomia is a rare autosomal recessive disorder affecting infants and children of Jewish Ashkenazi population which has a high carrier rate (1:30). It is caused by a mutation in the *ELP1* gene that encodes scaffold proteins and regulators of different kinases. The discovery of this mutation made prenatal diagnosis possible and resulted in a dramatic reduction in new patients. The pathophysiology is due to progressive autonomic neuropathy (blood pressure and heart rate instability, impaired sensation, swallowing dysfunction, ataxia) associated with progressive loss of small myelinated and unmyelinated fibers. The clinical manifestations may be present at birth. Over time, affected children and adults suffer from cardiovascular, respiratory, gastrointestinal, musculoskeletal, renal dysfunction, and developmental abnormalities. Patients have abnormal ventilatory responses to hypoxia and hypercapnia. Breath-holding spells appear during infancy and persist throughout life. Overall, 91% of pediatric patients and 85% of adults have some degree of SDB (obstructive apnea, central apnea, desaturation, hypoventilation). SDB is a consequence of chemoreflex failure causing impaired ventilatory drive, neuromuscular dysfunction causing or aggravating upper airway obstruction, scoliosis, and chronic lung disease. Untreated sleep apnea is a risk factor for sudden unexpected death during sleep in these patients.

Rett Syndrome [110–114]

Rett syndrome is a rare X-linked genetic disorder (1:10,000 female infants) that typically appears after 6–18 months of age. Symptoms and signs include loss of acquired speech; stereotypic hand movements; deceleration of head and brain growth; autistic behaviors; seizures; scoliosis; dysautonomia in the form of respiratory, cardiac, and gastrointestinal dysfunction; and sleeping problems. More than 95% of girls show a de novo loss of function mutation in the gene for the *MECP2* protein involved in transcriptional silencing and epigenetic regulation of methylated DNA.

Breathing abnormalities are a prominent clinical feature and included in the diagnostic criteria. The classic breathing abnormality in girls with Rett syndrome occurs during wakefulness. It is characterized by rapid shallow breathing (causing hyperventilation), followed by central apnea with breath holding, often followed by profound desaturation and cyanosis. Rett girls can have daily severe breathing abnormalities while awake but breathe more normally when asleep. This unexpected finding suggests an imbalance between the behavioral and metabolic control of respiratory. Rett girls also have markedly impaired sleep–wake patterns (delayed sleep onset, more night waking, and excessive daytime sleep) which may worsen over time but may be amenable to behavioral modification and melatonin. Other night behaviors include nighttime laughter, night screaming, nighttime seizures, and severe bruxism. Approximately 25% of patients die prematurely of cardiorespiratory failure.

Hindbrain Malformations (Chiari I and Spina Bifida) [29, 115]

Chiari I [86, 116–121]

Chiari I malformation, occurring in 1 per 1000–5000 births, includes malformations of the cerebellum and brainstem in which the cerebellar tonsils are displaced below the foramen magnum. Patients with Chiari I malformation may present with headaches, snoring, apnea, and dysphagia. SDB, including obstructive sleep apnea, central sleep apnea, and central alveolar hypoventilation, is estimated to occur in one-quarter of non-syndromic patients. SDB prevalence increases when Chiari I is part of a syndrome with other malformations. SDB is more severe when cervicome-dullary compression and/or syringomyelia is present. Compression of the brainstem and respiratory centers is thought to be the mechanism involved in producing central apneas while compression of cranial nerves IX and X leads to decreased upper airway patency and OSA.

Chiari II [92, 122–124]

Spina bifida includes a Chiari II malformation with herniation of the cerebellum and medulla into the spinal canal in association with a myelomeningocele. Over one-half of the children have SDB which is associated with sudden death in young adults. SDB includes central respiratory control abnormalities [apnea (central and/or obstructive), bradypnea, hypoventilation, impaired ventilatory and arousal responses to CO_2 and O_2, breathing holding spells] and restrictive lung disease due to neuromuscular weakness and scoliosis.

CNS Tumors [89]

Medulloblastoma and brainstem gliomas are tumors that can cause both central and obstructive apnea by compression of the respiratory nuclei or cranial nerves that innervate the tongue and pharynx. Tumors that affect the hypothalamus can affect sleep–wake patterns and produce fragmented sleep, increased daytime sleepiness, obesity, and secondary narcolepsy. Medullary nuclei involved in breathing include the dorsal respiratory nucleus (inspiration), the ventral respiratory nucleus (inspiration and expiation), the pre-Bötzinger complex and retrotrapezoid nucleus (respiratory pacemaker), and the nucleus of the tractus solitarius (vagal afferents). Cranial nerves that innervate the tongue and pharyngeal muscles emerge from nuclei in the medulla (hypoglossal nucleus and nucleus ambiguous). Damage to these nuclei by tumor compression or as a complication of surgical resection can affect breathing, producing central or obstructive apnea. Patients treated for CNS tumors may also present with more daytime sleepiness compared to patient treated for other malignancies.

Sleep-Disordered Breathing in Infants [125]

Infants can show a wide range of SDB patterns including: [1] apnea of prematurity, [2] apnea of infancy with central apnea, [3] periodic breathing, and [4] obstructive sleep apnea. Apnea is extremely common in infants decreasing in frequency as central control of breathing matures during the first year of life [126]. Immaturity of the central respiratory control system is a major factor underlying apnea in infants. Fig. 11.2 shows multiple factors that can trigger apnea in infants.

Infants and young children have more variable breathing during REM, including normal central apneas and central events that even occasionally last longer than 20 s [127]. Among healthy full-term infants recorded at home, 43% had central apneas longer than 20 s and 2% had apnea longer than 30 s. Regular breathing is seen in NREM sleep while irregular breathing is typical of REM sleep. Thoracoabdominal asynchrony in REM sleep is normal up to age 2–3 years [128]. Desaturations following these central apneas are typically brief, but can be associated with SpO_2 nadirs below 90%, even in healthy infants [129, 130]. Other factors that predispose infants to respiratory instability include low functional residual capacity, neuronal instability, increase time in REM sleep stage, and lower apneic threshold.

Apnea of Prematurity [131–134]

Immaturity of central control of breathing is major factor in apnea of prematurity. Almost 100% of infants born less than 28-week gestational age will have apnea of prematurity, 25–30% of infants born at 34 weeks, but it is rare in infants born after 38-week gestational age. The earlier the gestational age, the longer apnea of prematurity persists [135]. In former preterm infants, it disappears by the time the infant reaches 44-week postmenstrual age. Especially in former preterm or low-birthweight infants, external events can trigger apnea spells in infants who were previously stable. For example, there is an increased risk of apnea events within 2–3 days of routine 2-month immunizations, post anesthesia, and in association with RSV infection.

Premature infants have impaired ventilatory and arousal responses to hypercapnia and hypoxia as well as more compliant chest walls, lower end-expiratory volumes, greater distal airway closure, and greater bradycardia in response to stimulation of the carotid bodies by hypoxia. Although apnea of prematurity is often considered a centrally mediated problem with cessation of respiratory effort, pharyngeal upper airway obstruction can precipitate up to 50% of the central apneas. Upper airway collapse can appear at the end of a prolonged central apnea. The infant's highly compliant airway and relative ventilatory instability contribute to the propensity for upper airway obstruction during sleep. Of note, infants have a robust laryngeal chemoreceptor reflex in response to upper airway collapse which is characterized by repeated swallows, central apnea, and bradycardia.

For diagnostic purposes, the American Academy of Sleep Medicine's latest International Classification of Sleep Disorders (ICSD-3) defines "apnea of prematurity" as observed apnea or cyanosis or a detected central apnea, bradycardia, or desaturation on a hospital's cardiorespiratory monitoring, when the infant is <37-week postmenstrual age at the time of presentation [136]. The term "apnea of infancy" uses the same cardiorespiratory signs, but applied to an infant who is now

Fig. 11.2 Factors that precipitate apnea in infants

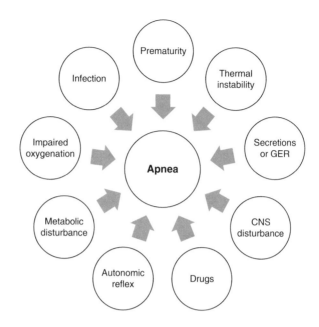

≥37-week gestational or postmenstrual age. Caffeine is effective in the treatment of apnea of prematurity with evidence of long-term safety [137]. Home cardiorespiratory monitoring may be useful as part of an individualized plan for some infants with persistent apnea of prematurity [138].

Periodic Breathing [139]

Periodic breathing, repetitive short cycles of respiratory pauses and breathing, is a normal pattern of breathing that occurs during sleep in most newborns. It is distinct from apnea of prematurity in that it occurs in term as well as preterm infants, peaks later, and lasts longer. Periodic breathing is absent in the first days of life, becomes more frequent at 2–4 weeks postnatal age, then decreases, but may continue for up to 6 months or longer. A major contributing factor to this immature breathing pattern is altered sensitivity to changes in blood oxygen and carbon dioxide content with increased gain in the receptors. In newborns, the PCO_2 apneic threshold is only slightly below the eupneic PCO_2 making these infants more prone to respiratory oscillations and favoring the appearance of periodic breathing [140]. Supplemental oxygen reduces percent time spent in periodic breathing and respiratory instability even in preterm infants with normal baseline SpO_2 values [141]. Of note, oxygen desaturations frequently occur during sleep, and the majority of desaturations are associated with periodic breathing [129, 130, 142]. Periodic breathing is also associated with low lung volumes which predispose toward decreased oxygen reserves and increased intrapulmonary shunting.

Periodic breathing persists longer in infants born at lower gestational age and lower birth weight, but rarely occupies more than 10% of recording time once term postmenstrual age is reached [125, 126, 142]. While periodic breathing is a normal immature breathing pattern in neonates, excessive periodic breathing or an abrupt increase over prior baseline warrants consideration for potential pathology. In older infants and children, elevated periodic breathing outside of wake–sleep transitions can also be a marker for a CNS pathology, hindbrain malformation, or metabolic disorder. Finally, periodic breathing is elevated in any age group at high altitude.

For PSG scoring purposes, periodic breathing is defined as clusters of three or more episodes of central apneas lasting for at least 3 seconds each and separated by ≤20 seconds of normal breathing [143]. Periodic breathing occurs in both REM and NREM sleep. In NREM, periodic breathing is characterized by a regular pattern of pauses separated by consistent intervals of respiratory efforts, while in REM, both irregular and regular patterns are seen. In infants, periodic breathing is more common in REM sleep. In adults (and some children), periodic breathing is most often seen during NREM sleep at sleep onset or sleep-wake transitions.

Apnea of Infancy with Central Apnea [125]

Breathing is irregular in newborns whose respiratory rates are faster and more variable than in older children. Distinguishing between normal and abnormal breathing during sleep can be challenging, especially in infants born prematurely or with congenital abnormalities. For PSG scoring purposes in infants, a central apnea is defined as a prolonged pause in breathing (≥ 20 s) or a shorter pause with physiological corroboration ($\geq 3\%$ desaturation, arousal, or bradycardia with heart rate < 60 bpm for at least 15 s). Hypopneas have similar duration and physiological corroboration and require a 30% reduction in airflow or its estimate. Obstructive apneas in infants and children are defined by >90% reduction in airflow lasting at least a two missed breaths in duration (compared with the baseline respiratory rate), but no physiological corroboration is required [143]. Central apneas are common in newborns and infants and central apnea indices are higher, so age appropriate normative data are required to interpret PSG data [144–147].

Terminology: Apnea of Infancy, ALTE, and BRUE

The terminology and the approach to evaluation and management of apnea of infancy has evolved over the last decade. In 1986, NIH Consensus Conference on Infantile Apnea coined the term "apparent life-threatening event (ALTE)" to replace the term "near miss sudden infant death syndrome (SIDS)." [148] An ALTE was defined as an episode that is frightening to the observer and that is characterized by some combination of apnea (central or occasionally obstructive), color change (usually cyanotic or pallid, but occasionally erythematous or plethoric), marked change in muscle tone (usually marked limpness), choking, or gagging. In some cases, the observer fears that the infant has died. A broad range of disorders can present as an ALTE including arrhythmias, child abuse, congenital abnormalities, epilepsy, inborn errors of metabolism, and infections. This term was problematic for several reasons. First, for most well-appearing infants with ALTE-like symptoms, the risk of recurrent events or a serious underlying disorder was extremely low. It created a feeling of uncertainty for both the caregiver and clinician. Clinicians felt compelled to perform costly, sometimes risky, often unnecessary tests (including PSG) and to hospitalize the patient even though this management plan often was unlikely to lead to a treatable diagnosis or prevent future events.

In 2016, the American Academy of Pediatrics (AAP) published a clinical practice guideline that recommended replacement of the term ALTE with a new term, "brief resolved unexplained event" (BRUE) [149]. This term describes an event in an infant less than 1 year when the observer reports a sudden, brief, and now resolved episode of at least one of the following: (1) cyanosis or pallor; (2) absent, decreased, or irregular breathing; (3) marked change in tone (hyper- or hypotonia); and (4) altered level of responsiveness. Clinicians should diagnosis a BRUE only when there is no explanation for a qualifying event after conducting a history and physical examination. This newer guideline shows an approach to evaluation and management that is based on the risk that the infant will have a repeat event or has a serious underlying disorder. It identifies (1) lower-risk patients based on history and physical examination, for whom evidence-based guidelines for evaluation and management are offered and (2) higher-risk patient, whose history and physical examination suggest the need for further investigation, monitoring, and/or treatment. Overnight PSG was not recommended for the management for infants who met criteria for having experienced a low-risk BRUE. The criteria for a higher-risk BRUE are listed in Table 11.7.

In an updated clinical practice guideline to provide a framework for evaluation of in the higher-risk group, PSG may be considered to characterize and quantify apnea type and is indicated in select patients with prematurity, noisy respirations, or recurrent and/or severe BRUE in whom SDB is suspected [150].

Table 11.7 Higher-risk BRUE criteria [150]

Age < 60 days
Prematurity: Gestational <32 weeks and postmenstrual age < 45 weeks
Recurrent event or occurring in clusters
Duration of event ≥1 min
CPR required by trained medical professional
Concerning historical features
Concerning physical examination findings

SUID, SIDS and Other Sleep-Related Infant Deaths [151, 152]

Each year, 3500 infants die in the US from sleep-related infant deaths, including the following ICD-10 diagnosis categories: sudden infant death syndrome (SIDS), ill-defined deaths, and accidental suffocation and strangulation in bed. SIDS is a sub-category of sudden unexpected infant death (SUID) and a cause assigned to infant deaths that cannot be explained after a through case investigations including autopsy, a scene investigation, and review of clinical history. In 2018, the SUID rate was 90.9 per 100,000 live births with about 1300 deaths due to SIDS, about 1300 deaths due to unknown causes, and about 800 deaths due to accidental suffocation and strangulation in bed. SIDS rates declined significantly from 130.3 deaths per 100,000 live births in 1990 to 35.2 deaths per 100,000 live births in 2018 [153]. After this first decrease in SIDS deaths by more than 50% through several public health initiatives, the overall death rate attributable to sleep-related infant deaths has not declined further. SIDS is still the leading cause of post-neonatal (28 days to 1 year of age) death. These SIDS and SUID mortality rates, like other causes of infant mortality, have notable and persistent racial and ethnic disparities. The rates in non-Hispanic black and American Indian/Alaska Native infant were more than double the rate in non-Hispanic white infants.

The American Academy of Pediatrics updated recommendations for a safe sleep environment (Fig. 11.3) that can reduce the risk of all sleep-related infant deaths includes supine position, the use of a firm sleep surface, room-sharing without bed-sharing, and the avoidance of soft bedding and overheating. Other recommendations for SIDS risk reduction include the avoidance of exposure to environmental tobacco smoke, alcohol, or illicit drugs; breastfeeding; routine immunizations; and use of a pacifier.

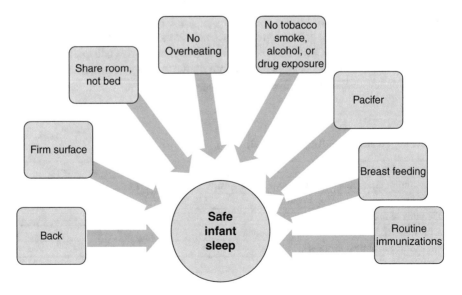

Fig. 11.3 Safe infant sleep

OSA and oSDB Presenting in Infants [3, 19, 154, 155]

Obstructive sleep apnea in infants has a distinctive pathophysiology, natural history, and treatment that is different from older children and adults. Infants are particularly vulnerable to obstructive SDB related to their upper airway structure, adverse pulmonary mechanics, ventilatory control, arousal threshold, laryngeal chemoreflex, and a REM-predominant sleep state distribution. OSA in infants can arise from diverse airway abnormalities extending from the nose to the larynx. Especially in infants, the highly compliant airway and the relative ventilatory instability further contribute to a propensity for upper airway obstruction during sleep. In addition to history of prematurity, other abnormalities that predispose to OSA and obstructive SDB in infants are summarized in Table 11.8.

Table 11.8 Predisposing factors and medical conditions associated with OSA in infants [125, 155]

Craniofacial	**Neurological**
Maxillary hypoplasia	Cerebral palsy
Down syndrome	Chiari malformations
Achondroplasia	Spinal muscular atrophy
Craniosynostosis	Nemaline rod myopathy
Treacher Collins	Mitochondrial disorders
Micrognathia and/or retrognathia	**Respiratory mechanics/ventilatory control**
Non-syndromic Pierre Robin sequence (cleft palate)	High chest wall compliance
Syndromic Pierre Robin sequence (Stickler, Treacher Collins)	Rib configuration round/horizontal
Hemifacial microsomia	Small diaphragmatic zone of apposition
Nager syndrome (acrofacial dysostosis)	High metabolic rate
Macroglossia	NREM apneic threshold close to eupneic CO_2 level
Down syndrome	Ventilation-perfusion mismatch
Achondroplasia	**Miscellaneous**
Beckwith-Wiedemann	Prader-Willi syndrome
Hemangioma, lymphangioma	Mucopolysaccharidoses
Laryngeal	Gastroesophageal reflux
Laryngomalacia	Chronic lung disease of infancy
Vocal cord paralysis	Obesity
Laryngeal webs/cysts; edema	Adenotonsillar hypertrophy
Congenital or acquired subglottic stenosis	Increased REM sleep
Hemangiomas	Neck flexion
Nasal obstruction	Respiratory infection
Choanal atresia or stenosis	Sleep deprivation
Nasogastric tube	Sedating medications
Allergic rhinitis	Maternal smoking during gestation
Upper respiratory tract infection	
Septal deviation	
Nasolacrimal duct cysts	

OSA in infants has been associated with failure to thrive, behavioral deficits, and sudden unexpected death. Especially in infants, the clinical history and physical examination alone are poor predictors of objectively measured upper airway obstruction. Many otherwise healthy infants without obstructive sleep apnea will snore [156]. Snoring has not been found to be predictive of OSA presence or severity in infants with cleft palate and micrognathia [157, 158]. The presence and severity of the OSA can be confirmed by PSG. Infants with severe OSA can have marked hypoxemia, hypoventilation, and/or sleep fragmentation. PSG can be challenging in infants and interpretation requires comparison with normative infant data and consideration of the infant's gestational and postmenstrual ages [159]. Direct endoscopic visualization is essential to show the specific cause of airway collapsibility and critical to selecting the optimal therapy. The management plan should be patient-centered and consider the natural history of the disorder, severity of the OSA, and other co-occurring medical problems and family preferences. A high percentage of infants diagnosed with OSA have a history of prematurity or underlying congenital conditions and require coordination of care by multiple subspecialties [160]. Nonsurgical treatment options can include nasopharyngeal stents, PAP therapy, supplemental oxygen, positional therapy, and treatment of reflux. Surgical options should target the underlying anatomic etiology. Examples include supraglottoplasty for severe laryngomalacia, mandibular distraction for micrognathia, tonsillectomy and/or adenoidectomy for lymphoid hyperplasia, choanal atresia repair, laryngeal reconstruction, and/or tracheostomy. A recent review provides diagnostic and management guidance for obstructive SDB in infants and toddlers less than 2 years of age, including those with complex conditions like Down's and Prader–Willi syndromes [3].

Polysomnography and Diagnostic Testing: Special Considerations in Children [161]

The American Academy of Sleep Medicine (AASM) endorses the usefulness of PSG in the evaluation of SDB in children of all ages. [7, 8] The AASM Scoring Manual supplies guidance for technical PSG performance standards and respiratory and non-respiratory signal scoring rules for infants and children [143]. Table 11.9 takes an updated look at the respiratory indications for PSG in children.

In laboratory, attended PSG has been the "gold standard" for the diagnosis of OSA in children. The American Academy of Pediatrics also recommends that PSG be performed in children with snoring and symptoms or signs of OSA [1] and for high-risk BRUE infants in whom there are clinical concerns for SDB [150]. PSG is also the "gold standard" for diagnosis of pediatric SDB including nocturnal hypoventilation in need of ventilatory support with the goal of identification of SDB before patients become symptomatic [162]. PSG is also helpful in assessing for residual SDB prior to removing a tracheostomy [163].

Table 11.10 summarizes the differences for acquisition, scoring, and reporting of respiratory parameters in children versus adults [143]. In brief, carbon dioxide is measured, respiratory events shorter than 10 s are scored, and periodic breathing and hypoventilation are reported in children. In children, central apneas are scored if they are at least 2 breaths in duration (compared to the child's baseline respiratory rate) and are associated with a $\geq 3\%$ desaturation, an arousal or bradycardia, or are ≥ 20 second in duration. This differs from adult criteria for scoring central apneas where the duration of the pause must be ≥ 10 seconds, and

Table 11.9 Updated view of respiratory indications for PSG assessment in children

Diagnosis	Management
OSA	Reevaluate residual OSA, s/p adenotonsillectomy or craniofacial surgery
Central sleep apnea ± hypoventilation[a]	Initiate PAP titration or PAP respiratory support[a]
CCHS or other control of breathing disorders	Evaluate oral appliance
Sleep-related hypoxemia/hypoventilation due to other disorders[a]	Prior to tracheostomy decannulation[a]
Apnea of infancy Higher risk BRUE with concerns for SDB	Reassess adequacy of ventilatory support therapies, noninvasive or via trach[a]

aWith these diagnostic concerns, the sleep laboratory will need CO_2 monitoring equipment (both end-tidal CO_2 and transcutaneous CO_2) and must be prepared to accommodate ventilatory support either noninvasively or via tracheostomy in medically stable patients

Table 11.10 Differences for acquisition, scoring, and reporting respiratory parameters in children versus adults [143]

	Child	Adult
Obstructive	2 missed breaths duration No corroboration required	≥ 10 s duration No corroboration required
Central	2 missed breaths duration associated with $\geq 3\%$ desaturation, arousal, or HR <50 for 5 s* If ≥ 20 s duration, no corroboration needed Score/report periodic breathing * If age < 1 yr., use <60 bpm for 15 s	≥ 10 s duration Score/report Cheyne–stokes respiratory pattern if criteria met
Hypopnea	2 missed breaths duration $\geq 30\%$ ↓nasal pressure or back-up associated with $\geq 3\%$ desaturation or arousal	≥ 10 sec duration $\geq 30\%$ ↓nasal pressure + $\geq 3\%$ desaturation or arousal or $\geq 30\%$ ↓nasal pressure + $\geq 4\%$ desaturation
Hypoventilation	>25% total sleep time with CO_2 > 50 mmHg $EtCO_2$ or $tcCO_2$ or arterial Measure/report hypoventilation recommended	↑ CO_2 > 55 mmHg for ≥ 10 min ↑ $CO_2 \geq 10$ mmHg from wake supine to sleep with values >50 mmHg for ≥ 10 min Report hypoventilation: optional

there is no requirement for associated desaturation, arousal, or bradycardia. Desaturation with central apneas usually shows a decreased pulmonary reserve, while prolonged central apneas are more likely to indicate a CNS abnormality or immature control of breathing. Central apneas are also more common in infants and children because of a vigorous Hering–Breuer reflex characterized by compensatory central respiratory pauses after stimulation of pulmonary stretch receptors following a large breath, such as with a sigh or body movement. Normative respiratory and sleep PSG data are available for infants and children [145–147, 164–170].

When assessing the severity of OSA in children, it is useful to consider the obstructive apnea and hypopneas indices together and separate from the central apnea index. Since central events can be frequent and normal in children (especially post movement, post sigh, in REM sleep, and in transition from waking), they should not contribute to measuring the severity of the obstruction, unless they are clearly related to unmasking of the apnea–hypocapnia phenomenon sometimes seen post arousal or waking after an obstructive event. It is also important to capture baseline cardiorespiratory data in quiet wakefulness prior to the sleep recording to confirm that any abnormal cardiorespiratory findings are truly sleep related, and not just related to the patient's chronic health problems.

PSG, long considered to be the "gold standard" for diagnosis of OSA in children, allows for simultaneous, continuous comprehensive monitoring of sleep, breathing, and other signals and can detect the presence and severity of physiological disturbances. Comprehensive assessment and attended studies may be more important when testing children with complex medication conditions. On the downside, it is expensive, burdensome for families, may not be tolerated by all children, and access is limited to facilities with pediatric expertise.

In the COVID era, pediatric sleep medicine was thrust into telemedicine and HSAT quickly became a safer "option" for selected patients with other options were simply not available. The future role for HSAT in the diagnosis of OSA in children is a topic of active investigation and keen interest to improve disparities in diagnosis, access to care, and treatment outcomes [171–175].

PSG Interpretation in Pediatrics

Compared to adults, healthy children are much better defenders of upper airway patency and have many more normal central pauses. They have healthier lungs with higher baseline oxyhemoglobin saturation values, more robust chemo- and mechano-reflexes, and are less arousable during sleep [19]. These protective factors result in lower obstructive apnea hypopnea indices, higher central apnea indices (especially in infants), less sleep-related hypoxemia, and less sleep fragmentation. In terms of OSA thresholds in children, many pediatric sleep specialists consider an oAHI <1 as "normal," 1–1.99 as "very mild," 2–4.99 as "mild," 5–9.99 as "moderate," and ≥ 10 as "severe."

The obstructive AHI derived from the PSG has been the primary disease defining metric to decide the presence and severity of OSA. However, in the presence of medical comorbidities (e.g., chronic pulmonary conditions, neuromuscular weakness, thoracic cage deformities) some of the respiratory events that meet scoring criteria for hypopneas may not be true signs of upper airway obstruction. Failure to recognize the contribution that lower respiratory tract problems make to scoreable hypopneas in the AHI can lead to overestimation of upper airway obstruction, misdiagnosis of OSA, and inappropriate therapies.

In children, when reviewing all the comprehensive physiologic data contained in a PSG, it is important to "read beyond the AHI." The reader should not only confirm obstructive AHI, but look for other markers of respiratory dysfunction: oximetry metrics (lower baseline SpO_2 values, frequency of desaturation events, time spent with low saturation values); the presence of paradoxical respiratory efforts, tachypnea, or loss of nasal airflow/mouth breathing; determine whether REM supine time was captured, track hypoventilation, unexpected central apneas, respiratory-related arousals or movements; sleep disruption or abnormal sleep architecture; and sinus tachycardia for age or other cardiac arrhythmias. When reviewing PSG studies in children, focusing on the AHI alone as the primary disease-defining metric can lead to an underestimation of sleep disordered breathing especially in the presence of comorbid medical condition. SDB can also be overestimated if normal central pauses that meet AHI scoring criteria are counted as evidence of disease.

Finally, in terms of clinical utility, the read should understand that the oAHI metric has not been the best predictor of OSA-related impairments or their response to treatments like adenotonsillectomy. In fact, OSA symptom scores were better than the oAHI at reflecting OSA-related impairments of behavior, quality of life, and sleepiness and better at predicting improvements after adenotonsillectomy [176].

Accommodating Children in the Sleep Laboratory

Most sleep laboratories are adult-oriented with more than half of AASM accredited sleep center only performing studies in children aged 13 years and above and very few dedicated solely to pediatrics [177]. Specifically for young children or older children and adults with intellectual or developmental disabilities, initiation of PAP therapy will likely require mask desensitization techniques prior to scheduling a titration study [178]. Several references describe best practices for accommodating children and families in the sleep lab [179–181]. Table 11.11 summarizes some of those basics.

Table 11.11 Basics of accommodating children in the sleep laboratory

Know all about the patient who is coming for testing   Comorbidities, medications, wake–sleep schedule, mobility concerns, special needs

Create protocols to offer child-friendly and family-centered services
  For example, allow earlier arrival and later sleep times; lower staff-to-patient ratios,
  accommodate caregiver

Prepare the child and family for the PSG procedure prior to their arrival
Train staff to work with children and families
Offer comfortable, in-room sleeping arrangements for the parent
Assure availability of pediatric-sized sensors, CO_2 monitoring, PAP masks
Engage the children and caregiver with the PSG procedure
Interpret studies using pediatric normative data
Improve quality by following up with families about their experience

Summary of Key Points

- Sleep-disordered breathing (SDB) in children includes not only obstructive sleep apnea (OSA) related to adenotonsillar hypertrophy in otherwise healthy children, but also OSA in children with complex medical conditions, control of breathing problems (central sleep apnea, hypoventilation), and worsening breathing in sleep in children with genetic, craniofacial, central nervous system, neuromuscular, chest wall, or other chronic pulmonary disorders.
- There are important differences in the clinical presentation, evaluation, PSG approach, and management of OSA between children and adults.

    – The nature of SDB changes in preterm neonates, term neonates, and infants depending on gestational age, chronological age, and postmenstrual age as control of breathing matures and stabilizes over the first year of life.

- The sleep medicine specialist and sleep center should be prepared to comprehensively assess and manage a broad range of sleep-related breathing problems across the age spectrum, from infants to young adults.
- A child-focused and family-centered approach to PSG evaluation of SDB in children is part of best practices for diagnosis and treatment.

References

1. Marcus CL, Brooks LJ, Draper KA, et al. Diagnosis and management of childhood obstructive sleep apnea syndrome. Pediatrics. 2012;130(3):576–84.
2. Marcus CL, Brooks LJ, Draper KA, et al. Diagnosis and management of childhood obstructive sleep apnea syndrome. Pediatrics. 2012;130(3):e714–55.
3. Kaditis AG, Alonso Alvarez ML, Boudewyns A, et al. ERS statement on obstructive sleep disordered breathing in 1- to 23-month-old children. Eur Respir J. 2017;50(6):1700985.

4. Kaditis AG, Alonso Alvarez ML, Boudewyns A, et al. Obstructive sleep disordered breathing in 2- to 18-year-old children: diagnosis and management. Eur Respir J. 2016;47(1):69–94.
5. Marcus CL, Moore RH, Rosen CL, et al. A randomized trial of adenotonsillectomy for childhood sleep apnea. N Engl J Med. 2013;368(25):2366–76.
6. Mitchell RB, Garetz S, Moore RH, et al. The use of clinical parameters to predict obstructive sleep apnea syndrome severity in children: the childhood Adenotonsillectomy (CHAT) study randomized clinical trial. JAMA Otolaryngol Head Neck Surg. 2015;141(2):130–6.
7. Aurora RN, Zak RS, Karippot A, et al. Practice parameters for the respiratory indications for polysomnography in children. Sleep. 2011;34(3):379–88.
8. Wise MS, Nichols CD, Grigg-Damberger MM, et al. Executive summary of respiratory indications for polysomnography in children: an evidence-based review. Sleep. 2011;34(3):389–398aw.
9. Kothare SV, Rosen CL, Lloyd RM, et al. Quality measures for the care of pediatric patients with obstructive sleep apnea. J Clin Sleep Med. 2015;11(3):385–404.
10. Mitchell RB, Archer SM, Ishman SL, et al. Clinical practice guideline: tonsillectomy in children (update)—executive summary. Otolaryngology Head Neck Surg (United States). 2019;160(2):187–205.
11. Mitchell RB, Archer SM, Ishman SL, et al. Clinical practice guideline: tonsillectomy in children (update). Otolaryngol Head Neck Surg. 2019;160(1_suppl):S1–S42.
12. Lloyd R, Kirsch DB, Carden KA, Malhotra RK, Rosen IM, Ramar K. Letter to the editor regarding the updated American Academy of Otolaryngology-Head and Neck Surgery Foundation clinical practice guideline on tonsillectomy in children. J Clin Sleep Med. 2019;15(2):363–5.
13. Garetz SL, Mitchell RB, Parker PD, et al. Quality of life and obstructive sleep apnea symptoms after pediatric adenotonsillectomy. Pediatrics. 2015;135(2):e477–86.
14. Paruthi S, Buchanan P, Weng J, et al. Effect of adenotonsillectomy on parent-reported sleepiness in children with obstructive sleep apnea. Sleep. 2016;39(11):2005–12.
15. Thomas NH, Xanthopoulos MS, Kim JY, et al. Effects of adenotonsillectomy on parent-reported behavior in children with obstructive sleep apnea. Sleep. 2017;40(4):zsx018.
16. Amin R, Holler T, Narang I, Cushing SL, Propst EJ, Al-Saleh S. Adenotonsillectomy for obstructive sleep apnea in children with complex chronic conditions. Otolaryngol Head Neck Surg. 2018;158(4):760–6.
17. Parmar A, Baker A, Narang I. Positive airway pressure in pediatric obstructive sleep apnea. Paediatr Respir Rev. 2019;31:43–51.
18. Khaytin I, Tapia IE, Xanthopoulos MS, et al. Auto-titrating CPAP for the treatment of obstructive sleep apnea in children. J Clin Sleep Med. 2020;16(6):871–8.
19. Arens R, Marcus CL. Pathophysiology of upper airway obstruction: a developmental perspective. Sleep. 2004;27(5):997–1019.
20. Katz ES, Moore RH, Rosen CL, et al. Growth after adenotonsillectomy for obstructive sleep apnea: an RCT. Pediatrics. 2014;134(2):282–9.
21. Mitchell RB, Kelly J. Outcome of adenotonsillectomy for obstructive sleep apnea in obese and normal-weight children. Otolaryngol Head Neck Surg. 2007;137(1):43–8.
22. Schwab RJ, Kim C, Bagchi S, et al. Understanding the anatomic basis for obstructive sleep apnea syndrome in adolescents. Am J Respir Crit Care Med. 2015;191(11):1295–309.
23. Gadoth N, Oksenberg A. Sleep and sleep disorders in rare hereditary diseases: a reminder for the pediatrician, pediatric and adult neurologist, general practitioner, and sleep specialist. Front Neurol. 2014;5:133.
24. Cielo CM, Marcus CL. Obstructive sleep apnoea in children with craniofacial syndromes. Paediatr Respir Rev. 2015;16(3):189–96.
25. Cielo CM, Konstantinopoulou S, Hoque R. OSAS in specific pediatric populations. Curr Probl Pediatr Adolesc Health Care. 2016;46(1):11–8.
26. Tan HL, Kheirandish-Gozal L, Abel F, Gozal D. Craniofacial syndromes and sleep-related breathing disorders. Sleep Med Rev. 2016;27:74–88.

27. Dosier LBM, Vaughn BV, Fan Z. Sleep disorders in childhood neurogenetic disorders. Children (Basel). 2017;4(9):children4090082.
28. ElMallah M, Bailey E, Trivedi M, Kremer T, Rhein LM. Pediatric obstructive sleep apnea in high-risk populations: clinical implications. Pediatr Ann. 2017;46(9):e336–9.
29. Yates JF, Troester MM, Ingram DG. Sleep in children with congenital malformations of the central nervous system. Curr Neurol Neurosci Rep. 2018;18(7):38.
30. Zaffanello M, Antoniazzi F, Tenero L, Nosetti L, Piazza M, Piacentini G. Sleep-disordered breathing in paediatric setting: existing and upcoming of the genetic disorders. Ann Transl Med. 2018;6(17):343.
31. Lal C, White DR, Joseph JE, van Bakergem K, LaRosa A. Sleep-disordered breathing in down syndrome. Chest. 2015;147(2):570–9.
32. Nation J, Brigger M. The efficacy of adenotonsillectomy for obstructive sleep apnea in children with down syndrome: a systematic review. Otolaryngol Head Neck Surg. 2017;157(3):401–8.
33. Horne RS, Wijayaratne P, Nixon GM, Walter LM. Sleep and sleep disordered breathing in children with down syndrome: effects on behaviour, neurocognition and the cardiovascular system. Sleep Med Rev. 2019;44:1–11.
34. Waters KA, Castro C, Chawla J. The spectrum of obstructive sleep apnea in infants and children with Down Syndrome. Int J Pediatr Otorhinolaryngol. 2020;129:109763.
35. Bull MJ, Committee on G. Health supervision for children with Down syndrome. Pediatrics. 2011;128(2):393–406.
36. Nixon GM, Brouillette RT. Sleep and breathing in Prader-Willi syndrome. Pediatr Pulmonol. 2002;34(3):209–17.
37. McCandless SE, Committee on G. Clinical report-health supervision for children with Prader-Willi syndrome. Pediatrics. 2011;127(1):195–204.
38. Sedky K, Bennett DS, Pumariega A. Prader Willi syndrome and obstructive sleep apnea: co-occurrence in the pediatric population. J Clin Sleep Med. 2014;10(4):403–9.
39. Pavone M, Caldarelli V, Khirani S, et al. Sleep disordered breathing in patients with Prader-Willi syndrome: a multicenter study. Pediatr Pulmonol. 2015;50(12):1354–9.
40. Gillett ES, Perez IA. Disorders of sleep and ventilatory control in Prader-Willi syndrome. Diseases. 2016;4(3):diseases4030023.
41. Tan HL, Urquhart DS. Respiratory complications in children with Prader Willi syndrome. Paediatr Respir Rev. 2017;22:52–9.
42. Zimmermann M, Laemmer C, Woelfle J, Fimmers R, Gohlke B. Sleep-disordered breathing in children with Prader-Willi syndrome in relation to growth hormone therapy onset. Horm Res Paediatr. 2020;93(2):85–93.
43. MacLean JE. Sleep frequently asked questions: question 1: what abnormalities do babies with cleft lip and/or palate have on polysomnography? Paediatr Respir Rev. 2018;27:44–7.
44. Afsharpaiman S, Saburi A, Waters KA. Respiratory difficulties and breathing disorders in achondroplasia. Paediatr Respir Rev. 2013;14(4):250–5.
45. Tenconi R, Khirani S, Amaddeo A, et al. Sleep-disordered breathing and its management in children with achondroplasia. Am J Med Genet A. 2017;173(4):868–78.
46. Pauli RM. Achondroplasia: a comprehensive clinical review. Orphanet J Rare Dis. 2019;14(1):1.
47. Trotter TL, Hall JG, American Academy of Pediatrics Committee on G. Health supervision for children with achondroplasia. Pediatrics. 2005;116(3):771–83.
48. Raghunathan VM, Whitesell PL, Lim SH. Sleep-disordered breathing in patients with sickle cell disease. Ann Hematol. 2018;97(5):755–62.
49. Katz T, Schatz J, Roberts CW. Comorbid obstructive sleep apnea and increased risk for sickle cell disease morbidity. Sleep Breath. 2018;22(3):797–804.
50. Rosen CL, Debaun MR, Strunk RC, et al. Obstructive sleep apnea and sickle cell anemia. Pediatrics. 2014;134(2):273–81.
51. Shi J, Al-Shamli N, Chiang J, Amin R. Management of rare causes of pediatric chronic respiratory failure. Sleep Med Clin. 2020;15(4):511–26.

52. Bach JR, Turcios NL, Wang L. Respiratory complications of pediatric neuromuscular diseases. Pediatr Clin N Am. 2021;68(1):177–91.
53. Iftikhar M, Frey J, Shohan MJ, Malek S, Mousa SA. Current and emerging therapies for Duchenne muscular dystrophy and spinal muscular atrophy. Pharmacol Ther. 2020;220:107719.
54. Abreu NJ, Waledrop MA. Overview of gene therapy in spinal muscular atrophy and Duchenne muscular dystrophy. Pediatr Pulmonol. 2020;56:710.
55. Fay AJ, Knox R, Neil EE, Strober J. Targeted treatments for inherited neuromuscular diseases of childhood. Semin Neurol. 2020;40(3):335–41.
56. Roy B, Griggs R. Advances in treatments in muscular dystrophies and motor neuron disorders. Neurol Clin. 2021;39(1):87–112.
57. Fauroux B, Griffon L, Amaddeo A, et al. Respiratory management of children with spinal muscular atrophy (SMA). Arch Pediatr. 2020;27(7s):7s29–27s34.
58. Gurbani N, Pascoe JE, Katz S, Sawnani H. Sleep disordered breathing: assessment and therapy in the age of emerging neuromuscular therapies. Pediatr Pulmonol. 2020;56:700.
59. Waldrop MA, Elsheikh BH. Spinal muscular atrophy in the treatment era. Neurol Clin. 2020;38(3):505–18.
60. Hoque R. Sleep-disordered breathing in Duchenne muscular dystrophy: an assessment of the literature. J Clin Sleep Med. 2016;12(6):905–11.
61. LoMauro A, D'Angelo MG, Aliverti A. Sleep disordered breathing in Duchenne muscular dystrophy. Curr Neurol Neurosci Rep. 2017;17(5):44.
62. Birnkrant DJ, Bushby K, Bann CM, et al. Diagnosis and management of Duchenne muscular dystrophy, part 2: respiratory, cardiac, bone health, and orthopaedic management. Lancet Neurol. 2018;17(4):347–61.
63. Sawnani H. Sleep disordered breathing in Duchenne muscular dystrophy. Paediatr Respir Rev. 2019;30:2–8.
64. Bianchi ML, Losurdo A, Di Blasi C, et al. Prevalence and clinical correlates of sleep disordered breathing in myotonic dystrophy types 1 and 2. Sleep Breath. 2014;18(3):579–89.
65. West SD, Lochmuller H, Hughes J, et al. Sleepiness and sleep-related breathing disorders in myotonic dystrophy and responses to treatment: a prospective cohort study. J Neuromuscul Dis. 2016;3(4):529–37.
66. Ho G, Carey KA, Cardamone M, Farrar MA. Myotonic dystrophy type 1: clinical manifestations in children and adolescents. Arch Dis Child. 2019;104(1):48–52.
67. Harlaar L, Hogrel JY, Perniconi B, et al. Large variation in effects during 10 years of enzyme therapy in adults with Pompe disease. Neurology. 2019;93(19):e1756–67.
68. Kansagra S, Austin S, DeArmey S, Kishnani PS, Kravitz RM. Polysomnographic findings in infantile Pompe disease. Am J Med Genet Part A. 2013;161a(12):3196–3200.
69. Kansagra S, Austin S, DeArmey S, Kazi Z, Kravitz RM, Kishnani PS. Longitudinal polysomnographic findings in infantile Pompe disease. Am J Med Genet Part A. 2015;167a(4):858–61.
70. Amdani SM, Sanil Y. Infantile Pompe disease and enzyme replacement therapy. J Paediatr Child Health. 2017;53(12):1242–3.
71. van der Meijden JC, Kruijshaar ME, Harlaar L, Rizopoulos D, van der Beek N, van der Ploeg AT. Long-term follow-up of 17 patients with childhood Pompe disease treated with enzyme replacement therapy. J Inherit Metab Dis. 2018;41(6):1205–14.
72. van Capelle CI, Poelman E, Frohn-Mulder IM, et al. Cardiac outcome in classic infantile Pompe disease after 13 years of treatment with recombinant human acid alpha-glucosidase. Int J Cardiol. 2018;269:104–10.
73. Baba S, Yoshinaga D, Akagi K, et al. Enzyme replacement therapy provides effective, long-term treatment of cardiomyopathy in Pompe disease. Circ J. 2018;82(12):3100–1.
74. ElMallah MK, Desai AK, Nading EB, DeArmey S, Kravitz RM, Kishnani PS. Pulmonary outcome measures in long-term survivors of infantile Pompe disease on enzyme replacement therapy: a case series. Pediatr Pulmonol. 2020;55(3):674–81.
75. Hsieh T, Chen M, McAfee A, Kifle Y. Sleep-related breathing disorder in children with vagal nerve stimulators. Pediatr Neurol. 2008;38(2):99–103.

76. Kritzinger FE, Al-Saleh S, Narang I. Descriptive analysis of central sleep apnea in childhood at a single center. Pediatr Pulmonol. 2011;46(10):1023–30.
77. Felix O, Amaddeo A, Olmo Arroyo J, et al. Central sleep apnea in children: experience at a single center. Sleep Med. 2016;25:24–8.
78. McLaren AT, Bin-Hasan S, Narang I. Diagnosis, management and pathophysiology of central sleep apnea in children. Paediatr Respir Rev. 2019;30:49–57.
79. Burg CJ, Montgomery-Downs HE, Mettler P, Gozal D, Halbower AC. Respiratory and polysomnographic values in 3- to 5-year-old normal children at higher altitude. Sleep. 2013;36(11):1707–14.
80. Duenas-Meza E, Bazurto-Zapata MA, Gozal D, González-García M, Durán-Cantolla J, Torres-Duque CA. Overnight polysomnographic characteristics and oxygen saturation of healthy infants, 1 to 18 months of age, born and residing at high altitude (2,640 meters). Chest. 2015;148(1):120–7.
81. Hill CM, Carroll A, Dimitriou D, et al. Polysomnography in Bolivian children native to high altitude compared to children native to low altitude. Sleep. 2016;39(12):2149–55.
82. Hughes BH, Brinton JT, Ingram DG, Halbower AC. The impact of altitude on sleep-disordered breathing in children dwelling at high altitude: a crossover study. Sleep. 2017;40(9):zsx120.
83. DelRosso LM, Martin K, Marcos M, Ferri R. Transient central sleep apnea runs triggered by disorder of arousal in a child. J Clin Sleep Med. 2018;14(6):1075–8.
84. d'Orsi G, Demaio V, Scarpelli F, Calvario T, Minervini MG. Central sleep apnoea in Rett syndrome. Neurol Sci. 2009;30(5):389–91.
85. Wolfe L, Lakadamyali H, Mutlu GM. Joubert syndrome associated with severe central sleep apnea. J Clin Sleep Med. 2010;6(4):384–8.
86. Losurdo A, Dittoni S, Testani E, et al. Sleep disordered breathing in children and adolescents with Chiari malformation type I. J Clin Sleep Med. 2013;9(4):371–7.
87. Ramezani RJ, Stacpoole PW. Sleep disorders associated with primary mitochondrial diseases. J Clin Sleep Med. 2014;10(11):1233–9.
88. Khayat A, Narang I, Bin-Hasan S, Amin R, Al-Saleh S. Longitudinal evaluation of sleep disordered breathing in infants with Prader-Willi syndrome. Arch Dis Child. 2017;102(7):634–8.
89. Rosen G, Brand SR. Sleep in children with cancer: case review of 70 children evaluated in a comprehensive pediatric sleep center. Support Care Cancer. 2011;19(7):985–94.
90. White KK, Parnell SE, Kifle Y, Blackledge M, Bompadre V. Is there a correlation between sleep disordered breathing and foramen magnum stenosis in children with achondroplasia? Am J Med Genet Part A. 2016;170a(1):32–41.
91. Zaffanello M, Sala F, Sacchetto L, Gasperi E, Piacentini G. Evaluation of the central sleep apnea in asymptomatic children with Chiari 1 malformation: an open question. Childs Nerv Syst. 2017;33(5):829–32.
92. Shellhaas RA, Kenia PV, Hassan F, Barks JDE, Kaciroti N, Chervin RD. Sleep-disordered breathing among newborns with myelomeningocele. J Pediatr. 2018;194:244–247.e241.
93. Al-Saleh S, Kantor PF, Chadha NK, Tirado Y, James AL, Narang I. Sleep-disordered breathing in children with cardiomyopathy. Ann Am Thorac Soc. 2014;11(5):770–6.
94. Amos LB, D'Andrea LA. Severe central sleep apnea in a child with leukemia on chronic methadone therapy. Pediatr Pulmonol. 2013;48(1):85–7.
95. Guichard K, Micoulaud-Franchi JA, McGonigal A, et al. Association of valproic acid with central sleep apnea syndrome: two case reports. J Clin Psychopharmacol. 2019;39(6):681–4.
96. Locatelli F, Formica F, Galbiati S, et al. Polysomnographic analysis of a pediatric case of baclofen-induced central sleep apnea. J Clin Sleep Med. 2019;15(2):351–4.
97. Gurbani N, Verhulst SL, Tan C, Simakajornboon N. Sleep complaints and sleep architecture in children with idiopathic central sleep apnea. J Clin Sleep Med. 2017;13(6):777–83.
98. Cielo C, Marcus CL. Central hypoventilation syndromes. Sleep Med Clin. 2014;9(1):105–18.
99. Weese-Mayer DE, Berry-Kravis EM, Ceccherini I, et al. An official ATS clinical policy statement: congenital central hypoventilation syndrome: genetic basis, diagnosis, and management. Am J Respir Crit Care Med. 2010;181(6):626–44.

100. Weese-Mayer DE, Rand CM, Zhou A, Carroll MS, Hunt CE. Congenital central hypoventilation syndrome: a bedside-to-bench success story for advancing early diagnosis and treatment and improved survival and quality of life. Pediatr Res. 2017;81(1–2):192–201.
101. Trang H, Samuels M, Ceccherini I, et al. Guidelines for diagnosis and management of congenital central hypoventilation syndrome. Orphanet J Rare Dis. 2020;15(1):252.
102. Mellins RB, Balfour HH Jr, Turino GM, Winters RW. Failure of automatic control of ventilation (Ondine's curse). Report of an infant born with this syndrome and review of the literature. Medicine (Baltimore). 1970;49(6):487–504.
103. Ize-Ludlow D, Gray JA, Sperling MA, et al. Rapid-onset obesity with hypothalamic dysfunction, hypoventilation, and autonomic dysregulation presenting in childhood. Pediatrics. 2007;120(1):e179–88.
104. Carroll MS, Patwari PP, Kenny AS, Brogadir CD, Stewart TM, Weese-Mayer DE. Rapid-onset obesity with hypothalamic dysfunction, hypoventilation, and autonomic dysregulation (ROHHAD): response to ventilatory challenges. Pediatr Pulmonol. 2015;50(12):1336–45.
105. Reppucci D, Hamilton J, Yeh EA, Katz S, Al-Saleh S, Narang I. ROHHAD syndrome and evolution of sleep disordered breathing. Orphanet J Rare Dis. 2016;11(1):106.
106. Harvengt J, Gernay C, Mastouri M, et al. ROHHAD(NET) syndrome: systematic review of the clinical timeline and recommendations for diagnosis and prognosis. J Clin Endocrinol Metab. 2020;105(7):2119–31.
107. Palma JA, Norcliffe-Kaufmann L, Perez MA, Spalink CL, Kaufmann H. Sudden unexpected death during sleep in familial dysautonomia: a case-control study. Sleep. 2017;40(8):zsx083.
108. Singh K, Palma JA, Kaufmann H, et al. Prevalence and characteristics of sleep-disordered breathing in familial dysautonomia. Sleep Med. 2018;45:33–8.
109. Kazachkov M, Palma JA, Norcliffe-Kaufmann L, et al. Respiratory care in familial dysautonomia: systematic review and expert consensus recommendations. Respir Med. 2018;141:37–46.
110. Marcus CL, Carroll JL, McColley SA, et al. Polysomnographic characteristics of patients with Rett syndrome. J Pediatr. 1994;125(2):218–24.
111. Weese-Mayer DE, Lieske SP, Boothby CM, Kenny AS, Bennett HL, Ramirez JM. Autonomic dysregulation in young girls with Rett syndrome during nighttime in-home recordings. Pediatr Pulmonol. 2008;43(11):1045–60.
112. Katz DM, Dutschmann M, Ramirez JM, Hilaire G. Breathing disorders in Rett syndrome: progressive neurochemical dysfunction in the respiratory network after birth. Respir Physiol Neurobiol. 2009;168(1–2):101–8.
113. Amaddeo A, De Sanctis L, Arroyo JO, Khirani S, Bahi-Buisson N, Fauroux B. Polysomnographic findings in Rett syndrome. Eur J Paediatr Neurol. 2019;23(1):214–21.
114. Sarber KM, Howard JJM, Dye TJ, Pascoe JE, Simakajornboon N. Sleep-disordered breathing in pediatric patients with Rett syndrome. J Clin Sleep Med. 2019;15(10):1451–7.
115. Dauvilliers Y, Stal V, Abril B, et al. Chiari malformation and sleep related breathing disorders. J Neurol Neurosurg Psychiatry. 2007;78(12):1344–8.
116. Gosalakkal JA. Sleep-disordered breathing in Chiari malformation type 1. Pediatr Neurol. 2008;39(3):207–8.
117. Dhamija R, Wetjen NM, Slocumb NL, Mandrekar J, Kotagal S. The role of nocturnal polysomnography in assessing children with Chiari type I malformation. Clin Neurol Neurosurg. 2013;115(9):1837–41.
118. Losurdo A, Testani E, Scarano E, Massimi L, Della MG. What causes sleep-disordered breathing in Chiari I malformation? Comment on: "MRI findings and sleep apnea in children with Chiari I malformation". Pediatr Neurol. 2013;49(5):e11–3.
119. Khatwa U, Ramgopal S, Mylavarapu A, et al. MRI findings and sleep apnea in children with Chiari I malformation. Pediatr Neurol. 2013;48(4):299–307.
120. Pomeraniec IJ, Ksendzovsky A, Awad AJ, Fezeu F, Jane JA Jr. Natural and surgical history of Chiari malformation type I in the pediatric population. J Neurosurg Pediatr. 2016;17(3):343–52.

121. Ferre A, Poca MA, de la Calzada MD, et al. Sleep-related breathing disorders in chiari malformation type 1: a Prospective Study of 90 patients. Sleep. 2017;40(6).
122. Waters KA, Forbes P, Morielli A, et al. Sleep-disordered breathing in children with myelomeningocele. J Pediatr. 1998;132(4):672–81.
123. Kirk VG, Morielli A, Gozal D, et al. Treatment of sleep-disordered breathing in children with myelomeningocele. Pediatr Pulmonol. 2000;30(6):445–52.
124. Patel DM, Rocque BG, Hopson B, et al. Sleep-disordered breathing in patients with myclomeningocele. J Neurosurg Pediatr. 2015;16(1):30–5.
125. Katz ES. Chapter 34 – Disorders of central respiratory control during sleep in children. In: Barkoukis TJ, Matheson JK, Ferber R, Doghramji K, editors. Therapy in sleep medicine. Philadelphia: W.B. Saunders; 2012. p. 434–47.
126. MacLean JE, Fitzgerald DA, Waters KA. Developmental changes in sleep and breathing across infancy and childhood. Paediatr Respir Rev. 2015;16(4):276–84.
127. Ramanathan R, Corwin MJ, Hunt CE, et al. Cardiorespiratory events recorded on home monitors: comparison of healthy infants with those at increased risk for SIDS. JAMA. 2001;285(17):2199–207.
128. Gaultier C, Praud JP, Canet E, Delaperche MF, D'Allest AM. Paradoxical inward rib cage motion during rapid eye movement sleep in infants and young children. J Dev Physiol. 1987;9(5):391–7.
129. Hunt CE, Corwin MJ, Lister G, et al. Longitudinal assessment of hemoglobin oxygen saturation in healthy infants during the first 6 months of age. Collaborative Home Infant Monitoring Evaluation (CHIME) Study Group. J Pediatr. 1999;135(5):580–6.
130. Hunt CE, Corwin MJ, Weese-Mayer DE, et al. Longitudinal assessment of hemoglobin oxygen saturation in preterm and term infants in the first six months of life. J Pediatr. 2011;159(3):377–383 e371.
131. Martin RJ, Abu-Shaweesh JM. Control of breathing and neonatal apnea. Biol Neonate. 2005;87(4):288–95.
132. Edwards BA, Sands SA, Berger PJ. Postnatal maturation of breathing stability and loop gain: the role of carotid chemoreceptor development. Respir Physiol Neurobiol. 2013;185(1):144–55.
133. Di Fiore JM, Martin RJ, Gauda EB. Apnea of prematurity–perfect storm. Respir Physiol Neurobiol. 2013;189(2):213–22.
134. Eichenwald EC, Committee on F, Newborn AAoP. Apnea of prematurity. Pediatrics. 2016;137(1):e20153757.
135. Eichenwald EC, Aina A, Stark AR. Apnea frequently persists beyond term gestation in infants delivered at 24 to 28 weeks. Pediatrics. 1997;100(3 Pt 1):354–9.
136. American Academy of Sleep Medicine. International classification of sleep disorders. 3rd ed. Darien: American Academy of Sleep Medicine; 2014.
137. Marcus CL, Meltzer LJ, Roberts RS, et al. Long-term effects of caffeine therapy for apnea of prematurity on sleep at school age. Am J Respir Crit Care Med. 2014;190(7):791–9.
138. Committee on Fetus and Newborn. American Academy of Pediatrics. Apnea, sudden infant death syndrome, and home monitoring. Pediatrics. 2003;111(4 Pt 1):914–7.
139. Patel M, Mohr M, Lake D, et al. Clinical associations with immature breathing in preterm infants: part 2-periodic breathing. Pediatr Res. 2016;80(1):28–34.
140. Khan A, Qurashi M, Kwiatkowski K, Cates D, Rigatto H. Measurement of the CO_2 apneic threshold in newborn infants: possible relevance for periodic breathing and apnea. J Appl Physiol (1985). 2005;98(4):1171–6.
141. Simakajornboon N, Beckerman RC, Mack C, Sharon D, Gozal D. Effect of supplemental oxygen on sleep architecture and cardiorespiratory events in preterm infants. Pediatrics. 2002;110(5):884–8.
142. Hunt CE, Corwin MJ, Lister G, et al. Precursors of cardiorespiratory events in infants detected by home memory monitor. Pediatr Pulmonol. 2008;43(1):87–98.
143. Berry RB, Quan SF, Abreu AR, et al. for the American Academy of Sleep Medicine. The AASM manual for the scoring of sleep and associated events: rules, terminology, and technical specifications, version 2.6. American Academy of Sleep Medicine: Darien; 2020.

144. Brockmann PE, Poets A, Urschitz MS, Sokollik C, Poets CF. Reference values for pulse oximetry recordings in healthy term neonates during their first 5 days of life. Arch Dis Child Fetal Neonatal Ed. 2011;96(5):F335–8.
145. Brockmann PE, Poets A, Poets CF. Reference values for respiratory events in overnight polygraphy from infants aged 1 and 3months. Sleep Med. 2013;14(12):1323–7.
146. Daftary AS, Jalou HE, Shively L, Slaven JE, Davis SD. Polysomnography reference values in healthy newborns. J Clin Sleep Med. 2019;15(3):437–43.
147. Ng DK, Chan CH. A review of normal values of infant sleep polysomnography. Pediatr Neonatol. 2013;54(2):82–7.
148. National Institutes of Health Consensus Development Conference on Infantile Apnea and Home Monitoring, Sept 29 to Oct 1, 1986. Pediatrics. 1987;79(2):292–9.
149. Tieder JS, Bonkowsky JL, Etzel RA, et al. Brief resolved unexplained events (Formerly Apparent Life-Threatening Events) and evaluation of lower-risk infants: executive summary. Pediatrics. 2016;137(5):e20160591.
150. Merritt JL, 2nd, Quinonez RA, Bonkowsky JL, et al. A framework for evaluation of the higher-risk infant after a brief resolved unexplained event. Pediatrics. 2019;144(2):e20184101.
151. Moon RY, Task Force On Sudden Infant Death S. SIDS and other sleep-related infant deaths: evidence base for 2016 updated recommendations for a safe Infant sleeping environment. Pediatrics. 2016, 138(5):e20162940.
152. Task Force On Sudden Infant Death S. SIDS and other sleep-related infant deaths: updated 2016 recommendations for a safe Infant sleeping environment. Pediatrics. 2016:138(5).
153. CDC Centers for Disease Control and Prevention. Sudden Unexpected Infant Death and Sudden Infant Death Syndrome 2014–2018. https://www.cdc.gov/sids/data.htm.
154. Katz ES, Mitchell RB, D'Ambrosio CM. Obstructive sleep apnea in infants. Am J Respir Crit Care Med. 2012;185(8):805–16.
155. Mehta B, Waters K, Fitzgerald D, Badawi N. Sleep disordered breathing (SDB) in neonates and implications for its long-term impact. Paediatr Respir Rev. 2020;34:3–8.
156. Kahn A, Groswasser J, Sottiaux M, et al. Clinical symptoms associated with brief obstructive sleep apnea in normal infants. Sleep. 1993;16(5):409–13.
157. MacLean JE, Fitzsimons D, Fitzgerald DA, Waters KA. The spectrum of sleep-disordered breathing symptoms and respiratory events in infants with cleft lip and/or palate. Arch Dis Child. 2012;97(12):1058–63.
158. Anderson IC, Sedaghat AR, McGinley BM, Redett RJ, Boss EF, Ishman SL. Prevalence and severity of obstructive sleep apnea and snoring in infants with Pierre Robin sequence. Cleft Palate-Craniofac J. 2011;48(5):614–8.
159. Cielo CM. Question 3: what are the indications for and challenges in performing polysomnography in infants? Paediatr Respir Rev. 2019;30:27–9.
160. Qubty WF, Mrelashvili A, Kotagal S, Lloyd RM. Comorbidities in infants with obstructive sleep apnea. J Clin Sleep Med. 2014;10(11):1213–6.
161. Stowe RC, Afolabi-Brown O. Pediatric polysomnography—a review of indications, technical aspects, and interpretation. Paediatr Respir Rev. 2019;34:9.
162. Berry RB, Budhiraja R, Gottlieb DJ, et al. Rules for scoring respiratory events in sleep: update of the 2007 AASM manual for the scoring of sleep and associated events. Deliberations of the sleep apnea definitions Task Force of the American Academy of sleep medicine. J Clin Sleep Med. 2012;8(5):597–619.
163. Lee J, Soma MA, Teng AY, Thambipillay G, Waters KA, Cheng AT. The role of polysomnography in tracheostomy decannulation of the paediatric patient. Int J Pediatr Otorhinolaryngol. 2016;83:132–6.
164. Montgomery-Downs HE, O'Brien LM, Gulliver TE, Gozal D. Polysomnographic characteristics in normal preschool and early school-aged children. Pediatrics. 2006;117(3):741–53.
165. Tapia IE, Karamessinis L, Bandla P, et al. Polysomnographic values in children undergoing puberty: pediatric vs. adult respiratory rules in adolescents. Sleep. 2008;31(12):1737–44.
166. Beck SE, Marcus CL. Pediatric polysomnography. Sleep Med Clin. 2009;4(3):393–406.

167. Accardo JA, Shults J, Leonard MB, Traylor J, Marcus CL. Differences in overnight polysomnography scores using the adult and pediatric criteria for respiratory events in adolescents. Sleep. 2010;33(10):1333–9.
168. Scholle S, Beyer U, Bernhard M, et al. Normative values of polysomnographic parameters in childhood and adolescence: quantitative sleep parameters. Sleep Med. 2011;12(6):542–9.
169. Scholle S, Wiater A, Scholle HC. Normative values of polysomnographic parameters in childhood and adolescence: cardiorespiratory parameters. Sleep Med. 2011;12(10):988–96.
170. Scholle S, Wiater A, Scholle HC. Normative values of polysomnographic parameters in childhood and adolescence: arousal events. Sleep Med. 2012;13(3):243–51.
171. Certal V, Camacho M, Winck JC, Capasso R, Azevedo I, Costa-Pereira A. Unattended sleep studies in pediatric OSA: a systematic review and meta-analysis. Laryngoscope. 2015;125(1):255–62.
172. Kirk V, Baughn J, D'Andrea L, et al. American Academy of sleep medicine position paper for the use of a home sleep apnea test for the diagnosis of OSA in children. J Clin Sleep Med. 2017;13(10):1199–203.
173. Brockmann PE, Alonso-Alvarez ML, Gozal D. Diagnosing sleep apnea-hypopnea syndrome in children: past, present, and future. Arch Bronconeumol. 2018;54(6):303–5.
174. Hassan F, D'Andrea LA. Best and safest care versus care closer to home. J Clin Sleep Med. 2018;14(12):1973–4.
175. Ross KR, Redline S. Is it time to head home for the night? Home sleep testing in young children. Ann Am Thorac Soc. 2020;17(10):1207–9.
176. Rosen CL, Wang R, Taylor HG, et al. Utility of symptoms to predict treatment outcomes in obstructive sleep apnea syndrome. Pediatrics. 2015;135(3):e662–71.
177. Gregus M. Written communication, AASM unpublished data. In:Feb 2020.
178. Berry RB, Chediak A, Brown LK, et al. Best clinical practices for the sleep center adjustment of noninvasive positive pressure ventilation (NPPV) in stable chronic alveolar hypoventilation syndromes. J Clin Sleep Med. 2010;6(5):491–509.
179. Das S, Mindell J, Millet GC, et al. Pediatric polysomnography: the patient and family perspective. J Clin Sleep Med. 2011;7(1):81–7.
180. Zaremba EK, Barkey ME, Mesa C, Sanniti K, Rosen CL. Making polysomnography more "child friendly:" a family-centered care approach. J Clin Sleep Med. 2005;1(2):189–98.
181. Ibrahim S, Stone J, Rosen CL. Best practices for accommodating children in the polysomnography lab: enhancing quality and patient experience (in press). In: Gozal D, Kheirandish-Gozal L, editors. Pediatric sleep medicine. SpringerNature; 2021.

Part III
Non-respiratory Sleep Disorders

Chapter 12
Diagnosis of Insomnia Disorder

Rachel Atkinson and Christopher Drake

Keywords Insomnia · Hyperarousal · Depression · Sleep reactivity · Circadian rhythm · CBT-I

Introduction

Insomnia disorder is one of the most prevalent sleep disorders and is characterized by trouble falling asleep, staying asleep, or awakening earlier than desired, and experiencing related daytime dysfunction [1, 2]. It is estimated that approximately one-third of adults experience insomnia symptoms, and 10% or more of the general population have insomnia disorder [3–5]. In addition to the high prevalence of insomnia disorder, this condition is characterized by *its chronicity*, with approximately three-quarters of individuals experiencing symptoms for at least 1 year, and almost half of individuals experiencing symptoms for over 3 years [5]. Although there are effective treatments for insomnia, almost a quarter of individuals who enter remission will go on to experience a relapse of symptoms [5]. Insomnia is also a risk factor for a variety of chronic illnesses if left untreated, particularly cardiovascular disease, hypertension, type 2 diabetes, and neurodegenerative diseases such as dementia and cortical atrophy [6–13]. Moreover, the strong bidirectional relationship between insomnia and depression is now well established [14–17]. The odds of an individual with insomnia developing depression are 2.6 times higher than those of an individual with good sleep [14]. Regardless of the presence of depression,

R. Atkinson
University of Toledo College of Medicine and Life Sciences, Toledo, OH, USA

C. Drake (✉)
Henry Ford Sleep Disorders and Research Center, Detroit, MI, USA
e-mail: CDRAKE1@hfhs.org

© Springer Nature Switzerland AG 2022
M. S. Badr, J. L. Martin (eds.), *Essentials of Sleep Medicine*,
Respiratory Medicine, https://doi.org/10.1007/978-3-030-93739-3_12

insomnia symptoms are associated with suicidal ideation, particularly in younger individuals [17]. Compounding the physical and mental effects of insomnia disorder on the patient are the consequences of untreated insomnia on the public, particularly in terms of healthcare costs, reduced productivity, and risk of accidents. Chronic untreated insomnia can lead to decreased productivity at work and increased use of sick leave, as well as increased physician visits and an increased risk of motor vehicle accidents [18, 19]. Furthermore, the economic burden of insomnia is immense, with the annual direct cost of healthcare for patients with insomnia averaging $851 more than those without insomnia and the nationwide cost due to decreased work performance is estimated at $63.2 billion [20, 21].

For these reasons, it is essential for healthcare providers to be able to recognize the symptoms of insomnia disorder across both specialty and primary care settings in order to properly diagnose insomnia disorder and recommend appropriate treatments to prevent the downstream deleterious effects of insomnia on both the patient and society. This chapter will focus on the current diagnostic criteria for insomnia disorder, various biopsychosocial contributors to insomnia, challenges in insomnia assessment, appropriate evaluation tools, and briefly discuss goals for treatment. The purpose of this chapter is to prepare health care providers with the tools and guidance necessary to efficiently and successfully evaluate and consider treatments for insomnia disorder.

Pathophysiology and Neuropsychology of Insomnia

A characteristic feature of insomnia disorder is hyperarousal, which involves a pathological increase in the physiologic, affective, or cognitive activities of the body and mind, subsequently leading to difficulty disengaging from one's surroundings and significantly disrupting sleep [22]. At the cognitive level, hyperarousal can present in the form of racing thoughts, rumination, and perseverative thinking. Hyperarousal can also manifest at other levels, including increased high-frequency electroencephalogram (EEG) activation (e.g., elevated beta frequency activity during sleep), dysregulation of hormone secretion (e.g., cortisol), increased metabolic rate, and elevated sympathetic nervous system activity, including increased heart rate and blood pressure [23]. On a molecular basis, insomnia is reflected in a dysregulation of the molecules involved in regulating the sleep–wake cycle, such as gamma-amino-butyric acid (GABA), as evidenced by widespread depletion of GABA in the brains of people with insomnia [22, 24]. From an integrative lens of sleep psychophysiology, hyperarousal can stimulate emotional and cognitive systems, which results in activation of wake-promoting brain regions but also suppression of sleep-promoting regions of the brain [22, 25]. As sleep-promoting regions are suppressed, wake-promoting regions may become disinhibited leading to increased wakefulness [22, 25, 26]. Thus, the balance between wake-promoting and sleep-promoting brain regions is disturbed. However, the exact nature of this dysregulation remains poorly understood, in terms of which specific brain system(s) and neuropeptides represent differences underlying the pathophysiology of insomnia in contrast to those differences which are a consequence of the chronic sleep disruption and comorbid disorders associated with insomnia.

In addition to the role of hyperarousal in insomnia disorder, changes in the normal two-process model of sleep regulation involving processes S (wake-dependent process, or homeostatic "sleep drive") and C (wake-independent process, or circadian rhythm) plays a similarly important role in sleep–wake cycle regulation [27, 28]. Normally, processes S and C are synchronized with each other leading to a regular sleep–wake rhythm. However, in individuals with insomnia, it is suggested that dysfunction in process C, which controls an individual's circadian rhythm, may lead to desynchronization between process S and C, resulting in the symptoms observed in insomnia disorder [22]. However, direct evidence supporting this role for circadian dysregulation as a pathophysiological process involved in insomnia remains scant.

Several studies provide evidence for a moderate genetic component of insomnia disorder. However, current evidence points to the potential role of multiple genes involved with a variety of physiological processes such as brain function and regulation of arousal and sleep–wake cycle pathways in insomnia emphasizing the complexity and heterogeneity of the molecular aspects of insomnia disorder [22, 29].

At the psychological level, one of the most prominent models of insomnia is the 3-P model which emphasizes predisposing, precipitating, and perpetuating factors that play a role in the progression and prolongation of insomnia [30, 31]. Of relevance to hyperarousal, specifically, are predisposing and perpetuating factors. Predisposing factors include individual traits or attributes such as female gender or a family history of insomnia that increase the likelihood of developing insomnia disorder, while perpetuating factors are those that further the development and maintenance of insomnia once it occurs [30]. For example, with regard to perpetuating factors, remaining in bed awake when unable to fall asleep may lead to increased anxiety about insomnia and unfavorable associations with the bedroom, leading to maintenance and exacerbation of insomnia symptoms. Precipitating factors can be severely stressful or anxiety-provoking events such as divorce or the death of a loved one that serve as the "tipping point" for the onset of insomnia and lead to overactivation of the stress response, leading to hyperarousal [30]. It is also important to understand that predisposing factors can interact with stressful precipitating events, which can significantly elevate the risk of developing insomnia for certain individuals [32].

One predisposing factor, sleep reactivity, plays a crucial role in understanding the onset and course of insomnia disorder. Sleep reactivity is defined as the degree to which an individual's sleep is disrupted during exposure to an external stressor [33]. Sleep reactivity has recently been shown to be a major predictive factor for the development of insomnia disorder, and its interaction with cognitive and emotional factors such as rumination and worry has been increasingly explored [33]. Specifically, there appears to be a synergistic relationship between sleep reactivity and cognitive-emotional arousal such that as stress progressively disrupts sleep patterns in vulnerable individuals, the cognitive-emotional response is further exacerbated due to additional time awake that permits continued rumination in bed [33, 34]. Thus, as stress heightens the cognitive-emotional response, the sleep system responds with increased wakefulness and a vicious cycle ensues [33].

While our knowledge of the neurobiology and psychology of insomnia is still evolving, the advances in the field that have been made over the last several decades have led us to a point where we are able to use this knowledge to better evaluate patients in the clinic and point them toward appropriate treatment options. Understanding the biopsychosocial aspects that contribute to the development and maintenance of insomnia disorder is fundamental to understanding how to assess and treat patients with this chronic and challenging condition. The remainder of this chapter will outline how to appropriately use diagnostic criteria to evaluate insomnia patients in the clinical setting.

Diagnostic Criteria

The diagnosis of insomnia disorder is symptom based, with objective sleep measurements recommended only in cases of suspected comorbid sleep conditions (e.g., obstructive sleep apnea). There are myriad reasons for the reliance on patient-reported symptoms rather than objective polysomnographic (PSG) electroencephalogram-based laboratory measures of sleep for insomnia diagnostic criteria. One critical element is that cortical EEG assessment of sleep (usually based on limited cortical brain sites) does not necessarily reflect the subcortical-limbic hyperarousal that is observed in insomnia using more sophisticated imaging approaches, nor is PSG assessment always reflective of insomnia symptoms at home [35]. The purely clinical aspect of the diagnosis stresses the significance of being familiar with the appropriate clinical assessments and information to gather from the patient, as more often than not, there will be a lack of objective PSG sleep data to support a diagnosis.

Patients with insomnia disorder will typically present with a straightforward list of chief nocturnal complaints. These include trouble falling asleep or staying asleep, increased early morning awakenings, and impaired daytime function [1, 2]. Importantly, diagnostic criteria from the *Diagnostic and Statistical Manual of Mental Disorders, Fifth Edition* (DSM-5) and the *International Classification of Sleep Disorders, Third Edition* (ICSD-3) emphasize the daytime dysfunction and distress to the patient caused by their sleeping difficulties, as well as the duration and frequency of their insomnia symptoms [1, 2]. Both the DSM-5 and ICSD-3 require an insomnia diagnosis to be made on the basis that symptoms cause distress to the patient and interfere with their daily functioning, in addition to nocturnal symptoms having occurred at least 3 days per week for at least 3 months [1, 2]. In addition to the distress experienced by the patient, the sleeping difficulties must occur despite adequate opportunity for sleep; individuals who have decreased opportunities for sleep exclusively due to scheduling constraints, for example, do not meet criteria for insomnia disorder [1, 2]. Similar to other disorders listed in the

DSM-5 and ICSD-3, the sleeping difficulties must not be explained more completely by another sleep disorder (e.g., obstructive sleep apnea, restless legs syndrome), although the presence of another sleep disorder does not preclude diagnosis of insomnia disorder [1, 2]. Table 12.1 provides a complete review of all diagnostic criteria for insomnia disorder from the DSM-5 and ICSD-3.

A point of confusion for many healthcare providers may be the outdated categorization of primary versus secondary insomnia disorder. Prior to 2005, the DSM-5 separated secondary insomnia, or insomnia due to other physical/mental disorders, from primary insomnia [36]. The DSM-5 now emphasizes that diagnostic criteria for insomnia disorder may only be met if coexisting physical and mental conditions do not sufficiently explain the patient's insomnia symptoms [1]. This union of primary and secondary insomnia diagnoses takes into account the comorbid nature of the disorder and encourages treatment of insomnia symptoms even in the context of a comorbid condition [37]. In terms of comorbidities, obstructive sleep apnea treatment with continuous positive airway pressure (CPAP) may precipitate significant sleep disturbance that may require separate treatment for sleep and may be a precipitating factor for more chronic sleep disturbance leading to insomnia disorder.

Although the role of objective PSG sleep assessment in evaluating insomnia has been debated, recent research points to its utility in differentiating a particular phenotype of insomnia disorder termed insomnia with objective short sleep duration (< 6 hours of sleep per night), which is the most severe phenotype of insomnia disorder in terms of morbidity [10]. It is associated with increased cognitive-emotional and cortical arousal, as well as activation of both the hypothalamic–pituitary–adrenal (HPA) and sympatho-adrenal-medullary (SAM) axes of the stress response system as compared to insomnia with objectively normal sleep duration [10, 38]. The objective short sleep phenotype of insomnia may respond better to medications, while insomnia with objective normal sleep duration may be successfully treated with cognitive behavioral therapy for insomnia (CBT-I) [10], which is the first-line recommended treatment for insomnia disorder. While the use of PSG assessment may be valuable in detecting objective short sleep in an insomnia patient and therefore selecting the most beneficial treatment, there is no current consensus for this approach and it remains an active area of study [39]. Even if PSG is able to provide specific and sensitive objective data, there remains a lack of consensus regarding quantitative cutoffs for sleep parameters that should be used for making an insomnia diagnosis [40]. Nevertheless, for accurate objective assessment PSG would need to be combined with longer-term objective monitoring as insomnia disorder has a characteristic longstanding pattern of sleep disruption that cannot be accurately determined from one or even two nights in the sleep laboratory.

For the reasons outlined above, it is not advantageous to either the patient or the provider to employ the use of PSG data in the insomnia disorder diagnosis. The expenses to both the patient and the healthcare system are too great, and there is not satisfactory evidence to support the finding that the objective data offered by PSG studies is necessary in making an insomnia disorder diagnosis. The subjective complaints proffered by the patient are sufficient for the proper diagnosis of insomnia, given that the provider is able to accurately elicit the appropriate information and

Table 12.1 Comparison of diagnostic criteria for insomnia disorder based on the *Diagnostic and Statistical Manual, 5th edition* (DSM-5), the *International Classification of Sleep Disorders, 3rd edition* (ICSD-3), and the *International Classification of Diseases, 10th edition* (ICD-10)

DSM-5 [1]	ICSD-3 [2]	ICD-10 [76]
A. A predominant complaint of dissatisfaction with sleep quantity or quality, associated with one (or more) of the following symptoms: 1. Difficulty initiating sleep. (In children, this may manifest as difficulty initiating sleep without caregiver intervention) 2. Difficulty maintaining sleep, characterized by frequent awakenings or problems returning to sleep after awakenings. (In children, this may manifest as difficulty returning to sleep without caregiver intervention) 3. Early-morning awakening with inability to return to sleep.	A. The patient reports, or the patient's parent or caregiver observes, one or more of the following: 1. Difficulty initiating sleep 2. Difficulty maintaining sleep 3. Waking up earlier than desired 4. Resistance to going to bed on appropriate schedule Difficulty sleeping without parent or caregiver intervention	Disturbance of sleep onset or sleep maintenance, or poor sleep quality
B. The sleep disturbance causes clinically significant distress or impairment in social, occupational, educational, academic, behavioral, or other important areas of functioning	B. The patient reports, or the patient's parent or caregiver observes, one or more of the following related to the nighttime sleep difficulty: 1. Fatigue/malaise 2. Attention, concentration or memory impairment 3. Impaired social, family, occupational or academic performance 4. Mood disturbance/ irritability 5. Daytime sleepiness 6. Behavioral problems (e.g., hyperactivity, impulsivity, aggression) 7. Reduced motivation/energy/ initiative 8. Proneness for errors/ accidents 9. Concerns about or dissatisfaction with sleep	The afflicted individuals focus extremely on their sleep disorder (especially during the night) and worry about the negative consequences of insomnia. The insufficient sleep duration and quality is coupled with a high degree of suffering or impairs daily activities.

Table 12.1 (continued)

DSM-5 [1]	ICSD-3 [2]	ICD-10 [76]
E. The sleep difficulty occurs despite adequate opportunity for sleep	C. The reported sleep–wake complaints cannot be explained purely by inadequate opportunity (i.e., enough time is allotted for sleep) or inadequate circumstances (i.e., the environment is safe, dark, quiet, and comfortable) for sleep	
C. The sleep difficulty occurs at least 3 nights per week	D. The sleep disturbance and associated daytime symptoms occur at least three times per week	Sleep disturbances occur at least three times a week over a period of 1 month
D. The sleep difficulty is present for at least 3 months	E. The sleep disturbance and associated daytime symptoms have been present for at least 3 months	
F. The insomnia is not better explained by and does not occur exclusively during the course of another sleep–wake disorder (e.g., narcolepsy, a breathing-related sleep disorder, a circadian rhythm sleep–wake disorder, a parasomnia)	F. The sleep/wake difficulty is not explained more clearly by another sleep disorder	
G. The insomnia is not attributable to the physiological effects of a substance (e.g., a drug of abuse, a medication)		
H. Coexisting mental disorders and medical conditions do not adequately explain the predominant complaint of insomnia		

rule out other causes. The following section will detail the information that must be gathered from the patient and will outline an appropriate patient encounter when insomnia disorder is suspected.

Clinical Evaluation of Insomnia Disorder

Challenges in Insomnia Assessment

When evaluating patients for insomnia disorder, it is important for practitioners to be aware of common challenges they may experience during the office visit. The primary issue that practitioners may face will be the time it takes to properly assess a patient with insomnia symptoms, as practitioners are frequently pressed on time and have a myriad of other important factors to address during the visit. Therefore, it is imperative for practitioners to have a solid roadmap in place when evaluating insomnia symptoms in order to conduct the interview in the most efficient manner possible. The Structured Clinical Interview for Diagnostic and Statistical Manual of Mental Disorders, Fifth Edition (DSM-5) Sleep Disorders (SCISD) has been shown to have excellent interrater reliability and is a reasonable tool for clinicians to utilize as it takes approximately 10–20 minutes to administer [41].

An additional challenge that practitioners may face is lacking assurance of the most appropriate treatment option for their patients, as these guidelines have recently changed. Cognitive behavioral therapy for insomnia (CBT-I) has recently been recommended as the first-line treatment for insomnia disorder, and it is no longer recommended that medications be used as an initial treatment approach for most patients [42]. However, approved hypnotics may be acceptable in combination with CBT-I, as a second-line therapy, or in circumstances where CBT-I may not be feasible (e.g., cognitively impaired patients) or desirable for a given patient. As discussed above, insomnia disorder typically has both psychological and physiological elements, and CBT-I has been shown to be highly effective in providing long-term benefits for insomnia disorder in comparison to pharmacotherapy with fewer potential risks [43].

Most importantly, the rapport that a practitioner has with their patient is paramount in uncovering insomnia symptoms as well as encouraging the patient to adhere to appropriate insomnia treatment. Practitioners may struggle to form a genuine connection with their patients during short office visits, especially with new patients. Compounding this issue, many patients are unsure of how to discuss insomnia symptoms with their practitioner; therefore, practitioners should actively create a welcoming space to discuss their patients' sleep habits. As many physicians' offices are now administering the Patient Health Questionnaire-9 (PHQ-9) to detect symptoms of depression in patients, a logical opening to the conversation of sleep difficulties may be the patient's answer to item three on the PHQ-9 ("Trouble falling or staying asleep, or sleeping too much") [44]. If the patient has endorsed this item ("Several days," "More than half the days," "Nearly every day"), the practitioner has a natural opportunity to address this sleep concern with the patient even if the patient does not have depression. If the office does not offer the PHQ-9 or the patient has not endorsed item three, the practitioner still ought to inquire about the patient's sleep [44]. While the use of an open-ended question such as "How is your sleep?" is a sufficient opening into a conversation about sleep, it must be followed with more definitive, closed-ended questions that address more specific aspects of the patient's sleep. Examples of apt follow-up questions include "How many hours of sleep did you get on average over the past 2 weeks?", "When you get into bed, how long does it take you to fall asleep?", "On a typical night, how many times do you wake up? And how long does it take to fall back asleep?" These closed-ended questions that address explicit characteristics of the patient's sleep allow ample opportunity for the patient to discuss any sleep difficulties they may be suffering from as well as help the patient to feel that the practitioner genuinely cares about their health and well-being, thereby building rapport. Finally, this type of quantitative assessment of insomnia (i.e., minutes to fall asleep, sleep duration, etc.) will allow the health provider to [1] assess the patients sleep relative to others with insomnia in terms of severity and [2] provide a good basis for assessing response to treatment.

Identifying Patients to Evaluate for Insomnia Disorder

Sleep is a vital aspect of a patient's physical and emotional well-being and ought to be, at a minimum, briefly discussed with the practitioner at every visit. However, there are particular social, psychological, and biological conditions that practitioners ought to pay special attention to, as these may be predisposing factors for patients to develop insomnia disorder. In particular, older adults and women are at heightened risk for developing insomnia disorder, as well as patients with significant life stressors or comorbid disorders such as chronic pain, psychiatric illnesses, and substance abuse problems [45]. The latter is particularly important as alcohol is frequently used by patients to address sleep problems and this pattern can lead to increased risk for exacerbation of substance use problems. The practitioner should take extra care to assess pregnant and peri-menopausal women for insomnia disorder, as these are transient periods where women are vulnerable to developing insomnia symptoms that can develop into insomnia disorder as well as an increased risk of depression and suicidal ideation [46, 47]. Recent data suggest CBT-I is highly efficacious in these populations of pregnant and peri-menopausal women [48, 49]. Additionally, it is of principal importance that the practitioner gathers a full social history for each patient, as patients who work the night shift are unemployed, have lower socioeconomic status, reside in dangerous neighborhoods, or experience discrimination are also at risk of developing insomnia disorder [50, 51]. While there is no known gene directly responsible for insomnia disorder, individuals with past or current diagnosis of insomnia disorder are more likely to report having a family history of insomnia than individuals without a past or current insomnia diagnosis, and these individuals rate their insomnia as more severe than those without a family history [52]. This points to the significance of gathering a family insomnia history from patients, as it may lead to increased support for an insomnia disorder diagnosis. Taken together, these "red flags" for insomnia disorder susceptibility can help guide the practitioner toward an insomnia disorder diagnosis and will aid in prevention efforts and early intervention.

Approach to Assessment of Insomnia Disorder

When weighing an insomnia disorder diagnosis, having a standardized format for the patient interview will allow for consistency across patients, as well as efficiency during the office visit. The assessment of insomnia disorder can be viewed similarly to the evaluation of any routine complaint, as the practitioner should conduct a history of present illness for the chief complaint followed by sleep-specific follow-up questions. The characterization of each type of complaint – difficulty falling asleep, nighttime awakenings, time to fall back asleep, early morning awakenings, and daytime functioning – should be addressed in full, followed by the onset, duration, frequency, severity, course (progressive, intermittent, chronic), and remitting or exacerbating factors related to the specific symptoms.

Patients often pursue insomnia treatments on their own before talking with a healthcare provider, and inquiring about these attempts can inform the clinical picture. When evaluating self-treatments, it is critical to inquire about the use of alcohol or other substances of abuse, over-the-counter sleep medications, and off-label medications. These substances are common methods of self-medication for insomnia symptoms that are often maladaptive and may be harmful to the patient. As one becomes tolerant to many medications or substances over time, dose escalation can occur leading to additional risks such as substance abuse. Additionally, withdrawal symptoms from these substances, particularly alcohol, may contribute to the patient's insomnia symptoms and continued use of alcohol for sleep [53]. Of note, the impact of the insomnia symptoms on the patient's daytime function should be evaluated, as the patient may instead simply be a short sleeper if they do not experience any dissatisfaction or daytime dysfunction as a result of their sleep problems. Information regarding the patient's past or current treatment attempts for insomnia disorder should also be gathered, as this may affect the future course of treatment and it is not always clear if a patient's previous treatment(s) were appropriately selected and implemented [50, 54].

Following the history of present illness portion of the interview, practitioners should gauge the pre-sleep conditions of their patients, including their sleeping environments, bedtime routines, and states of mind prior to sleep. If a practitioner uncovers that their patient is sleeping in a noisy, light-filled environment and eats a large meal or exercises directly before bedtime, this is an appropriate time to educate the patient on proper sleep hygiene. However, it should be recognized that sleep hygiene is not a suitable standalone treatment for patients with insomnia disorder and should only be used as a primary treatment for insomnia symptoms if the practitioner determines that the patient's poor sleep habits are the major factor in the patients presenting complaint [50]. The practitioner should also assess the patient's perspective of why they may be experiencing insomnia symptoms, as this may uncover any potential stressors in the patient's life or maladaptive beliefs that could be countered through cognitively focused treatment [55, 56]. Additionally, inquiring about the patient's coping responses when they are unable to sleep (e.g., watching television, remaining in bed, moving to a different room) can be useful in informing the treatment approach.

Uncovering the sleep–wake schedule of the patient is valuable in narrowing the differential diagnosis and distinguishing insomnia disorder from circadian rhythm disorders (advanced/delayed sleep phase type) and behaviorally induced insufficient sleep due to restricted time in bed. If a patient works several jobs and does not have a sufficient amount of opportunity to sleep, they will not meet criteria for an insomnia diagnosis. Similarly, if a patient's natural sleep–wake schedule is significantly advanced or delayed, leaving them with a constrained amount of time for sleep due to social responsibilities such as work or school, a diagnosis of a circadian rhythm disorder may be more appropriate along with a referral to a sleep specialist for the application of circadian interventions. When assessing the sleep–wake schedule, the practitioner should determine the patient's time to bed, estimated time to fall asleep, number and length of awakenings, wake time, time out of bed during the night, and any naps during the daytime. Use of a sleep diary or sleep log can be an effective approach to gathering reliable information on these and other sleep habits. Patients who take frequent daytime naps will have a decreased sleep drive in the evening which can manifest as an increased sleep onset latency or a later time to bed. Counseling the patient against frequent daytime napping can be a beneficial recommendation in the outpatient setting before referring the patient for more intensive treatment such as CBT-I. Additionally, the practitioner should ask the patient to differentiate between their sleep–wake schedules on work and school days versus weekend and vacation days. This may allow the practitioner to clue in on maladaptive behaviors such as "catching up on sleep" or may point to a circadian rhythm disorder if the patient's sleep–wake schedule varies drastically between weekdays and weekends or vacation days [50, 54, 57].

Inquiring about the nocturnal behaviors that the patient engages in when they are unable to sleep can point to comorbid conditions that the patient may have. For example, if a patient reports that they lie awake in bed allowing their thoughts to race or engages in rumination, there is cause for suspicion that they may respond well to a course of CBT-I. Similarly, if a patient endorses severe snoring, gasping or choking, or frequent leg movements or discomfort, comorbid diagnoses of OSA or restless legs syndrome (RLS), respectively, is appropriate to consider. Bed partner reports, if possible, are also critical to include in the evaluation of nocturnal behaviors, as a bed partner may report snoring that the patient themselves is unaware of, leading to consideration of OSA, or may counter the patient's reports that they do not sleep at night, pointing toward a potential paradoxical insomnia diagnosis [50, 54].

To thoroughly assess the patient's daytime functioning, there are an assortment of aspects that must be considered. In addition to feeling a lack of energy during the day or the presenting complaint of "fatigue," patients may endorse problems with their work or school, difficulties with concentration and memory, and cognitive-emotional problems such as irritability or mental health conditions [58, 59]. Notably, most patients with insomnia disorder will present with feelings of fatigue rather than sleepiness, so it is essential to consider these two facets of insomnia separately. The eight-item Epworth Sleepiness Scale (ESS) should be used to assess daytime sleepiness, as this questionnaire can also be used to support an OSA diagnosis when scores are elevated [60]. If a patient scores 10 or greater on the ESS, the patient should be educated about the risks of excessive sleepiness while driving or operating heavy machinery, as the patient is exhibiting excessive sleepiness [60]. The number, length, and timing (morning, afternoon, evening) of naps is also a useful indicator of a patient's daytime sleepiness and provides an additional opportunity for sleep hygiene education. On the contrary, the nine-item Fatigue Severity Scale

(FSS) is useful in evaluating fatigue as opposed to sleepiness [61]. Assessing the patient's mood disturbances and cognitive difficulties as well as the effect of their insomnia symptoms on their overall quality of life is also critical when evaluating the patient's daytime function. The fatigue, irritability, and cognitive challenges associated with insomnia disorder may result in an inability to engage in one's normal daytime activities, leading to decreased quality of life. Finally, the bidirectional relationship between comorbid conditions and insomnia disorder (e.g., depression, pain disorders) may result in the exacerbation of comorbid conditions such as depression, anxiety, or joint pain. Therefore, if applicable, the practitioner ought to ask the patient how their insomnia symptoms have impacted their comorbid conditions. As the symptom-based nature of insomnia disorder requires evidence for daytime impairment, appropriate evaluation of the effect of the patient's insomnia symptoms on their daily activities is a critical element of the assessment [50, 54].

To conclude the patient interview, obtaining a detailed medical history, social and psychiatric history, and medication list can provide important supplemental information to support or detract from a potential insomnia disorder diagnosis. Information attained from a detailed medical history, particularly for new patients, may inform the practitioner of comorbid conditions that may impact the patient's insomnia symptoms. Understanding these comorbid conditions can ensure that the chosen treatment method will optimize the reduction of both the symptoms of insomnia and those of the patient's comorbid conditions. Inquiring about the patient's social and psychiatric history will allow the practitioner to learn that the patient may be a shift worker or have a concomitant anxiety or depression diagnosis, which may alter the diagnosis and treatment approach. Similarly, discussing the patient's work or school hours as well as any current stressors in their life will provide the practitioner with useful information for formulating a differential diagnosis. Examining the patient's current medications (including route of administration, dosage, frequency, timing, and side effects) and inquiring specifically about caffeine and alcohol use may also point to a contributor of the patient's insomnia symptoms and may provide an initial option for symptom relief from reduction of these substances [62, 63]. Beyond caffeine and alcohol use, the use of antidepressants ought to be considered, as medications such as imipramine, desipramine, fluoxetine, paroxetine, venlafaxine, reboxetine, and bupropion can have either sedating or activating effects on the patient that must be addressed by moving the medication dose from evening to morning or transitioning to a more appropriate antidepressant that has fewer sleep disrupting side effects [64]. Over-the-counter allergy medications such as pseudoephedrine or phenylephrine as well as asthma medications such as albuterol have stimulatory properties that may also contribute to insomnia symptoms, and patients need to be advised not to take these medications within at least several hours of bedtime. Finally, the use of beta-blockers should be assessed and moved to morning administration as these medications can suppress melatonin and disrupt sleep [65].

Due to the symptom-based nature of the insomnia disorder diagnosis, it is vital that the patient interview be conducted in a manner that emphasizes the concerns of the patient in a trusted environment, while also maintaining logical order and efficiency for the practicality of an outpatient office visit. The following section on useful tools for insomnia disorder diagnosis will provide strategies for both building rapport with the patient without compromising efficiency.

Tools for Assessment of Insomnia Disorder

Utilizing a variety of tools and questionnaires may drastically expedite obtaining information necessary to make an insomnia disorder diagnosis. The Insomnia Severity Index (ISI) is useful in questioning the patient about their insomnia-specific symptoms such as their sleep onset latency and nighttime awakenings [66]. It is common for patients to have a sleep onset latency of ≤35 minutes; however, sleep onset latencies of >30–35 minutes should be broached by the clinician [57]. Similarly, several brief nighttime awakenings are benign, but the clinician should address nighttime awakenings that lead to prolonged wakefulness during the night known as wake after sleep onset (WASO). A duration of wakefulness >40 minutes is outside the normal range and indicates potential insomnia if occurring on a frequent basis [67]. In addition to measures such as sleep onset latency and WASO, the Pittsburgh Sleep Quality Index (PSQI) asks questions such as "During the past month, how often have you taken medicine (prescribed or 'over the counter') to help you sleep?" in order to ascertain aspects of the patient's sleep problem that may otherwise not be addressed by the patient interview [68]. Both of these instruments allow for the evaluation of the patient's insomnia complaints in the context of normative data so that a clear picture of the severity of the sleep disturbance can be obtained. Normative cutoffs for the ISI vary, but a frequently used cutoff in the community setting is ≥ 10 while the cutoff for the PSQI is >5 [68, 69].

Sleep Diary

A valuable tool for the practitioner is a 2-week "sleep diary" that the patient completes each morning immediately after awakening. The sleep diary includes the patient's self-reported bedtime, "lights out time," sleep onset latency, number and duration of nighttime awakenings, amount of wake after sleep onset, time in bed, total sleep time, sleep efficiency (total sleep time divided by time in bed), self-reported sleep quality, number and duration of naps, and any caffeine, alcohol, or sleep aid use (prescription or over the counter). The sleep diary allows the practitioner to gain an accurate picture of the patient's sleep habits and sense any trends in the patient's sleep schedule, such as a phase advance/delay or excessive use of caffeine or alcohol. The advantage to using the sleep diary as opposed to asking the patient to recall this information during the office visit is that the patient may struggle to recollect information about their sleep or may misperceive their long-term sleep habits. Having a patient fill out a sleep diary each morning for 2 weeks provides the most accurate picture of their sleep and should be utilized prior to full clinical evaluation whenever possible. If the practitioner is aware in advance that a patient is scheduling a visit for insomnia symptoms, they may request office staff to send a sleep diary worksheet or recommend app-based sleep diaries to the patient to fill out for 2 weeks prior to the visit. Alternatively, it may be beneficial to schedule a 2-week follow-up visit with the patient and request that they fill out the sleep diary during this 2-week interval to better ascertain their sleep habits and develop a successful treatment plan. When used properly, sleep diaries are a valuable part of the treatment process as they allow both the patient and the practitioner to track the progress of the treatment and adjust the treatment as needed. The National Sleep Foundation is an excellent source for obtaining a free to use standardized sleep diary [70].

Despite the rise in popularity of "wearable" devices such as Fitbits, Apple watches, etc., their questionable validity makes them less than ideal methods for tracking the sleep of insomnia patients. When compared to PSG sleep measures, wearable technology demonstrated a high sensitivity of over 90% for detecting sleep; however, its specificity for detecting wake was substantially diminished, leading to an artificially inflated total sleep time and diminished WASO [71]. Sleep onset also tended to be delayed when measured with wearable technology, with a typical delay of about 20 minutes when compared to PSG [71]. While results remained consistent across various categories of body mass indices and sexes, results tended to vary across age groups [71]. Additionally, wearable technology is generally programmed to detect a certain amount of sleep, typically at least an hour, leading to extreme inaccuracies in detecting napping [71]. Therefore, it is important for practitioners evaluating patients for insomnia disorder to not rely only on data from wearable devices but rather on information presented from sleep diaries filled out by patients themselves. In most cases, patient reports of symptoms should be taken at face value given the frequent discrepancy between subjective and objective sleep assessments (including actigraphy) in insomnia disorder. However, wearable devices are particularly useful for tracking sleep in patients who may be unable to provide accurate self-assessments (e.g., young children, cognitively impaired) or for those with widely varying sleep schedules such as night shift workers.

Taken together, the information provided through validated questionnaires such as the ESS, ISI, and PSQI in combination with sleep diary worksheets that track the patient's sleep habits will provide the practitioner with the most accurate depiction of the patient's insomnia symptoms.

Differential Diagnosis

In the differential diagnosis for insomnia disorder, a variety of other sleep and non-sleep-related disorders should be considered. Primarily, depression often presents with symptoms of insomnia, so it is imperative that the practitioner utilizes screening questionnaires such as the PHQ-9 and ISI to establish whether the patient is experiencing symptoms of depression, insomnia, or both. In many cases, due to the high comorbidity between insomnia and mental illness, the patient may be experiencing both depression and insomnia, and the patient ought to have both conditions treated at the time of the office visit. Although certain atypical antidepressants such as trazodone and mirtazapine have been used to treat insomnia, they are off-label and guidance on efficacy and appropriate doses for treatment of insomnia disorder are limited [72].

The symptoms of OSA may also present similarly to insomnia disorder, with patients reporting fatigue during the daytime and frequent awakenings at night. To differentiate between insomnia disorder and OSA, the practitioner should use tools that assess risks and symptoms of sleep-disordered breathing and OSA, such as the ESS and the four-item STOP/STOP-BANG [73, 74]. If a patient screens positive on either or both of these questionnaires, the practitioner should schedule a diagnostic study (home sleep apnea test or PSG) or make an appropriate referral to further investigate a potential diagnosis of OSA.

Movement disorders such as RLS may also present similarly to insomnia disorder, as the unpleasant sensations and urge to move at nighttime may prevent the patient from falling asleep. Questioning the patient about the symptoms of RLS and following up with a PSG study if positive symptoms are endorsed will help the practitioner to differentiate RLS from insomnia disorder. There are several unique characteristics of RLS that facilitate this process including a circadian rhythm of symptoms, unpleasant sensations in the legs, and the patient reports some relief with movement.

As previously mentioned, circadian rhythm disorders may also present as insomnia disorder, as a patient with phase delay may be unable to fall asleep until far past the patient's usual bedtime. Patients with a circadian rhythm disorder can show either a phase delay (i.e., delayed sleep onset and waketime) or a phase advance (i.e., earlier sleep onset than desired and early morning awakenings). Therefore, closely examining a patient's sleep diary and paying particular attention to weekday and weekend, holiday, or vacation data will inform the practitioner of a possible circadian rhythm disorder. When a patient presents with a consistently extreme early or consistently extreme late bedtime additional assessment is warranted by a sleep specialist to rule out a circadian rhythm disorder. If there is substantive discord between the objective and subjective data and all other disorders have been ruled out, paradoxical insomnia could be considered [75].

In summary, insomnia disorder has a host of comorbid conditions that can contribute to insomnia symptoms or that may present similarly to insomnia disorder. If the practitioner is uncertain that an insomnia disorder diagnosis is the most appropriate for a given patient, a variety of screening questionnaires and the use of a PSG study in conjunction to sleep specialist referral are important aspects for obtaining an accurate diagnosis.

Treatment Options and Goals

Evaluation of insomnia should conclude with a discussion of treatment options and the patient's treatment goals. The primary goals in treating patients with insomnia disorder are typically to improve their sleep quality, thereby improving the patient's subjective experience of their sleep [50] and improving their daytime functioning. For patients wishing to discontinue the use of sleep medications, tapering and eventual discontinuation of pharmacological treatment may occur in concert with CBT-I once the patient's insomnia symptoms are below the threshold for severe insomnia for several weeks (ISI < 22) [50, 66]. Secondary goals of insomnia disorder treatment should be to reduce any psychological distress or correct any maladaptive belief systems that the patient has regarding sleep by referring the patient to a CBT-I provider [42, 50]. Importantly, when discussing treatment goals with the patient, the practitioner ought to ask the patient for their desired outcome and any treatment preferences they may have. Engaging in shared decision-making and goal formulation in this way will not only help to guide treatment options but also help the patient to be actively engaged in their treatment and build rapport [42].

Assessment of insomnia remission after initiation of treatment should include the same measures and questionnaires used for the initial evaluation of the diagnosis rather than exclusively asking the patient if their symptoms have improved. Of note, many patients will learn to tolerate their symptoms or believe that poor sleep is acceptable yet will still be displaying insomnia symptoms and experiencing daytime impairment [40]. Repeating the initial measures and questionnaires will provide a more accurate picture of the progression of the patient's sleep pattern before and after treatment. Importantly, emphasis should be placed on if the patient's daytime functioning has improved, as this is one foundation of the insomnia disorder diagnosis. If the patient is still exhibiting impaired daytime functioning or displaying other symptoms of insomnia, the practitioner should question the patient about treatment adherence (both behavioral and pharmacological), or consider if a different diagnosis is more appropriate. In some cases where remission does not occur, it can be effective to have the patient to use an alternative or additional treatment approach. Furthermore, as over a quarter of individuals in remission will relapse within 3 years, it is essential that the practitioner follow-up with the patient at all future appointments [5]. Thorough documentation in the medical record of the insomnia disorder diagnosis and treatment efforts will help in future visits with the patient and will aid other providers if insomnia recurrence occurs.

Summary

Insomnia disorder is a highly pervasive and persistent sleep disorder that negatively impacts both the patient and society as a whole. The clinical management of insomnia disorder in a primary care setting can be challenging, but given the proper tools, any practitioner can be prepared to efficiently and effectively treat insomnia disorder. Keeping in mind the potential etiology of the disorder, the practitioner will be able to understand the myriad underlying reasons for the patient's symptom presentation and use this knowledge to inform the patient of their appropriate treatment options. Being familiar with the signs, symptoms, and treatments of insomnia disorder will allow general practitioners including those in primary care to be optimal first-line interventionists for these patients and deliver high-quality, compassionate care to those suffering from this debilitating disorder.

Key Summary Points
1. Insomnia disorder is a common clinical condition impacting at least 10% of adults.
2. Insomnia disorder is diagnosed based on a thorough clinical history; diagnosis does not require the patient to undergo polysomnography.
3. First-line treatment for insomnia disorder is cognitive behavioral therapy for insomnia (CBT-I).
4. If left untreated, insomnia disorder can contribute to the development of depression and increase a patient's risk of suicidality.
5. Insomnia disorder can often present similarly to other sleep disorders such as obstructive sleep apnea (OSA), restless legs syndrome (RLS), and circadian rhythm disorders; therefore, the practitioner must consider these alternate diagnoses in patients presenting with sleep difficulties.

References

1. DSMTF, editor. Diagnostic and statistical manual of mental disorders: DSM-5. American Psychiatric A, American Psychiatric Association. Arlington: American Psychiatric Association; 2013.
2. Medicine AAoS. International classification of sleep disorders—third edition (ICSD-3) online version. Westchester: American Academy of Sleep Medicine; 2014.
3. Roth T, Coulouvrat C, Hajak G, Lakoma MD, Sampson NA, Shahly V, et al. Prevalence and perceived health associated with insomnia based on DSM-IV-TR; international statistical classification of diseases and related health problems, tenth revision; and research diagnostic criteria/international classification of sleep disorders, second edition criteria: results from the America insomnia survey. Biol Psychiatry. 2011;69(6):592–600.
4. Ohayon MM. Epidemiology of insomnia: what we know and what we still need to learn. Sleep Med Rev. 2002;6(2):97–111.
5. Morin CM, Belanger L, LeBlanc M, Ivers H, Savard J, Espie CA, et al. The natural history of insomnia: a population-based 3-year longitudinal study. Arch Intern Med. 2009;169(5):447–53.
6. Sofi F, Cesari F, Casini A, Macchi C, Abbate R, Gensini GF. Insomnia and risk of cardiovascular disease: a meta-analysis. Eur J Prev Cardiol. 2014;21(1):57–64.
7. Fernandez-Mendoza J, He F, Vgontzas AN, Liao D, Bixler EO. Interplay of objective sleep duration and cardiovascular and cerebrovascular diseases on cause-specific mortality. J Am Heart Assoc. 2019;8(20):e013043.

8. Cheng P, Pillai V, Mengel H, Roth T, Drake CL. Sleep maintenance difficulties in insomnia are associated with increased incidence of hypertension. Sleep Health. 2015;1(1):50–4.

9. Jarrin DC, Alvaro PK, Bouchard MA, Jarrin SD, Drake CL, Morin CM. Insomnia and hypertension: a systematic review. Sleep Med Rev. 2018;41:3–38.

10. Vgontzas AN, Fernandez-Mendoza J, Liao D, Bixler EO. Insomnia with objective short sleep duration: the most biologically severe phenotype of the disorder. Sleep Med Rev. 2013;17(4):241–54.

11. Lin CL, Chien WC, Chung CH, Wu FL. Risk of type 2 diabetes in patients with insomnia: a population-based historical cohort study. Diabetes Metab Res Rev. 2018;34(1)

12. Sexton CE, Storsve AB, Walhovd KB, Johansen-Berg H, Fjell AM. Poor sleep quality is associated with increased cortical atrophy in community-dwelling adults. Neurology. 2014;83(11):967–73.

13. Hung CM, Li YC, Chen HJ, Lu K, Liang CL, Liliang PC, et al. Risk of dementia in patients with primary insomnia: a nationwide population-based case-control study. BMC Psychiatry. 2018;18(1):38.

14. Baglioni C, Battagliese G, Feige B, Spiegelhalder K, Nissen C, Voderholzer U, et al. Insomnia as a predictor of depression: a meta-analytic evaluation of longitudinal epidemiological studies. J Affect Disord. 2011;135(1–3):10–9.

15. Cheng P, Kalmbach DA, Tallent G, Joseph CL, Espie CA, Drake CL. Depression prevention via digital cognitive behavioral therapy for insomnia: a randomized controlled trial. Sleep. 2019;42(10)

16. Bishop TM, Crean HF, Hoff RA, Pigeon WR. Suicidal ideation among recently returned veterans and its relationship to insomnia and depression. Psychiatry Res. 2019;276:250–61.

17. Russell K, Rasmussen S, Hunter SC. Insomnia and nightmares as markers of risk for suicidal ideation in young people: investigating the role of defeat and entrapment. J Clin Sleep Med. 2018;14(5):775–84.

18. Kucharczyk ER, Morgan K, Hall AP. The occupational impact of sleep quality and insomnia symptoms. Sleep Med Rev. 2012;16(6):547–59.

19. Brossoit RM, Crain TL, Leslie JJ, Hammer LB, Truxillo DM, Bodner TE. The effects of sleep on workplace cognitive failure and safety. J Occup Health Psychol. 2019;24(4):411–22.

20. Asche CV, Joish VN, Camacho F, Drake CL. The direct costs of untreated comorbid insomnia in a managed care population with major depressive disorder. Curr Med Res Opin. 2010;26(8):1843–53.

21. Klemas N. Clinical Economics. Insomnia Med Econ. 2015;92(6):24–5, 30

22. Levenson JC, Kay DB, Buysse DJ. The pathophysiology of insomnia. Chest. 2015;147(4):1179–92.

23. Bonnet MH, Arand DL. Hyperarousal and insomnia: state of the science. Sleep Med Rev. 2010;14(1):9–15.

24. Winkelman JW, Buxton OM, Jensen JE, Benson KL, O'Connor SP, Wang W, et al. Reduced brain GABA in primary insomnia: preliminary data from 4T proton magnetic resonance spectroscopy (1H-MRS). Sleep. 2008;31(11):1499–506.

25. Saito YC, Maejima T, Nishitani M, Hasegawa E, Yanagawa Y, Mieda M, et al. Monoamines inhibit GABAergic neurons in ventrolateral preoptic area that make direct synaptic connections to hypothalamic arousal neurons. J Neurosci. 2018;38(28):6366–78.

26. Mazzocchi G, Malendowicz LK, Gottardo L, Aragona F, Nussdorfer GG. Orexin a stimulates cortisol secretion from human adrenocortical cells through activation of the adenylate cyclase-dependent signaling cascade. J Clin Endocrinol Metabol. 2001;86(2):778–82.

27. Borbely AA, Daan S, Wirz-Justice A, Deboer T. The two-process model of sleep regulation: a reappraisal. J Sleep Res. 2016;25(2):131–43.

28. Achermann P, Borbély AA. Chapter 37 - Sleep homeostasis and models of sleep regulation. In: Kryger MH, Roth T, Dement WC, editors. Principles and practice of sleep medicine. 5th ed. Philadelphia: W.B. Saunders; 2011. p. 431–44.

29. Drake CL, Friedman NP, Wright KP Jr, Roth T. Sleep reactivity and insomnia: genetic and environmental influences. Sleep. 2011;34(9):1179–88.
30. Spielman AJ, Caruso LS, Glovinsky PB. A behavioral perspective on insomnia treatment. Psychiatr Clin North Am. 1987;10(4):541–53.
31. Perlis M, Shaw PJ, Cano G, Espie CA. Chapter 78 – Models of insomnia. In: Kryger MH, Roth T, Dement WC, editors. Principles and practice of sleep medicine. 5th ed. Philadelphia: W.B. Saunders; 2011. p. 850–65.
32. Drake CL, Pillai V, Roth T. Stress and sleep reactivity: a prospective investigation of the stress-diathesis model of insomnia. Sleep. 2014;37(8):1295–304.
33. Kalmbach DA, Anderson JR, Drake CL. The impact of stress on sleep: pathogenic sleep reactivity as a vulnerability to insomnia and circadian disorders. J Sleep Res. 2018;27(6):e12710-e.
34. Kalmbach DA, Buysse DJ, Cheng P, Roth T, Yang A, Drake CL. Nocturnal cognitive arousal is associated with objective sleep disturbance and indicators of physiologic hyperarousal in good sleepers and individuals with insomnia disorder. Sleep Med. 2020;71:151–60.
35. Nofzinger EA, Buysse DJ, Germain A, Price JC, Miewald JM, Kupfer DJ. Functional neuroimaging evidence for hyperarousal in insomnia. Am J Psychiatry. 2004;161(11):2126–8.
36. Riemann D, Baglioni C, Bassetti C, Bjorvatn B, Dolenc Groselj L, Ellis JG, et al. European guideline for the diagnosis and treatment of insomnia. J Sleep Res. 2017;26(6):675–700.
37. Seow LSE, Verma SK, Mok YM, Kumar S, Chang S, Satghare P, et al. Evaluating DSM-5 insomnia disorder and the treatment of sleep problems in a psychiatric population. J Clin Sleep Med JCSM. 2018;14(2):237–44.
38. Vgontzas AN, Bixler EO, Lin HM, Prolo P, Mastorakos G, Vela-Bueno A, et al. Chronic insomnia is associated with nyctohemeral activation of the hypothalamic-pituitary-adrenal axis: clinical implications. J Clin Endocrinol Metab. 2001;86(8):3787–94.
39. Edinger JD, Ulmer CS, Means MK. Sensitivity and specificity of polysomnographic criteria for defining insomnia. J Clin Sleep Med. 2013;9(5):481–91.
40. Pillai V, Roth T, Drake CL. Towards quantitative cutoffs for insomnia: how current diagnostic criteria mischaracterize remission. Sleep Med. 2016;26:62–8.
41. Taylor DJ, Wilkerson AK, Pruiksma KE, Williams JM, Ruggero CJ, Hale W, et al. Reliability of the structured clinical interview for DSM-5 sleep disorders module. J Clin Sleep Med. 2018;14(3):459–64.
42. Qaseem A, Kansagara D, Forciea MA, Cooke M, Denberg TD. Management of chronic insomnia disorder in adults: a clinical practice guideline from the American College of Physicians. Ann Intern Med. 2016;165(2):125–33.
43. Mitchell MD, Gehrman P, Perlis M, Umscheid CA. Comparative effectiveness of cognitive behavioral therapy for insomnia: a systematic review. BMC Fam Pract. 2012;13:40.
44. Kroenke K, Spitzer RL, Williams JB. The PHQ-9: validity of a brief depression severity measure. J Gen Intern Med. 2001;16(9):606–13.
45. Klink ME, Quan SF, Kaltenborn WT, Lebowitz MD. Risk factors associated with complaints of insomnia in a general adult population. Influence of previous complaints of insomnia. Arch Intern Med. 1992;152(8):1634–7.
46. Kalmbach DA, Cheng P, Ong JC, Ciesla JA, Kingsberg SA, Sangha R, et al. Depression and suicidal ideation in pregnancy: exploring relationships with insomnia, short sleep, and nocturnal rumination. Sleep Med. 2020;65:62–73.
47. Kalmbach DA, Cheng P, Arnedt JT, Cuamatzi-Castelan A, Atkinson RL, Fellman-Couture C, et al. Improving daytime functioning, work performance, and quality of life in postmenopausal women with insomnia: comparing cognitive behavioral therapy for insomnia, sleep restriction therapy, and sleep hygiene education. J Clin Sleep Med. 2019;15(7):999–1010.
48. Drake CL, Kalmbach DA, Arnedt JT, Cheng P, Tonnu CV, Cuamatzi-Castelan A, et al. Treating chronic insomnia in postmenopausal women: a randomized clinical trial comparing cognitive-behavioral therapy for insomnia, sleep restriction therapy, and sleep hygiene education. Sleep. 2019;42(2)

49. Kalmbach DA, Cheng P, O'Brien LM, Swanson LM, Sangha R, Sen S, et al. A randomized controlled trial of digital cognitive behavioral therapy for insomnia in pregnant women. Sleep Med. 2020;72:82–92.
50. Schutte-Rodin S, Broch L, Buysse D, Dorsey C, Sateia M. Clinical guideline for the evaluation and management of chronic insomnia in adults. J Clin Sleep Med. 2008;4(5):487–504.
51. Grandner MA, Williams NJ, Knutson KL, Roberts D, Jean-Louis G. Sleep disparity, race/ethnicity, and socioeconomic position. Sleep Med. 2016;18:7–18.
52. Beaulieu-Bonneau S, LeBlanc M, Merette C, Dauvilliers Y, Morin CM. Family history of insomnia in a population-based sample. Sleep. 2007;30(12):1739–45.
53. Hodges CJ, Ogeil RP, Lubman DI. The effects of acute alcohol withdrawal on sleep. Hum Psychopharmacol. 2018;33(3):e2657.
54. Krystal AD, Prather AA, Ashbrook LH. The assessment and management of insomnia: an update. World Psychiatry. 2019;18(3):337–52.
55. Harvey AG. A cognitive model of insomnia. Behav Res Ther. 2002;40(8):869–93.
56. Harvey AG, Tang NK, Browning L. Cognitive approaches to insomnia. Clin Psychol Rev. 2005;25(5):593–611.
57. Drake CL, Vargas I, Roth T, Friedman NP. Quantitative measures of nocturnal insomnia symptoms predict greater deficits across multiple daytime impairment domains. Behav Sleep Med. 2015;13(1):73–87.
58. Zammit GK. Subjective ratings of the characteristics and sequelae of good and poor sleep in normals. J Clin Psychol. 1988;44(2):123–30.
59. Carey TJ, Moul DE, Pilkonis P, Germain A, Buysse DJ. Focusing on the experience of insomnia. Behav Sleep Med. 2005;3(2):73–86.
60. Johns MW. A new method for measuring daytime sleepiness: the Epworth sleepiness scale. Sleep. 1991;14(6):540–5.
61. Lerdal A. Fatigue severity scale. In: Michalos AC, editor. Encyclopedia of quality of life and well-being research. Dordrecht: Springer Netherlands; 2014. p. 2218–21.
62. Treur JL, Gibson M, Taylor AE, Rogers PJ, Munafo MR. Investigating genetic correlations and causal effects between caffeine consumption and sleep behaviours. J Sleep Res. 2018;27(5):e12695.
63. Thakkar MM, Sharma R, Sahota P. Alcohol disrupts sleep homeostasis. Alcohol. 2015;49(4):299–310.
64. Wichniak A, Wierzbicka A, Jernajczyk W. Sleep and antidepressant treatment. Curr Pharm Des. 2012;18(36):5802–17.
65. Stoschitzky K, Sakotnik A, Lercher P, Zweiker R, Maier R, Liebmann P, et al. Influence of beta-blockers on melatonin release. Eur J Clin Pharmacol. 1999;55(2):111–5.
66. Bastien CH, Vallieres A, Morin CM. Validation of the Insomnia Severity Index as an outcome measure for insomnia research. Sleep Med. 2001;2(4):297–307.
67. Lineberger MD, Carney CE, Edinger JD, Means MK. Defining insomnia: quantitative criteria for insomnia severity and frequency. Sleep. 2006;29(4):479–85.
68. Buysse DJ, Reynolds CF 3rd, Monk TH, Berman SR, Kupfer DJ. The Pittsburgh Sleep Quality Index: a new instrument for psychiatric practice and research. Psychiatry Res. 1989;28(2):193–213.
69. Morin CM, Belleville G, Bélanger L, Ivers H. The Insomnia Severity Index: psychometric indicators to detect insomnia cases and evaluate treatment response. Sleep. 2011;34(5):601–8.
70. National Sleep Foundation. Sleep Diary 2020 [Available from: https://www.sleepfoundation.org/sites/default/files/inline-files/SleepDiaryv6.pdf.
71. de Zambotti M, Cellini N, Goldstone A, Colrain IM, Baker FC. Wearable sleep technology in clinical and research settings. Med Sci Sports Exerc. 2019;51(7):1538–57.
72. Atkin T, Comai S, Gobbi G. Drugs for insomnia beyond benzodiazepines: pharmacology, clinical applications, and discovery. Pharmacol Rev. 2018;70(2):197–245.

73. Silva GE, Vana KD, Goodwin JL, Sherrill DL, Quan SF. Identification of patients with sleep disordered breathing: comparing the four-variable screening tool, STOP, STOP-Bang, and Epworth sleepiness scales. J Clin Sleep Med. 2011;7(5):467–72.
74. Vana KD, Silva GE, Goldberg R. Predictive abilities of the STOP-Bang and Epworth sleepiness Scale in identifying sleep clinic patients at high risk for obstructive sleep apnea. Res Nurs Health. 2013;36(1):84–94.
75. Castelnovo A, Ferri R, Punjabi NM, Castronovo V, Garbazza C, Zucconi M, et al. The paradox of paradoxical insomnia: a theoretical review towards a unifying evidence-based definition. Sleep Med Rev. 2019;44:70–82.
76. World Health O. ICD-10 : international statistical classification of diseases and related health problems: tenth revision. 2nd ed. Geneva: World Health Organization; 2004.

Chapter 13
Management of Insomnia Disorder

Gwendolyn C. Carlson, Michelle R. Zeidler, and Jennifer L. Martin

Keywords Insomnia · Sleep medicine · Clinical practice guidelines · CBT-I

Management of Insomnia Disorder

Insomnia disorder is characterized by difficulty initiating and maintaining sleep. It is estimated that 10–30% of the population experiences insomnia [1–3]. There are two primary diagnostic systems for the identification of clinically significant insomnia symptoms: (1) the American Psychiatric Association's (APA) Diagnostic and Statistical Manual of Mental Disorder-fifth Edition (DSM-5) [4] and (2) the *International Classification of Sleep Disorders*-Third *Edition* (ICSD-3) of the American Academy of Sleep Medicine (AASM) [5]. A diagnosis of insomnia

G. C. Carlson
Department of Mental Health, VA Greater Los Angeles Healthcare System, VA Health Services Research and Development Service (HSR&D) Center for the Study of Healthcare Innovation, Implementation and Policy, Los Angeles, CA, USA

Department of Psychiatry and Biobehavioral Sciences, David Geffen School of Medicine, University of California, Los Angeles, Los Angeles, CA, USA

M. R. Zeidler
Sleep Disorders Center, VA Greater Los Angeles VA Healthcare System, Department of Medicine, David Geffen School of Medicine, University of California, Los Angeles, Los Angeles, CA, USA

J. L. Martin (✉)
Geriatric Research, Education and Clinical Center, Veteran Affairs Greater Los Angeles Healthcare System, Department of Medicine, David Geffen School of Medicine, University of California, Los Angeles, Los Angeles, CA, USA
e-mail: Jennifer.martin@va.gov

© Springer Nature Switzerland AG 2022
M. S. Badr, J. L. Martin (eds.), *Essentials of Sleep Medicine*,
Respiratory Medicine, https://doi.org/10.1007/978-3-030-93739-3_13

disorder is characterized by poor sleep, with daytime consequences, that persists for 3 months and occurs at least three times per week. Per the ICSD-3, a diagnosis of chronic insomnia requires that a patient report sleep disturbance for at least 3 months, with short-term insomnia characterized by sleep disturbance that is less than 3 months in duration [5]. Consequences associated with sleep disturbance include increased risk for other medical and mental health comorbidities, lost productivity and increased absenteeism, and increase risk for accident, injury, and death [6].

Given the prevalence of and impairment associated with poor sleep, interventions have been developed to treat the symptoms of insomnia disorder [2, 7, 8]. Interventions include both behavioral (i.e., non-medication) treatments and medication treatments. This chapter describes the best practices for the treatment of insomnia disorder. Based on the AASM Clinical Practice Guidelines [8], Fig. 13.1 describes a decision-making framework for the treatment of insomnia disorder. Evidence-based treatments, patients' preferences, sleep disorder comorbidities, and treatment responses will inform decision-making. The following sections describe the treatments included in this framework and factors that may influence treatment delivery and referral.

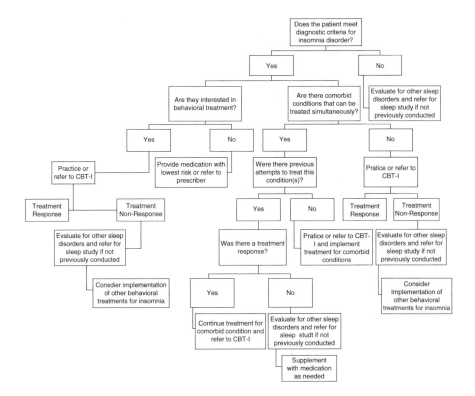

Fig. 13.1 Treatment decision-making framework for the treatment of insomnia disorder

Behavioral Interventions

Cognitive behavioral therapy for insomnia The first line treatment for insomnia is cognitive behavioral therapy for insomnia (CBT-I) [7]. The AASM Clinical Practice Guidelines strongly recommend clinicians use multicomponent CBT-I for the treatment of chronic insomnia disorder in adults [9]. A "strong recommendation" indicates that clinicians should implement or refer to this treatment under most circumstances. A "conditional" recommendation indicates that clinicians should consider knowledge of the patient (i.e., patient values and preferences) and clinical knowledge and experience to determine the best intervention. While multicomponent CBT-I is strongly recommended, individual components of CBT-I are also conditionally recommended for the treatment of chronic insomnia disorder in adults. The following sections will describe the components of CBT-I.

The "3-Ps" model underlies the rationale for CBT-I. This model proposes that insomnia develops from and is maintained by predisposing factors, precipitating factors, and perpetuating factors [10]. Predisposing factors increase an individual's risk of developing insomnia (e.g., family history of sleep disorders). Precipitating factors include circumstances or events that lead patients to experience clinically significant sleep difficulties (e.g., injuries/medical conditions, interpersonal events) [11]. Attempts to cope with precipitating factors can lead to perpetuating factors (e.g., compensatory daytime napping, prolonged time awake in bed at night, caffeine use during that day). According to the 3-Ps model, perpetuating factors lead to chronic insomnia [10]. Insomnia is maintained by the interrelations among problematic emotions, thoughts, and behaviors. Patients can develop anxiety or other emotions regarding their sleep difficulties, experience inaccurate and unhelpful thoughts about their sleep difficulties, and engage in maladaptive behaviors to cope with difficulties initiating and maintaining sleep [12, 13]. CBT-I intervenes on this problematic cycle by changing problematic behaviors and thoughts [8]. CBT-I sessions typically incorporate the following intervention components: (1) stimulus control, (2) sleep restriction, (3) sleep hygiene recommendations, (4) relaxation strategies, and (5) cognitive therapy exercises. Of these components, the strongest evidence supports stimulus control and sleep restriction as stand-alone treatments, while evidence for the other components remains more modest [14, 15].

Stimulus control Stimulus control is a behavioral phenomenon that underlies multiple behaviors, including sleep [16]. In basic terms, sleep is considered an instrumental behavior, and cues (or stimuli) in a patient's environment provide information about whether sleep will be reinforced or not [17, 18]. Example of discriminative stimuli for sleep include darkness/nighttime or being in bed. However, if these stimuli are inconsistently paired with sleep, difficulty sleeping may be the result of inadequate discriminative stimulus control. Patients who undergo CBT-I are provided with education about classical and operant conditioning to ensure they understand the rationale for stimulus control therapy [19]. The provider and patient discuss the associations that can develop between the bed (i.e., place of sleep) and anxiety and/

or other non-sleep behaviors/activities and how these associations lead to conditioned insomnia [14]. The intervention of stimulus control involves using the sleep area only for sleeping, refraining from doing other activities in the sleep area, and avoiding sleeping in areas other than the designated sleep area. Per the AASM Clinical Practice Guidelines, it conditionally recommended that clinicians implement stimulus control as a single-component therapy for the treatment of insomnia disorder.

Sleep restriction In addition to stimulus control, patients are oriented to the rationale for tracking sleep. Behavior monitoring is a common component of many behavioral therapies [20]. Patients are oriented to the sleep diary and are asked to complete a weekly sleep diary, which includes daily bedtimes, sleep onset latencies, wake times after sleep onset, number of nighttime awakenings, rise times, and daytime awakenings (see Fig. 13.2 for an example of sleep diary information). Based on data on the sleep diary, patients are oriented to the concept of sleep efficiency. Sleep efficiency is calculated by dividing total sleep time by total time in bed (minutes from bedtime to rise time) and converting the quotient to a percentage. Patients and providers discuss how low sleep efficiency can exacerbate problematic associations between bed and wakefulness, maintaining insomnia symptoms [15]. Patients may develop inaccurate beliefs that more time in bed provides a greater opportunity for sleep. In fact, excessive time in bed not sleeping can further contribute to inadequate stimulus control. Sleep restriction involves reducing the amount of time a patient spends in bed in an effort to improve sleep efficiency [18, 21]. This involves setting a sleep window based on a patient's sleep diary total time in bed. Patients are

Complete on: *Sun Mon Tues Wed Thurs Fri Sat [date]* _____
      Day 1

Morning questions		
1. What time did you got to bod last night?	__:__ am/pm	
2. How long did it take you to fall asleep last night?	minutes	
3. Did you wake up during the night last night?	☐ No	☐ Yes
a. *If yes,* How many times did you wake up?	times	
b. *If yes,* What was the total amount of time that you wereawake?	minutes	
4. Last night, did you take any medication to help you sleep?	☐ No	☐ Yes
a. *If yes,* What did you take? (*write down any sleep aid below*)		
b. What time did you take this?	__:__ am/pm	
5. What time did you wake up for the last time this morning?	__:__ am/pm	
6. This morning, what time did you get up for the day?	__:__ am/pm	

Bedtime questions		
7. Did you take any naps or doze off at any time today before getting into bed for the night?	☐ No	☐ Yes
a. *If yes,* How many times did you spend napping or dozing?	minutes	
8. Did you drink any beverages containing caffeine today?	☐ No	☐ Yes
a. *If yes,* About how many cups or glasses?	__ cups/glasses	
b. *If yes,* What time did you have your last one?	__:__ am/pm	
9. Did you drink any beverages containing alcohol today?	☐ No	☐ Yes
a. *If yes,* About how many drinks did you have? (*Please refer to the "Drink Conversion Table" on the inside back cover*)	drinks	
b. What time did you have your last drink?	__:__ am/pm	
10. Did you remove the sleep watch for any reason today?	☐ No	☐ Yes
a. *If yes,* what time?		
Time off __:__ am/pm Time on: __:__ am/pm		
b. Reason removed _____		

Fig. 13.2 Example of information collected in sleep diary

instructed to only sleep within this window of time (i.e., between prescribed bedtime and rise time). Patients should not go to bed earlier than their prescribed bedtime or wake up later than their prescribed rise time, and should avoid napping outside of their sleep window [15, 22]. It is conditionally recommended that providers implement sleep restriction as a single-component treatment for insomnia disorder [9].

Sleep hygiene recommendations CBT-I providers present information about daytime and nighttime activities that can help or hinder good sleep. Patients receive information about how factors (e.g., light exposure, alcohol/substances, medications, caffeine, food intake, and exercise) can impact wakefulness and sleepiness [23]. The patient and provider also discuss the sleep environment and what environmental factors can help or hinder sleep (e.g., temperature, noise, light, bodily discomfort, bed partner, etc.). The patient and provider discuss changes the patient can implement to improve their sleep [23]. Sleep hygiene education, as a standalone intervention, has been shown to be less effective than multicomponent CBT-I [24]; however, sleep hygiene is conditionally recommended as a single-component treatment for insomnia disorder [8].

Relaxation strategies Anxiety and hyperarousal at bedtime serve as barriers to sleep initiation. CBT-I providers educate patients about the problematic relationships among thoughts, emotions, and sleep behaviors that occur in the context of insomnia. The goal of relaxation strategies in the context of insomnia is to reduce hyperarousal at bedtime. Consistent with the principle of counter-conditioning, an undesired response (i.e., arousal) is reduced as the stimulus (i.e., place of sleep) is consistently paired with a more desired response (i.e., relaxation) [25]. Relaxation strategies, including breathing exercises [26] and progressive muscle relaxation [27], are often presented as part of CBT-I protocols [28]. Additionally, patients are encouraged to implement a relaxing bedtime routine (i.e., buffer zone) each night in an effort to (1) reduce anxious thoughts at bedtime [22] and (2) weaken the association between hyperarousal and bedtime that may have developed due to poor sleep habits. Relaxation therapy is conditionally recommended as a single-component treatment for insomnia disorder [8].

Cognitive therapy techniques As a form of cognitive behavioral therapy, CBT-I incorporates cognitive techniques to challenge unhelpful and inaccurate thoughts that lead to problematic sleep behavior (i.e., "I have to go to bed early, and then I will sleep more tonight") [29]. To identify and adapt problematic thoughts related to sleep, providers will utilize Socratic questioning [30]. Additionally, providers may ask patients to examine their thoughts by looking at their sleep diary data (i.e., "Do you actually sleep more if you spend more time in your bed?") or encourage patients to test these thoughts by engaging in a behavioral experiment. Sleep diary information can also help to challenge inaccurate or problematic thoughts about daytime functioning (e.g., "If I don't get eight hours of sleep, I will not be able to function the next day"). By providing evidence to the contrary regarding the relationship between total sleep time and daytime functioning, data gathered during CBT-I sessions can lessen anxiety about sleep difficulties and the perceived consequences of insomnia. Additionally, cognitive techniques can be used if patients express reluctance to engage in other components of CBT-I (e.g., sleep restriction). Other cognitive techniques include but are not limited to (1) evaluating the evidence for or against a thought, (2) exploring alternative explanations or interpretation, (3) and/or presenting new information to patients [31].

Multiple meta-analyses have demonstrated the effectiveness of CBT-I at improving wake/sleep patterns among patients with insomnia, including patients with comorbid medical and psychiatric conditions [28, 32, 33]. The intervention components of CBT-I and their implementation are described in Table 13.1. It should be noted that the delivery of CBT-I is individualized for each patient, with the emphasis and timing of each intervention component depending on the clinical presentation of each individual patient.

Individual format CBT-I interventions have been most commonly studied using a one-on-one, in person therapy format [28, 32]. Most protocols consist of four to six, 60-minute sessions with a trained CBT-I provider. However, CBT-I has also been delivered using telemedicine platforms, with high feasibility and acceptability reported by patients and providers [34]. Meta-analyses have consistently found individual-based CBT-I to be an effective treatment for insomnia symptoms [32, 33]. As previously stated, the multicomponent, individual-based form of CBT-I is strongly recommended by the AASM Clinical Practice Guidelines for the Treatment of Insomnia [8]. This means that under most circumstances (or when possible), providers should refer patients to or implement individual-based CBT-I [8].

Group format Despite the efficacy of this intervention, we recognize that there are circumstances when one-on-one CBT-I may not be readily available or accessible to patients [35]. Fortunately, there is also research demonstrating the efficacy for group-based CBT-I, though there is less evidence for group-based CBT-I compared to one-on-one CBT-I [36]. This form of CBT-I involves providing psychoeducation about sleep, including the rationales for stimulus control, sleep restriction, and the other intervention components of CBT-I to a group of patients [37]. Each patient tracks their sleep using a sleep diary, and sleep windows are prescribed to each patient based on individual data from patients' respective sleep diaries.

Telehealth Telehealth modalities have been used to deliver CBT-I in several studies and can increase access to treatment for patients with insomnia disorder who many find it difficult to travel to in-person sessions or to navigate a self-guided treatment without provider support. There is evidence that CBT-I can be delivered via telehealth in both individual and group format, and it is non-inferior to in-person delivery [38, 39]; however, there are challenges to group delivery including privacy consideration and technological challenges.

Table 13.1 Typical intervention components of cognitive behavioral therapy for insomnia (CBT-I)

Topics covered	Session activities	Homework
Getting started with CBT-I (sleep education, sleep hygiene, and stimulus control)		
Sleep education: sleep regulation, insomnia (3P model), sleep stages and macrostructure Introduce stimulus control concepts Lifestyle habits that enhance or hinder sleep Introduce and explain daily sleep diary	Discuss classical conditioning and insomnia Action plan: sleep hygiene changes, stimulus control	Implement action plan (sleep hygiene practices, stimulus control) Daily sleep diary
Scheduling sleep (sleep restriction therapy)		
Learn about the homeostatic and circadian sleep processes Introduce sleep restriction	Review/discuss sleep diary Action plan: daily sleep schedule	Implement action plan (sleep schedule) Daily sleep diary
Thoughts about sleep (cognitive therapy)		
Adjust time in bed Discuss validity and utility of unhelpful sleep-related thoughts	Review/discuss sleep diary Action plan: revise sleep schedule, develop coping cards	Implement action plan (sleep schedule, coping cards) Daily sleep diary
CBT-I: progress and obstacles (cognitive therapy)		
Adjust time in bed Review progress and obstacles Use cognitive strategies to address barriers to adherence	Review/discuss sleep diary Addressing barriers and obstacles using cognitive-therapy methods Action plan: identify obstacles and strategies to address them	Implement action plan (sleep schedule, strategies to address obstacles) Daily sleep diary
CBT-I: sleeping well over the long-term (relapse prevention)		
Adjust time in bed Discuss relapse prevention and coping	Review/discuss sleep diary Action plan for relapse prevention	Use tools/skills for future sleepless nights

Self-guided formats To increase access to CBT-I, online, self-guided protocols and CBT-I informed apps have been developed. Evidence-based examples include the Veteran Health Administration's (VHA) "Path to Better Sleep" [40] and "CBT-I Coach." [41] Online behavioral interventions for insomnia have been shown to improve sleep outcomes [42–44]. There is also evidence that face-to-face CBT-I is more effective than guided online interventions [45]. That being said, CBT-I providers report using CBT-I Coach when delivering one-on-one CBT-I, and research demonstrates that the app is viewed favorably by patients [46, 47]. It should be noted that use of CBT-I Coach or other apps alone is not comparable to the delivery of CBT-I by a trained provider.

Brief behavioral treatment for insomnia Given that stimulus control and sleep restriction are the intervention components of CBT-I with the strongest evidence, brief behavioral treatment for insomnia (BBT-I) was derived from CBT-I. BBT-I is shorter than CBT-I [48, 49], typically involving four sessions, and focuses on helping patients to make behavioral changes to improve their sleep. BBT-I provides education about homeostatic (i.e., sleep drive) and circadian drives (i.e., biological clock) and how waking behaviors associated with insomnia disorder can interfere with these processes [50]. Similar education is provided in CBT-I protocols as well [22]. Intervention components of BBT-I include (1) sleep restriction to increase sleepiness at the prescribed bedtime, (2) stimulus control to reduce time spent awake in bed, (3) adherence to prescribed bedtimes and rise times, (4) and elimination/reduction of bad sleep hygiene behaviors and promotion of good sleep hygiene behaviors. BBT-I encourages patients to modify waking behaviors to normalize homeostatic and circadian drives. BBT-I does not target sleep-related thoughts and does not incorporate cognitive strategies [50]. While CBT-I remains the first line treatment for insomnia disorder, a recent noninferiority clinical trial found no significant differences between BBT-I and CBT-I on sleep-related outcomes [51]. The AASM Clinical Practice Guidelines recommend that providers may use multicomponent brief therapies for insomnia [9].

Consistent with CBT-I, patients who undergo BBT-I complete a sleep diary each week, which guides treatment recommendations. If a patient's sleep onset latency is >20 minutes, it is recommended they leave their sleeping area and engage in a low-stimulating activity until they are sleepy, at which point they are instructed to return to bed. Generally, if a patient is taking >30 minutes to fall asleep or they are awake >30 minutes after sleep onset, it is recommended that the patient reduce their time in bed by 15 minutes. Alternatively, if the patient is taking <30 minutes to fall asleep or they are awake <30 minutes after sleep onset, it is recommended that the patient increase their time in bed by 15 minutes [22, 50]. This is known as the 30/30 rule in BBT-I [50, 52].

Due to the high incidence and persistence of untreated insomnia [53], an important part of both CBT-I and BBT-I is relapse prevention. Patients are encouraged to consider the strategies they have learned in insomnia treatment and to identify a plan for how they will intervene on their own behavior in the future should they have trouble initiating or maintaining sleep again. A recent meta-analysis showed the effects of CBT-I remain significant a year after therapy [54]. The focus on relapse prevention in the termination session highlights the importance of patient education in both CBT-I and BBT-I, ensuring that patients understand the treatment rationales and develop a sense of agency regarding their sleep.

Novel behavioral approaches Despite the body of research demonstrating the efficacy and effectiveness of CBT-I, challenges with treatment completion remain. Estimates of treatment dropout in clinical settings range from 13.7% to 34.0% [55, 56]. Shorter total sleep time and greater depression symptoms at baseline predict treatment attrition in clinical trials of CBT-I. Adherence challenges have also led practitioners and researchers to explore adaptations of CBT-I [57]. Mindfulness and acceptance-based approaches (so-called third-wave cognitive behavioral therapies) are receiving growing attention. Kabat-Zinn (1994) defined mindfulness as "paying attention in a particular way: on purpose, in the present moment, and nonjudgmentally" (p. 4) [58]. Components of mindfulness (e.g., present moment awareness, observation, description) have been incorporated into cognitive behavioral therapies, with the goal of noticing thoughts, rather than challenging or changing said thoughts [59].

Mindfulness-based   Ong et al. (2012) proposed a model of insomnia consist with third-wave approaches. The model suggests that sleep-related arousal is caused first by sleep difficulties and their consequences, and then the arousal is exacerbated by "meta-cognitive" factors, such as distress about concerns regarding the insomnia [60]. Addressing meta-cognitive factors may improve the general effectiveness of treatment and reduce non-adherence through increased tolerance of discomfort [60]. Mindfulness-based therapy for insomnia (MBTI) incorporates (1) experiential mindfulness practices (e.g., body scan, sitting meditation), (2) education about mindfulness, and (3) behavioral strategies to improve insomnia (i.e., stimulus control, sleep restriction, and targeted sleep hygiene recommendations). Similar to CBT-I and BBT-I, patients undergoing MBTI are asked to keep a sleep diary, but they are also asked to keep a meditation diary [61]. MBTI has been found to be effective at improving insomnia symptoms [62].

Acceptance-based   A third-wave cognitive behavioral therapy that incorporates mindfulness is Acceptance and Commitment Therapy (ACT) [63, 64]. CBT and ACT have similarities and distinct differences. Both emphasize the role of cognition in psychopathology, but each model proposes different mechanisms of change [65]. In CBT, adaptive changes in thoughts and behaviors contribute to therapeutic change [66]. The ACT model suggests that thoughts do not directly cause problematic behaviors and a decrease in dysfunctional thoughts is not a prerequisite for therapeutic change [67]. Therapeutic change occurs by changing the relationship one has with "dysfunctional thoughts" through contacting the present moment, and, based on what that situation affords, acting in accordance with one's chosen values. This process is referred to as psychological flexibility [64].

Within the ACT framework, there are six interrelated processes which promote psychological flexibility including (1) present moment awareness, (2) acceptance of current experience, (3) self as context (i.e., non-identification with thoughts), (4) cognitive defusion (i.e., creating "space" between self and thoughts), (5) values (i.e., activities that give lives meaning), and (6) committed actions (i.e., behaviors in service of these values) [63, 64]. While ACT has been used to treat multiple psychiatric conditions and improve distress among individual with multiple comorbid medical conditions, few studies have examined insomnia as a primary outcome variable [68]. However, there was a recent meta-analysis that examined the impact of ACT on insomnia and sleep quality, and findings indicated that engagement in ACT was associated with improved sleep outcomes [69]. While case studies and developmental study findings for ACT-based insomnia treatment are promising [70, 71], additional clinical trials are needed.

Behavioral Treatment for Insomnia: Safety Considerations

The risks associated with participation in CBT-I or other behavioral treatments for insomnia are minimal [8]. However, there are times when sleep restriction is contraindicated. For instance, if a patient has a history of bipolar disorder, disruptions to the sleep schedule can trigger hypomanic/manic symptoms [72, 73]. Generally, it is not recommended that providers prescribe a sleep window less than 5 hours [22], even when patients are reporting total sleep time of less than 5 hours. BBT-I guidelines recommend a sleep window of no less than 6 hours [50]. CBT-I providers and patients should also discuss the utility of sleep outside of the prescribed sleep window when patients are sleepy and they must engage in activities where sleep deprivation is dangerous (e.g., driving).

Additionally, while CBT-I has been shown to be effective at treating insomnia in patients with comorbid sleep conditions, assessment of sleep disorders (e.g., obstructive sleep apnea [OSA], restless leg syndrome) [8, 74, 75] is recommended prior to initiation of behavioral insomnia treatment. This ensures that patients receive treatments for their other sleep disorders (e.g., continues positive airway pressure [CPAP], medications/supplements) and optimizes the effectiveness of behavior treatments for insomnia. Research has also shown that participation in CBT-I increases CPAP use in patients with comorbid insomnia and OSA [76]. Finally, research has demonstrated that insomnia is a risk factor for suicidal ideation [77, 78]. While research has shown CBT-I and attendance of sleep medicine appointments reduces depression symptoms and lowers risk of suicide [79, 80], risk assessment and safety planning should be conducted prior to initiating CBT-I with patients to ensure that patients are not a harm to themselves or others.

Behavioral Treatments for Insomnia: Considerations for Special Populations

Since insomnia disorder is highly comorbid with a variety of medical and mental health disorders [3, 81], special considerations should be made with some patients. Providers should involve caregivers when patients with insomnia present with cognitive impairment or are dependent on caregivers to complete activities of daily living. Caregivers may also benefit from components of CBT-I to both optimize their sleep and caregiving abilities [82]. Additionally, patients with limited mobility or pain may require modification to traditional stimulus control recommendations. Understanding the unique factors that contribute to nighttime awakenings (e.g., pain, need to urinate, hot flashes) is critical in developing effective behavioral treatment plans [3, 83, 84]. Patients with psychiatric comorbidities may require greater emphasis on interventions for problematic thoughts related to sleep and avoidance of sleep (e.g., patients with posttraumatic stress disorder [PTSD] may avoid sleep due to fear of nightmares) [85]. Finally, for a patient to be diagnosed with insomnia, the patient must report sleep problems, despite having the opportunity to sleep [4]. This differentiation is important when assessing patients who may not have a consistent opportunity to sleep (e.g., parents of infants) and/or patients who do not have a consistent/safe place to sleep (i.e., individual with unstable housing). In these circumstances, it may be best to delay initiation of behavioral treatments for insomnia and first address barriers to consistent and safe opportunities for sleep.

Medication Treatments for Insomnia

While CBT-I is the gold standard first line treatment for insomnia disorder, pharmacotherapy plays a role in several clinical situations. Medications are often used for short-term insomnia, for individuals who cannot or choose not to undergo CBT-I, for individuals who did not respond fully to CBT-I treatment, and for individuals who require intermittent medication in addition to CBT-I. A limited number of medications are FDA approved for treatment of insomnia (Table 13.2), although many other prescription medications, dietary supplements, and over-the-counter medications with sedating properties are used off-label in clinical practice. Importantly, off-label use of medications to treat insomnia but that are not FDA approved is also not recommended for use in clinical practice guidelines, generally due to the fact that the potential side effects from these medications outweigh the potential benefits for treating insomnia disorder [86, 87].

Table 13.2 FDA medications approved for treatment of insomnia disorder in adults

Prescription medications	Over-the-counter agents
Ambien (zolpidem)	Benadryl (diphenhydramine)[a]
Belsomra (suvorexant)	Unisom (doxylamine)[a]
Butisol (butabarbital)	
Doral (quazepam)	
Edluar (zolpidem)	
Estazolam	
Flurazepam	
Halcion (triazolam)	
Hetlioz (tasimelteon)	
Intermezzo (zolpidem)	
Lunesta (eszopiclone)	
Restoril (temazepam)	
Rozerem (ramelteon)	
Seconal (secobarbital)	
Silenor (doxepin)	
Sonata (zaleplon)	
Zolpimist (zolpidem)	

Source: US Food and Drug Administration [104]
[a]Note: agents also in many cold and headache combination products

The choice of pharmacotherapy agent should be made using a shared decision-making approach. Factors to consider include type of insomnia (sleep onset, maintenance, or early awakening), consideration of the patients' age, comorbidities inclusive of renal and hepatic dysfunction, additional medications including polypharmacy, response to prior therapy, cost and availability of medications, prior history of dependence on controlled substances, and patient and clinician preferences. Medication alone rarely results in a full remission of insomnia disorder, and over time increased dosage is needed to obtain the same efficacy. In addition, unlike CBT-I, where the effects of treatment are long lasting, discontinuation of pharmacotherapy for insomnia results in return of the insomnia symptoms.

Several randomized controlled studies comparing pharmacotherapy vs. CBT-I have been performed with consistent findings that behavioral therapies are superior in treating insomnia when compared to medication and that the effects achieved with behavioral therapy are long lasting. Morin et al. compared CBT-I with temazepam for an 8-week treatment period and then a 2-year follow-up [88]. In this study, CBT-I was superior to temazepam in improving sleep time after sleep onset immediately post-treatment, and at 24 months follow-up, CBT-I gains in sleep time were sustained while the temazepam group was similar to the placebo group. Similar results were noted by Jacobs et al. using CBT-I compared to zolpidem when using sleep latency as a primary outcome [89]. CBT-I resulted in more sustained benefits than medications in both studies.

Non-Benzodiazepine receptor agonists (non-BZRAs) Non-BZRAs are commonly used to treat insomnia and include eszopiclone, zaleplon, and zolpidem. Middle of the night formulations (dissolving tablets or spray) of zolpidem are available. The mechanism of action is enhancement of the neurotransmitter gamma-aminobutyric acid (GABA) function at the GABA-A receptor within the central nervous system (CNS). These medications are FDA approved for sleep onset and sleep maintenance insomnia and, due to their shorter half-life (1–6 hours), are considered to have a better safety profile and less daytime impairment when compared with benzodiazepines. They are all Schedule IV controlled substances although appear to have less potential for abuse when compared with traditional benzodiazepines. All the non-BZRAs are metabolized by CYP enzymes resulting in potential drug interactions and in reduced recommended dosages in older patients. For middle of the night awakenings, zolpidem spray and sublingual dissolving tablets offer a faster onset of action. Zaleplon can also be considered due to its very short half-life (1 hour). For middle of night awakening, these medications can be used if there is remaining 4 hours of sleep after the awakening. Zolpidem extended release has the longest half-life and can be considered in patients where the other non-BZRAs wane in efficacy over the course of the night. In addition to the usual central nervous system impairment noted with all insomnia medication, the non-BZRAs carry an FDA box warning for sleep behaviors such as sleepwalking, sleep driving, sexsomnia, and sleep eating among others. They should not be prescribed in patient with preexisting parasomnias. According to a meta-analytic review, these medications decrease sleep latency by 10–20 minutes and increase sleep time by 10–30 minutes [90].

Benzodiazepine receptor agonists (BZRAs) BZRAs with FDA approval for insomnia include estazolam, flurazepam, quazepam, temazepam, and triazolam. All are Schedule IV controlled substances and tend to be avoided for treatment of insomnia due to their longer half-life when compared with non-BZRAs, increased potential for dependence, and increased risk for side effects with abrupt discontinuation. Benzodiazepines also function by enhancing GABA at the GABA receptor within the CNS but have less affinity for the GABA-A receptor, and thus tend to cause more sedation than their non-BZRA counterparts. They are metabolized by CYP-34A, and like the non-BZRA medications, adjustments must be made for age and polypharmacy. Due to the long half-life of these sedatives, the FDA has placed a box warning to avoid with use of narcotics due to the concern for respiratory suppression. Studies on the efficacy of BZRAs use both self-reported and polysomnography data, and the results vary. On average this class of medication reduces sleep latency by 10–20 minutes and increases nighttime sleep by 30–60 minutes [90].

Melatonin receptor agonists Ramelteon is a MT1 and MT2 melatonin receptor agonist which is FDA approved for the treatment of sleep onset insomnia. Ramelteon is cleared by CYP1A2 and CYP2C9 and should be avoided in individuals with severe liver disease and those on medications inhibiting these enzymes (i.e., fluvoxamine). Effect size of ramelteon is small, but a meta-analysis showed a reduction in sleep latency of approximately 5 minutes and increase in overall sleep time of 7 minutes [91].

Orexin receptor antagonists Lemborexant and suvorexant are dual orexin receptor antagonists (DORAs) which function at the OX1R and OX2R receptors. Both are FDA approved for sleep onset and sleep maintenance insomnia. The orexin/hypocretin system initiates at the hypothalamus and communicates with multiple wake-promoting regions of the brain responsible for secreting acetylcholine, dopamine, histamine, norepinephrine, and serotonin. As with other insomnia medications, DORAs cause somnolence. This class should specifically be avoided in individuals with narcolepsy and individuals on medications which inhibit CYP3A and those with hepatic impairment. Both medications improve sleep onset latency and increase sleep time [92].

Antidepressants Trazadone is one of the most commonly prescribed antidepressants for insomnia, and it improves some sleep parameters over the short-term [93]. Its mechanism of action is via antagonism of 5-HT2A, 5-HT2B, alpha-1A, and 2C receptors, agonism of 5-HT1, and inhibition of serotonin reuptake. The AASM clinical practice guidelines recommend against use of trazadone for insomnia as there is minimal data regarding its efficacy and a very small size effect which was not sustained over time noted in the one randomized trial available for inclusion in the guidelines [87]. There are many potential side effects of trazadone including QT prolongation, orthostatic hypotension, priapism, increased suicidal ideation, mania and hypomania, closed-angle glaucoma, and serotonin syndrome, among others. Due to the potential side effects at higher doses, it is not recommended to increase doses over 150 mg nightly for the treatment of insomnia. Trazadone also has a long half-life (10–12 hours) leading to the risk of increased daytime sleepiness in patients [94].

Low-dose doxepin (3 or 6 mg tablets) is FDA approved for the treatment of sleep maintenance insomnia. Doxepin is a tricyclic antidepressant with primarily antihistamine antagonist (H1 receptor) features at a low dose. As with all other tricyclic antidepressants, MAOI inhibitors need to be avoided, and it should not be used in patients with urinary retention or those with untreated closed-angle glaucoma. Due to the cost of the low-dose tablets, providers may sometimes prescribe the liquid formulation or the 10 mg tablets, which are significantly lower priced in the USA. On average doxepin increases sleep time by 25–40 minutes.

Antipsychotics Quetiapine is a commonly prescribed anti-psychotic medication for insomnia although there is minimal data on its effect on sleep in patients without psychiatric disease, and it poses significant side effect risks [87]. Its mechanism of action is not wholly understood but is known to be a D2 and 5-HT2 antagonist, and it is metabolized by CYP3A4. It has a high side effect profile including orthostatic hypotension, dizziness, suicidality in younger patients, and extrapyramidal symptoms, among others. Due to its high side effect profile and the paucity of data on sleep, it is not recommended for the treatment of insomnia, especially in individuals without mood disorders or schizophrenia [95].

Nutritional Supplements

Several dietary supplements are marketed for insomnia. Dietary supplements are not FDA regulated, resulting in variability of concentration and purity of active ingredients [96]. Although there is scant evidence for the efficacy of supplements for the treatment of insomnia, overall, the risk for adverse effects is low. Hepatic failure, however, has been reported with valerian root and kava root.

Melatonin Melatonin is a commonly used dietary supplement for the treatment of insomnia. It is a melatonin receptor agonist acting at the suprachiasmatic nucleus, among other areas. As with endogenous melatonin, exogenous melatonin assists with sleep onset by reducing arousal caused by the suprachiasmatic nucleus. It is typically dosed between 1 and 5 mg for insomnia. Studies of efficacy of melatonin for the treatment of insomnia show a minimal effect on sleep onset and total sleep time, which may not be clinically meaningful [97]. Potential side effects include headache, nightmares, dizziness, and daytime sleepiness. Exogenous melatonin is not recommended for use by AASM clinical practice guidelines due to the lack of efficacy data [87].

Medication Treatments for Insomnia: Safety Considerations

All medications for treatment of insomnia can result in depression of the central nervous system and motor impairment leading to increased risk of falls, motor vehicle accidents, and occupational accidents. This is confounded in individuals with polypharmacy inclusive of other sedating medications, individuals with cognitive impairment, individuals with obstructive sleep apnea, and in those who drink alcohol. The benzodiazepines can also suppress respiratory drive. This is enhanced by addition of opiates and other sedating medications leading to a potential deadly combination.

Special consideration in the pharmacologic treatment of insomnia needs to occur in individuals where side effects are particularly problematic or may increase risk for adverse outcomes. This includes:

- Advanced age
- Cognitive impairment
- Fall risk
- Obstructive sleep apnea or hypoventilation
- Hepatic and renal impairment
- Concomitant medications which induce or inhibit CYP P450 3
- Polypharmacy inclusive of opiates or other sedating medications
- History of dependence on controlled or illicit substances
- History of significant depression, especially in those with active or historical suicidal ideation or attempts
- Abnormal sleep behaviors

There is also extensive epidemiological data indicating increased mortality with hypnotic use. Kripke et al. [98] reviewed 10,529 patients who received hypnotic prescriptions in the USA (mean age 54) and 23,676 matched controls between 2002 and 2007. After controlling for other co-factors associated with increased mortality the group prescribed hypnotics had a mortality hazard ratio (HR) from 3.6 to 5.32 compared to controls, with increasing HR in individuals with higher number of prescriptions for hypnotics. Similar findings were reported in a later study by Linnet et al. in multi-morbid and non-multi-morbid patients with increasing mortality noted in individuals with high numbers of hypnotic prescriptions [99]. Although the specific cause of death is not delineated in these cohort studies, there is ample evidence to suggest increased mortality with increasing number of prescriptions for hypnotics.

Summary of Key Points

Insomnia is highly prevalent with the population [100]. CBT-I is the first line treatment for insomnia disorder, and a large body of research shows that CBT-I is highly effective for the treatment of insomnia in patients with multiple medical and psychiatric comorbidities [8, 32]. The strongest research is for the delivery of CBT-I in an individual treatment format, but there is also research demonstrating the helpfulness of group-based CBT-I, self-guided CBT-I, and apps as a supplement to traditional CBT-I treatment [45, 47]. There is also research support for BBT-I and mindfulness-based intervention for insomnia [51, 62]. The risks associated with behavioral treatments for insomnia are minimal, though there are circumstances in which some intervention components (e.g., sleep restriction) may be contraindicated [72, 73]. It is important to thoroughly assess daytime activities, comorbid sleep disorders, medical conditions, and mental health conditions, as well as potential safety concerns prior to initiating behavioral treatments with patients endorsing insomnia symptoms. CBT-I has been shown to be superior for the treatment of insomnia when compared with pharmacologic treatment in terms of immediate effect on sleep and longevity of treatment. Ideally, pharmacotherapy should not be used without a behavioral component to address factors that contribute to insomnia maintenance over time; however, pharmacotherapy can be used in specific situations with emphasis on a time-limited treatment plan and monitoring of side effects.

Patient preferences are important considerations when providers collaborate with patients to develop a treatment plan. The shared decision-making model of clinical practice involves presenting evidence-based treatment options to the patient [101]. In the case of insomnia, this would involve educating patient about the strong recommendation for the use of CBT-I to treat insomnia disorder and conditional recommendations for behavioral components of CBT-I to treat insomnia disorder. Providers should also describe the risks associated with CBT-I relative to medication treatments for insomnia and the impact of CBT-I and/or medications on any comorbid conditions (e.g., sleep apnea) and their corresponding treatments (e.g., CPAP). This information will allow patients to make informed choices about their treatment. While each patient is unique, research suggests that patients prefer non-medication treatment for insomnia over medication treatment [102]. Additionally, when patients with comorbid insomnia, depression, and PTSD are presented with evidence-based treatments for each condition, a study found that patients report preference for CBT-I [103]. Figure 13.1 includes a decision-making framework for providers to follow after they have educated patients about evidence-based treatments for insomnia. Through a collaborative and transparent process, providers can connect patients with insomnia symptoms to the most effective interventions available.

References

1. Buysse DJ, Angst J, Gamma A, Ajdacic V, Eich D, Rössler W. Prevalence, course, and comorbidity of insomnia and depression in young adults. Sleep. 2008;31(4):473–80.
2. Schutte-Rodin S, Broch L, Buysse D, Dorsey C, Sateia M. Clinical guideline for the evaluation and management of chronic insomnia in adults. J Clin Sleep Med. 2008;4(5):487–504.
3. Taylor DJ, Mallory LJ, Lichstein KL, Durrence HH, Riedel BW, Bush AJ. Comorbidity of chronic insomnia with medical problems. Sleep. 2007;30(2):213–8.
4. American Psychiatric Association. Diagnostic and statistical manual of mental disorders (DSM-5®). Arlington: American Psychiatric Pub; 2013.
5. American Academy of Sleep Medicine. International classification of sleep disorders, Diagnostic and coding manual. Darien: American Academy of Sleep Medicine; 2005. p. 51–5.
6. Medic G, Wille M, Hemels ME. Short-and long-term health consequences of sleep disruption. Nat Sci Sleep. 2017;9:151.
7. Qaseem A, Kansagara D, Forciea MA, Cooke M, Denberg TD. Management of chronic insomnia disorder in adults: a clinical practice guideline from the American College of Physicians. Ann Intern Med. 2016;165(2):125–33.
8. Edinger JD, Arnedt JT, Bertisch SM, et al. Behavioral and psychological treatments for chronic insomnia disorder in adults: an American Academy of Sleep Medicine clinical practice guideline. J Clin Sleep Med. 2021;17(2):255–62.
9. Edinger JD, Arnedt JT, Bertisch SM, et al. Behavioral and psychological treatments for chronic insomnia disorder in adults: an American Academy of Sleep Medicine systematic review, meta-analysis and GRADE assessment. J Clin Sleep Med. 2020;0(0):jcsm.8988.
10. Spielman AJ, Caruso LS, Glovinsky PB. A behavioral perspective on insomnia treatment. Psychiatr Clin. 1987;10(4):541–53.
11. Carlson GC, Kelly MR, Grinberg AM, Mitchell MN, McGowan S, Culver NC, Kay M, Alessi CA, Washington DL, Yano EM, Martin JL. Insomnia precipitating events among Women Veterans: the impact of traumatic and nontraumatic events on sleep and mental health symptoms. Behav Sleep Med. 2020;19(5):672–88.
12. Singareddy R, Vgontzas AN, Fernandez-Mendoza J, et al. Risk factors for incident chronic insomnia: a general population prospective study. Sleep Med. 2012;13(4):346–53.
13. Levenson JC, Benca RM, Rumble ME. Sleep related cognitions in individuals with symptoms of insomnia and depression. J Clin Sleep Med. 2015;11(8):847–54.
14. Morgenthaler T, Kramer M, Alessi C, et al. Amer ican academy of sleep medicine. Practice parameters for the psychological and behavioral treatment of insomnia: an update. An american academy of sleep medicine report. Sleep. 2006;29(11):1415.
15. Miller CB, Espie CA, Epstein DR, et al. The evidence base of sleep restriction therapy for treating insomnia disorder. Sleep Med Rev. 2014;18(5):415–24.
16. Embry DD, Biglan A. Evidence-based kernels: fundamental units of behavioral influence. Clin Child Fam Psychol Rev. 2008;11(3):75–113.
17. Bootzin RR, Epstein D, Wood JM. Stimulus control instructions. In: Case studies in insomnia. Boston: Springer; 1991. p. 19–28.
18. Bootzin RR. Stimulus control treatment for insomnia. Proc Am Psychol Assoc. 1972;7:395–6.
19. Sharma MP, Andrade C. Behavioral interventions for insomnia: theory and practice. Indian J Psychiatry. 2012;54(4):359.
20. Cohen JS, Edmunds JM, Brodman DM, Benjamin CL, Kendall PC. Using self-monitoring: implementation of collaborative empiricism in cognitive-behavioral therapy. Cogn Behav Pract. 2013;20(4):419–28.
21. Spielman AJ, Saskin P, Thorpy MJ. Treatment of chronic insomnia by restriction of time in bed. Sleep. 1987;10(1):45–56.
22. Manber R. Cognitive behavioral therapy for insomnia guide to overcoming your insomnia. In: Affairs USDoV, ed. Washington, D.C. 2010.

23. Stepanski EJ, Wyatt JK. Use of sleep hygiene in the treatment of insomnia. Sleep Med Rev. 2003;7(3):215–25.

24. Chung K-F, Lee C-T, Yeung W-F, Chan M-S, Chung EW-Y, Lin W-L. Sleep hygiene education as a treatment of insomnia: a systematic review and meta-analysis. Fam Pract. 2018;35(4):365–75.

25. Davison GC. Systematic desensitization as a counterconditioning process. J Abnorm Psychol. 1968;73(2):91.

26. Tsai H, Kuo TB, Lee GS, Yang CC. Efficacy of paced breathing for insomnia: enhances vagal activity and improves sleep quality. Psychophysiology. 2015;52(3):388–96.

27. Alexandru BV, Róbert B, Viorel L, Vasile B. Treating primary insomnia: a comparative study of self-help methods and progressive muscle relaxation. J Evid Based Psychother. 2009;9(1):67.

28. Taylor DJ, Pruiksma KE. Cognitive and behavioural therapy for insomnia (CBT-I) in psychiatric populations: a systematic review. Int Rev Psychiatry. 2014;26(2):205–13.

29. Beck AT. Cognitive therapy: past, present, and future. J Consult Clin Psychol. 1993;61(2):194.

30. Carey TA, Mullan RJ. What is Socratic questioning? Psychoth: Theory Res Pract Train. 2004;41(3):217.

31. Beck AT, Haigh EA. Advances in cognitive theory and therapy: the generic cognitive model. Annu Rev Clin Psychol. 2014;10:1–24.

32. Wu JQ, Appleman ER, Salazar RD, Ong JC. Cognitive behavioral therapy for insomnia comorbid with psychiatric and medical conditions: a meta-analysis. JAMA Intern Med. 2015;175(9):1461–72.

33. Okajima I, Komada Y, Inoue Y. A meta-analysis on the treatment effectiveness of cognitive behavioral therapy for primary insomnia. Sleep Biol Rhythms. 2011;9(1):24–34.

34. Gehrman P, Shah MT, Miles A, Kuna S, Godleski L. Feasibility of group cognitive-behavioral treatment of insomnia delivered by clinical video telehealth. Telemed e-Health. 2016;22(12):1041–6.

35. Koffel E, Bramoweth AD, Ulmer CS. Increasing access to and utilization of cognitive behavioral therapy for insomnia (CBT-I): a narrative review. J Gen Intern Med. 2018;33(6):955–62.

36. Koffel EA, Koffel JB, Gehrman PR. A meta-analysis of group cognitive behavioral therapy for insomnia. Sleep Med Rev. 2015;19:6–16.

37. Espie CA, MacMahon KM, Kelly H-L, et al. Randomized clinical effectiveness trial of nurse-administered small-group cognitive behavior therapy for persistent insomnia in general practice. Sleep. 2007;30(5):574–84.

38. Gehrman P, Gunter P, Findley J, et al. Randomized noninferiority trial of telehealth delivery of cognitive behavioral treatment of insomnia compared to in-person care. J Clin Psychiatry. 2021;82(5):20m13723.

39. Arnedt JT, Conroy DA, Mooney A, Furgal A, Sen A, Eisenberg D. Telemedicine versus face-to-face delivery of cognitive behavioral therapy for insomnia: a randomized controlled non-inferiority trial. Sleep. 2021;44(1):zsaa136.

40. Ulmer C, Bosworth H, Voils C, et al. 0403 Tele-self CBTI: provider supported self-management cognitive behavioral therapy for insomnia. Sleep. 2018;41:A153.

41. Kuhn E, Weiss BJ, Taylor KL, et al. CBT-I coach: a description and clinician perceptions of a mobile app for cognitive behavioral therapy for insomnia. J Clin Sleep Med. 2016;12(4):597–606.

42. Batterham PJ, Christensen H, Mackinnon AJ, et al. Trajectories of change and long-term outcomes in a randomised controlled trial of internet-based insomnia treatment to prevent depression. BJPsych Open. 2017;3(5):228–35.

43. Espie CA, Kyle SD, Williams C, et al. A randomized, placebo-controlled trial of online cognitive behavioral therapy for chronic insomnia disorder delivered via an automated media-rich web application. Sleep. 2012;35(6):769–81.

44. Ritterband LM, Thorndike FP, Ingersoll KS, et al. Effect of a web-based cognitive behavior therapy for insomnia intervention with 1-year follow-up: a randomized clinical trial. JAMA Psychiat. 2017;74(1):68–75.

45. Lancee J, van Straten A, Morina N, Kaldo V, Kamphuis JH. Guided online or face-to-face cognitive behavioral treatment for insomnia: a randomized wait-list controlled trial. Sleep. 2016;39(1):183–91.
46. Miller KE, Kuhn E, Owen JE, et al. Clinician perceptions related to the use of the CBT-I coach mobile app. Behav Sleep Med. 2019;17(4):481–91.
47. Koffel E, Kuhn E, Petsoulis N, et al. A randomized controlled pilot study of CBT-I Coach: feasibility, acceptability, and potential impact of a mobile phone application for patients in cognitive behavioral therapy for insomnia. Health Informatics J. 2018;24(1):3–13.
48. Germain A, Moul DE, Franzen PL, et al. Effects of a brief behavioral treatment for late-life insomnia: preliminary findings. J Clin Sleep Med. 2006;2(04):407–8.
49. Buysse DJ, Germain A, Moul DE, et al. Efficacy of brief behavioral treatment for chronic insomnia in older adults. Arch Intern Med. 2011;171(10):887–95.
50. Troxel WM, Germain A, Buysse DJ. Clinical management of insomnia with brief behavioral treatment (BBTI). Behav Sleep Med. 2012;10(4):266–79.
51. Bramoweth AD, Lederer LG, Youk AO, Germain A, Chinman MJ. Brief behavioral treatment for insomnia vs. cognitive behavioral therapy for insomnia: results of a randomized noninferiority clinical trial among veterans. Behav Ther. 2020;51(4):535–47.
52. Lichstein K, Durrence H, Taylor D, Bush A, Riedel B. Quantitative criteria for insomnia. Behav Res Ther. 2003;41(4):427–45.
53. Morin CM, Jarrin DC, Ivers H, Mérette C, LeBlanc M, Savard J. Incidence, persistence, and remission rates of insomnia over 5 years. JAMA Netw Open. 2020;3(11):–e2018782.
54. van der Zweerde T, Bisdounis L, Kyle SD, Lancee J, van Straten A. Cognitive behavioral therapy for insomnia: a meta-analysis of long-term effects in controlled studies. Sleep Med Rev. 2019;48:101208.
55. Espie CA, Inglis SJ, Tessier S, Harvey L. The clinical effectiveness of cognitive behaviour therapy for chronic insomnia: implementation and evaluation of a sleep clinic in general medical practice. Behav Res Ther. 2001;39(1):45–60.
56. Morgan K, Thompson J, Dixon S, Tomeny M, Mathers N. Predicting longer-term outcomes following psychological treatment for hypnotic-dependent chronic insomnia. J Psychosom Res. 2003;54(1):21–9.
57. Matthews EE, Arnedt JT, McCarthy MS, Cuddihy LJ, Aloia MS. Adherence to cognitive behavioral therapy for insomnia: a systematic review. Sleep Med Rev. 2013;17(6):453–64.
58. Kabat-Zinn J. Wherever you go, there you are: mindfulness meditation in everyday life. Hachette Books; 2009.
59. Keng S-L, Smoski MJ, Robins CJ. Effects of mindfulness on psychological health: a review of empirical studies. Clin Psychol Rev. 2011;31(6):1041–56.
60. Ong JC, Ulmer CS, Manber R. Improving sleep with mindfulness and acceptance: a metacognitive model of insomnia. Behav Res Ther. 2012;50(11):651–60.
61. Ong JC, Shapiro SL, Manber R. Combining mindfulness meditation with cognitive-behavior therapy for insomnia: a treatment-development study. Behav Ther. 2008;39(2):171–82.
62. Ong JC, Manber R, Segal Z, Xia Y, Shapiro S, Wyatt JK. A randomized controlled trial of mindfulness meditation for chronic insomnia. Sleep. 2014;37(9):1553–63.
63. Hayes SC, Strosahl KD, Bunting K, Twohig M, Wilson KG. What is acceptance and commitment therapy? In: A practical guide to acceptance and commitment therapy. New York: Springer; 2004. p. 3–29.
64. Hayes SC, Luoma JB, Bond FW, Masuda A, Lillis J. Acceptance and commitment therapy: model, processes and outcomes. Behav Res Ther. 2006;44(1):1–25.
65. Jiménez FJR. Acceptance and commitment therapy versus traditional cognitive behavioral therapy: a systematic review and meta-analysis of current empirical evidence. Int J Psychol Psychol Ther. 2012;12(3):333–58.
66. David D, Cristea I, Hofmann SG. Why cognitive behavioral therapy is the current gold standard of psychotherapy. Front Psych. 2018;9:4.

67. Ruiz FJ. A review of Acceptance and Commitment Therapy (ACT) empirical evidence: correlational, experimental psychopathology, component and outcome studies. Int J Psychol Psychol Ther. 2010;10(1):125–62.

68. A-tjak JG, Davis ML, Morina N, Powers MB, Smits JA, Emmelkamp PM. A meta-analysis of the efficacy of acceptance and commitment therapy for clinically relevant mental and physical health problems. Psychother Psychosom. 2015;84(1):30–6.

69. Salari N, Khazaie H, Hosseinian-Far A, et al. The effect of acceptance and commitment therapy on insomnia and sleep quality: a systematic review. BMC Neurol. 2020;20(1):1–18.

70. Fiorentino L, Martin JL, Alessi CA. The ABCs of insomnia (ABC-I): an acceptance commitment therapy (ACT)-based insomnia treatment development study: pilot results and future directions. In: Sleep medicine and mental health. Cham: Springer; 2020. p. 85–100.

71. Dalrymple KL, Fiorentino L, Politi MC, Posner D. Incorporating principles from acceptance and commitment therapy into cognitive-behavioral therapy for insomnia: a case example. J Contemp Psychother. 2010;40(4):209–17.

72. Barbini B, Bertelli S, Colombo C, Smeraldi E. Sleep loss, a possible factor in augmenting manic episode. Psychiatry Res. 1996;65(2):121–5.

73. Harvey AG. Sleep and circadian rhythms in bipolar disorder: seeking synchrony, harmony, and regulation. Am J Psychiatr. 2008;165(7):820–9.

74. Sweetman A, Lack L, Lambert S, Gradisar M, Harris J. Does comorbid obstructive sleep apnea impair the effectiveness of cognitive and behavioral therapy for insomnia? Sleep Med. 2017;39:38–46.

75. Einollahi B, Izadianmehr N. Restless leg syndrome: a neglected diagnosis. Nephro-urology Monthly. 2014;6(5):e22009.

76. Sweetman A, Lack L, Catcheside PG, et al. Cognitive and behavioral therapy for insomnia increases the use of continuous positive airway pressure therapy in obstructive sleep apnea participants with comorbid insomnia: a randomized clinical trial. Sleep. 2019;42(12):zsz178.

77. Woznica AA, Carney CE, Kuo JR, Moss TG. The insomnia and suicide link: toward an enhanced understanding of this relationship. Sleep Med Rev. 2015;22:37–46.

78. Pigeon WR, Pinquart M, Conner K. Meta-analysis of sleep disturbance and suicidal thoughts and behaviors. J Clin Psychiatry. 2012;73(9):0.

79. Bishop TM, Walsh PG, Ashrafioun L, Lavigne JE, Pigeon WR. Sleep, suicide behaviors, and the protective role of sleep medicine. Sleep Med. 2020;66:264–70.

80. Trockel M, Karlin BE, Taylor CB, Brown GK, Manber R. Effects of cognitive behavioral therapy for insomnia on suicidal ideation in veterans. Sleep. 2015;38(2):259–65.

81. Khurshid KA. Comorbid insomnia and psychiatric disorders: an update. Innov Clin Neurosci. 2018;15(3–4):28.

82. McCurry SM, Song Y, Martin JL. Sleep in caregivers: what we know and what we need to learn. Curr Opin Psychiatry. 2015;28(6):497–503.

83. Husak AJ, Bair MJ. Chronic pain and sleep disturbances: a pragmatic review of their relationships, comorbidities, and treatments. Pain Med. 2020;21(6):1142–52.

84. Guthrie KA, Larson JC, Ensrud KE, et al. Effects of pharmacologic and nonpharmacologic interventions on insomnia symptoms and self-reported sleep quality in women with hot flashes: a pooled analysis of individual participant data from four MsFLASH trials. Sleep. 2018;41(1):zsx190.

85. Miller KE, Brownlow JA, Gehrman PR. Sleep in PTSD: treatment approaches and outcomes. Curr Opin Psychol. 2020;34:12–7.

86. Mysliwiec V, Martin JL, Ulmer CS, et al. The management of chronic insomnia disorder and obstructive sleep apnea: synopsis of the 2019 U.S. Department of Veterans Affairs and U.S. Department of Defense Clinical Practice Guidelines. Ann Intern Med. 2020;172(5):325–36.

87. Sateia MJ, Buysse DJ, Krystal AD, Neubauer DN, Heald JL. Clinical practice guideline for the pharmacologic treatment of chronic insomnia in adults: an American Academy of Sleep Medicine Clinical Practice Guideline. J Clin Sleep Med. 2017;13(2):307–49.

88. Morin CM, Colecchi C, Stone J, Sood R, Brink D. Behavioral and pharmacological therapies for late life insomnia: a randomized controlled trial. JAMA. 1999;281(11):991–9.

89. Jacobs GD, Pace-Schott EF, Stickgold R, Otto MW. Cognitive behavioral therapy and pharmacotherapy for insomnia: a randomized controlled trial and direct comparison. Arch Intern Med. 2004;164(17):1888–96.

90. Buscemi N, Vandermeer B, Friesen C, et al. The efficacy and safety of drug treatments for chronic insomnia in adults: a meta-analysis of RCTs. J Gen Intern Med. 2007;22:1335–50.

91. Kuriyama A, Honda M, Hayashino Y. Ramelteon for the treatment of insomnia in adults: a systematic review and meta-analysis. Sleep Med. 2014;15(4):385–92.

92. Kishi T, Nomura I, Matsuda Y, et al. Lemborexant vs suvorexant for insomnia: a systematic review and network meta-analysis. J Psychiatr Res. 2020;128:68–74.

93. Yi XY, Ni SF, Ghadami MR, et al. Trazodone for the treatment of insomnia: a meta-analysis of randomized placebo-controlled trials. Sleep Med. 2018;45:25–32.

94. Rojas-Fernandez CH, Chen Y. Use of ultra-low-dose ($\leq$6 mg) doxepin for treatment of insomnia in older people. Can Pharm J (Ott). 2014;147(5):281–9.

95. Anderson SL, Vande Griend JP. Quetiapine for insomnia: a review of the literature. Am J Health Syst Pharm. 2014;71(5):394–402.

96. Leach MJ, Page AT. Herbal medicine for insomnia: a systematic review and meta-analysis. Sleep Med Rev. 2015;24:1–12.

97. Low TL, Choo FN, Tan SM. The efficacy of melatonin and melatonin agonists in insomnia – an umbrella review. J Psychiatr Res. 2020;121:10–23.

98. Kripke DF, Langer RD, Kline LE. Hypnotics' association with mortality or cancer: a matched cohort study. BMJ Open. 2012;2(1):e000850.

99. Linnet K, Sigurdsson JA, Tomasdottir MO, Sigurdsson EL, Gudmundsson LS. Association between prescription of hypnotics/anxiolytics and mortality in multimorbid and non-multimorbid patients: a longitudinal cohort study in primary care. BMJ Open. 2019;9(12):e033545.

100. Calhoun SL, Fernandez-Mendoza J, Vgontzas AN, Liao D, Bixler EO. Prevalence of insomnia symptoms in a general population sample of young children and preadolescents: gender effects. Sleep Med. 2014;15(1):91–5.

101. Elwyn G, Frosch D, Thomson R, et al. Shared decision making: a model for clinical practice. J Gen Intern Med. 2012;27(10):1361–7.

102. Culver NC, Song Y, McGowan SK, et al. Acceptability of medication and nonmedication treatment for insomnia among female veterans: effects of age, insomnia severity, and psychiatric symptoms. Clin Ther. 2016;38(11):2373–85.

103. Gutner CA, Pedersen ER, Drummond SP. Going direct to the consumer: examining treatment preferences for veterans with insomnia, PTSD, and depression. Psychiatry Res. 2018;263:108–14.

104. United States Food and Drug Administration. Sleep Disorder (Sedative-Hypnotic) Drug Information (https://www.fda.gov/drugs/postmarket-drug-safety-information-patients-and-providers/sleep-disorder-sedative-hypnotic-druginformation). https://www.fda.gov/drugs/postmarket-drug-safety-information-patients-and-providers/sleep-disorder-sedativehyp-notic-drug-information. Published 2019. Updated 4/30/2019. Accessed 9/8/2021.

Chapter 14
Circadian Rhythm Sleep-Wake Disorders

Mia Y. Bothwell and Sabra M. Abbott

Keywords Circadian · Light · Melatonin · Sleep · Delayed sleep-wake phase · Advanced sleep-wake phase · Non-24 · Irregular · Shift work · Jet lag

Introduction

All life forms have intrinsic daily rhythms in cellular activity, physiology, and behavior. These self-sustained biological rhythms are near-24-hour oscillations that allow organisms to coordinate their internal processes to anticipate the environment so that physiological functions occur at the appropriate times. Misalignment of the internal circadian clock with the external 24-hour day-night cycle and/or social behavior can lead to sleep disturbances, daytime impairments, mood disturbances, and increase the risk for chronic disease [1–3].

Circadian properties are determined by both genetic and environmental influences. On a molecular level, circadian rhythms are generated by a transcriptional-translational feedback loop of clock genes and proteins. At its core, the molecular clock consists of a heterodimeric complex of proteins of the genes *CLOCK* and *BMAL1*, which positively regulate the expression of *Period (PER 1,2,3)* and *Cryptochrome (CRY 1, 2)* genes which, in turn, form their own transcription repressor complex to inhibit the activity of CLOCK and BMAL1. This feedback loop is further regulated by kinases like casein kinase 1 (CK1) which contribute to timekeeping through the destabilization of PER proteins [4]. The cycle takes

M. Y. Bothwell
University of Illinois at Urbana-Champaign Medical Scholars Program, Champaign, IL, USA

S. M. Abbott (✉)
Northwestern University Feinberg School of Medicine, Department of Neurology, Chicago, IL, USA
e-mail: sabra.abbott@northwestern.edu

© Springer Nature Switzerland AG 2022
M. S. Badr, J. L. Martin (eds.), *Essentials of Sleep Medicine*,
Respiratory Medicine, https://doi.org/10.1007/978-3-030-93739-3_14

approximately 24 hours to complete, and disruptions to this molecular system can alter the period and amplitude of circadian rhythms.

On an organismal level, the mammalian circadian system is organized hierarchically. The suprachiasmatic nucleus (SCN) of the hypothalamus is the master clock that not only organizes and synchronizes peripheral clocks to other tissues but also to the 24-hour external environment [5–7]. If humans are isolated from all environmental time cues, their intrinsic circadian rhythms will "free run" with a period slightly longer than 24 hours. In sighted people, the average circadian period is 24.18 hours [8]. Thus, synchronization of the endogenous circadian system to the 24-hour day requires frequent adjustments in response to time cues (zeitgebers) in a process known as entrainment. Light is the most powerful zeitgeber, but a number of external stimuli such as food availability, exercise, social activity, and internal stimuli such as melatonin secretion can also influence this process [9].

Photic information is conveyed from the eyes by melanopsin-expressing intrinsically photosensitive retinal ganglion cells (ipRGCs) that send projections to the SCN via the retinohypothalamic tract [10, 11]. The timing of light exposure is an important aspect of the entrainment process, producing shifts of the circadian rhythm, as demonstrated by the phase response curve (Fig. 14.1). Light exposure in the first half of the night before the nadir of core body temperature will delay circadian timing. Light exposure in the latter half/early morning will advance circadian timing [12]. The magnitude of phase shifting in response to light depends on the time of exposure, intensity, and wavelength as ipRGCs are most sensitive to short-wavelength light [10]. Although light is the strongest signal, non-photic cues can also regulate circadian rhythm timing. Melatonin is a hormone secreted by the pineal gland and regulated by the SCN to be released in a circadian pattern, with endogenous levels rising at night and declining before morning [13]. Opposite of the light exposure phase response curve, administration of exogenous melatonin at night will advance the circadian rhythm, and melatonin given in the early morning will delay the rhythm [14].

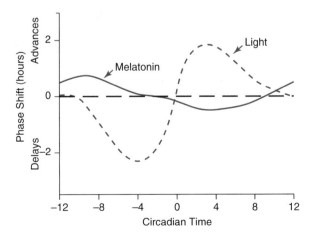

Fig. 14.1 Phase-response curve to light and melatonin. Circadian time 0 = time of temperature nadir. (Reprinted with permission from Essentials of Sleep Medicine (first edition))

One of the many patterns generated by the circadian system is a rhythm in sleep/ wake timing. The current understanding of sleep timing and regulation lies within the two-process model of continuous interaction between circadian rhythmicity (Process C) and sleep homeostasis (Process S) proposed more than three decades ago [15, 16]. Process S represents the homeostatic sleep drive and accumulates during wakefulness and declines during sleep. Process C is the endogenous biological rhythm oscillating between day and night in response to external time cues to oppose and balance the homeostatic drive to facilitate wakefulness during the day and continuous sleep during the night [17].

Circadian rhythm sleep-wake disorders (CRSWDs) arise from disruption of the circadian system or mismatch between the external sleep/wake schedule and the intrinsic circadian rhythm. This chapter focuses on the diagnosis and treatment of CRSWDs as well as providing a general overview of each disorder. The International Classification of Sleep Disorders (ICSD-3) describes six CRSWD subtypes: delayed sleep-wake phase disorder (DSWPD), advanced sleep-wake phase disorder (ASWPD), non-24-hour sleep-wake rhythm disorder (N24SWD), irregular sleep-wake rhythm disorder (ISWRD), shift work disorder, and jet lag disorder. DSWPD, ASWPD, N24SWD, and ISWRD are considered intrinsic circadian disorders, resulting from physiologic circadian disruption or misalignment. Shift work and jet lag disorders are considered extrinsic circadian disorders because they result from misalignment secondary to externally imposed schedules. Per ICSD-3 diagnostic criteria, CRSWDs must meet the following three requirements: A) Sleep complaint is chronic and primarily due to misalignment between endogenous circadian rhythm, sleep-wake schedule, and/or social schedule. B) Circadian rhythm disruption leads to symptoms of insomnia, excessive sleepiness, or both. C) Symptoms cause clinically significant distress or impairment in functioning [18]. Each CRSWD has an additional set of specific diagnostic criteria that must be met. Assessment of sleep-wake patterns and endogenous circadian timing is important for the accurate diagnosis and treatment of CRSWDs. Sleep logs and actigraphy are essential tools for diagnosis, and measurement of circadian phase markers such as melatonin rhythms can provide additional useful information for diagnosis and treatment. Effective treatment often requires a multimodal and individualized approach of strategically timed light exposure and/or melatonin as well as behavioral modification aimed to adjust circadian misalignment.

Delayed Sleep-Wake Phase Disorder

Delayed Sleep-Wake Phase Disorder (DSWPD) is the most commonly diagnosed CRSWD and can be challenging to differentiate from sleep-onset insomnia. It was first described in 1981 by Weitzman et al. and is characterized by sleep-wake timing that is significantly delayed compared to a conventional schedule [19]. These individuals have circadian rhythms that are entrained to 24 hours but are out of phase with the environment. Symptoms manifest as difficulty initiating sleep with delayed sleep onset and excessive daytime sleepiness. It typically presents in adolescence and persists into adulthood [18].

Prevalence

The prevalence of DSWPD has not been well-documented and is estimated between 0.1 and 9% depending on the population sampled and diagnostic criteria used. An early Norwegian study among adults aged 18–67 calculated a prevalence of 0.17% [20]. A study of New Zealand adults aged 20–59 estimated prevalence between 1.51% and 8.90% depending on the definition used [21]. The prevalence of delayed sleep phase is estimated to be between 3.3% and 8.4% in the adolescent population [22, 23]. DSWPD is extremely rare in older adults as circadian timing advances with age [24]. Approximately 10% of patients presenting with insomnia have DSWPD, and a detailed sleep history is important to differentiate the two [18].

Pathophysiology

The etiology of DSWPD is unclear, and the pathophysiology may be multifactorial and include biological, psychological, behavioral, and genetic elements. Several possible mechanisms include differences in properties of the circadian oscillator, altered homeostatic regulation of sleep, increased sensitivity to light, and genetics.

Intrinsic circadian timing plays an important role in sleep-timing preference [25]. A prolonged circadian period (tau) has been found in those with evening preference, indicating a longer amount of time to complete the circadian cycle which can contribute to a delay in circadian phase [25–27]. Multiple studies have found delays in circadian timing in patients with DSWPD compared to normal sleepers as evidenced by delays in physiologic markers of circadian phase such as body temperature and melatonin rhythms [28–31]. In addition to circadian dysfunction, there may be a difference in homeostatic sleep mechanisms in these patients. Studies have found that those with DSWPD are less able to accumulate compensatory sleep drive than controls and are slower to wake [30, 32]. Environmental factors also contribute to the pathogenesis of DSWPD. Patients are exposed to more light at night and less light in the morning, which may perpetuate the delayed sleep/wake timing [33]. There is also evidence that they are more sensitive to light and have altered circadian phase shifting with larger delays in response to light exposure [34, 35]. A recent study showed that patients with DSWPD had decreased exposure to light during the phase advancing window, increasing the tendency to delay [36].

While there are multiple genetic variations that shorten the circadian period linked to a familial type of Advanced Sleep-Wake Phase Disorder (FASPD), the genetic component of DSWPD is less clear. Twin studies indicate there is a strong hereditary influence on chronotype, and the heritability of bedtime preference is estimated to be approximately 50% [37–39]. A UK study found that a four-repeat allele length polymorphism in *Per3* is associated with DSWPD, while the five-repeat allele is linked to morning preference [40]. However, a South American study showed the opposite effect linking the five-repeat allele to DSWPD and speculate the difference may be due to variables related to latitude such as day length and temperature [41]. A familial form of DSWPD has been identified with a gain-of-function mutation of the *CRY1* gene resulting in lengthened circadian period and inheritance of DSWPD in an autosomal dominant pattern. This allele has a frequency between 0.1% and 0.6% [42]. Most recently a study of Japanese patients has shown that a low-frequency missense variant in *PER2* within the CRY-binding domain is associated with DSWPD [43].

Clinical Features

DSWPD is characterized by a persistent inability to fall asleep until late in the evening and excessive sleep inertia (difficulty waking) in the morning. These patients have great difficulty adhering to conventional sleep-wake schedules and typically follow a sleep-wake schedule delayed by more than 2 hours [44]. Typical bedtimes range from 2:00 AM to 6:00 AM or even later. Patients frequently have complaints of insomnia, morning drowsiness, and tend to be more alert in the evening [19]. When patients can set their own schedules, such as during weekends or on vacation, they no longer have difficulty sleeping or waking but will prefer a later schedule. This is a fundamental feature that differentiates DSWPD from sleep-onset insomnia.

Diagnosis

The ICSD-3 requires five essential diagnostic criteria that must be met to be diagnosed with true DSWPD: (A) significant delay in sleep phase that manifests as an inability to fall asleep and difficulty waking in relation to a desired or required time; (B) symptoms are present for at least 3 months; (C) patients experience improved sleep quality and duration for age when allowed to dictate their own schedule and will exhibit a delayed sleep-wake pattern; (D) sleep log and/or actigraphy for at least 7 days (preferably 14 days) including school/work days and free days that demonstrate a delayed sleep-wake pattern; (E) sleep disturbance is not better explained by other causes of insomnia and daytime sleepiness such as another sleep disorder, psychiatric disorder, or medical disorder [18].

Clinical assessment should involve a detailed sleep history and include information regarding the patient's sleep-wake schedule on work/school days as well as free days and their preferred schedule if given the opportunity to choose. To aid in the diagnosis, obtain sleep logs for at least 7–14 days, with wrist actigraphy if possible. Measurement of circadian phase biomarkers such as salivary dim light melatonin onset (DLMO) is helpful to confirm intrinsic circadian timing and can be used to time treatments. However, it is important to note that not all patients with clinically diagnosed DSWPD will have delayed DLMO. In an Australian study of 182 DSWPD patients sampled, 57% had delayed DLMO occurring at or after desired bedtime, and 43% did not show misaligned timing of melatonin rhythm with DLMO occurring before desired bedtime [45]. The Morningness-Eveningness Questionnaire is a self-assessment of the patient's preferred sleep-wake and activity timing and can provide a reasonable estimate of chronotype and demonstrate an evening preference [46]. Polysomnography is not indicated for diagnosis and should demonstrate normal sleep architecture other than possible prolonged sleep onset latency and decreased duration if conducted during typical laboratory times [47]. Insomnia may co-occur with DSWPD secondary to conditioned arousal from time spent in bed unable to fall asleep at standard bedtimes [48]. Comorbid psychiatric disorders are common, and a thorough mental health history should be obtained [45]. Diagnosis of DSWPDs should be made only after the exclusion of other sleep disorders, psychiatric disorders, or medical disorders that can lead to the presenting sleep disturbance.

Treatment

Treatment of DSWPD is primarily focused on advancing the patient's biological clock to better align with their imposed environment. Current treatment primarily relies on a combination of appropriately timed melatonin and bright light therapy. Shortly after the discovery of DSWPD, chronotherapy was developed as a therapeutic technique by progressively delaying sleep time further until the sleep period circles around the clock and reaches the desired bedtime [49]. However, caution is advised, as there have been some reports of adult patients who subsequently developed a non-24-hour sleep-wake pattern after treatment [50]. Chronotherapy is not currently a recommended treatment per the most recent American Academy of Sleep Medicine (AASM) guidelines as there have been insufficient published trials showing efficacy. Sleep-promoting agents and wakefulness-promoting agents are also not currently recommended for DSWPD, as there is little data showing efficacy [44].

The mainstay of DSWPD treatment is strategically timed administration of exogenous melatonin in the evening as recommended by AASM guidelines [44]. Low doses (0.5–3 mg) of melatonin are most effective with less concern for the residual elevation of melatonin, causing further phase delay [51, 52]. A recent randomized, placebo-controlled, double-blind trial of 0.5 mg melatonin taken 1 hour before the desired bedtime resulted in an average sleep onset advance of 34 min in patients diagnosed with DSWPD [53]. The magnitude of the phase advance response is dependent upon the timing of melatonin administration, and maximum advances occurred at 2 to 4 hours before DLMO, making the ideal time for melatonin 5 to 6 hours before habitual bedtime [48, 54].

Although there is no specific AASM recommendation for timed light therapy for adults, morning light can provide an additional benefit in entrainment when administered at the optimal time for phase advance. A combination of bright light therapy and melatonin is often used in the clinical setting. It is imperative for light therapy to be administered at the correct time to avoid further phase delay. To appropriately phase advance the patient, bright light should be delivered after the nadir of core body temperature (referred to as CBTmin), which occurs approximately 2 to 3 hours before habitual wake time [55, 56]. Exposure to light before the CBTmin can cause further delay and evening light should be restricted. Combination therapy of low dose melatonin (0.5–3 mg) 5 to 6 hours before bedtime and bright light (>5000 lux) for 30 min to 2 hours on awakening with a gradually advancing schedule results in greater long-term phase-advancing capacity than either alone [48, 57–59]. Large-scale randomized trials are still needed to fully determine the efficacy of combined light and melatonin.

Advanced Sleep-Wake Phase Disorder

Advanced Sleep-Wake Phase Disorder (ASWPD) is characterized by sleep-wake timing that is advanced in relation to conventional schedules. These individuals typically present with an earlier natural sleep phase than the general population with earlier bedtime and wake-up time. There is also a familial subtype of ASWPD in which a strong family history of advanced sleep phase is present, and multiple causative mutations have been identified [60–62].

Prevalence

There are few population studies on the prevalence of ASWPD, and true ASWPD by stringent diagnostic criteria is thought to be rare. Of 10,000 randomly sampled Norwegian adults aged 18–67 who received screening questionnaires, there were zero cases of ASWPD detected [20]. A sample of 9100 New Zealand adults aged 20–59 was surveyed, and the calculated prevalence of ASPWD ranged from 0.25% to 7.12% depending on the definition used, with a higher prevalence in older adults [21]. A recent study of 2422 new patients presenting to a North American sleep center over 10 years calculated an advanced sleep phase (ASP) prevalence of 0.33%, familial ASP prevalence of 0.21%, and estimated prevalence of ASPWD by strict definition of chronic circadian dysfunction to be at least 0.04%. Most cases presenting in young people were due to familial ASP [63]. One possible explanation for the low prevalence of ASPWD may be that it is minimally disruptive, or even advantageous, to daily life and affected individuals are less likely to seek medical attention.

Pathophysiology

There is a strong genetic component to ASWPD, and those with reports of advanced sleep phase in a first-degree relative can be considered to have a familial form [64]. The first report of a familial subtype was in 1999 when three families were identified with members experiencing significant phase advances of almost 4 hours in sleep-wake, melatonin, and temperature rhythms inherited in an autosomal dominant pattern [60]. One family was found to have a missense mutation in the *PER2* gene, which disrupts the casein kinase Iε (CKIε) binding region, resulting in a shortened endogenous circadian period [62]. Multiple additional mutations have been identified in *CKIδ*, *CRY2*, *PER3*, and *TIMELESS* [61, 65–67]. Additional mechanisms include dysregulated phase resetting in response to light with a blunted phase-delay response to evening light [67].

Clinical Features

Patients with ASWPD usually present with an advance of sleep-wake schedule by at least 2 hours in relation to desired or required times [44]. These individuals usually have difficulty staying awake between 6:00 PM and 9:00 PM and wake up between 2:00 AM and 5:00 AM with complaints of excessive late afternoon/early evening sleepiness and morning insomnia [48]. They also may experience chronic sleep loss due to early morning awakenings and sleep maintenance insomnia (ICSD-3). When patients are allowed to set their own sleep-wake schedule, they experience good age-appropriate sleep quality and quantity and will prefer an early schedule. The onset of ASWPD usually occurs later in life and is more common in older adults due to age-related advancing of circadian timing. However, familial types typically present with earlier age of onset.

Diagnosis

The diagnostic process of ASWPD is similar to that of DSWPD. The ICSD-3 requires five essential criteria: (A) significant advance in sleep phase episode that manifests as an inability to stay awake and inability to remain asleep until desired or required conventional bedtime and wake-up time; (B) symptoms are present for at least 3 months; (C) patients experience improved sleep quality and duration for age when allowed to dictate their own schedule and will exhibit an advanced sleep-wake pattern; (D) sleep log and/or actigraphy for at least 7 days (preferably 14 days) including school/work days and free days that demonstrate an advanced sleep-wake pattern; (E) sleep disturbance is not better explained by other causes of insomnia and daytime sleepiness such as another sleep disorder, psychiatric disorder, or medical disorder [18].

Clinical assessment should involve a detailed sleep history, including the patient's sleep-wake schedule on work/school days as well as free/vacation days and their preferred schedule if given the opportunity to choose. Diagnosis can be made based on sleep logs and actigraphy data, if feasible, for at least 7–14 days. Circadian phase biomarkers such as DLMO should demonstrate an advanced phase, and standardized chronotype questionnaires such as the Morningness-Eveningness Questionnaire should show a morning preference. These tools can be helpful in diagnosis and treatment. Diagnosis of ASWPD must be made only after the exclusion of other causes of sleep disruption, such as major depressive disorder.

Treatment

The primary goal of treatment is to delay the circadian clock to the desired schedule. The AASM practice guidelines recommend light therapy as treatment. Bright light before the nadir of core body temperature results in a delay of circadian phase, and several studies have shown some efficacy with evening light treatment. In an early study, exposure to bright white light (2500 lux) for two consecutive nights in nine patients with early morning insomnia resulted in 1 to 2-hour delays in circadian biomarkers including melatonin and temperature [68]. Similarly, treatment of 24 patients with 2500 lux light for 4 hours between 8:00 PM and 9:00 PM on two consecutive nights resulted in average phase delays of 2 hours [69]. It is important to note that patients in these cohorts were not formally diagnosed with ASWPD. A study testing exposure to bright white light (4000 lux) against dim red light control (50 lux) for 2 hours before habitual bedtime in older subjects meeting ICSD criteria for ASWPD resulted in a delay in wake time of 1 hour and improved sleep efficiency and sleep time [70]. Per AASM guidelines, the largest phase-delay effects were achieved after a 12-day treatment of 2 hours of bright, broad-spectrum light (4000 lux) between 20:00 and 23:00, before habitual bedtime [44].

Exogenous melatonin administered in the morning results in circadian phase delay, and low dose melatonin upon early morning awakening can be considered as an option [71]. However, there has been no evidence demonstrating its efficacy and administration of melatonin in the morning may cause drowsiness. Therefore, morning melatonin is not currently recommended by the AASM [44]. One case study reported a patient with ASWPD who responded to chronotherapy with scheduled bedtime and wake time advancing 3 hours every 2 days until goal bedtime was reached [72]. There have been no further investigations of the efficacy of chronotherapy to date, and it is currently not a recommended treatment [44].

Non-24-Hour Sleep-Wake Disorder

The human circadian pacemaker has an average endogenous period of slightly longer than 24 hours at approximately 24.18 hours, and entrainment of the endogenous clock to the 24-hour day-night cycle requires daily tuning to environmental cues [8]. Non-24-hour sleep-wake rhythm disorder (N24SWD) is characterized by cycles that are typically longer than 24 hours and are not synchronized to the environment, leading to a daily drift of progressively delayed sleep-wake timing. Symptoms are often cyclical as they resolve during the time that the individual's sleep-wake schedule lines up with the 24-hour environment before continuing to drift. N24SWD primarily affects blind individuals with no light perception and, although rare, has been reported in sighted patients as well.

Prevalence

N24SWD affects both blind and sighted patients. It is most common in those who are blind due to a lack of external light signals and rare in sighted individuals. The prevalence of N24SWD in either population has not been well studied. There is a high frequency of sleep disturbances in individuals who are blind and can be as high as 66% in those with complete loss of light perception [73]. In a study of 20 totally blind subjects, approximately 50% were found to have free running endogenous rhythms with a high incidence of N24SWD [74]. In a study of 127 blind female subjects, 2/3 of those with no light perception were not entrained to the 24-hour environmental cycle compared to 1/3 in those with some light perception [75]. In a cohort of sighted patients with N24SWD, 63% developed symptoms during their teenage years, and 72% were male [76].

Pathophysiology

The average endogenous circadian period in humans is slightly longer than 24 hours and requires daily tuning in response to external cues to synchronize to the 24-hour environmental cycle. The strongest of these external influences is light, but other daily cues include food intake, social activity, and exercise. In blind patients who have no photic input to the central circadian pacemaker, light signaling to the SCN is disrupted, and the circadian phase resetting response to light is absent. Interestingly, not all of those who are totally blind are free-running, and this is most strikingly illustrated by evidence of some bilaterally enucleated subjects who are normally entrained [77]. This is perhaps because these individuals have endogenous rhythms that are closer to 24 hours to begin with or are more responsive to entrainment by non-photic time cues [78].

The pathophysiology of N24SWD in sighted patients is less well understood and likely multifactorial. In sighted patients with N24SWD subjected to a forced desynchrony protocol (i.e. a reasearch protocol designed to uncouple sleep-wake timing from circadian timing), it was found that they had significantly lengthened periods with a mean melatonin rhythm of 24.48 ± 0.05 hours [79]. Many individuals initially present with complaints similar to that of DSWPD but eventually develop N24SWD [76, 80]. There are reports of patients with DSWPD who subsequently developed a non-24-hour pattern after chronotherapy [50]. There may also be a decreased ability to suppress melatonin in response to bright light and blunted plasma melatonin rhythm in sighted patients with N24SWD [81, 82]. This may be due to decreased sensitivity to light, although it is unclear if phase shifting is affected in these patients. Inappropriately timed light exposure may also contribute to the development of a non-24-hour pattern. These patients often initiate sleep at a later phase than normal patients and expose themselves to light at a time in the circadian cycle that causes further phase delay.

Lastly, there are reports of N24SWD in the context of traumatic brain injury or schizophrenia, suggesting congenital or acquired lesions that disrupt circadian structures or pathways can contribute to the development of non-24-hour sleep/wake patterns [83, 84]. No familial patterns have been observed in N24SWD, and genetic associations have not been explored.

Clinical Features

Patients with N24SWD present with a progressive daily delay in the sleep-wake pattern, often with complaints of nighttime insomnia and/or excessive daytime sleepiness that alternate with periods of normal sleep. Symptomatic periods are most severe when the intrinsic biological rhythm and the extrinsic 24-hour environmental cycle are most out of phase, and sleep is occurring during the daytime. The frequency and duration of symptomatic periods depend on the magnitude of the daily delay. For example, a patient with an intrinsic period of closer to 25 hours would have a greater magnitude of delay and experience more frequent symptoms than a patient with an intrinsic period closer to 24 hours. These patients frequently have severe social disruption and may not be able to complete school or hold down a job. For most sighted patients, the average age of onset was in adolescence [76, 80]. These patients commonly start with a delayed sleep-wake phenotype and then progress to a N24 pattern [80].

Diagnosis

The ICSD-3 requires four essential diagnostic criteria that must be met: (A) history of insomnia, excessive daytime sleepiness, or both, due to circadian misalignment. Sleep disturbances alternate with asymptomatic episodes of normal sleep. (B) Symptoms persist for at least 3 months. (C) Daily sleep log and actigraphy for at least 14 days (longer for blind individuals) demonstrating a sleep-wake pattern that delays each day. The circadian period is longer than 24 hours. (D) Sleep disturbance is not better explained by other causes of insomnia and daytime sleepiness such as another sleep disorder, psychiatric disorder, or medical disorder [18].

Documentation of a non-24-hour sleep-wake pattern is essential for diagnosis. Thus, sleep log and/or actigraphy must be adequately long to capture the progressively delaying pattern and should be continued for at least 14 days. Circadian biomarkers such as DLMO or the urinary melatonin metabolite 6-sulfatoxymelatonin should be obtained at two time points 2–4 weeks apart (enough time for drift to be apparent) to confirm a non-entrained rhythm. Chronotype questionnaires are less helpful as sleep-wake preferences may vary depending on which stage of the cycle.

Treatment

Treatment varies depending on the underlying cause of the disorder with the common goal of entraining to a 24-hour cycle and maintenance of synchronization. For blind individuals, strategically timed melatonin is the mainstay of treatment and has been relatively well-studied [44]. The first demonstration of the efficacy of exogenous melatonin was in blind subjects with N24SWD who received placebo or 5 mg melatonin at 21:00 for 35–71 days. Four of the seven subjects receiving melatonin exhibited shortening of circadian period similar to entrainment [85]. In a crossover study with seven totally blind subjects with free-running rhythms given 10 mg melatonin or placebo 1 hour before preferred bedtime, six of seven were entrained to 24-hr cycle with daily melatonin compared to zero entrained with placebo. Entrainment persisted even once the daily dose was lowered to 0.5 mg [86]. Subsequent studies demonstrated that 0.5 mg melatonin was sufficient to initiate synchronization and was as effective as higher doses at shortening the circadian period [87, 88]. An alternative to melatonin, the selective melatonin receptor agonist Tasimelteon is approved for the treatment of N24SWD by the Food and Drug Administration. Two consecutive placebo-controlled trials in blind adults with N24SWD showed daily administration 1 hour before target bedtime for 6 months showed circadian entrainment and improved clinical outcome measures [89].

Treatment of sighted patients is less established and relies on a combination of light and melatonin based on known phase response curves. The usage of melatonin in the treatment of sighted patients has been demonstrated in several case reports with the administration of evening low dose melatonin (0.5 mg) or high dose melatonin (5 mg) with vitamin B_{12} showing evidence of entrainment [81, 90]. Morning bright light therapy upon awakening has also been shown to be effective in restoring a 24-hour rhythm [91, 92]. Combination therapy with bright light upon awakening and 2 mg melatonin 2 to 3 hours before habitual bedtime or 3 mg 1 hour before bedtime successfully entrained the rhythm with a delayed phase [93, 94]. A recent case series demonstrated a combination treatment algorithm of bright light and melatonin initiated when the predicted bedtime aligns with the target bedtime. Treatment consisted of low dose melatonin (0.5–1 mg) given 2 hours before predicted bedtime and bright light therapy (10,000 lux) given for 1 hour after predicted wake time. The goal was to maintain timing, rather than inducing large phase shifts, to achieve target sleep-wake timing [80].

Irregular Sleep-Wake Rhythm Disorder

Irregular sleep-wake rhythm disorder (ISWRD) is characterized by the lack of a clearly discernable circadian pattern in sleep-wake behavior. This typically manifests as chronic complaints of fragmented periods of sleep that occur both during the day and night with no major sleep episode. ISWRD is more commonly observed in adults with neurodegenerative disorders or children with developmental delays.

Prevalence

The exact prevalence of ISWRD is unknown, but is generally considered to be rare and mostly observed in those with neurodevelopmental or neurodegenerative disorders. It is more common in older adults, as the incidence of dementia increases [24]. There have been no reports of gender differences in ISWRD.

Pathophysiology

The pathogenesis of ISWRD is not entirely understood and is likely multifactorial. It may depend on the underlying neuropathological cause of sleep disruption associated with the patient. Those affected include older patients with neurodegenerative diseases, such as Alzheimer's, adults with psychiatric disorders including schizophrenia, and children with neurodevelopmental disorders such as Angelman syndrome, Smith-Magenis syndrome, and Autism spectrum disorder [48]. One important underlying causative factor is thought to be the degeneration or disruption of SCN neurons in the circadian system. Disruptive lesions can be congenital or result from neurodegeneration or traumatic injury. This is supported by SCN ablation studies in the diurnal squirrel monkey, which resulted in the fragmentation of sleep, similar to an irregular sleep-wake pattern [95].

In the older adult population, insufficient exposure to entrainment cues such as light can contribute to the development of ISWRD. Older adults are exposed to significantly less environmental bright light relative to healthy younger adults. Those who are institutionalized are exposed to even less light overall. Older patients are also at risk of decreased transmission of light to the retina due to age-related changes such as cataracts, glaucoma, macular degeneration, and diabetic retinopathy [96]. In Alzheimer's disease, there is evidence of a reduction in numbers of vasopressin-expressing neurons in the SCN as well as an age-related decrease in melatonin secretion that can contribute to the loss of cohesive rhythms [97]. Furthermore, sleep abnormalities may precede dementia and may be an early sign of neurodegeneration as well as accelerate pathology [98].

Clinical Features

ISWRD typically presents as a lack of a discernable circadian sleep-wake rhythm in which the patient sleeps in multiple short bursts lasting less than 4 hours throughout the day and night. ICSD-3 diagnostic criteria require at least three short sleep episodes with no extended sleep period during the 24-hour cycle. The longest sleep episode usually occurs between 2 and 6 AM with multiple naps throughout the day. However, total sleep time over 24 hours is typically appropriate for age [99]. Patients or their caretakers may report chronic symptoms of sleep maintenance insomnia, excessive daytime sleepiness, or both. ISWRD is more common in the setting of neurodegenerative disorders, neurodevelopmental disorders, and psychiatric disorders and can be quite challenging for caregivers.

Diagnosis

Per ICSD-3, four diagnostic criteria must be met to be diagnosed with ISWRD: (A) chronic or recurrent pattern of irregular sleep and wake periods throughout the 24-hour day with symptoms of insomnia during normal sleep period at nighttime, excessive sleepiness or napping during the daytime, or both. (B) Symptoms present for at least 3 months. (C) Sleep log and/or actigraphy for at least 7 days (preferably 14 days) showing no extended sleep period and at least 3 irregular sleep episodes during a 24-hour period. (D) Sleep disturbance is not better explained by other causes of insomnia and daytime sleepiness such as another sleep disorder, poor sleep hygiene, psychiatric disorder, or medical disorder [18].

Clinical assessment should involve a detailed sleep history, and sleep logs should be obtained for at least 7–14 days and with wrist actigraphy, if available. Actigraphy may show low amplitude activity rhythms and at least three short sleep episodes throughout the day and night in a 24-hour period [48]. Caregivers may also provide valuable information regarding sleep-wake timing if the patient is unable to give accurate information. Polysomnography is not required for diagnosis. Measurement of circadian biomarkers such as melatonin and core body temperature may reveal loss of circadian rhythmicity or a low amplitude rhythm [18].

Treatment

The goal of ISWRD treatment is to consolidate sleep and enhance circadian entrainment to the day/night cycle. Treatment is multimodal and includes light therapy, exogenous melatonin, and behavioral interventions. The AASM practice guidelines recommend bright light therapy for the treatment of ISWRD in older adults with dementia. In early trials, patients with dementia treated with 2 hours of 3000–5000 lux broad-spectrum light each morning for 4 weeks consolidated nocturnal sleep, decreased daytime napping, and improved behavioral symptoms [100]. Bright light exposure of 2500 lux for 2 hours in either morning or evening is beneficial in patients with dementia and resulted in increased consolidated sleep [101]. Exogenous melatonin alone is not recommended in older patients with dementia due to the lack of evidence for efficacy and possible exacerbation of mood symptoms but may be effective in combination with light [44]. A randomized study of assisted living facilities with common areas lit with bright white broad-spectrum light (1000 lux) or dim light (300 lux) with evening melatonin (2.5 mg) or placebo found that a combination of bright light and melatonin led to improved sleep efficiency, nocturnal restlessness, and less aggressive behavior [102]. For adults with dementia, a non-pharmacological mixed modality approach consisting of morning bright light exposure (>10,000 lux), daytime physical activity, minimizing noise and light at night, and a structured bedtime routine was effective in reducing nighttime awakenings and improving daytime sleepiness [48, 103, 104]. The AASM currently does not recommend the use of sleep-promoting medications for older patients with dementia due to the high potential for adverse effects [44].

In children with neurodevelopmental delay and sleep disturbances, bright light exposure of a minimum of 4000 lux resulted in normalization of sleep in some of the children treated [105]. In a randomized controlled trial of children with autism spectrum disorder and sleep disturbances, 2 mg–10 mg of melatonin 30–40 min before bedtime improved sleep latency and total sleep time by 45 min compared to placebo [106].

Shift Work Disorder

Shift work disorder (SWD) is a consequence of shift work that prevents individuals from adhering to a normal sleep-wake schedule. Shifts outside of the traditional 9-to-5 workday may require the worker to sleep during the day and be awake at the times of night typically reserved for sleep. Some workers may have trouble adapting to this schedule, leading to chronic circadian misalignment and impairments in sleep and wakefulness with significant negative consequences impacting health and quality of life. Shift workers suffer increased rates of cancer, higher incidence of cardiovascular and metabolic disorders, and are at a significantly higher risk for psychiatric disorders [107, 108]. Other adverse consequences of SWD include increased risk of workplace injuries and errors as well as auto accidents, which incur a high societal cost.

Prevalence

Recent calculations approximate that 15–30% of the European and American workforce are shift workers [107]. An estimated 20% of US workers are engaged in shift work, and the numbers are rising in an increasingly 24/7 global economy [109].

While some workers may be able to adapt to their schedules, others experience chronic sleep disturbance and impaired function. Data obtained from the US National Health and Nutrition Examination Survey estimated a 62% prevalence of short sleep duration (< 7 hours/day) and 31% prevalence of poor sleep quality among night-shift workers with impaired activities of daily living (ADL) score and insomnia in 36% [110]. In a study of 2570 US workers, the prevalence of SWD meeting ICSD diagnostic criteria was estimated to be 10% in night and rotating shift workers [111].

Pathophysiology

Shift workers live within the confines of an imposed schedule that conflicts with their endogenous circadian rhythm and the external environment. Shift schedules vary depending on industry, and overnight work is especially common in service and healthcare occupations. Common examples include night shifts, early morning shifts, evening shifts, rotating shifts, on-call overnight duty, and extended shifts of 24 hours or longer [18]. There is wide variability in the adaptability of shift workers to their schedules. It is not completely clear why some people are more affected than others, but individuals do vary in their sleep requirements and preferences for timing. For example, those with evening-oriented chronotype may prefer night shifts and be more challenged by early morning shifts, and those with morning chronotypes may be more challenged by night shifts. Age may be a risk factor for SWD, as young people are able to recover more quickly from shifts [112]. Other factors that can influence tolerance of shift work include sex, health status, and lifestyle choices [113]. The type of shift may contribute to the development of SWD. Rapidly rotating shift rotations are associated with a greater reduction in total sleep time compared to slowly rotating or permanent shifts [114]. There may also be a genetic predisposition for excessive sleepiness in some shift workers. Shift workers who reported insomnia and sleepiness during wake hours were found to be more likely to carry a long polymorphism of PER3 than those who were less sleepy [115].

Clinical Features

Shift work disorder is characterized by insomnia, excessive sleepiness, or both, as a consequence of shift work with hours that interfere with conventional sleep times. Patients experience chronically decreased total sleep time due to sleep disruption and may report worsening function during waking hours. The effects of chronic sleep deprivation compounded with circadian misalignment leave many shift workers vulnerable to depression, anxiety, chronic fatigue, substance use, and cognitive deficits [116]. Symptoms usually only last for the duration of the shift work, but some sleep difficulties may persist as shift work can be a precipitant of insomnia in certain individuals [117].

Diagnosis

The ICSD-3 requires the four following criteria must be met to be diagnosed with shift work disorder: (A) symptoms of insomnia and/or excessive sleepiness, or both, accompanied by decreased total sleep time associated with a work schedule that overlaps with the usual time for sleep. (B) Symptoms have been present and associated with shift work schedule for at least 3 months. (C) Sleep log and wrist actigraphy (preferably with light exposure measurement) for at least 14 days (including work and free days) demonstrate a disturbed sleep/wake pattern. (D) Sleep disturbance is not better explained by other causes of insomnia and excessive sleepiness such as another sleep disorder, poor sleep hygiene, psychiatric disorder, or medical disorder [18].

Diagnosis is made based primarily on history. Clinical assessment should involve a detailed sleep history, including sleep schedule and habits before and after the initiation of shift work. Work history should be obtained that includes occupation with a detailed work schedule, and sleep patterns should be assessed for working and non-working periods. Cognitive difficulties, performance deficits, and safety concerns are important to identify as there is an increased risk of fatigue-related motor vehicle accidents in shift workers [118, 119]. It is imperative to assess safety risks such as excessive sleepiness while driving or operating machinery. The Epworth Sleepiness Scale is a validated and commonly used method to assess sleepiness during waking hours. Polysomnography is not required for diagnosis but can be helpful if there is a need to rule out other causes of poor sleep, such as sleep apnea.

Treatment

The goal of SWD treatment is to improve sleep quality and reduce wake-time sleepiness. A multifaceted approach is most effective in addressing symptoms and promoting stable circadian entrainment, and should be tailored to the patient's individual needs and circumstance.

Non-pharmacological approaches aim to maintain circadian alignment and include keeping a comfortable sleeping environment, adhering to a regular sleep/wake and dietary schedule, scheduled napping, and strategic light exposure. There is strong evidence for napping before or during a night shift, which has been shown to improve performance and decrease accidents [120–122]. Appropriately timed light may be effective in targeting circadian misalignment and aid in adaptation to shift work schedules. Several studies have shown that exposure to bright light (2000–12,000 lux) administered in constant or intermittent schedules for various durations before or during the first half of night shift was effective in improving alertness and tolerance of night shift [123, 124]. Avoidance of light at times that may interfere with sleep is also an important part of optimizing entrainment to night shifts. Patients can reduce bright light exposure in the morning, for example, on the drive home, with dark sunglasses [47]. Exogenous melatonin can be used to enhance daytime sleep. A meta-analysis found that administration of 1–10 mg of melatonin before bedtime is associated with increased daytime sleep duration in those who work night shifts but does not affect sleep latency time [125].

Wake-promoting agents that increase alertness may be prescribed to improve function during work hours. Modafinil and armodafinil are FDA approved for the treatment of excessive wake time sleepiness with modest improvement. In randomized trials of patients with SWD, 150 mg armodafinil taken 30–60 min before the start of the night shift improved work shift sleepiness compared with placebo regardless of shift duration [126–128]. Treatment with 200 mg modafinil before the start of night shift is more effective in reducing sleepiness than a placebo [129, 130]. Caffeine can also be an effective agent for improving alertness during work hours and has significantly fewer side effects than stimulant-type medications [109].

For patients who have trouble initiating daytime sleep, short-acting hypnotics may be used to treat insomnia and promote sleep at the desired time [109]. Benzodiazepine and non-benzodiazepine hypnotics have been found to be effective in inducing sleep in the setting of chronic insomnia, although with a risk of significant side effects such as dependence, withdrawal, and rebound insomnia [130, 131]. Short-acting hypnotics such as zolpidem and intermediate-acting benzodiazepines such as triazolam have been shown to increase daytime sleep in shift workers [132, 133]. However, these medications do not address circadian misalignment and may have serious side effects. There is evidence that suggest matching individual employee chronotypes to shift schedules reduces circadian disruption and improves sleep and general wellbeing [134]. However, this may not be practical in most work environments but should be taken into consideration, if feasible. When possible, pharmacologic agents should be used in combination with non-pharmacologic therapy, and good sleep hygiene should be a key element of any treatment regimen. Lastly, all patients should be educated on the dangers of fatigue and drowsiness while driving and should be counseled on how to recognize when they are unable to operate a vehicle.

Jet Lag Disorder

Jet lag disorder (JLD) is characterized by temporary symptoms of insomnia and/or excessive daytime sleepiness, with a decrease in total sleep time as a consequence of circadian misalignment associated with air travel across at least two time zones. Under these circumstances, the circadian system is not given enough time to catch up to the current time zone, and there is a lag in the entrainment of the intrinsic rhythms relative to the new environment. Although JLD is generally self-limited, it can be extremely disruptive to travelers, and severe symptoms warrant treatment.

Treatment and prevention of jet lag are of particular interest to professional athletes, business travelers, and the military.

Prevalence

The prevalence of JLD is unknown but likely affects many people, considering the large proportion of the population who engage in air travel globally. International and frequent travelers are especially vulnerable, especially if crossing five or more time zones [135]. All age groups and genders are at risk for jet lag. Some studies suggest that middle-aged and older individuals are more prone to having symptoms and take a longer time to recuperate [24, 136] while others have found older subjects were less likely to experience jet lag and fatigue [137]. More studies are needed to better establish a relationship between age and jet lag.

Pathophysiology

The pathophysiology of JLD is relatively straightforward. Insomnia and daytime somnolence are caused by a misalignment between the endogenous circadian rhythm, homeostatic sleep drive, and local sleep-wake schedule caused by the rapid changing of time zones. A period of desynchrony persists until the circadian system is re-entrained. Symptom severity and duration are dependent on the number of time zones crossed, the direction of the time change, the extent of travel-related sleep deprivation, and individual differences in circadian adaptability [138]. Because the human endogenous rhythm is longer than 24 hours, it is easier for the circadian system to phase delay than to advance. Thus, individuals are more likely to experience jet lag and take longer to resynchronize with eastward travel due to the requirement to advance rather than delay the body's intrinsic rhythm [18].

Clinical Features

Patients suffering from jet lag usually present with symptoms of insomnia and daytime drowsiness with impaired functioning within a day or two of air travel across at least two time zones. Many may also experience fatigue, headaches, irritability, cognitive difficulties, and gastrointestinal dysfunction such as indigestion, appetite changes, and inconsistent bowel function [139]. Eastward travel is associated with sleep onset difficulty as the traveler's biological time is behind the local time. Westward travel is associated with daytime and early evening sleepiness as the traveler's biological time is ahead of the local time. Symptoms tend to be more severe going from West to East and are typically compounded by general fatigue and stress caused by travel [18]. Unlike typical travel fatigue, jet lag symptoms typically do not resolve after a good night's sleep and can take several days to re-adjust.

Diagnosis

The ICSD-3 requires three essential diagnostic criteria that must be met: (A) complaint of insomnia and/or excessive daytime sleepiness, accompanied by reduced total sleep time in the setting of air travel across at least two time zones. (B) Presence of associated impairment of daytime function, fatigue, or somatic symptoms such as gastrointestinal disturbance within one to two days after travel. (C) Sleep disturbance is not better explained by other causes of insomnia and daytime somnolence such as another sleep disorder, psychiatric disorder, or medical disorder [18].

The diagnosis can be made based on sleep and travel history alone, and laboratory testing is usually not indicated. However, a thorough history and physical exam may help exclude underlying sleep or medical conditions, especially in the setting of gastrointestinal complaints. In some cases of international travel across multiple time zones, prophylactic treatment can be initiated before travel to blunt the effects of jet lag, and a diagnosis will not be required.

Treatment

Treatment for JLD differs for eastward or westward travel but has a shared focus on reducing symptoms of insomnia and excessive sleepiness as well as speeding up the adjustment process. Therapy is tailored to facilitate phase advances for travel eastward and delays for travel westward. Treatment for international trips across multiple time zones may begin before travel to shift the patient's schedule preemptively or after travel to accelerate entrainment.

For eastbound travel, a combination of timed morning bright light, evening low dose melatonin, and gradually advancing sleep scheduling starting 3 days before the day of travel can be employed to phase advance the circadian clock preemptively. Both light and melatonin have advancing effects when used alone and can be used together with an additive effect [140]. In one study, continuous bright light (>3000 lux) for 3 hours each day for 3 days was sufficient to produce a 2-hour phase advance [141]. Another found that four 30 min pulses of 5000 lux light alternating with 30 min ambient light produced phase advances of 1 hour per day with the addition of 0.5–3.0 mg melatonin 5 hours before bedtime [142, 143]. As sitting in front of bright light for an extended period of time can be difficult, a study determined that a single 30 min exposure of 5000 lux light with 0.5 mg melatonin 5 hours before bedtime produced phase advances of similar magnitude as longer light treatments (approximately 2 hours) [59]. If treatment is initiated after travel, melatonin can decrease the effects of jet lag and is recommended for travelers crossing five or more time zones. A comprehensive meta-analysis found melatonin doses ranging from 0.5 mg to 5 mg taken near target bedtime are similarly effective, but higher doses had greater sleep-inducing effects [144]. There are fewer studies pertaining to westbound travel, and it is much easier to phase delay than to advance. Maximizing evening light exposure and avoiding morning light may be useful in facilitating phase delay [145]. Administration of morning melatonin could help delay timing, but its hypnotic effects may cause daytime drowsiness.

If travel is short (2 days or less), the sleep/wake schedule can be kept unchanged, and short-term use of hypnotics or wake-enhancing agents such as caffeine can be considered for the alleviation of symptoms, as circadian realignment may not be necessary or practical [109]. These agents can be used for symptom relief for more extended travel as well, but it should be kept in mind that they do not address the underlying circadian desynchrony.

Conclusion

The circadian system regulates and synchronizes many important physiologic functions, including the sleep/wake cycle. CRSWDs arise as a consequence of the misalignment between the endogenous rhythm and the external environment. This may result from biological modifications within the circadian system or from behavioral and societal pressure that imposes a mismatched schedule. In an increasingly globalized 24-hour economy in which people are surrounded by artificial lighting and bright screens, it is more important than ever to recognize the importance of circadian disorders. Early identification and treatment are important in prevention of the negative health impacts of chronic circadian misalignment and improving patient quality of life.

Key Summary Points
1. The primary circadian pacemaker is located in the suprachiasmatic nucleus in the hypothalamus.
2. Most humans have an endogenous circadian period that is slightly longer than 24 hours.
3. Light is the strongest regulator of the mammalian circadian clock, and timed light exposure can be used to either advance or delay circadian timing.
4. Other non-photic time cues such as melatonin, activity, and food timing provide weaker time signals than light, but can also be used to adjust circadian timing.
5. Circadian rhythm sleep-wake disorders result when the endogenous circadian clock is misaligned with the external environment. This can occur either secondary to endogenous differences in circadian timing creating misalignment with the external environment (DSWPD, ASWPD, N24SWD, and ISWRD) or because of extrinsic factors requiring an individual to be awake during their biological night (SWD and JLD).

References

1. Menet JS, Rosbash M. When brain clocks lose track of time: cause or consequence of neuropsychiatric disorders. Curr Opin Neurobiol. 2011;21(6):849–57. https://doi.org/10.1016/j.conb.2011.06.008.
2. Abbott SM, Malkani RG, Zee PC. Circadian disruption and human health: a bidirectional relationship. Eur J Neurosci. 2020;51(1):567–83. https://doi.org/10.1111/ejn.14298.
3. Foster RG. Sleep, circadian rhythms and health. Interface Focus. 2020;10(3):20190098. https://doi.org/10.1098/rsfs.2019.0098.
4. Ko CH, Takahashi JS. Molecular components of the mammalian circadian clock. Hum Mol genet. 2006;15(2):R271–7. https://doi.org/10.1093/hmg/ddl207.
5. Moore RY, Eichler VB. Loss of a circadian adrenal corticosterone rhythm following suprachiasmatic lesions in the rat. Brain Res. 1972;42(1):201–6. https://doi.org/10.1016/0006-8993(72)90054-6.
6. Stephan FK, Zucker I. Circadian rhythms in drinking behavior and locomotor activity of rats are eliminated by hypothalamic lesions. Proc Natl Acad Sci U S A. 1972;69(6):1583–6. https://doi.org/10.1073/pnas.69.6.1583.
7. Lehman MN, Silver R, Gladstone WR, Kahn RM, Gibson M, Bittman EL. Circadian rhythmicity restored by neural transplant. Immunocytochemical characterization of the graft and its integration with the host brain. J Neurosci. 1987;7(6):1626–38.
8. Czeisler CA, Duffy JF, Shanahan TL, Brown EN, Mitchell JF, Rimmer DW, Ronda JM, Silva EJ, Allan JS, Emens JS, Dijk DJ, Kronauer RE. Stability, precision, and near-24-hour period of the human circadian pacemaker. Science. 1999;284(5423):2177–81. https://doi.org/10.1126/science.284.5423.2177.
9. Golombek DA, Rosenstein RE. Physiology of circadian entrainment. Physiol Rev. 2010;90(3):1063–102. https://doi.org/10.1152/physrev.00009.2009.
10. Berson DM, Dunn FA, Takao M. Phototransduction by retinal ganglion cells that set the circadian clock. Science. 2002;295(5557):1070–3. https://doi.org/10.1126/science.1067262.
11. Hattar S, Liao HW, Takao M, Berson DM, Yau KW. Melanopsin-containing retinal ganglion cells: architecture, projections, and intrinsic photosensitivity. Science. 2002;295(5557):1065–70. https://doi.org/10.1126/science.1069609.
12. Czeisler CA, Allan JS, Strogatz SH, Ronda JM, Sanchez R, Rios CD, Freitag WO, Richardson GS, Kronauer RE. Bright light resets the human circadian pacemaker independent of the timing of the sleep-wake cycle. Science. 1986;233(4764):667–71. https://doi.org/10.1126/science.3726555.
13. Benloucif S, Guico MJ, Reid KJ, Wolfe LF, L'Hermite-Baleriaux M, Zee PC. Stability of melatonin and temperature as circadian phase markers and their relation to sleep times in humans. J Biol Rhythm. 2005;20(2):178–88. https://doi.org/10.1177/0748730404273983.
14. Burgess HJ, Revell VL, Eastman CI. A three pulse phase response curve to three milligrams of melatonin in humans. J Physiol. 2008;586(2):639–47. https://doi.org/10.1113/jphysiol.2007.143180.
15. Borbely AA. A two process model of sleep regulation. Hum Neurobiol. 1982;1(3):195–204.
16. Daan S, Beersma DG, Borbely AA. Timing of human sleep: recovery process gated by a circadian pacemaker. Am J Phys. 1984;246(2 Pt 2):R161–83. https://doi.org/10.1152/ajpregu.1984.246.2.R161.
17. Borbely AA, Daan S, Wirz-Justice A, Deboer T. The two-process model of sleep regulation: a reappraisal. J Sleep Res. 2016;25(2):131–43. https://doi.org/10.1111/jsr.12371.
18. Sateia MJ. International classification of sleep disorders-third edition: highlights and modifications. Chest. 2014;146(5):1387–94. https://doi.org/10.1378/chest.14-0970.
19. Weitzman ED, Czeisler CA, Coleman RM, Spielman AJ, Zimmerman JC, Dement W, Richardson G, Pollak CP. Delayed sleep phase syndrome. A chronobiological disorder with sleep-onset insomnia. Arch Gen Psychiatry. 1981;38(7):737–46. https://doi.org/10.1001/archpsyc.1981.01780320017001.

20. Schrader H, Bovim G, Sand T. The prevalence of delayed and advanced sleep phase syndromes. J Sleep Res. 1993;2(1):51–5. https://doi.org/10.1111/j.1365-2869.1993.tb00061.x.
21. Paine SJ, Fink J, Gander PH, Warman GR. Identifying advanced and delayed sleep phase disorders in the general population: a national survey of New Zealand adults. Chronobiol Int. 2014;31(5):627–36. https://doi.org/10.3109/07420528.2014.885036.
22. Saxvig IW, Pallesen S, Wilhelmsen-Langeland A, Molde H, Bjorvatn B. Prevalence and correlates of delayed sleep phase in high school students. Sleep Med. 2012;13(2):193–9. https://doi.org/10.1016/j.sleep.2011.10.024.
23. Sivertsen B, Pallesen S, Stormark KM, Boe T, Lundervold AJ, Hysing M. Delayed sleep phase syndrome in adolescents: prevalence and correlates in a large population based study. BMC Public Health. 2013;13:1163. https://doi.org/10.1186/1471-2458-13-1163.
24. Kim JH, Duffy JF. Circadian rhythm sleep-wake disorders in older adults. Sleep Med Clin. 2018;13(1):39–50. https://doi.org/10.1016/j.jsmc.2017.09.004.
25. Duffy JF, Rimmer DW, Czeisler CA. Association of intrinsic circadian period with morningness-eveningness, usual wake time, and circadian phase. Behav Neurosci. 2001;115(4):895–9. https://doi.org/10.1037//0735-7044.115.4.895.
26. Emens JS, Yuhas K, Rough J, Kochar N, Peters D, Lewy AJ. Phase angle of entrainment in morning- and evening-types under naturalistic conditions. Chronobiol Int. 2009;26(3):474–93. https://doi.org/10.1080/07420520902821077.
27. Lazar AS, Santhi N, Hasan S, Lo JC, Johnston JD, Von Schantz M, Archer SN, Dijk DJ. Circadian period and the timing of melatonin onset in men and women: predictors of sleep during the weekend and in the laboratory. J Sleep Res. 2013;22(2):155–9. https://doi.org/10.1111/jsr.12001.
28. Ozaki S, Uchiyama M, Shirakawa S, Okawa M. Prolonged interval from body temperature nadir to sleep offset in patients with delayed sleep phase syndrome. Sleep. 1996;19(1):36–40.
29. Shibui K, Uchiyama M, Okawa M. Melatonin rhythms in delayed sleep phase syndrome. J Biol Rhythm. 1999;14(1):72–6. https://doi.org/10.1177/074873049901400110.
30. Uchiyama M, Okawa M, Shibui K, Kim K, Tagaya H, Kudo Y, Kamei Y, Hayakawa T, Urata J, Takahashi K. Altered phase relation between sleep timing and core body temperature rhythm in delayed sleep phase syndrome and non-24-hour sleep-wake syndrome in humans. Neurosci Lett. 2000;294(2):101–4. https://doi.org/10.1016/s0304-3940(00)01551-2.
31. Wyatt JK, Stepanski EJ, Kirkby J. Circadian phase in delayed sleep phase syndrome: predictors and temporal stability across multiple assessments. Sleep. 2006;29(8):1075–80. https://doi.org/10.1093/sleep/29.8.1075.
32. Uchiyama M, Okawa M, Shibui K, Liu X, Hayakawa T, Kamei Y, Takahashi K. Poor compensatory function for sleep loss as a pathogenic factor in patients with delayed sleep phase syndrome. Sleep. 2000;23(4):553–8.
33. Joo EY, Abbott SM, Reid KJ, Wu D, Kang J, Wilson J, Zee PC. Timing of light exposure and activity in adults with delayed sleep-wake phase disorder. Sleep Med. 2017;32:259–65. https://doi.org/10.1016/j.sleep.2016.09.009.
34. Aoki H, Ozeki Y, Yamada N. Hypersensitivity of melatonin suppression in response to light in patients with delayed sleep phase syndrome. Chronobiol Int. 2001;18(2):263–71. https://doi.org/10.1081/cbi-100103190.
35. Watson LA, Phillips AJK, Hosken IT, McGlashan EM, Anderson C, Lack LC, Lockley SW, Rajaratnam SMW, Cain SW. Increased sensitivity of the circadian system to light in delayed sleep-wake phase disorder. J Physiol. 2018;596(24):6249–61. https://doi.org/10.1113/JP275917.
36. Wilson J, Reid KJ, Braun RI, Abbott SM, Zee PC. Habitual light exposure relative to circadian timing in delayed sleep-wake phase disorder. Sleep. 2018;41(11) https://doi.org/10.1093/sleep/zsy166.
37. Heath AC, Kendler KS, Eaves LJ, Martin NG. Evidence for genetic influences on sleep disturbance and sleep pattern in twins. Sleep. 1990;13(4):318–35. https://doi.org/10.1093/sleep/13.4.318.

38. Hur YM. Stability of genetic influence on morningness-eveningness: a cross-sectional examination of south Korean twins from preadolescence to young adulthood. J Sleep Res. 2007;16(1):17–23. https://doi.org/10.1111/j.1365-2869.2007.00562.x.

39. Koskenvuo M, Hublin C, Partinen M, Heikkila K, Kaprio J. Heritability of diurnal type: a nationwide study of 8753 adult twin pairs. J Sleep Res. 2007;16(2):156–62. https://doi.org/10.1111/j.1365-2869.2007.00580.x.

40. Archer SN, Robilliard DL, Skene DJ, Smits M, Williams A, Arendt J, von Schantz M. A length polymorphism in the circadian clock gene Per3 is linked to delayed sleep phase syndrome and extreme diurnal preference. Sleep. 2003;26(4):413–5. https://doi.org/10.1093/sleep/26.4.413.

41. Pereira DS, Tufik S, Louzada FM, Benedito-Silva AA, Lopez AR, Lemos NA, Korczak AL, D'Almeida V, Pedrazzoli M. Association of the length polymorphism in the human Per3 gene with the delayed sleep-phase syndrome: does latitude have an influence upon it? Sleep. 2005;28(1):29–32.

42. Patke A, Murphy PJ, Onat OE, Krieger AC, Ozcelik T, Campbell SS, Young MW. Mutation of the human circadian clock gene CRY1 in familial delayed sleep phase disorder. Cell. 2017;169(2):203–215 e213. https://doi.org/10.1016/j.cell.2017.03.027.

43. Miyagawa T, Hida A, Shimada M, Uehara C, Nishino Y, Kadotani H, Uchiyama M, Ebisawa T, Inoue Y, Kamei Y, Tokunaga K, Mishima K, Honda M. A missense variant in PER2 is associated with delayed sleep-wake phase disorder in a Japanese population. J Hum Genet. 2019;64(12):1219–25. https://doi.org/10.1038/s10038-019-0665-6.

44. Auger RR, Burgess HJ, Emens JS, Deriy LV, Thomas SM, Sharkey KM (2015) Clinical Practice Guideline for the Treatment of Intrinsic Circadian Rhythm Sleep-Wake Disorders: Advanced Sleep-Wake Phase Disorder (ASWPD), Delayed Sleep-Wake Phase Disorder (DSWPD), Non-24-Hour Sleep-Wake Rhythm Disorder (N24SWD), and Irregular Sleep-Wake Rhythm Disorder (ISWRD). An Update for 2015: An American Academy of sleep medicine clinical practice guideline. J Clin Sleep Med 11 (10):1199–1236. doi:https://doi.org/10.5664/jcsm.5100.

45. Murray JM, Sletten TL, Magee M, Gordon C, Lovato N, Bartlett DJ, Kennaway DJ, Lack LC, Grunstein RR, Lockley SW, Rajaratnam SM, Delayed Sleep on Melatonin Study G. Prevalence of circadian misalignment and its association with depressive symptoms in delayed sleep phase disorder. Sleep. 2017;40(1) https://doi.org/10.1093/sleep/zsw002.

46. Horne JA, Ostberg O. A self-assessment questionnaire to determine morningness-eveningness in human circadian rhythms. Int J Chronobiol. 1976;4(2):97–110.

47. Sack RL, Auckley D, Auger RR, Carskadon MA, Wright KP Jr, Vitiello MV, Zhdanova IV, American Academy of Sleep M. Circadian rhythm sleep disorders: part II, advanced sleep phase disorder, delayed sleep phase disorder, free-running disorder, and irregular sleep-wake rhythm. An American Academy of sleep medicine review. Sleep. 2007;30(11):1484–501. https://doi.org/10.1093/sleep/30.11.1484.

48. Abbott SM, Reid KJ, Zee PC. Circadian rhythm sleep-wake disorders. Psychiatr Clin North Am. 2015;38(4):805–23. https://doi.org/10.1016/j.psc.2015.07.012.

49. Czeisler CA, Richardson GS, Coleman RM, Zimmerman JC, Moore-Ede MC, Dement WC, Weitzman ED. Chronotherapy: resetting the circadian clocks of patients with delayed sleep phase insomnia. Sleep. 1981;4(1):1–21. https://doi.org/10.1093/sleep/4.1.1.

50. Oren DA, Wehr TA. Hypernyctohemeral syndrome after chronotherapy for delayed sleep phase syndrome. N Engl J Med. 1992;327(24):1762. https://doi.org/10.1056/NEJM199212103272417.

51. van Geijlswijk IM, Korzilius HP, Smits MG. The use of exogenous melatonin in delayed sleep phase disorder: a meta-analysis. Sleep. 2010;33(12):1605–14. https://doi.org/10.1093/sleep/33.12.1605.

52. Mundey K, Benloucif S, Harsanyi K, Dubocovich ML, Zee PC. Phase-dependent treatment of delayed sleep phase syndrome with melatonin. Sleep. 2005;28(10):1271–8. https://doi.org/10.1093/sleep/28.10.1271.

53. Sletten TL, Magee M, Murray JM, Gordon CJ, Lovato N, Kennaway DJ, Gwini SM, Bartlett DJ, Lockley SW, Lack LC, Grunstein RR, Rajaratnam SMW, Delayed Sleep on Melatonin Study G. Efficacy of melatonin with behavioural sleep-wake scheduling for delayed sleep-wake phase disorder: a double-blind, randomised clinical trial. PLoS Med. 2018;15(6):e1002587. https://doi.org/10.1371/journal.pmed.1002587.
54. Burgess HJ, Swanson GR, Keshavarzian A. Endogenous melatonin profiles in asymptomatic inflammatory bowel disease. Scand J Gastroenterol. 2010;45(6):759–61. https://doi.org/10.3109/00365521003749818.
55. Rosenthal NE, Joseph-Vanderpool JR, Levendosky AA, Johnston SH, Allen R, Kelly KA, Souetre E, Schultz PM, Starz KE. Phase-shifting effects of bright morning light as treatment for delayed sleep phase syndrome. Sleep. 1990;13(4):354–61.
56. Minors DS, Waterhouse JM, Wirz-Justice A. A human phase-response curve to light. Neurosci Lett. 1991;133(1):36–40. https://doi.org/10.1016/0304-3940(91)90051-t.
57. Burke TM, Markwald RR, Chinoy ED, Snider JA, Bessman SC, Jung CM, Wright KP Jr. Combination of light and melatonin time cues for phase advancing the human circadian clock. Sleep. 2013;36(11):1617–24. https://doi.org/10.5665/sleep.3110.
58. Wilhelmsen-Langeland A, Saxvig IW, Pallesen S, Nordhus IH, Vedaa O, Lundervold AJ, Bjorvatn B. A randomized controlled trial with bright light and melatonin for the treatment of delayed sleep phase disorder: effects on subjective and objective sleepiness and cognitive function. J Biol Rhythm. 2013;28(5):306–21. https://doi.org/10.1177/0748730413500126.
59. Crowley SJ, Eastman CI. Phase advancing human circadian rhythms with morning bright light, afternoon melatonin, and gradually shifted sleep: can we reduce morning bright-light duration? Sleep Med. 2015;16(2):288–97. https://doi.org/10.1016/j.sleep.2014.12.004.
60. Jones CR, Campbell SS, Zone SE, Cooper F, DeSano A, Murphy PJ, Jones B, Czajkowski L, Ptacek LJ. Familial advanced sleep-phase syndrome: a short-period circadian rhythm variant in humans. Nat Med. 1999;5(9):1062–5. https://doi.org/10.1038/12502.
61. Kurien P, Hsu PK, Leon J, Wu D, McMahon T, Shi G, Xu Y, Lipzen A, Pennacchio LA, Jones CR, Fu YH, Ptacek LJ. TIMELESS mutation alters phase responsiveness and causes advanced sleep phase. Proc Natl Acad Sci U S A. 2019;116(24):12045–53. https://doi.org/10.1073/pnas.1819110116.
62. Toh KL, Jones CR, He Y, Eide EJ, Hinz WA, Virshup DM, Ptacek LJ, Fu YH. An hPer2 phosphorylation site mutation in familial advanced sleep phase syndrome. Science. 2001;291(5506):1040–3. https://doi.org/10.1126/science.1057499.
63. Curtis BJ, Ashbrook LH, Young T, Finn LA, Fu YH, Ptacek LJ, Jones CR. Extreme morning chronotypes are often familial and not exceedingly rare: the estimated prevalence of advanced sleep phase, familial advanced sleep phase, and advanced sleep-wake phase disorder in a sleep clinic population. Sleep. 2019;42(10) https://doi.org/10.1093/sleep/zsz148.
64. Ashbrook LH, Krystal AD, Fu YH, Ptacek LJ. Genetics of the human circadian clock and sleep homeostat. Neuropsychopharmacology. 2020;45(1):45–54. https://doi.org/10.1038/s41386-019-0476-7.
65. Xu Y, Padiath QS, Shapiro RE, Jones CR, Wu SC, Saigoh N, Saigoh K, Ptacek LJ, Fu YH. Functional consequences of a CKIdelta mutation causing familial advanced sleep phase syndrome. Nature. 2005;434(7033):640–4. https://doi.org/10.1038/nature03453.
66. Zhang L, Hirano A, Hsu PK, Jones CR, Sakai N, Okuro M, McMahon T, Yamazaki M, Xu Y, Saigoh N, Saigoh K, Lin ST, Kaasik K, Nishino S, Ptacek LJ, Fu YH. A PERIOD3 variant causes a circadian phenotype and is associated with a seasonal mood trait. Proc Natl Acad Sci U S A. 2016;113(11):E1536–44. https://doi.org/10.1073/pnas.1600039113.
67. Hirano A, Shi G, Jones CR, Lipzen A, Pennacchio LA, Xu Y, Hallows WC, McMahon T, Yamazaki M, Ptacek LJ, Fu YH. A Cryptochrome 2 mutation yields advanced sleep phase in humans. Elife. 2016;5 https://doi.org/10.7554/eLife.16695.
68. Lack L, Wright H. The effect of evening bright light in delaying the circadian rhythms and lengthening the sleep of early morning awakening insomniacs. Sleep. 1993;16(5):436–43. https://doi.org/10.1093/sleep/16.5.436.

69. Lack L, Wright H, Kemp K, Gibbon S. The treatment of early-morning awakening insomnia with 2 evenings of bright light. Sleep. 2005;28(5):616–23. https://doi.org/10.1093/sleep/28.5.616.

70. Campbell SS, Dawson D, Anderson MW. Alleviation of sleep maintenance insomnia with timed exposure to bright light. J Am Geriatr Soc. 1993;41(8):829–36. https://doi.org/10.1111/j.1532-5415.1993.tb06179.x.

71. Lewy AJ, Bauer VK, Ahmed S, Thomas KH, Cutler NL, Singer CM, Moffit MT, Sack RL. The human phase response curve (PRC) to melatonin is about 12 hours out of phase with the PRC to light. Chronobiol Int. 1998;15(1):71–83. https://doi.org/10.3109/07420529808998671.

72. Moldofsky H, Musisi S, Phillipson EA. Treatment of a case of advanced sleep phase syndrome by phase advance chronotherapy. Sleep. 1986;9(1):61–5. https://doi.org/10.1093/sleep/9.1.61.

73. Tabandeh H, Lockley SW, Buttery R, Skene DJ, Defrance R, Arendt J, Bird AC. Disturbance of sleep in blindness. Am J Ophthalmol. 1998;126(5):707–12. https://doi.org/10.1016/s0002-9394(98)00133-0.

74. Sack RL, Lewy AJ, Blood ML, Keith LD, Nakagawa H. Circadian rhythm abnormalities in totally blind people: incidence and clinical significance. J Clin Endocrinol Metab. 1992;75(1):127–34. https://doi.org/10.1210/jcem.75.1.1619000.

75. Flynn-Evans EE, Tabandeh H, Skene DJ, Lockley SW. Circadian rhythm disorders and melatonin production in 127 blind women with and without light perception. J Biol Rhythm. 2014;29(3):215–24. https://doi.org/10.1177/0748730414536852.

76. Hayakawa T, Uchiyama M, Kamei Y, Shibui K, Tagaya H, Asada T, Okawa M, Urata J, Takahashi K. Clinical analyses of sighted patients with non-24-hour sleep-wake syndrome: a study of 57 consecutively diagnosed cases. Sleep. 2005;28(8):945–52. https://doi.org/10.1093/sleep/28.8.945.

77. Lockley SW, Skene DJ, Arendt J, Tabandeh H, Bird AC, Defrance R. Relationship between melatonin rhythms and visual loss in the blind. J Clin Endocrinol Metab. 1997;82(11):3763–70. https://doi.org/10.1210/jcem.82.11.4355.

78. Emens JS, Lewy AJ, Lefler BJ, Sack RL. Relative coordination to unknown "weak zeitgebers" in free-running blind individuals. J Biol Rhythm. 2005;20(2):159–67. https://doi.org/10.1177/0748730404273294.

79. Kitamura S, Hida A, Enomoto M, Watanabe M, Katayose Y, Nozaki K, Aritake S, Higuchi S, Moriguchi Y, Kamei Y, Mishima K. Intrinsic circadian period of sighted patients with circadian rhythm sleep disorder, free-running type. Biol Psychiatry. 2013;73(1):63–9. https://doi.org/10.1016/j.biopsych.2012.06.027.

80. Malkani RG, Abbott SM, Reid KJ, Zee PC. Diagnostic and treatment challenges of sighted Non-24-hour sleep-wake disorder. J Clin Sleep Med. 2018;14(4):603–13. https://doi.org/10.5664/jcsm.7054.

81. McArthur AJ, Lewy AJ, Sack RL. Non-24-hour sleep-wake syndrome in a sighted man: circadian rhythm studies and efficacy of melatonin treatment. Sleep. 1996;19(7):544–53. https://doi.org/10.1093/sleep/19.7.544.

82. Nakamura K, Hashimoto S, Honma S, Honma K. Daily melatonin intake resets circadian rhythms of a sighted man with non-24-hour sleep-wake syndrome who lacks the nocturnal melatonin rise. Psychiatry Clin Neurosci. 1997;51(3):121–7. https://doi.org/10.1111/j.1440-1819.1997.tb02373.x.

83. Boivin DB, James FO, Santo JB, Caliyurt O, Chalk C. Non-24-hour sleep-wake syndrome following a car accident. Neurology. 2003;60(11):1841–3. https://doi.org/10.1212/01.wnl.0000061482.24750.7c.

84. Wulff K, Dijk DJ, Middleton B, Foster RG, Joyce EM. Sleep and circadian rhythm disruption in schizophrenia. Br J Psychiatry. 2012;200(4):308–16. https://doi.org/10.1192/bjp.bp.111.096321.

85. Lockley SW, Skene DJ, James K, Thapan K, Wright J, Arendt J. Melatonin administration can entrain the free-running circadian system of blind subjects. J Endocrinol. 2000;164(1):R1–6. https://doi.org/10.1677/joe.0.164r001.

86. Sack RL, Brandes RW, Kendall AR, Lewy AJ. Entrainment of free-running circadian rhythms by melatonin in blind people. N Engl J Med. 2000;343(15):1070–7. https://doi.org/10.1056/NEJM200010123431503.

87. Lewy AJ, Bauer VK, Hasler BP, Kendall AR, Pires ML, Sack RL. Capturing the circadian rhythms of free-running blind people with 0.5 mg melatonin. Brain Res. 2001;918(1–2):96–100. https://doi.org/10.1016/s0006-8993(01)02964-x.

88. Hack LM, Lockley SW, Arendt J, Skene DJ. The effects of low-dose 0.5-mg melatonin on the free-running circadian rhythms of blind subjects. J Biol Rhythm. 2003;18(5):420–9. https://doi.org/10.1177/0748730403256796.

89. Lockley SW, Dressman MA, Licamele L, Xiao C, Fisher DM, Flynn-Evans EE, Hull JT, Torres R, Lavedan C, Polymeropoulos MH. Tasimelteon for non-24-hour sleep-wake disorder in totally blind people (SET and RESET): two multicentre, randomised, double-masked, placebo-controlled phase 3 trials. Lancet. 2015;386(10005):1754–64. https://doi.org/10.1016/S0140-6736(15)60031-9.

90. Tomoda A, Miike T, Uezono K, Kawasaki T. A school refusal case with biological rhythm disturbance and melatonin therapy. Brain and Development. 1994;16(1):71–6. https://doi.org/10.1016/0387-7604(94)90117-1.

91. Hoban TM, Sack RL, Lewy AJ, Miller LS, Singer CM. Entrainment of a free-running human with bright light? Chronobiol Int. 1989;6(4):347–53. https://doi.org/10.3109/07420528909056941.

92. Oren DA, Giesen HA, Wehr TA. Restoration of detectable melatonin after entrainment to a 24-hour schedule in a 'free-running' man. Psychoneuroendocrinology. 1997;22(1):39–52. https://doi.org/10.1016/s0306-4530(96)00038-8.

93. Brown MA, Quan SF, Eichling PS. Circadian rhythm sleep disorder, free-running type in a sighted male with severe depression, anxiety, and agoraphobia. J Clin Sleep Med. 2011;7(1):93–4.

94. Kuzniar TJ, Kovacevic-Ristanovic R, Nierodzik CL, Smith LC. Free-running (non-entrained to 24-h period) circadian sleep disorder in a patient with obstructive sleep apnea, delayed sleep phase tendency, and lack of social interaction. Sleep Breath. 2012;16(2):313–5. https://doi.org/10.1007/s11325-011-0535-8.

95. Edgar DM, Miller JD, Prosser RA, Dean RR, Dement WC. Serotonin and the mammalian circadian system: II. Phase-shifting rat behavioral rhythms with serotonergic agonists. J Biol Rhythm. 1993;8(1):17–31. https://doi.org/10.1177/074873049300800102.

96. Van Someren EJ, Riemersma RF, Swaab DF. Functional plasticity of the circadian timing system in old age: light exposure. Prog Brain Res. 2002;138:205–31. https://doi.org/10.1016/S0079-6123(02)38080-4.

97. Swaab DF, Dubelaar EJ, Hofman MA, Scherder EJ, van Someren EJ, Verwer RW. Brain aging and Alzheimer's disease; use it or lose it. Prog Brain Res. 2002;138:343–73. https://doi.org/10.1016/S0079-6123(02)38086-5.

98. Havekes R, Heckman PRA, Wams EJ, Stasiukonyte N, Meerlo P, Eisel ULM. Alzheimer's disease pathogenesis: the role of disturbed sleep in attenuated brain plasticity and neurodegenerative processes. Cell Signal. 2019;64:109420. https://doi.org/10.1016/j.cellsig.2019.109420.

99. Zee PC, Vitiello MV. Circadian rhythm sleep disorder: irregular sleep wake rhythm type. Sleep Med Clin. 2009;4(2):213–8. https://doi.org/10.1016/j.jsmc.2009.01.009.

100. Mishima K, Okawa M, Hishikawa Y, Hozumi S, Hori H, Takahashi K. Morning bright light therapy for sleep and behavior disorders in elderly patients with dementia. Acta Psychiatr Scand. 1994;89(1):1–7. https://doi.org/10.1111/j.1600-0447.1994.tb01477.x.

101. Ancoli-Israel S, Gehrman P, Martin JL, Shochat T, Marler M, Corey-Bloom J, Levi L. Increased light exposure consolidates sleep and strengthens circadian rhythms in severe

Alzheimer's disease patients. Behav Sleep Med. 2003;1(1):22–36. https://doi.org/10.1207/S15402010BSM0101_4.

102. Riemersma-van der Lek RF, Swaab DF, Twisk J, Hol EM, Hoogendijk WJ, Van Someren EJ. Effect of bright light and melatonin on cognitive and noncognitive function in elderly residents of group care facilities: a randomized controlled trial. JAMA. 2008;299(22):2642–55. https://doi.org/10.1001/jama.299.22.2642.

103. McCurry SM, Gibbons LE, Logsdon RG, Vitiello MV, Teri L. Nighttime insomnia treatment and education for Alzheimer's disease: a randomized, controlled trial. J Am Geriatr Soc. 2005;53(5):793–802. https://doi.org/10.1111/j.1532-5415.2005.53252.x.

104. Alessi CA, Martin JL, Webber AP, Cynthia Kim E, Harker JO, Josephson KR. Randomized, controlled trial of a nonpharmacological intervention to improve abnormal sleep/wake patterns in nursing home residents. J Am Geriatr Soc. 2005;53(5):803–10. https://doi.org/10.1111/j.1532-5415.2005.53251.x.

105. Guilleminault C, McCann CC, Quera-Salva M, Cetel M. Light therapy as treatment of dyschronosis in brain impaired children. Eur J Pediatr. 1993;152(9):754–9. https://doi.org/10.1007/BF01953995.

106. Wright B, Sims D, Smart S, Alwazeer A, Alderson-Day B, Allgar V, Whitton C, Tomlinson H, Bennett S, Jardine J, McCaffrey N, Leyland C, Jakeman C, Miles J. Melatonin versus placebo in children with autism spectrum conditions and severe sleep problems not amenable to behaviour management strategies: a randomised controlled crossover trial. J Autism Dev Disord. 2011;41(2):175–84. https://doi.org/10.1007/s10803-010-1036-5.

107. Cheng P, Drake CL. Psychological impact of shift Work. Curr Sleep Med Rep. 2018;4(2):104–9.

108. Brown JP, Martin D, Nagaria Z, Verceles AC, Jobe SL, Wickwire EM. Mental health consequences of shift Work: an updated review. Curr Psychiatry Rep. 2020;22(2):7. https://doi.org/10.1007/s11920-020-1131-z.

109. Morgenthaler T, Alessi C, Friedman L, Owens J, Kapur V, Boehlecke B, Brown T, Chesson A Jr, Coleman J, Lee-Chiong T, Pancer J, Swick TJ, Standards of Practice C, American Academy of Sleep M. Practice parameters for the use of actigraphy in the assessment of sleep and sleep disorders: an update for 2007. Sleep. 2007;30(4):519–29. https://doi.org/10.1093/sleep/30.4.519.

110. Yong LC, Li J, Calvert GM. Sleep-related problems in the US working population: prevalence and association with shiftwork status. Occup Environ Med. 2017;74(2):93–104. https://doi.org/10.1136/oemed-2016-103638.

111. Drake CL, Roehrs T, Richardson G, Walsh JK, Roth T. Shift work sleep disorder: prevalence and consequences beyond that of symptomatic day workers. Sleep. 2004;27(8):1453–62. https://doi.org/10.1093/sleep/27.8.1453.

112. Harma MI, Hakola T, Akerstedt T, Laitinen JT. Age and adjustment to night work. Occup Environ Med. 1994;51(8):568–73. https://doi.org/10.1136/oem.51.8.568.

113. Ritonja J, Aronson KJ, Matthews RW, Boivin DB, Kantermann T. Working time society consensus statements: individual differences in shift work tolerance and recommendations for research and practice. Ind Health. 2019;57(2):201–12. https://doi.org/10.2486/indhealth.SW-5.

114. Pilcher JJ, Lambert BJ, Huffcutt AI. Differential effects of permanent and rotating shifts on self-report sleep length: a meta-analytic review. Sleep. 2000;23(2):155–63.

115. Gumenyuk V, Belcher R, Drake CL, Roth T. Differential sleep, sleepiness, and neurophysiology in the insomnia phenotypes of shift work disorder. Sleep. 2015;38(1):119–26. https://doi.org/10.5665/sleep.4336.

116. Zee PC, Attarian H, Videnovic A. Circadian rhythm abnormalities. Continuum (Minneap Minn). 2013;19(1 Sleep Disorders):132–47. https://doi.org/10.1212/01.CON.0000427209.21177.aa.

117. Booker LA, Magee M, Rajaratnam SMW, Sletten TL, Howard ME. Individual vulnerability to insomnia, excessive sleepiness and shift work disorder amongst healthcare shift

workers. A systematic review. Sleep Med Rev. 2018;41:220–33. https://doi.org/10.1016/j. smrv.2018.03.005.

118. Barger LK, Cade BE, Ayas NT, Cronin JW, Rosner B, Speizer FE, Czeisler CA, Harvard Work Hours H, Safety G. Extended work shifts and the risk of motor vehicle crashes among interns. N Engl J Med. 2005;352(2):125–34. https://doi.org/10.1056/NEJMoa041401.

119. Ftouni S, Sletten TL, Howard M, Anderson C, Lenne MG, Lockley SW, Rajaratnam SM. Objective and subjective measures of sleepiness, and their associations with on-road driving events in shift workers. J Sleep Res. 2013;22(1):58–69. https://doi.org/10.1111/j.1365-2869.2012.01038.x.

120. Purnell MT, Feyer AM, Herbison GP. The impact of a nap opportunity during the night shift on the performance and alertness of 12-h shift workers. J Sleep Res. 2002;11(3):219–27. https://doi.org/10.1046/j.1365-2869.2002.00309.x.

121. Garbarino S, Mascialino B, Penco MA, Squarcia S, De Carli F, Nobili L, Beelke M, Cuomo G, Ferrillo F. Professional shift-work drivers who adopt prophylactic naps can reduce the risk of car accidents during night work. Sleep. 2004;27(7):1295–302. https://doi.org/10.1093/sleep/27.7.1295.

122. Schweitzer PK, Randazzo AC, Stone K, Erman M, Walsh JK. Laboratory and field studies of naps and caffeine as practical countermeasures for sleep-wake problems associated with night work. Sleep. 2006;29(1):39–50. https://doi.org/10.1093/sleep/29.1.39.

123. Burgess HJ, Sharkey KM, Eastman CI. Bright light, dark and melatonin can promote circadian adaptation in night shift workers. Sleep Med Rev. 2002;6(5):407–20.

124. Lowden A, Ozturk G, Reynolds A, Bjorvatn B. Working time society consensus statements: evidence based interventions using light to improve circadian adaptation to working hours. Ind Health. 2019;57(2):213–27. https://doi.org/10.2486/indhealth.SW-9.

125. Liira J, Verbeek J, Ruotsalainen J. Pharmacological interventions for sleepiness and sleep disturbances caused by shift work. JAMA. 2015;313(9):961–2. https://doi.org/10.1001/jama.2014.18422.

126. Czeisler CA, Walsh JK, Wesnes KA, Arora S, Roth T. Armodafinil for treatment of excessive sleepiness associated with shift work disorder: a randomized controlled study. Mayo Clin Proc. 2009;84(11):958–72. https://doi.org/10.1016/S0025-6196(11)60666-6.

127. Erman MK, Seiden DJ, Yang R, Dammerman R. Efficacy and tolerability of armodafinil: effect on clinical condition late in the shift and overall functioning of patients with excessive sleepiness associated with shift work disorder. J Occup Environ Med. 2011;53(12):1460–5. https://doi.org/10.1097/JOM.0b013e318237a17e.

128. Drake C, Gumenyuk V, Roth T, Howard R. Effects of armodafinil on simulated driving and alertness in shift work disorder. Sleep. 2014;37(12):1987–94. https://doi.org/10.5665/sleep.4256.

129. Czeisler CA, Walsh JK, Roth T, Hughes RJ, Wright KP, Kingsbury L, Arora S, Schwartz JR, Niebler GE, Dinges DF, Group USMiSWSDS. Modafinil for excessive sleepiness associated with shift-work sleep disorder. N Engl J Med. 2005;353(5):476–86. https://doi.org/10.1056/NEJMoa041292.

130. Huedo-Medina TB, Kirsch I, Middlemass J, Klonizakis M, Siriwardena AN. Effectiveness of non-benzodiazepine hypnotics in treatment of adult insomnia: meta-analysis of data submitted to the Food and Drug Administration. BMJ. 2012;345:e8343. https://doi.org/10.1136/bmj.e8343.

131. Buscemi N, Vandermeer B, Friesen C, Bialy L, Tubman M, Ospina M, Klassen TP, Witmans M. The efficacy and safety of drug treatments for chronic insomnia in adults: a meta-analysis of RCTs. J Gen Intern Med. 2007;22(9):1335–50. https://doi.org/10.1007/s11606-007-0251-z.

132. Walsh JK, Schweitzer PK, Anch AM, Muehlbach MJ, Jenkins NA, Dickins QS. Sleepiness/alertness on a simulated night shift following sleep at home with triazolam. Sleep. 1991;14(2):140–6.

133. Balkin TJ, O'Donnell VM, Wesensten N, McCann U, Belenky G. Comparison of the daytime sleep and performance effects of zolpidem versus triazolam. Psychopharmacology. 1992;107(1):83–8. https://doi.org/10.1007/BF02244970.
134. Vetter C, Fischer D, Matera JL, Roenneberg T. Aligning work and circadian time in shift workers improves sleep and reduces circadian disruption. Curr Biol. 2015;25(7):907–11. https://doi.org/10.1016/j.cub.2015.01.064.
135. Herxheimer A. Jet lag. BMJ Clin Evid. 2014;2014
136. Moline ML, Pollak CP, Monk TH, Lester LS, Wagner DR, Zendell SM, Graeber RC, Salter CA, Hirsch E. Age-related differences in recovery from simulated jet lag. Sleep. 1992;15(1):28–40. https://doi.org/10.1093/sleep/15.1.28.
137. Waterhouse J, Edwards B, Nevill A, Carvalho S, Atkinson G, Buckley P, Reilly T, Godfrey R, Ramsay R. Identifying some determinants of "jet lag" and its symptoms: a study of athletes and other travellers. Br J Sports Med. 2002;36(1):54–60. https://doi.org/10.1136/bjsm.36.1.54.
138. Sack RL. The pathophysiology of jet lag. Travel Med Infect Dis. 2009;7(2):102–10. https://doi.org/10.1016/j.tmaid.2009.01.006.
139. Waterhouse J, Reilly T, Atkinson G, Edwards B. Jet lag: trends and coping strategies. Lancet. 2007;369(9567):1117–29. https://doi.org/10.1016/S0140-6736(07)60529-7.
140. Paul MA, Gray GW, Lieberman HR, Love RJ, Miller JC, Trouborst M, Arendt J. Phase advance with separate and combined melatonin and light treatment. Psychopharmacology. 2011;214(2):515–23. https://doi.org/10.1007/s00213-010-2059-5.
141. Burgess HJ, Crowley SJ, Gazda CJ, Fogg LF, Eastman CI. Preflight adjustment to eastward travel: 3 days of advancing sleep with and without morning bright light. J Biol Rhythm. 2003;18(4):318–28. https://doi.org/10.1177/0748730403253585.
142. Eastman CI, Gazda CJ, Burgess HJ, Crowley SJ, Fogg LF. Advancing circadian rhythms before eastward flight: a strategy to prevent or reduce jet lag. Sleep. 2005;28(1):33–44. https://doi.org/10.1093/sleep/28.1.33.
143. Revell VL, Burgess HJ, Gazda CJ, Smith MR, Fogg LF, Eastman CI. Advancing human circadian rhythms with afternoon melatonin and morning intermittent bright light. J Clin Endocrinol Metab. 2006;91(1):54–9. https://doi.org/10.1210/jc.2005-1009.
144. Herxheimer A, Petrie KJ. Melatonin for the prevention and treatment of jet lag. Cochrane Database Syst Rev. 2002;2:CD001520. https://doi.org/10.1002/14651858.CD001520.
145. Lu Z, Klein-Cardena K, Lee S, Antonsen TM, Girvan M, Ott E. Resynchronization of circadian oscillators and the east-west asymmetry of jet-lag. Chaos. 2016;26(9):094811. https://doi.org/10.1063/1.4954275.

Chapter 15
Narcolepsy and Idiopathic Hypersomnia

Imran Ahmed and Michael Thorpy

Keywords Narcolepsy · Idiopathic hypersomnia · Symptoms · Epidemiology Pathophysiology · Diagnosis · Differential · Pediatric · Treatment

Introduction

Narcolepsy was originally described by Gelineau in 1880 as a disorder involving excessive sleepiness and sleep attacks associated with a variety of emotional states. He also described episodes of falls or "astasia" which was later termed cataplexy. Our understanding of narcolepsy has since advanced. In the 1950s sleep onset REM periods were identified as a prominent feature in narcolepsy. In the latter part of the 1900s, the discovery of the association between narcolepsy and the Human Leukocyte antigens (HLA) DRB1*1501/DRB1*1503 and with DQB1*0602 suggested an autoimmune process. Also, the discovery by two independent groups in 2005 of a reduction in the neuropeptide, hypocretin/orexin, is now strongly believed to be responsible for many of the symptoms of narcolepsy. Around 2010, our understanding of the genetic factors and environmental factors (e.g., vaccines, infections) associated with narcolepsy has given us a window into the pathophysiology of the disorder.

Additionally, in 2013, the *International Classification of Sleep Disorders*, third edition (ICSD-3), categorized narcolepsy into two different types: narcolepsy type 1 and narcolepsy type 2 based on cataplexy and the deficiency, or non-deficiency, of hypocretin/orexin, respectively. The terms that classified narcolepsy based on the presence or absence of cataplexy, as used by the *International Classification of*

I. Ahmed (✉) · M. Thorpy
Sleep-Wake Disorders Center, Montefiore Medical Center, and Albert Einstein College of Medicine, Bronx, NY, USA
e-mail: iahmed@montefiore.org

© Springer Nature Switzerland AG 2022
M. S. Badr, J. L. Martin (eds.), *Essentials of Sleep Medicine*,
Respiratory Medicine, https://doi.org/10.1007/978-3-030-93739-3_15

Sleep Disorders, second edition, were deemed inappropriate as some patients without cataplexy will also have low cerebrospinal fluid hypocretin levels.

The term "idiopathic hypersomnia" was first used in 1976 by Bedrich Roth to describe a disorder with both a monosymptomatic and a polysymptomatic form. The monosymptomatic form exhibits only EDS, whereas the polysymptomatic form manifests not only symptoms of EDS but also a long duration of the major sleep period and a prominent sleep inertia upon awakening. Accordingly, in 2005, the ICSD-2 classified idiopathic hypersomnia into two types, one associated with a prolonged sleep episode at night, which was called idiopathic hypersomnia with long sleep time, and another that has a normal duration of sleep at night called idiopathic hypersomnia without long sleep time. The ICSD-3 eliminated the division of the idiopathic hypersomnia's classification based on the sleep duration because of the lack of validity for such a division based on sleep duration and classifies it only as idiopathic hypersomnia.

Clinical Features

Narcolepsy

Narcolepsy is described as a syndrome consisting of EDS (including periods of irresistible sleep), cataplexy, sleep paralysis, and hypnagogic hallucinations; additional features include frequent and vivid dreams, automatic behaviors, and fragmented or disrupted nighttime sleep. The effects of narcolepsy can be considered a manifestation of REM sleep dissociation, with features of REM sleep that intrude into sleep and wakefulness.

Narcolepsy typically begins with the symptom of excessive sleepiness, and other symptoms of variable severity can develop slowly, suddenly, or not at all. Occasionally, cataplexy can develop first and then later be followed by the development of excessive sleepiness; this is especially true in children, where sleepiness is disguised as behavioral abnormalities [1]. Narcolepsy patients often have an irresistible urge to sleep, which often occurs at inopportune times whether it is during monotonous sedentary tasks or while performing mentally or physically demanding activities. For instance, they can fall asleep while eating, while sitting at a meeting, during phone conversations, during sexual intercourse, or while driving a car. These sleep episodes occur about 3–5 times/day in most patients and usually vary from a few minutes to several hours in duration [2]. Patients often report that after these sleep episodes or after taking scheduled naps, they wake up feeling refreshed and may not feel sleepy again for up to a few hours later; however, there are also many patients who indicate persistent (although perhaps somewhat improved) sleepiness despite taking these naps. Patients can also experience microsleep events, which are seconds or less of sleep that intrude into the waking state. Patients are not aware of the microsleep episodes and continue the activities they were performing. It is likely that such episodes are at least partially associated with patients' complaints of difficulty concentrating, inattention, or memory impairment.

In children, it is difficult to identify classic narcolepsy symptoms since many are not able to provide an accurate history of cataplexy, sleep-related hallucinations, or sleep paralysis. Sleepiness may also manifest as behavioral problems (e.g., irritability, hyperactivity), decreased performance, inattentiveness, lack of energy, or bizarre hallucinations that makes it even more difficult to diagnose narcolepsy. Furthermore, when excessive sleepiness is present, it can often be mistaken for normal behaviors in children of preschool age, as they usually take habitual naps. Occasionally in school-aged children, excessive sleepiness can be identified when there is a reappearance of daytime naps in a child who had previously discontinued regular napping [3].

Cataplexy is the most specific symptom of narcolepsy consisting of an abrupt, bilateral (occasionally unilateral) loss of skeletal muscle tone; it is associated with narcolepsy type 1. It is usually triggered by the occurrence of sudden emotion such as laughter or humorous experiences; sometimes even the memory of a humorous event can precipitate an attack. Other triggers for cataplexy include anger, embarrassment, surprise, stress, or even sexual arousal [4]. During a cataplexy attack, which can last up to several minutes, the patient is unable to move; however, the diaphragm and ocular muscles are unaffected. During this time, the patient remains awake, aware of their surroundings and able to remember the details of the event and comments or questions that were made to them. If the attack is prolonged, however, sleep can follow. More commonly, attacks of cataplexy are partial, affecting only certain muscle groups, such as the arms, neck, or face. During partial cataplexy attacks, the jaw may sag, the head can droop, and speech may become garbled [5]. Deep tendon reflexes are usually absent during generalized cataplexy episodes; however, they have been reported to be persistent during partial attacks [6]. In children, atypical manifestations of cataplexy can include blurred vision, irregular breathing, sudden loss of smiling, or "semipermanent eyelid and jaw weakness." Additionally, children's cataplexy may also manifest as subtle and unusual facial expressions or choreic-like movements which are not seen in adults [7, 8].

Sleep-related hallucinations, sleep paralysis, and automatic behaviors are common manifestations of many disorders that disrupt/fragment sleep and cause excessive sleepiness, including narcolepsy and idiopathic hypersomnia [9]. Similar to cataplexy, patients with sleep paralysis experience a brief loss of voluntary muscle control with an inability to move or speak, but retain awareness during the event. Unlike cataplexy, these episodes are not provoked by intense emotion or stress. The phenomena usually occur during sleep–wake transitions and are often associated with fearful sleep-related hallucinations, hypnopompic or hypnagogic. They are intense dream-like states that occur when falling asleep (hypnagogic) or when waking from sleep (hypnopompic) [10]. The events typically remit on their own within 1–10 min, but can also be terminated when someone touches the patient [10].

The sleep-related hallucinations can also occur independently of the sleep paralysis episodes and are usually visual or auditory and occasionally involve other senses, e.g., tactile or vestibular. They are occasionally pleasant, but quite often frightening or disturbing to the patient. The visual hallucinations can consist of simple forms, such as circles or multi-sided geometric figures or can be more intricate such as animals or people. Similarly, the auditory hallucinations can manifest as simple sounds, such as knocking on a door or a phone ring, or more complex tunes, such as a musical composition. Less often, patients report hallucinations such as smelling a scent/odor, or having a sense that one is falling, or feeling that someone or something is touching them.

Automatic behavior is the performance of simple or complex routine tasks by individuals who remain unaware of the activity. These behaviors range from activities such as talking on the phone or writing to walking, cooking, or driving. Some patients report that they have ordered items through the phone, or cooked a meal, and did not remember doing so. Some also report driving home from work and not realizing how they got there. The personal and public hazards of such behaviors are self-evident.

In addition to episodes of EDS, narcolepsy patients also report difficulty in maintaining sleep at night due to a dysfunction of central sleep regulation which causes frequent transitions between sleep and wakefulness throughout the entire 24-h cycle. Typically they can fall asleep quickly but report frequent nocturnal awakenings and occasionally indicate that they do not sleep for long periods during the night.

Idiopathic Hypersomnia

Similar to narcolepsy, patients with idiopathic hypersomnia also can have symptoms of excessive sleepiness. As mentioned earlier, it is no longer differentiated into subtypes based on sleep duration. It is characterized either by excessive sleep that usually is at least 11 hours in duration, but typically 12–14 hours, or daytime sleepiness with a mean sleep latency of less than or equal to 8 minutes with less than 2 sleep onset REM periods on a multiple sleep latency test (MSLT).

There is typically severe or prolonged sleep inertia with difficulty waking up that is often associated with irritability, automatic behaviors, and confusion. This sleep drunkenness is similar to the confusion and behaviors a normal person may experience if abruptly awoken from deep sleep. Patients are confused upon awakening and are unable to perform tasks or react appropriately [9, 11]. Accordingly, these patients also experience difficulty waking up in the morning and at the end of naps. They often never feel fully alert, even after their prolonged sleep period. They often require multiple alarm clocks to awaken in the morning or after naps, but usually end up becoming dependent on other people to awaken them. The naps are often irresistible, prolonged (up to 3–4 hours in duration) and unrefreshing [3, 9, 11].

In a report by Bassetti and Aldrich in 1997 [11], some patients with idiopathic hypersomnia were noted to have orthostatic hypotension, headaches, as well as cold hands and feet (Raynaud's type phenomena). A more recent study suggests that patients may have parasympathetic dysfunction during sleep and wake with altered autonomic responses to arousals [12]. Similar to narcolepsy (and sleep deprivation), other associated features in idiopathic hypersomnia include sleep-related hallucinations and sleep paralysis that are present in patients to a variable degree. Additionally, overnight polysomnograms may also demonstrate a high sleep efficiency ($\geq 90\%$) [3].

Epidemiology

Narcolepsy

Due to the overlap of clinical symptoms and polysomnographic/multiple sleep latency test (MSLT) features with other conditions such as depression, other sleep disorders, or even with normal individuals, it is difficult to make an accurate assessment of the true prevalence of narcolepsy. It is estimated that less than 50% of patients with narcolepsy have been diagnosed [13, 14]. Nevertheless, narcolepsy has been documented to begin at any age from infancy (rarely) to as late as old age, with a median age of 16 years but most commonly within the first two decades of life. Narcolepsy type 1 affects both men and women equally (perhaps a slight preponderance for males) with an approximate prevalence of 1 in 2000 people (0.05%) in the United States [15], less in Israel, and more in Japan.

There appears to be a genetic, racial, and ethnic predisposition for the development of narcolepsy [16]. The risk of a first-degree relative developing narcolepsy with cataplexy is approximately 1–2%, which is prominently higher than that estimated for the general population [17]. In addition, the HLA subtypes DR2 (DRB1*1501) and DQ (DQB1*0602) have also been found to be closely associated with narcolepsy. The HLA marker, DQB1*0602, has a prevalence ranging from 85 to 95% in patients with narcolepsy with cataplexy and about 40% in patients with narcolepsy without cataplexy vs. about 26% in the general population [18]. A review of the literature indicates that the prevalence of narcolepsy/cataplexy ranges from a low of 0.002% among Israeli Jews to a high of 0.15% among the Japanese general population. More recently, a general population study with a representative sample of over 18,000 subjects in five European countries estimated a prevalence of 0.047% [3].

The prevalence of cataplexy among patients with narcolepsy varies widely with estimates ranging from 60 to 90% [19]. Patients with cataplexy generally report that this symptom remains persistent with only minor fluctuations in severity; however, the severity and frequency of attacks may vary widely and range from occasional to multiple attacks daily. A few patients have reported spontaneous remission of cataplexy attacks. It has been suggested that a decline in cataplexy over time represents the ability of patients to adapt to their illness and learning to avoid those situations where cataplexy is most likely to occur.

The prevalence of narcolepsy type 2, on the other hand, is more uncertain. It is estimated that up to 36% of clinics' narcolepsy population have "narcolepsy without cataplexy." The ambiguity is at least partially attributed to population-based studies using MSLT diagnostic criteria for narcolepsy without the clinical symptom of cataplexy; these studies included individuals with sleep deprivation, shift work disorders, and even sleep apnea that likely contributed to false positive diagnoses [3]. It should be noted that the true prevalence of narcolepsy type 1 and narcolepsy type 2 are unknown as most epidemiologic studies were done prior to the publication of the ICSD 3.

Idiopathic Hypersomnia

More challenging than assessing the prevalence of narcolepsy is that of determining the prevalence of idiopathic hypersomnia. The reported prevalence in clinic populations when compared to narcolepsy patients widely varies depending upon the literature reviewed [7, 20–22]. At least part of the difficulty in determining idiopathic hypersomnia's prevalence is due to its nosological ambiguity. There has also been a propensity to label all difficult-to-classify cases of EDS as idiopathic hypersomnia [23]. Similar to narcolepsy type 1 and narcolepsy type 2, since the ICSD-3 classification scheme was developed, there have not been any systematic prevalence studies for idiopathic hypersomnia. Accordingly, it is safe to say that the true prevalence of idiopathic hypersomnia is unknown. What we do know is that there appears to be a female predominance [24] with the age of onset ranging from birth to early adulthood [25]. Some earlier studies also suggest an autosomal dominant mode of inheritance [26].

Pathophysiology

Narcolepsy

The discovery of the neuropeptide hypocretin [27, 28] has greatly enhanced our understanding of the pathophysiology of narcolepsy. It is thought that a deficiency of this arousal system (and perhaps other yet unknown arousal systems), rather than an overactivity of the sleep systems, underlies the pathogenesis of the symptoms in narcolepsy [29]. Hypocretin-containing neurons are located in the perifornical and lateral hypothalamus where they project widely to communicate with numerous brain nuclei including those responsible for the regulation of sleep, alertness, and muscle tone. Evidence suggests that most cases of narcolepsy are associated with loss of or partial loss of hypocretin-containing hypothalamic neurons and the development of cataplexy occurs when hypocretin is absent or nearly absent. Thannickal et al. [30] and Mignot et al. [31] reported an 85–95% loss of hypocretin-containing neurons in narcolepsy with cataplexy patients that corresponded to the finding of low or undetectable concentrations (≤ 110 pg/mL) of hypocretin in the cerebrospinal fluid (CSF) of these patients. Thannickal et al. [32] later found a loss of about a third of the hypothalamic hypocretin-containing cells in one patient with narcolepsy without cataplexy. An autoimmune process may be responsible for the loss of the hypocretin neurons; however, antibodies to hypocretin and hypocretin receptors have not been found [33–36].

As mentioned earlier, there is a higher occurrence of HLA DQB1*0602 in narcolepsy patients than in the general population. It is suspected that patients with this HLA marker (and likely other non-HLA genes associated with immune regulation or other currently unknown genetic links) may possess a genetic susceptibility for some event (e.g., environmental influences) that leads to the development of narcolepsy. This HLA association suggests a T-cell mediated autoimmunity. Researchers found a significant correlation between the degree of excessive sleepiness and the presence of activated T-cells in the central nervous system of narcolepsy type 1, narcolepsy type 2, and idiopathic hypersomnia patients lending further support to evidence of T-cell mediated autoimmunity [37].

Several studies have shown increased cases of narcolepsy in children and adolescents in relation to swine influenza A (H1N1). In Europe, the Pandemrix vaccination induced narcolepsy in patients who carried the HLA allele DQB1*0602, while in China infection with the virus was associated with the development of narcolepsy [38]. As mentioned above, polymorphisms in other non-HLA genes that may affect immune regulatory function are likely present as well. For example, the non-coding RNA gene GDNF-A51 was also significantly associated with the development of narcolepsy in the patients given the Pandemrix vaccination [39].

Environmental factors such as infections [40, 41], head trauma [42], neurotoxic metals, combustion smoke [43], or even a change in sleeping habits [41] have been associated with the onset of narcolepsy. While it is not known exactly how these environmental elements result in neurodegeneration of hypocretin neurons, Mori [43, 44] suggested these agents may cause release of proinflammatory cytokines in the olfactory bulb resulting in a breakdown of the blood-brain barrier; subsequently, this allows autoimmune cells access to the hypocretin neurons in the hypothalamus, which results in its degeneration.

Supporting evidence for the autoimmune etiology hypothesis continues to grow. Increased antistreptococcal antibodies were reported in patients with recent onset of narcolepsy, suggesting streptococcal infections may be an inciting event that is initiating an autoimmune process [40, 45]. Hallmayer et al. [46] also found a strong association between narcolepsy and a polymorphism in the T-cell receptor alpha locus (another indication that an autoimmune process has a role). Earlier in 2010, elevated Tribbles homolog 2 (Trib2) specific antibody levels were discovered in 16%–26% of patients with narcolepsy. Trib2 was previously known as an autoantigen in autoimmune uveitis; it has been identified in hypocretin neurons of a transgenic mouse model. In narcolepsy patients, titers of Trib2-specific antibodies were highest soon after narcolepsy onset and then decreased within the first 3 years of the disorder and finally stabilized at levels much higher than that of controls (normal controls and patients with idiopathic hypersomnia, multiple sclerosis, or other inflammatory neurologic disorders). Intracerebroventricular administration of immunoglobulin-G purified from anti-trib2 positive narcolepsy patients in subjects caused degeneration of hypocretin neurons [47, 48]. This finding provided support for an autoimmune etiology for narcolepsy; however, additional work by Tanaka S et al. in 2017 suggested that the anti-TRIB2 antibody seen in narcolepsy patients was a result rather than the cause of hypocretin cell degeneration [48].

Idiopathic Hypersomnia

In comparison to narcolepsy, less is known about the pathophysiology of idiopathic hypersomnia. One possible reason for this is that there are no specific criteria, clinical or polysomnographic, that is pathognomonic or even partially characteristic of the disorder, such as cataplexy or sleep onset REM periods in narcolepsy. There is no clear association with CSF hypocretin levels [49] as in narcolepsy. Although there appears to be a strong genetic component suggested by the high proportion of familial cases, no associated genes have been identified. Studies with HLAs have also found no connection [11].

Some studies suggested that dopamine and certain monoamine metabolites had a role in the etiology of idiopathic hypersomnia [50–53], but further studies have been inconclusive [3]. In some idiopathic hypersomnia patients, an endogenous hypnotic peptide stimulating GABA receptors during wakefulness is suspected to be at least partially etiologic [54]. Autoimmunity has also been suggested as etiologic in idiopathic hypersomnia [37]. Further studies to assess the validity of these hypotheses need to be done.

There is a possible common pathway between the pathophysiology of narcolepsy and idiopathic hypersomnia. A low CSF histamine level has been identified in both these disorders and has not been seen in patients with excessive sleepiness due to sleep apnea [55, 56]. Accordingly, it is hypothesized that low histamine may be specific to hypersomnias of central origin [56]; however, a more recent study failed to demonstrate this deficiency [57]. In addition, since idiopathic hypersomnia hypocretin levels are normal, it has been suggested that factors other than hypocretin deficiency are the cause of these low histamine levels. Further research still needs to be done to validate this hypothesis and to better understand the role of histamine in these disorders.

Diagnosis

Narcolepsy

There are three main types of narcolepsy: narcolepsy type 1, NT1, narcolepsy type 2, NT2, and secondary narcolepsy (Table 15.1). Narcolepsy type 1 is defined as excessive sleepiness that occurs for at least 3 months and is associated with definite cataplexy and/or a low CSF hypocretin level (≤110 pg/mL or one third of mean

Table 15.1 Diagnostic criteria for narcolepsy

Narcolepsy type 1
1. At least 3 months of excessive daytime sleepiness (EDS) as well as item 2 and/or item 3 below are present

2A. Cataplexy is present
2B. On a polysomnogram (PSG) followed by a multiple sleep latency test (MSLT):
    (a) The PSG rules out other causes of disrupted nocturnal sleep and demonstrates at least 7 h of sleep
    (b) The MSLT should show a sleep latency of ≤8 min and two or more sleep onset REM periods; if the PSG has a sleep onset REM period (i.e., within 15 minutes of sleep onset), then only 1 SOREMP is needed on the MSLT study.

3. A cerebrospinal fluid (CSF) hypocretin-1 level ≤110 pg/mL or < 1/3 of normal control values
Narcolepsy type 2
1. At least 3 months of EDS
2. Cataplexy is absent; however, questionable or atypical cataplexy-like episodes can be present

3. On a PSG followed by a MSLT:
    (a) The PSG rules out other causes of disrupted nocturnal sleep and demonstrate at least 7 h of sleep
    (b) The MSLT should show a sleep latency of ≤8 min and two or more sleep onset REM periods; if the PSG has a sleep onset REM period (i.e., within 15 minutes of sleep onset), then only 1 SOREMP is needed on the MSLT study.

4. CSF hypocretin-1 levels must be either unknown or ≥110 pg/mL (or 1/3 of normal control values)
5. The EDS or MSLT findings cannot be better explained by other causes, e.g., other sleep disorders, medication effect, or sleep deprivation

Adapted from American Academy of Sleep Medicine [3]

normal control values) [27]. In the presence of cataplexy, if CSF hypocretin level is unknown or ≥ 110 pg/ml, then a polysomnography followed by a MSLT is needed [58]. The polysomnography should confirm at least 7 h of sleep and exclude other sleep disorders that could account for the symptoms, such as obstructive sleep apnea syndrome. It usually demonstrates a short sleep latency and fragmented nocturnal sleep and may show increased stage 1 sleep and early REM sleep onset [59]. The MSLT should exhibit two or more sleep onset REM periods (SOREMP) with a mean sleep latency of ≤8 min [3]. If a sleep onset REM period occurs during the preceding polysomnogram (i.e., within 15 minutes of sleep onset), then only one SOREMP is needed in the MSLT [3]. Accordingly, a patient with hypersomnia without cataplexy can still meet criteria for a diagnosis of NT1 if CSF hypocretin levels are reduced as described above. Alternatively, a patient with hypersomnia with cataplexy can meet criteria for a diagnosis of NT1 if CSF hypocretin levels are "normal."

Patients with NT2 either do not have cataplexy or have atypical cataplexy-like events. The PSG followed by an MSLT should demonstrate features similar to that of NT1 as described above, and their CSF hypocretin-1 levels should be ≤110 pg/mL or one third of mean normal control values if measured [21, 27]. Other disorders that can explain the EDS and/or MSLT findings must be ruled out prior to making a diagnosis of NT2.

Secondary narcolepsy is classified as a subtype of NT1 and NT2 in the ICSD 3, namely, as narcolepsy type 1 due to a medical condition and narcolepsy type 2 due to a medical condition. Secondary narcolepsy can potentially occur after any lesion affecting the hypothalamus, including but not limited to tumors, autoimmune disorders, paraneoplastic disorders, sarcoidosis, multiple sclerosis, Parkinson's disease, or head trauma [3]. This condition is given the diagnosis of NT1 due to a medical condition or NT2 due to a medical condition, if the criteria for NT1 or NT2 are met, respectively, and is attributable to another medical disorder.

Similar to adults, the diagnosis of NT1 can be made in children if excessive sleepiness and definite cataplexy is present and the MSLT is diagnostic or if CSF hypocretin-1 deficiency is present. However, as mentioned earlier, it is difficult to identify classic narcolepsy symptoms in children. Additionally, normal values on sleep studies, especially for MSLTs, have not been standardized in subjects younger than 6 years of age and results should be interpreted with care. Carskadon [60] suggested using a child's Tanner stage of sexual development to compare sleep study results to normal values of nocturnal total sleep time, daytime sleep latency, and daytime REM sleep latency as these are closely linked to the Tanner stages. A more recent study showed that a MSLT with at least 2 SOREMPs and a mean sleep latency of ≤ 8.2 minutes was a reliable marker for the diagnosis of NT1 in the pediatric population [61]. Nevertheless, if the MSLT results are equivocal and there is still a high clinical suspicion for narcolepsy, a repeat study is warranted after a period of time.

Children with NT2 present similarly to those with NT1 except they do not have cataplexy and CSF hypocretin levels if measured are in the normal range. Occasionally, cataplexy may develop after the presenting symptom of excessive sleepiness. In this situation, the patient (typically a child, but also can be an adult) is given the diagnosis of NT2 until the onset of cataplexy at which time the diagnosis is changed to NT1.

As suggested earlier, HLA testing (in a child or adult) is not a useful screening or diagnostic tool; however, it might be useful in atypical narcolepsy with cataplexy presentations. A negative test should encourage the physician to make certain that other sleep disorders are excluded before assigning a diagnosis of NT1 narcolepsy.

Idiopathic Hypersomnia

In order to make the diagnosis of idiopathic hypersomnia (Table 15.2), the associated excessive sleepiness, similar to narcolepsy, needs to occur almost daily for at least 3 months and cataplexy is not present. There is often difficulty awaking from the sleep period including any naps. Polysomnography should rule out other causes of excessive sleepiness (e.g., sleep apnea), and a MSLT performed following the nocturnal polysomnography should show a mean sleep latency of ≤ 8 min with less than two sleep onset REM periods. If the preceding PSG has a SOREMP (i.e., within the initial 15 minutes of the study), then the MSLT should not have any SOREMPs [3]. Awaking patients with idiopathic hypersomnia in the morning

Table 15.2 Diagnostic criteria for idiopathic hypersomnia

Idiopathic hypersomnia
1. At least 3 months of EDS
2. Cataplexy is not present
3. The MSLT should show a sleep latency of ≤8 min and less than two sleep onset REM periods; if the preceding PSG has a sleep onset REM period (i.e., within 15 minutes of sleep onset), then there should not be a SOREMP on the MSLT.
4. If the mean sleep latency on the MSLT is >8 min, then a total sleep time of at least 11 hrs/24 hr. period should be demonstrated either with a 24 hr. polysomnogram or by wrist actigraphy and sleep log (averaged over at least 7 days)
5. Insufficient sleep syndrome should be ruled out
6. Other sleep, medical, or psychiatric disorders or medications/drugs should not better explain the EDS and/or MSLT findings

Adapted from American Academy of Sleep Medicine [3]

following an overnight polysomnogram to do a MSLT does not allow for the documentation of a prolonged sleep time. Additionally, the mean sleep latency on the MSLT may not always be diagnostic, and the short naps scheduled every 2 h do not allow for the demonstration of prolonged unrefreshing naps. Therefore, as an alternative to the MSLT showing a mean sleep latency of ≤8 min, the typical nocturnal sleep duration of at least 11 hours can be demonstrated with a 24 hr. polysomnographic recording or by wrist actigraphy and sleep logs over at least 7 days. Insufficient sleep syndrome and other sleep disorders should also be ruled out [3].

Similar to adults, before a diagnosis of idiopathic hypersomnia is made in children, other sleep disorders, especially insufficient sleep syndrome, and use of recreational drugs should be ruled out. If the sleep duration criteria is being used to diagnose idiopathic hypersomnia in the pediatric population, age appropriate normal values for total sleep time should be taken into account. A repeat MSLT study should be considered in patients diagnosed with idiopathic hypersomnia after a certain time interval, because SOREMPs may develop overtime in narcolepsy. If 2 or more SOREMP are present in the repeat PSG/MSLT study, then the patient should be reclassified as having NT2.

It is evident by many experts that the current diagnostic criteria have its limitations. It relies on ancillary testing such as the MSLT that is not well validated in all patient populations and is relatively nonspecific. The stability of repeated MSLT results is also in question with one study showing only 10–20% of patients with a positive initial MSLT being positive after the test was repeated in 4 years [62]. Additionally, although validated, the method for measurement of CSF hypocretin levels has some issues [63–65]. Sakai et al. showed that the typical method of hypocretin measurement actually measures hypocretin-1 metabolites believed to be inactive. Therefore, while standard testing would demonstrate deficiency of "hypocretin-1" in some NT1 patients, an alternative method of testing which measures the true active hypocretin-1 protein can actually demonstrate some degree of deficiency in NT1 and NT2 patients that were found to have no deficiency when tested with standard techniques [64].

Accordingly, it stands to reason that diagnostic tools utilizing other markers to aid in the diagnosis of narcolepsy are needed. For instance, Stephansen et al. demonstrated that a combination of a more thorough evaluation of the overnight polysomnogram and HLA testing yielded a high sensitivity and specificity for NT1 diagnosis. A PSG analysis revealing unusual sleep stage overlap alone achieved a sensitivity of 91% and specificity of 96%, and when combined with testing showing HLA-DQB1*0602, the specificity increased to 99% [66]. Identification of REM sleep without atonia (in at least 8% of stage REM sleep epochs) in the pediatric population has demonstrated high specificity for the diagnosis of narcolepsy [67]. Additionally, Murer et al. verified that sleep stage analysis with better characterization of REM sleep duration and sleep stage sequence during the PSG contributed to a higher MSLT specificity for narcolepsy [68].

Other features in patients with narcolepsy have been identified, and future tools utilizing these findings may aid in diagnosing narcolepsy or differentiating it from other hypersomnias. For instance, the frequency and distribution of eye movements during various sleep stages throughout the night as well as while awake was shown to be significantly different in NT1 patients compared to clinical controls as well as NT2 patients [69]. Furthermore, heart rate variability abnormalities during stage NREM 2 and non-dipping blood pressure patterns were found to be more prevalent in NT1 patients compared to control groups [70, 71]. Additionally, certain neuroanatomical correlates on neuroimaging studies may also contribute to diagnosing narcolepsy and other hypersomnias [72].

Differential Diagnosis

Excessive sleepiness is common to many sleep disorders, besides narcolepsy and idiopathic hypersomnia, and can also be a normal phenomenon in certain circumstances (e.g., sleep deprivation). Some of these sleep disorders can be differentiated from narcolepsy or idiopathic hypersomnia by history. For instance, identification of a disruptive environmental feature during sleep may lead one to the diagnosis of an environmental sleep disorder. A history of sleeping less than expected from age-adjusted normative data or having a sleep period that is delayed, advanced, or irregular would suggest behaviorally induced, insufficient sleep syndrome or a circadian rhythm disorder, respectively. A description of normal sleep between episodes of hypersomnia can suggest a diagnosis of recurrent hypersomnia. Certain psychiatric disorders (e.g., depression or substance abuse) can also be responsible for excessive sleepiness and are identifiable on history.

Narcolepsy is commonly comorbid with several medical and psychiatric disorders that can not only cause a misdiagnosis but can complicate narcolepsy treatment. Cardiac, mental, neurologic, gastrointestinal, renal, and pulmonary disorders are more common in narcolepsy [73]. Cardiac disorders can complicate therapy as some narcolepsy medications can cause cardiac arrhythmias or exacerbate fluid retention and add to hypertension or heart failure. Of the mental disorders, depression and anxiety are particularly prevalent and are common causes of delay in narcolepsy diagnosis. Anxiety disorders can contribute to stimulant medication failure due to exacerbating adverse effects [74]. In addition, concurrent sleep disorders, such as obstructive sleep apnea syndrome, sleep deprivation, restless legs syndrome, and circadian rhythm disorders, can contribute to, or mask, a narcolepsy diagnosis.

Disorders that cause excessive sleepiness cannot always be identified by history alone; additional studies to differentiate them from narcolepsy and idiopathic hypersomnia are often required. A polysomnogram will help identify sleep disordered breathing. Imaging studies may discover the presence of a brain tumor or stroke (although other findings on exam are also usually present). Blood work or CSF analysis can help identify metabolic abnormalities or encephalitis as a cause of sleepiness. There was a case report by Maestri et al. [75] on a patient that was diagnosed with idiopathic hypersomnia but after further evaluation was found to have an insulinoma. After management of the insulinoma, his symptoms of excessive sleepiness resolved. Another report by Shinno et al. [76] identified a patient with idiopathic hypersomnia who was subsequently found to have subclinical hypothyroidism; after management with levothyroxine his sleepiness improved.

History and additional laboratory studies are also useful in ruling out disorders that can mimic cataplexy. Transient weakness episodes can represent transient ischemic attacks (TIAs) if there is no history of an association with emotion or if there is a history of vascular risk factors and/or stroke. Seizures, syncope, and brainstem or diencephalic tumors can look like cataplexy; a positive EEG may suggest seizures; imaging studies can help identify tumors; and a history of loss of consciousness may help differentiate syncope or seizures from cataplexy.

Excessive Sleepiness Due to Head Trauma

Sleep disturbances, including excessive sleepiness, can occur as a result of traumatic brain injury (TBI); accordingly, TBI should be considered in the differential diagnosis of excessive sleepiness. Some researchers contend that the excessive sleepiness is due to the increased prevalence of obstructive sleep apnea and periodic limb movement disorder that is seen in TBI patients [77]. In addition, changes in nocturnal sleep pattern seen in TBI patients are similar to those of depressed patients, namely, increased nighttime awakenings and longer sleep onset latency [78]. It is speculated that the sleepiness is due in part to this disturbed nocturnal sleep and that treatment of concomitant mood disorders may improve the sleepiness in the TBI patients; however, further research needs to be done in this area.

Hypothalamic damage, not necessarily visible on imaging studies, may be responsible for the excessive sleepiness that is seen in many TBI patients. The ICSD-3 classified this group of TBI patients under several separate subtypes: NT1 or NT2 due to a medical condition and hypersomnia due to a medical condition (posttraumatic hypersomnia subtype). A 2007 study found that the CSF hypocretin-1 levels were decreased in these TBI patients, and a follow-up study in 2009 demonstrated the number of hypocretin neurons in the hypothalamus was significantly reduced [79, 80]. The loss of hypocretin is likely the etiology underlying TBI associated with narcolepsy and possibly post-traumatic hypersomnia.

Treatment

There is no known cure for either narcolepsy or idiopathic hypersomnia; however, with respect to idiopathic hypersomnia, there are reports of spontaneous remission [25]. For those with persistent disease, treatment is targeted at symptom management. Even with optimum management, the EDS in narcolepsy and idiopathic hypersomnia patients, and the cataplexy in narcolepsy patients, are seldom completely controlled.

Nonpharmacologic Management

Nonpharmacologic management should be initiated in all patients. Patient education is an important component of any treatment plan. Good sleep habits with avoidance of sleep deprivation and/or irregular sleep patterns should be emphasized. In narcolepsy patients, the scheduling of short naps (15–20 min) 2–3 times/day can help control EDS and improve alertness, but this is impractical in many settings. Napping, in contrast, is not recommended for management of sleepiness in patients with idiopathic hypersomnia as it usually does not help and may result in unpleasant sleep inertia. Patients and family members should also be warned about the potential dangers of sleepiness relative to driving and/or in other hazardous settings. Typically, lifestyle changes alone are not enough to adequately control the symptoms of either narcolepsy or idiopathic hypersomnia; most patients require lifelong medication.

Pharmacologic Management of Symptoms Common to Both Narcolepsy and Idiopathic Hypersomnia

Pharmacological management of EDS, with a few exceptions, is similar in both narcolepsy and idiopathic hypersomnia; however, it should be noted that randomized, double-blind, placebo-controlled clinical trials have not been done on idiopathic hypersomnia patients. Stimulants, such as methylphenidate or dextroamphetamine, have previously been used as first-line therapy. This transitioned to the use of modafinil and armodafinil as first-line treatment for most patients [81, 82], and more recently a newer agent, solriamfetol, might be the next agent that will gain acceptance as initial therapy for EDS treatment. Most clinical studies of stimulant medications report objective improvements in sleepiness in 65–85% of subjects.

Common adverse effects associated with stimulants include nervousness, headaches, irritability, tremor, insomnia, anorexia, gastrointestinal upset, and cardiovascular stimulation [83]. The development of drug tolerance or addiction can also occur; however, this risk is thought to be less than in other patient groups.

Modafinil is generally well tolerated, with headache and nausea being the most common side effects. Rarely, severe rashes and allergic reactions can occur. Modafinil also increases the metabolism of ethinylestradiol which lessens the efficacy of oral contraceptive agents. Armodafinil is the long-acting dextro-enantiomer component of racemic modafinil, which has equal amounts of S- and R-modafinil. It has a similar therapeutic and side effect profile to racemic modafinil, but with the advantage of having a longer elimination half-life ($t_{1/2}$) (3–4 h for S-modafinil vs. 10–15 h for armodafinil) [84]. Although comparative studies have not been done in narcolepsy or idiopathic hypersomnia, armodafinil has been shown to be effective and produce longer wakefulness than racemic modafinil in patients with sleepiness due to acute sleep loss [85].

Sodium oxybate, the sodium salt of gamma-hydroxybutyrate (GHB), an endogenous substance in the brain, is an effective medication in the treatment of daytime sleepiness cataplexy and sleep disruption in narcolepsy [81, 86, 87] and perhaps also the sleep-related hallucinations and sleep paralysis episodes prominent in this disorder. It is currently being studied in patients with idiopathic hypersomnia. Sodium oxybate's adverse effects include nausea (19%), dizziness (18% incidence), headache (18%), nasopharyngitis (6%), somnolence (6%), vomiting (8%), and urinary incontinence (6%) with most described as mild or moderate in severity. Dizziness, nausea, vomiting, and enuresis may be dose related [88].

Pitolisant is a medication that acts as an antagonist/inverse agonist on the histamine 3 receptors which results in increase of brain histamine levels that subsequently help maintain wakefulness. The more common adverse reactions include headaches, insomnia, nausea, and anxiety. Caution needs to be taken in patients at cardiac risk for prolonged QTc. As with modafinil, pitolisant also increases the metabolism of ethinylestradiol and therefore will lessen oral contraceptive efficacy. Although pitolisant does not currently have an FDA-approved indication to treat cataplexy, studies have also shown improvement in this symptom in treated NT1 patients [89, 90]. Alternative forms of H3 receptor inverse agonists are in investigation.

Solriamfetol works by inhibiting reuptake of both dopamine and norepinephrine. It has a similar adverse reaction profile to other medications with headache being most common followed by nausea, decreased appetite, nasopharyngitis, dry mouth, and anxiety. With its relatively unique mechanism of action, efficacy, and side effect profile, it has been increasingly used as first- or second-line therapy for the treatment of EDS [91]. It has an FDA-approved indication for the treatment of EDS in patients with narcolepsy.

Currently, sodium oxybate, amphetamines, methylphenidate, modafinil, armodafinil, solriamfetol, and pitolisant are the only medications FDA approved in the United States for the treatment of EDS in narcolepsy. Alterations of gamma amino butyric acid (GABA) levels in the brain with GABA-A receptor agonists (e.g., clarithromycin and flumazenil) have shown some efficacy in the treatment of EDS in narcolepsy patients [92]. Medications targeting the hypocretin receptors for the treatment of EDS are in development. One such medication currently undergoing clinical trials is TAK-994, which is a hypocretin-2 receptor selective agonist that has shown promise in preliminary studies. Other medications under investigation include a low sodium formulation of oxybate, and a new drug application (NDA) has been submitted for approval by the FDA. A long-acting, once-nightly formulation of sodium oxybate has been studied, and an NDA is about to be submitted. Reboxetine, a norepinephrine reuptake inhibitor, is currently undergoing evaluation in narcolepsy. Other medications have been reported to have beneficial results, but little data is available [93]. All medications are used "off-label" for the management of excessive sleepiness due to idiopathic hypersomnia.

Pharmacologic Management of Symptoms Specific to Narcolepsy

Cataplexy

Although treatment of sleepiness can have a mild beneficial effect on cataplexy, most wake-promoting agents/stimulants do not provide sufficient relief from cataplexy. Pitolisant, as mentioned earlier, has been shown to improve both EDS and cataplexy symptoms in patients with narcolepsy. Most medications used for the treatment of cataplexy have REM sleep suppressant properties and/or increase aminergic (mainly by blocking the norepinephrine (NE) transporter) activity [94]. Tricyclic antidepressants (TCAs), serotonin reuptake inhibitors, and NE reuptake inhibitors have demonstrated benefit in animal studies (which is believed to be a function of the NE reuptake inhibition). Sodium oxybate is highly efficacious for the treatment of cataplexy in narcolepsy and, as of the writing of this chapter, remains the only FDA-approved medication for its management.

Several small open-label studies and several decades of use have demonstrated that the TCAs desmethylimipramine, protriptyline, imipramine, and desipramine have beneficial anticataplectic effects [95]; however, clomipramine remains the most widely used. Adverse events commonly associated with TCA therapy include nausea, anorexia, dry mouth, urinary retention, and tachycardia. Men may encounter decreased libido, impotency, or delayed ejaculation. An unusual property of TCAs is the rebound cataplexy phenomenon that occurs upon abrupt discontinuation of TCA therapy. When severe, this is known as status cataplecticus and can be disabling for several days [96].

Similar to TCAs, the SSRIs including fluvoxamine, zimeldine, femoxetine, paroxetine, and fluoxetine have all demonstrated anticataplectic activity; however, fluoxetine appears to be the most commonly used of the SSRIs for the treatment of cataplexy [97]. As a class, the SSRIs are generally less efficacious than TCAs; however, they have a better safety profile and are better tolerated than the older antidepressants. Reported adverse events include headache, nausea, weight gain, dry mouth, and delayed ejaculation [97]. Other antidepressant medications have also been found to have some anticataplectic activity; these include monoamine oxidase inhibitors such as phenelzine and selegiline as well as other atypical antidepressants with pronounced NE reuptake inhibition, such as venlafaxine and atomoxetine.

Given the evidence supporting an autoimmune etiology of narcolepsy, intravenous immunoglobulin therapy (IVIG) has been used for the treatment of narcolepsy. Unfortunately, the studies evaluating its use are limited, and the few case reports have yielded conflicting results. Currently, it is not considered a valid treatment option [98].

Fragmented Nocturnal Sleep

As mentioned earlier, sodium oxybate taken at bedtime and again during the night increases slow wave sleep, decreases light sleep (stage N1 sleep), and decreases the number of arousals. REM sleep is initially increased, but then decreases after increasing dose and duration of therapy [87].

Other medications have also been tried in the management of the fragmented sleep of narcoleptics. A study evaluating 0.25 mg of triazolam taken at bedtime showed improved sleep efficiency and overall sleep quality, but had no beneficial effect on daytime sleepiness [99]. Unlike the GABA-A receptor agonists mentioned earlier, baclofen is actually a GABA B receptor agonist that has shown some efficacy in the treatment of EDS as well as sleep fragmentation in adolescent narcolepsy. Morse et al. described five patients that failed treatment with traditional narcolepsy medications, but reported subjective improvement in sleep maintenance and daytime sleepiness. Accordingly, baclofen may be an effective treatment option in narcolepsy that warrants further study [100]. Other medications such as zolpidem, eszopiclone, or clonazepam have been used with varying success in some patients (personal experience and conversations with other sleep medicine physicians). For symptoms of sleep paralysis and hypnagogic hallucinations, TCAs, other REM suppressant medications, and sodium oxybate have been successful.

Conclusion

Narcolepsy and idiopathic hypersomnia are primary central hypersomnias characterized by either EDS or prolonged nocturnal sleep. Whereas cataplexy is pathognomonic for narcolepsy, there is no pathognomonic symptom for idiopathic hypersomnia. Narcolepsy is believed to be due to a deficiency in hypocretin-producing neurons in the lateral hypothalamus, possibly as a result of an autoimmune disorder. The pathophysiology of idiopathic hypersomnia is currently unknown. The diagnosis is currently made by a combination of appropriate clinical symptoms, polysomnography followed by an MSLT and/or CSF hypocretin-1 testing. There are both nonpharmacologic and symptom directed pharmacologic treatments using medications targeting monoaminergic or GABA receptors. New formulations of oxybate and orexin receptor agonists are under investigation, as well as alternative NERIs and histaminergic medications. The effective pharmacologic management of narcolepsy is becoming a reality, although the treatment options are many and medication combinations are usually required for optimal management of cataplexy and excessive sleepiness.

Summary of Keypoints
- Narcolepsy is a syndrome consisting of EDS, cataplexy, sleep paralysis, and hypnagogic hallucinations. Additional features include automatic behaviors and fragmented or disrupted nighttime sleep.
- Classic narcolepsy symptoms are difficult to identify in children as sleepiness may manifest as inattentiveness, lack of energy, behavioral problems, or decreased performance.
- Cataplexy is the most specific symptom of narcolepsy consisting of an abrupt, bilateral loss of skeletal muscle tone, triggered by sudden emotion such as laughter. Cataplexy is seen in 60–90% of patients with narcolepsy.
- Poor nighttime sleep is also common in narcolepsy, due to a dysfunction of central sleep regulation which causes frequent transitions between sleep and wakefulness throughout the entire 24-h cycle.
- Most cases of NT1 are associated with reduced or absent csf hypocretin; cases of NT2 may be caused by a partial loss of hypocretin-containing hypothalamic neurons.
- Sleep disturbances, including excessive sleepiness, may occur following TBI. It is important to consider TBI among the causes of EDS.
- Appropriate sleep hygiene is critically important in patients with narcolepsy or idiopathic hypersomnia. Short naps (15–20 min) 2–3 times/day can help control sleepiness in narcolepsy and improve alertness. However, scheduled naps are not recommended in idiopathic hypersomnia.
- Alerting medications are the mainstay of management of daytime sleepiness in patients with narcolepsy or idiopathic hypersomnia, with most clinical studies reporting objective improvements in sleepiness in 65–85% of subjects. Cataplexy can be effectively treated with oxybate, H3 receptor inverse agonists, or NERIs.
- New formulations of current medications and orexin receptor agonists are currently under investigation and hold promise of greatly improving patient management.

References

1. Nevsimalova S. Narcolepsy in childhood. Sleep Med Rev. 2009;13(2):169–80.
2. Roth B. Narcolepsy and hypersomnia. Basel: Karger; 1980. p. 66–77.
3. American Academy of Sleep Medicine. International classification of sleep disorders. 3rd ed. Darien: American Academy of Sleep Medicine; 2014.
4. Krahn LE, Lymp JF, Moore WR, Slocumb N, Silber MH. Characterizing the emotions that trigger cataplexy. J Neuropsychiatry Clin Neurosci. 2005;17:45–50.
5. Overeem S, Mignot E, van Dijk JG, et al. Narcolepsy: clinical features, new pathological insights, and future perspectives. J Clin Neurophysiol. 2001;18:78–105.
6. Barateau L, Pizza F, Lopez R, et al. Persistence of deep-tendon reflexes during partial cataplexy. Sleep Med. 2018;45:80–2.
7. Serra L, Montagna P, Mignot E, et al. Cataplexy features in childhood narcolepsy. Mov Disord. 2008;23(6):858–65.
8. Plazzi G, Clawges HM, Owens J. Clinical characteristics and burden of illness in pediatric patients with narcolepsy. Pediatr Neurol. 2018;85:21–32.
9. Vernet C, Arnulf I. Idiopathic hypersomnia with and without long sleep time: a controlled series of 75 patients. Sleep. 2009;32:753–9.
10. Guilleminault C, Fromherz S. Narcolepsy: diagnosis and management. In: Kryger MH, Roth TA, Dement WC, editors. Principles and practice of sleep medicine. Philadelphia: WB Saunders; 2005. p. 780.
11. Bassetti C, Aldrich MS. Idiopathic hypersomnia: a series of 42 patients. Brain. 1997;120(8):1423–35.
12. Sforza E, Roche F, Barthelemy JC, et al. Diurnal and nocturnal cardiovascular variability and heart rate arousal response in idiopathic hypersomnia. Sleep Med. 2016;24:131–6.
13. Mayer G, Kesper K, Peter H, Ploch T, Leinweber T, et al. Comorbidity in narcoleptic patients. Dtsch Med Wochenschr. 2002;127(38):1942–6. German.
14. Kryger MH, Walid R, Manfreda J. Diagnoses received by narcolepsy patients in the year prior to diagnosis by a sleep specialist. Sleep. 2002;25(1):36–41.
15. Ohayon MM, Ferini-Strambi L, Plazzi G, et al. Frequency of narcolepsy symptoms and other sleep disorders in narcoleptic patients and their first-degree relatives. J Sleep Res. 2005;14(4):437–45.
16. Ohayon MM, Ferini-Strambi L, Plazzi G, et al. How age influences the expression of narcolepsy. J Psychosom Res. 2005;59(6):399–405.
17. Mignot E. Genetic and familial aspects of narcolepsy. Neurology. 1998;50(2 Suppl 1):S16–22.
18. Mignot E, Lin L, Rogers W, et al. Complex HLA-DR and -DQ interactions confer risk of narcolepsy-cataplexy in three ethnic groups. Am J Hum Genet. 2001;68:686–99.
19. Silber MH, Krahn LE, Olson EJ, et al. The epidemiology of narcolepsy in Olmsted County, Minnesota: a population-based study. Sleep. 2002;25(2):197–202.
20. Vignatelli L, d'Alessandro R, Mosconi P, et al. Health-related quality of life in Italian patients with narcolepsy: the SF-36 health survey. Sleep Med. 2004;5:467–75.
21. Heier MS, Evsiukova T, Vilming S, et al. CSF hypocretin-1 levels and clinical profiles in narcolepsy and idiopathic CNS hypersomnia in Norway. Sleep. 2007;30:969–73.
22. Dauvilliers Y, Paquereau J, Bastuji H, et al. Psychological health in central hypersomnias: the French Harmony Study. J Neurol Neurosurg Psychiatry. 2009;80:636–41.
23. Billiard M, Dauvilliers Y. Idiopathic hypersomnia. Sleep Med Rev. 2001;5(5):349–58.
24. Aldrich MS. The clinical spectrum of narcolepsy and idiopathic hypersomnia. Neurology. 1996;46:393–401.
25. Anderson KN, Pilsworth S, Sharples LD, et al. Idiopathic hypersomnia: a study of 77 cases. Sleep. 2007;30:1274–81.
26. Billiard M, Merle C, Carlander B, et al. Idiopathic hypersomnia. Psychiatry Clin Neurosci. 1998;52(2):125–9.

27. Nishino S, Ripley B, Overeem S, et al. Hypocretin (orexin) deficiency in human narcolepsy. Lancet. 2000;355:39–40.
28. Zeitzer JM, Nishino S, Mignot E. The neurobiology of hypocretins (orexins), narcolepsy and related therapeutic interventions. Trends Pharmacol Sci. 2006;27(7):368–74.
29. Barateau L, Lopez R, Dauvilliers Y. Clinical neurophysiology of CNS hypersomnias. Handb Clin Neurol. 2019;161:353–67.
30. Thannickal TC, Moore RY, Niehus R, et al. Reduced number of hypocretin neurons in human narcolepsy. Neuron. 2000;27:469–74.
31. Mignot E, Lammers GJ, Ripley B, et al. The role of cerebrospinal fluid hypocretin measurement in the diagnosis of narcolepsy and other hypersomnias. Arch Neurol. 2002;59:1553–62.
32. Thannickal TC, Nienhuis R, Siegel JM. Localized loss of hypocretin (orexin) cells in narcolepsy without cataplexy. Sleep. 2009;32(8):993–8.
33. Scammell TE. The frustrating and mostly fruitless search for an autoimmune cause of narcolepsy. Sleep. 2006;29(5):601–2.
34. Black JL III. Narcolepsy: a review of evidence for autoimmune diathesis. Int Rev Psychiatry. 2005;17(6):461–9.
35. Dauvilliers Y, Tafti M. Molecular genetics and treatment of narcolepsy. Ann Med. 2006;38(4):252–62.
36. Tanaka S, Honda Y, Inoue Y, et al. Detection of autoantibodies against hypocretin, hcrtrl, and hcrtr2 in narcolepsy: anti-Hcrt system antibody in narcolepsy. Sleep. 2006;29(5):633–8.
37. Lippert J, Young P, Gross C, et al. Specific T-celll activation in peripheral blood and cerebrospinal fluid in central disorders of hypersomnolence. Sleep. 2019;1:42(2).
38. Dye TJ, Gurbani N, Simakajornboon N. Epidemiology and pathophysiology of childhood narcolepsy. Paediatr Respir Rev. 2018;25:14–8.
39. Halberg P, Smedje H, Eriksson N, et al. Pandemrix-induced narcolepsy is associated with genes related to immunity and neuronal survival. EBioMedicine. 2019;40:595–604.
40. Aran A, Lin L, Nevsimalova S, et al. Elevated anti-streptococcal antibodies in patients with recent narcolepsy onset. Sleep. 2009;32(8):979–83.
41. Picchioni D, Hope CR, Harsh JR. A case-control study of the environmental risk factors for narcolepsy. Neuroepidemiology. 2007;29(3–4):185–92.
42. Castriotta RJ, Wilde MC, Lai JM, et al. Prevalence and consequences of sleep disorders in traumatic brain injury. J Clin Sleep Med. 2007;3(4):349–56.
43. Mori I. The olfactory bulb: A link between environmental agents and narcolepsy,from the standpoint of autoimmune etiology. Med Hypothesis. 2019;131:109294.
44. Mori I. The olfactory bulb: a link between environmental agents and narcolepsy. Med Hypothesis. 2019;126:66–8.
45. Longstreth WT Jr, Ton TG, Koepsell TD. Narcolepsy and streptococcal infections. Sleep. 2009;32(12):1548.
46. Hallmayer J, Faraco J, Lin L, et al. Narcolepsy is strongly associated with the T-cell receptor alpha locus. Nat Genet. 2009;41:708–11.
47. Cvetkovic V, Bayer L, Dorsaz S, et al. Tribbles homolog 2 as an autoantigen in human narcolepsy. J Clin Invest. 2010;120:713–9.
48. Tanaka S, Honda Y, Honda M, et al. Anti-Tribbles Pseudokinase 2 (TRIB2)-immunization modulates hypocretin/orexin neuronal functions. Sleep. 2017;40(1). https://doi.org/10.1093/sleep/zsw036.
49. Dauvilliers Y, Baumann CR, Carlander B, et al. CSF hypocretin-1 levels in narcolepsy, Kleine-Levin syndrome, and other hypersomnias and neurological conditions. J Neurol Neurosurg Psychiatry. 2003;74:1667–73.
50. Montplaisir J, de Champlain J, Young SN, et al. Narcolepsy and idiopathic hypersomnia: biogenic amines and related compounds in CSF. Neurology. 1982;32:1299–302.
51. Faull KF, Guilleminault C, Berger PA, et al. Cerebrospinal fluid monoamine metabolites in narcolepsy and hypersomnia. Ann Neurol. 1983;13:258–63.

52. Faull KF, Thiemann S, King RJ, et al. Monoamine interactions in narcolepsy and hypersomnia: a preliminary report. Sleep. 1986;9:246–9.
53. Bassetti CL, Khatami R, Poryazova R, et al. Idiopathic hypersomnia: a dopaminergic disorder. Sleep. 2009;32:A248–9.
54. Arnulf I, Leu-Semenescu S, Dodet P. Precision medicine for idiopathic hypersomnia. Sleep Med Clin. 2019;14(3):333–50.
55. Nishino S, Sakurai E, Nevsimalova S, et al. Decreased CSF histamine in narcolepsy with and without low CSF hypocretin-1 in comparison to healthy controls. Sleep. 2009;32:175–80.
56. Kanbayashi T, Kodama T, Kondo H, et al. CSF histamine contents in narcolepsy, idiopathic hypersomnia and obstructive sleep apnea syndrome. Sleep. 2009;32:181–7.
57. Dauvilliers Y, Delallee N, Jaussent I, et al. Normal cerebrospinal fluid histamine and tele-methylhistamine levels in hypersomnia conditions. Sleep. 2012;35:1359–66.
58. Rack M, Davis J, Roffwarg HP, et al. The multiple sleep latency test in the diagnosis of narcolepsy. Am J Psychiatry. 2005;162(11):2198–9.
59. Ferri R, Franceschini C, Zucconi M, et al. Sleep polygraphic study of children and adolescents with narcolepsy/cataplexy. Dev Neuropsychol. 2009;34(5):523–38.
60. Carskadon MA. The second decade. In: Guilleminault C, editor. Sleeping and waking disorders: indications and techniques. Menlo Park: Addison-Wesley; 1982. p. 99–125.
61. Pizza F, Barateau L, Jaussent I, et al. Validation of multiple sleep latency test for the diagnosis of pediatric narcolepsy type 1. Neurology. 2019;93(11):e1034–44.
62. Mayer G, Lammers GJ. The MSLT: more objections than benefits as a diagnostic gold standard? Sleep. 2014;37:1027–8.
63. Baumann CR. Bassetti CI Hypocretin (orexins) and sleep-wakedisorders. Lancet Neurol. 2005;10:673–82.
64. Sakai N, Matsumura M, Lin L, et al. HLPC analysis of CSF hypocretin-1 in type 1 and 2 narcolepsy. Sci Rep. 2019;9:477.
65. Basseti CL, Adamantidis A, Burdakov D, et al. Narcolepsy - clinical spectrum, aetiopathophysiology, diagnosis and treatment. Nat Rev Neurol. 2019;15(9):519–39.
66. Stephansen JB, Olesen AN, Olsen M, et al. Neural network analysis of sleep stages enables efficient diagnosis of narcolepsy. Nat Commun. 2018;9(1):5229.
67. Bin-Hasan S, Videnovic A, Maski K. Nocturnal REM sleep without atonia is a diagnostic biomarker of pediatric narcolepsy. J Clin Sleep Med. 2018;14(2):245–52.
68. Murer T, Imbach LL, Hackius M, et al. OptimizingMSLT specificity in narcolepsy with cataplexy. Sleep. 2017;1:40(12).
69. Chritensen JAE, Kempfner L, Leonthin HL, et al. Novel method for evaluation ofeye movements in patients with narcolepsy. Sleep Med. 2017;33:171–80.
70. Aslan S, Erbil N, Tezer FI. Heart rate variability during nocturnal sleep and daytime naps in patients with narcolepsy type 1 and type 2. J Clin Neurophysiol. 2019;36(2):104–11.
71. Sieminski M, Chwojnicki K, Sarkanen T, et al. The relationship between orexin levels and blood pressure changes in patients with narcolepsy. PLoS One. 2017;12(10):e0185975.
72. Hong SB. Neuroimaging of narcolepsy and Kleine-Levin syndrome. Sleep Med Clin. 2017;12(3):359–68.
73. Black J, Reaven NL, Funk SE. Medical comorbidity in narcolepsy: findings from the burden of narcolepsy disease (BOND) study. Sleep Med. 2017;33:13–8.
74. Ruoff CM, Reaven NL, Funk SE. High rates of psychiatric comorbidity in narcolepsy: findings from the burden of narcolepsy Dise ofase (BOND) study of 9312 patients in the United States. J Clin Psychiatry. 2017;78(2):171–6.
75. Maestri M, Monzani F, Bonanni E, et al. Insulinoma presenting as idiopathic hypersomnia. Neurol Sci. 2010;31(3):349–52.
76. Shinno H, Inami Y, Inagaki T, et al. Successful treatment with levothyroxine for idiopathic hypersomnia patients with subclinical hypothyroidism. Gen Hosp Psychiatry. 2009;31(2):190–3.

77. Masel BE, Scheibel RS, Kimbark T, et al. Excessive daytime sleepiness in adults with brain injuries. Arch Phys Med Rehabil. 2001;82(11):1526–32.

78. Dl P, Ponsford JL, Rajaratnam SM, et al. Self reported changes to nighttime sleep after traumatic brain injury. Arch Phys Med Rehabil. 2006;87(2):278–85.

79. Baumann CR, Werth E, Stocker R, et al. Sleep-wake disturbances 6 months after traumatic brain injury: a prospective study. Brain. 2007;130(Pt 7):1873–83.

80. Baumann CR, Bassetti CL, Valko PO, et al. Loss of hypocretin (orexin) neurons with traumatic brain injury. Ann Neurol. 2009;66(4):555–9.

81. Black J, Guilleminault C. Medications for the treatment of narcolepsy. Expert Opin Emerg Drugs. 2001;6(2):239–47.

82. Didato G, Nobili L. Treatment of narcolepsy. Expert Rev Neurother. 2009;9(6):897–910.

83. Mitler MM, Hayduk R. Benefits and risks of pharmacotherapy for narcolepsy. Drug Saf. 2002;25:791–809.

84. Harsh JR, Hayduk R, Rosenberg R, et al. The efficacy and safety of armodafinil as treatment for adults with excessive sleepiness associated with narcolepsy. Curr Med Res Opin. 2006;22(4):761–74.

85. Dinges DF, Arora S, Darwish M, et al. Pharmacodynamic effects on alertness of single doses of armodafinil in healthy subjects during a nocturnal period of acute sleep loss. Curr Med Res Opin. 2006;22(1):159–67.

86. U.S. Xyrem® International Study Group. A double blind placebo controlled study demonstrates sodium oxybate is effective for the treatment of excessive sleepiness in narcolepsy. J Clin Sleep Med. 2005;1(4):391–7.

87. U.S. Xyrem® Multicenter Study Group. Sodium oxybate demonstrates long-term efficacy for the treatment of cataplexy in patients with narcolepsy. Sleep Med. 2004;5:119–23.

88. Xyrem® Product Information, Orphan Medical, Inc.

89. Li S, Yang J. Pitolisant for treating patients with narcolepsy. Expert Rev Clin Pharmacol. 2020;13(2):79–84.

90. Dauvilliers Y, Arnulf I, Szakacs Z, et al. Long-term Use of Pitolisant to Treat Patients with Narcolepsy: Harmony III Study. Sleep. 2019;42(11):zsz174.

91. Thorpy MJ, Shapiro C, Mayer G, et al. A randomized study of solriamfetol for excessive daytime sleepiness in narcolepsy. Ann Neurol. 2019;85(3):359–70.

92. Abad VC. Guilleminault. New developments in the management of narcolepsy. Nat Sci Sleep. 2017;9:39–57.

93. Morgenthaler TI, Kapur VK, Brown T, et al. Practice parameters for the treatment of narcolepsy and other hypersomnias of central origin. Sleep. 2007;30(12):1705–11.

94. Guilleminault C, Raynal D, Takahashi S, et al. Evaluation of short-term and long-term treatment of the narcolepsy syndrome with clomipramine hydrochloride. Acta Neurol Scand. 1976;54:71–87.

95. Houghton WC, Scammell TE, Thorpy M. Pharmacotherapy for cataplexy. Sleep Med Rev. 2004;8:355–66.

96. Martinez-Rodriguez J, Iranzo A, Santamaria J, et al. Status cataplecticus induced by abrupt withdrawal of clomipramine. Neurologia. 2002;17:113–6.

97. Frey J, Darbonne C. Fluoxetine suppresses human cataplexy: a pilot study. Neurology. 1994;44:707–9.

98. Ruppert E, Zagalaa H, Chambe J, et al. Intravenous immunoglobulin therapy administered early after narcolepsy type 1 onset in three patients evaluated by clinical and polysomnographic follow-up. Behav Neurol. 2018;2018:1671–2.

99. Thorpy MJ, Snyder M, Aloe FS, et al. Short-term triazolam use improves nocturnal sleep of narcoleptics. Sleep. 1992;15(3):212–6.

100. Morse AM, Kelly-Pieper K, Kothare SV. Management of excessive daytime sleepiness in narcolepsy with baclofen. Pediatr Neurol. 2019;93:39–42.

Chapter 16
Non-REM Parasomnias

Nathan A. Walker and Bradley V. Vaughn

Keywords Parasomnia · Disorders of arousal · Sleepwalking · Sleep terror
Confusional arousal REM sleep behavior disorder · Sleep-related eating disorder
Exploding head syndrome

Introduction

Parasomnias are defined as "undesirable physical events or experiences that occur during entry into sleep, within sleep, or during arousal from sleep" [1]. As part of a larger collection of nocturnal events, parasomnias are included in the pathologies that produce behaviors and occurrences at night. Many envision these events as entertaining stories from family or roommates, or may be thought of as strange inexplicable incidents. The clinical symptoms of parasomnias include complex purposeful movements, unusual behaviors, perceptions, or emotional experiences. Many of the parasomnias are very common in the general population, especially in children. Although the majority of parasomnias are not harmful, injuries, sleep disruption, and psychosocial impairment can result from the events, and these events provide the opportunity to diagnose underlying sleep disorders or medical issues that may provoke the events. Therefore, it is useful to know the symptoms, clinical associations, and treatment options to guide patients.

In early nomenclature, parasomnias were categorized based upon the most prominent behavior. Some remnants of this convention still exist in terms such as sleepwalking and sleep-related eating. However, as we have furthered our understanding of the neuronal circuits determining the states of sleep and wake, we have grouped events toward the originating sleep-wake state while acknowledging pathologies

N. A. Walker · B. V. Vaughn (✉)
Department of Neurology, University of North Carolina, Chapel Hill, NC, USA
e-mail: vaughnb@neurology.unc.edu

© Springer Nature Switzerland AG 2022
M. S. Badr, J. L. Martin (eds.), *Essentials of Sleep Medicine*,
Respiratory Medicine, https://doi.org/10.1007/978-3-030-93739-3_16

that are held in common [1]. The brain's three distinct states of wake and NREM and REM sleep allow us to understand the starting physiological state that provides the substrate for some of these parasomnias. Thus parasomnias may be associated with NREM sleep, REM sleep, or the transitions between wake and sleep as a platform which demonstrates the underlying pathology. The current categorization in the International Classification of Sleep Disorders third edition (ICSD 3) divides the parasomnias into four main categories: NREM-related parasomnias, REM-related parasomnias, other parasomnias, and normal variants (Table 16.1). This context includes consideration of the drivers for the parasomnias as well as how to separate mimics that may present with similar behaviors.

This classification scheme also allows us to ultimately move toward a classification structure more aligned with physiology and subsequently underlying pathology. Several parasomnias represent a mixture of states [2]. This model is best demonstrated when considering the non-REM sleep-related parasomnias, disorders of arousals. The disorders of arousals (sleep terrors, sleepwalking, and confusional arousals) are associated with a mixture of features of NREM sleep with some wake-like behaviors. These disorders represent a continuum of complex behaviors that share features of NREM sleep, such as minimal cognitive functioning and amnesia for the events, with features of the awake state such as complex motor patterns and eyes open (Table 16.2) [1]. Commonly these events are triggered by stimuli during deeper NREM sleep and involve a variety of nonstereotyped behaviors. One REM-related parasomnia, recurrent isolated sleep paralysis, also represents a mixture of wake and REM sleep. Although many times associated with narcolepsy, these

Table 16.1 Outline of parasomnias

1. Non-REM parasomnias
(a) Disorders of arousal
(i) Confusional arousals
(ii) Sleepwalking
(iii) Sleep terrors
(b) Sleep-related eating disorder
2. REM-related parasomnias
(a) REM sleep behavior disorder
(b) Recurrent isolated sleep paralysis
(c) Nightmare disorder
3. Other parasomnias
(a) Exploding head syndrome
(b) Sleep-related hallucinations
(c) Sleep enuresis
(d) Parasomnia due to a medical disorder
(e) Parasomnia due to a medication or substance
(f) Parasomnia, unspecified
4. Isolated symptoms and normal variants
(a) Sleep talking

Table 16.2 Distinguishing features of nocturnal events. Reprinted with permission from Bradley Vaughn

Feature	Disorders of arousal	Sleep-related eating disorder	REM sleep behavior disorder	Recurrent isolated sleep paralysis	Exploding head syndrome	Psychogenic events	Nocturnal seizures
Behavior	Confused; semipurposeful movement with eyes open	Eating typically high-calorie foods; eyes open	Sometimes combative with eyes closed	Episodes of inability to move	Painless sensation of explosion inside the head	Variable	Dependent on the portion of brain involved
Age of onset	Childhood and adolescence	Variable	Older adult	Variable	Adult	Adolescence to adulthood	Variable
Time of occurrence	First third of night	First half of night	During REM	Typically on awakening	Usually near sleep onset but can be variable	Anytime	Anytime
Frequency of events	Less than one per night	Variable	Multiple per night	Variable less than weekly	Rare	Variable	Frontal seizures—multiple per night
Duration	Minutes	Minutes	Seconds to minute	Seconds to minutes	Seconds	Variable minutes or longer	Usually under 3 minutes
Memory of event	Usually none	Usually none or limited	Dream recall	Yes	Yes	None	Usually none
Eyes open or closed	Eyes open	Eyes open	Eyes closed	Eyes closed	Eyes closed but immediately open following the event	Variable	Variable
Stereotypical movements	No	No	No	No	Similar sensation	No	Yes
Polysomnogram findings	Arousals from slow wave sleep	Arousal from NREM sleep	Excessive electromyogram tone during REM sleep	Arousal from REM sleep	Usually occurs in light sleep	Occur from awake state	Potentially epileptiform activity

events in isolation are related to the intrusion of REM sleep-related paralysis into wakefulness [3, 4]. Other REM sleep parasomnias such as nightmare disorder and REM sleep behavior disorder are confined to the state. The latter is an example of neurological impairment of the circuitry that produces the REM sleep associated paralysis [5]. This disorder represents an example of how sleep dedicated neural circuitry may be uniquely more vulnerable to specific types of degeneration or injury.

Many of the "other parasomnias" represent events that occur during the transition between wake and sleep (Table 16.1). Some sensory events such as exploding head syndrome and sleep-related hallucinations are events that may occur as the patient enters light sleep, but may also occur upon awakening. Additionally, in this group are parasomnias that occur across the spectrum of sleep states or represent a loss of sleep-wake state distinction.

The goal of this chapter is to review the variety of disorders classified as parasomnias. This chapter provides a framework for parasomnias and outlines an overarching approach to patients with nocturnal events. The text reviews the known pathology and the possible drivers for the parasomnias as well as describes mimics that may present with similar behaviors. The challenge for the ardent clinician is to utilize historical and physical examination clues with the appropriate investigative tools to discern the underlying causes and propose appropriate therapy to improve the patient's condition.

Non-REM Related Parasomnias

As the name implicates, non-rapid eye movement (NREM) sleep-related parasomnias are parasomnia events that arise from NREM sleep. This group includes the disorders of arousal and sleep-related eating disorder. As a whole, the episodes may include a variety of complex movements that range a variety of basic behaviors. These parasomnias are classically thought of as partial triggered awakenings with retention of some features of sleep. Each of these disorders has their own criteria for diagnosis and unique features.

Disorders of Arousal

The International Classification of Sleep Disorders, 3rd edition (ICSD-3) defines disorders of arousal by specific universal features and then specific findings for the subdivisions of confusional arousals, and sleepwalking and sleep terrors. The disorders of arousal (DOA), as a group, have several common manifestations that define the cluster, while each also has unique features in behavior that allow their distinction. For the group of DOA, the ICSD-3 requires several features to be present to qualify as a DOA (Table 16.3).

Table 16.3 Features of disorders of arousal (adapted from ICSD-3)

1. Recurrent episodes of incomplete awakening from sleep
2. Inappropriate or absent responsiveness to intervention from observers or from others attempting to redirect the person during the episode
3. Limited or no associated cognition or dream imagery
4. Partial or complete amnesia for the episode
5. The disturbance is not better explained by other medical, psychiatric or sleep conditions or medications, or substance use

Furthermore, these three diagnoses share clinical features that help clinicians identify these as NREM sleep events. The majority of events occur in the first third of sleep and are relatively brief. Most of the events in disorders of arousal last for 30 seconds to a few minutes, but some may last up to 30 minutes. Many times, patients have their eyes open but have a glassy confused stare. They may be partially reactive to the environment and even may appear disoriented for several minutes following the events. During the events, patients lack higher cognitive processing and appear to be functioning unconsciously. These patients are difficult to awaken from the events, and stimulation may result in the patients becoming agitated. Following the event patients may have partial or total amnesia, although adults are more likely to remember portions of the episodes. These disorders are most common in children and typically improve with age. Males and females are equally represented in disorders of arousal, and family history of events is in nearly two thirds of carefully screened cases.

Pathology

The vast majority of patients with disorder of arousal are neurologically and psychologically normal. When examining the sleep physiology in these patients, the studies show relatively normal sleep architecture. On sleep studies the onset of NREM parasomnia is an abrupt arousal, usually from stage N3 sleep with the patients having a dull confused look on video. Some studies have shown increased spontaneous awakening or arousals from slow wave sleep, and some investigators have found increased runs of hypersynchronous delta waves just prior to events [6, 7]. These studies have suggested increased slow wave activity and slow oscillations in EEG patterns prior to sleepwalking events. These findings suggest that the pathology is related to incomplete switching of deeper NREM sleep to wake. Examination of the gross structure of the brain shows little differences between patients and control subjects. However, Heidbreder reported that subjects with NREM parasomnias had smaller gray volume of the dorsal posterior cingulate when compared to nonparasomnia controls using magnetic resonance imaging (MRI) and diffusion tensor imaging (DTI) [8]. Further studies using depth EEG electrode recordings showed that disorder of arousal events activated the motor and central cingulate cortex while deactivating the hippocampal and association cortices [9, 10]. This activation pattern of cingulate motor area while deactivation of other association cortices was seen using Single-Photon Emission Computed Tomography (SPECT) when tracer was injected during a sleepwalking episode [11]. Furthermore, studies of network function related to frontal inhibition elicited by transcranial magnetic stimulation (TMS) showed that sleepwalkers have an impaired efficiency of inhibitory circuits [12]. Based on their results, the authors postulated that sleepwalkers have a dysfunction of both GABA-A and cholinergic pathways leading to an inability to maintain slow wave sleep and suppress partial arousals in sleep. As part of testing this functional inhibition, another study of sleepwalkers showed they had greater impairment of inhibitory control resulting in increased errors on Stroop Color Word Test and errors of commission on Continuous Performance Test following 25 hours of sleep deprivation [13]. These studies appear to suggest that the typical processes that inhibit specific portions of the subclinical arousals are not sufficient in suppressing these partial arousals. Thus patients with disorders of arousal are more vulnerable to activity that produces arousals from NREM sleep.

Associated Conditions

Disorders of arousal have been reported with a variety of medical disorders including endocrinological, vascular, neurological, and sleep disorders. Case reports of new onset DOA have described right thalamic lesion, breathing disorder with Chiari I malformation, hyperthyroidism, and diabetes [14–16]. Historically, disorders of arousal were thought to be associated with depression and anxiety. However, more recent studies show no relationship of these disorders to psychopathology [17, 18]. One caveat is that sleep terrors in children do not usually present with psychopathology, but it may play a larger role in adults with sleep terrors [19].

The most common sleep disorder associated with NREM parasomnias is obstructive sleep apnea. Several studies have suggested the link of breathing disorders increasing the frequency of disorder of arousal events. Goodwin found that children with even mild upper airways disturbance were significantly more likely to have parasomnia events than those without any disturbance [20]. Similarly in adults, Lundetræ reported that sleepwalking has a higher prevalence in patients with severe OSA than those with mild OSA [21]. These reports highlight that disorders of arousal events may signal the presence of other sleep disorders and that patients with NREM parasomnias may benefit from investigation and treatment of these disorders.

Some disorder of arousal events appear to be elicited by specific medications. Medications such as antidepressants, antipsychotic agents, beta blockers, and GABA modulators have been reported as possible agents that can trigger events. Of these, the most well recognized are the short-acting hypnotic agents, such as zolpidem or sodium oxybate. These medications are linked to increase frequency of sleepwalking and confusional arousal events. This association raises the possible question that the mechanism is impairment of arousal circuitry caused by the medication [22].

Diagnosis

The gold standard for making the diagnosis of DOA is capturing an event arising from NREM sleep on polysomnography (PSG). This finding helps elucidate the key features of a mixture of wake and NREM sleep (Fig. 16.1). This testing also can shed some light if the patient is having other sleep issues, such as sleep apnea, that may be provoking the nocturnal events. Fois showed, in a study of 124 subjects, that PSG confirmed parasomnia diagnosis in up to 60% of their study group [23]. PSG was also helpful in identifying other diagnoses that may mimic the parasomnia. Video PSG can capture the events in detail, and these events may show a spectrum of behaviors from appearing awake and confused to non-agitated motor activity to events with extreme emotional distress. These events typically arise from stage N3 sleep but less commonly occur from N2 sleep. Although recording spontaneous

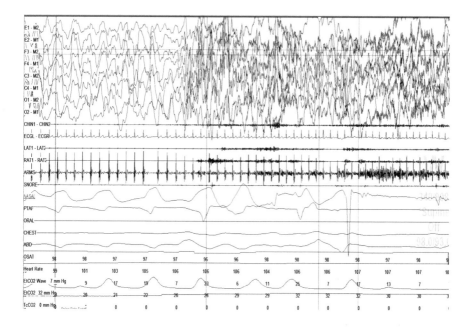

Fig. 16.1 This figure shows a standard polysomnogram during a confusional arousal in a 7-year-old boy. The patient is with eyes open during the event and has a confused look on his face. (Reprinted with permission from Bradley Vaughn MD)

parasomnia activity during PSG is uncommon, Pilon tested a technique that provoked events in nearly all of their subjects [24]. In their protocol, subjects with a history of sleepwalking were kept awake through the night and then allowed to sleep during the day. Once the subjects entered stage N3, an auditory stimulus was introduced to cause an arousal. Nearly all of the patients had a subsequent event. This study has yet to be repeated, but offers a possibility of a higher yield of events.

Management

Management of patients with disorders of arousal focuses on three major areas: safety, decreasing the frequency of events, and determining the possibility of other underlying provocative factors. The clinician initially needs to assess the possibility of harm from the events to the patient or family members. Many patients may have events without leaving the bed and have little chance of harm. For these patients reassurance is an important component in the treatment plan. For all cases, the patients and their families should be counselled on a safe sleeping environment and how to safely interact with the patient when they are having an event. For those at risk, placing the bed on the floor, securing windows and doors, and eliminating any access to sharp or dangerous objects are key. For some patients having their bedroom on the first floor to avoid falling or the use of door alarms is helpful.

Management may also focus on the predisposing, priming, and precipitating factors of what is called the three P model of NREM parasomnias [25]. The predisposing factors such as genetics, thus understanding family history, may help families be aware of the risks. Priming factors include medication that may increase the arousal threshold, e.g., Z-drugs; sleep deprivation which can increase the amount of SWS and increase arousal threshold; or substances that may increase arousals, caffeine or alcohol. Precipitating factors can include pain, a sleeping environment unconducive to sleep, and a myriad of other sleep disorders. Therefore, targeting good sleep hygiene, avoidance of priming substances/situations, and precipitating factors are useful tactics to reduce events. Tracking the frequency of events on a calendar may help identify patterns that lead to clues of provoking agents, as well as response to therapies.

Patients and their families may look for sources of arousals to reduce, such as environmental noise or stimuli as well as keeping a regular sleep schedule and avoiding sleep deprivation. Anticipatory awakening therapy is one behavioral therapy that is shown to be successful in children in reducing the frequency of events [26]. For this therapy the patient is allowed to go to sleep but awoken anywhere from 10 to 30 minutes prior to the typical time of the event. This is repeated for 2–3 weeks, and then the patient is assessed for further events. If the patient does resume having events, another round of awakenings can be performed. For a small minority of patients, medication is needed. Due to a lack of case control studies or randomized control trials, recommendations at times can be contradictory. Clinically, patients appear to respond to agents such as clonazepam or longer-acting benzodiazepines. In one series of 69 patients treated with these agents, 86% showed improvement [27]. Several case reports have suggested response to imipramine, trazadone, or paroxetine [28–30].

Confusional Arousals

Confusional arousals are the events of disorder of arousal in which the patient neither shows a prominent fear reaction nor ambulates. This diagnosis can include a
wide variety of behaviors that range from mild sitting with a confused look to complex actions appearing to meet a variety of basic needs. Patients may engage in a
range of emotions from amorous to aggressive outbursts, and behaviors can include
a variety of common everyday activities to more intrusive events including eating
and sexual behaviors.

Clinical Presentation

Confusional arousals are one of the disorders of arousal from NREM sleep [1].
Patients appear to be both asleep and awake. As the name implies, the patient
appears very confused. The patient is typically in bed, and the event commonly
involves the patient sitting upright with their eyes open and looking around. The
patient is often unresponsive or poorly responsive to questions or commands, and
some sleep talking may occur. The events are associated with partial or total amnesia and typically last only a few minutes with the person returning to sleep.
Confusional arousals occur in the first third of the night, predominantly from N3 or
slow wave sleep (SWS), when SWS is most likely to occur.

Epidemiology

Confusional arousals are more common in children than adults. Although these
events are nearly ubiquitous in children under the age of 3 years, the events are
noted to occur in 20–50% of preschool to school aged children [2]. These events are
present in up to 1–4% of young adults and as possibly as high as 7% in older adults
[26, 31]. The true incidence in all age groups is likely higher due to lack of reporting
and/or observation of events.

Pathophysiology

It is thought that confusional arousals and the other disorders of arousal (sleepwalking and night terrors) are due to a dissociation between the wake state and NREM
sleep. There is an incomplete arousal from NREM sleep that tends to occur in the
first third of the night when SWS predominates. However, 20% of cases may occur
from N2 or Stage 2 sleep [31, 32]. The preponderance of NREM parasomnias in
children may be due to the increased amounts of SWS as compared to adults.
Arousal thresholds are also at their highest during SWS. Substances or scenarios

that increase the arousal threshold can increase the likelihood of disorders of arousal, such as sleep aides and sleep deprivation, respectively [31]. Conversely, agents that increase arousals, such as a noisy sleeping environment or sleep apnea, can increase the occurrence of NREM-related parasomnias [32]. There is a strong genetic component to confusional arousals and the other disorders of arousals as there is usually a strong family history [31, 33].

Diagnosis

Currently, the diagnosis of confusional arousals is based on the clinical history. The ICSD-3 sets the specific characteristics for the diagnosis of confusional arousals as disorders of arousal:

1. The disorder meets the general criteria for NREM disorder of arousal.
2. The episodes are characterized by mental confusion or confused behavior that occurs while in bed.
3. An absence of terror or ambulation out of the bed.

The criteria specific for confusional arousal help differentiate these events from sleepwalking and sleep terrors. Video polysomnography (VPSG) is used for the diagnosis of confusional arousals when there is concern for the patient harming themselves or others or the other disorder of arousals except to differentiate from other disorders, i.e., seizures, in complex cases or to diagnose concomitant disorders, such as sleep apnea [1, 2, 33].

Treatment

Confusional arousals are usually self-resolving and usually resolve by adolescence. In children with little risk of harm, parents should be offered reassurance. Parents and bed partners should be counseled not to attempt to wake the patient during these events as it can result in worsening the confusion, increased agitation or aggressiveness, and prolonging the event. Treatment should focus on the priming and precipitating factors of the three P model (predisposing, priming and precipitating) of NREM parasomnias. Priming factors such as avoidance of actions such as sleep deprivation that increase the amount of slow wave sleep, and avoidance of substances that may increase arousals, such as caffeine or alcohol. Precipitating factors also need evaluation; thus the patient should be asked about things that cause arousals such as environmental noise and light as well as other symptoms suggestive of other sleep disorders. Therefore, targeting good sleep hygiene, avoidance of priming substances/situations, and precipitating factors are useful tactics to reduce events [2, 25, 33]. In the event that episodes are persistent despite the above or that the severity of the events is placing the patient or others at risk of harm, pharmacologic treatment may be necessary. Clonazepam is the medication with the most evidence for use, but melatonin, antidepressants, and even the hypnotic z-drugs have been used with reported effect [33].

Sleepwalking (Also Known as Somnambulism)

Sleepwalking or somnambulism is another disorder or arousal from NREM sleep. It is characterized by an incomplete arousal from NREM sleep with complex behavior and ambulation out of the bed. These events may go unnoticed as the sleepwalker may return to bed unnoticed and therefore not be reported. The main adverse outcome from sleepwalking is injury to the patient or others. Patients have limited ability to respond to the environment and thus are at risk for injury. As with other disorders of arousal, they occur mostly in children and usually improve with age; however onset in adulthood likely points to prior sleepwalking history or another underlying sleep disorder.

Clinical Presentation

Sleepwalking usually starts like a confusional arousal with the patient sitting up confused; however, unlike confusional arousal the patient gets out of bed. The events can be more complex than simple wandering about and involve opening locked doors or windows, dressing, and even urinating in inappropriate places. The episodes can end with the patient back in bed without reaching conscious awareness, or it may end suddenly in an inappropriate place, such as outdoors in inclement weather. Patients may have limited or no memory or vague dream like mentation of the event. Most events are relatively brief, but some patients have events that last several minutes [1, 2].

Epidemiology

Like the other disorders of arousal, sleepwalking is more common in children. The peak incidence is in the pre-teen to early teen years, 10–13, and resolves by adolescence in 75% of people. The lifetime prevalence is estimated to be between 22 and 29% [2, 34]. In roughly 13% of adults sleepwalking develops de novo, and the overall prevalence in adults is 4% [34]. Most adults with sleepwalking have a history of sleepwalking as children, and the de novo cases are most often associated with medications and neurodegenerative disorders [35].

Pathophysiology/Etiology

The basic pathophysiology of sleepwalking like other disorders of arousal is related to incomplete arousal from SWS. The patient has both features of being asleep and awake that evoke motor central pattern generators for complex motor behaviors. Several studies have shown that different brain regions have dissociative activity, that is, certain regions showing activity consistent with the waking state and others with activity consistent with the sleep state [10, 36]. Like the other disorders of arousal, there is a strong family history pointing to a genetic underpinning. There has been identification of chromosome 20q12-q13 as a possible locus as well as high frequency in patients with the HLA-DQB1 05:01 allele [2, 32]. Sleepwalking can be precipitated by increased arousals from SWS such as in the case of OSA, or it can be primed in the case of sleep deprivation. There are numerous reports of medications associated with somnambulism, particularly the z-drugs (zolpidem, zaleplon), but also for antidepressants of all classes, antipsychotics, and beta-blockers [22].

Diagnosis

The ICSD-3 criteria for sleepwalking include that the disorder meets the general criteria for a disorder of arousal and that the patient has events that are associated with ambulation or other complex behaviors out of bed. The ICDS-3 requires the following to establish the diagnosis:

1. The disorder meets the general criteria for NREM disorder of arousal.
2. The arousals are associated with ambulation and other complex behaviors out of bed.

The diagnosis of sleepwalking can usually be diagnosed based on clinical history, but since the patient is at inherent risk of harm by virtue of leaving the bed, video PSG is an important component of the evaluation. Patients need evaluation to determine if the events appear to be occurring from NREM sleep as well as other possible provoking factors such as sleep apnea.

Treatment

For most patients, therapy can focus on non-pharmacologic avenues unless the patient is at significant risk for harm. Reassurances should be given to parents that sleepwalking is not a sign of developmental disability nor other mental issues. The sleep environment should be made safe for the sleepwalker by removing sharp objects and sharp-edged furniture, locking doors and windows, and bed alarms. Parents and bed partners should be advised not to attempt to wake the patient as this can result in prolongation of the event, aggressive or violent behavior, or running away potentially causing harm to self and others. Additionally, efforts should be directed at avoiding or targeting priming and precipitating factors, such as sleep deprivation, sedative hypnotics, other sleep disorders, anxiety, etc. In the majority of childhood cases, sleepwalking is self-resolving, but adults may frequently need further intervention. Melatonin and clonazepam may be options [2, 6, 25, 33].

Sleep Terrors (Also Known as Night Terrors or Pavor Nocturnum)

Sleep terrors are the most dramatic of the disorders of arousal from NREM sleep. They often start with a piercing scream followed by consolable fear. These events are very impressive to the observer, but have little impact on the patient. Like the other disorders of arousal, they usually occur in the first part of the night and are more common in children. Sleep terrors resolve with age and rarely occur after age 7.

Clinical Presentation

Sleep terrors start abruptly, usually with an intense terrified scream, associated with intense fear and significant sympathetic outlay of the autonomic system. The patient can be found profusely diaphoretic with tachycardia, mydriasis, and tachypnea. The patient will be inconsolable and attempts to calm the patient can prolong the event. The patient is poorly responsive to observers and the environment but may look around or reach around. The episodes usually only last a few minutes, and then the patient will spontaneously return back to sleep. There is no memory for the event, and if the patient does wake at the end of the event, there is usually only a vague remembrance of fear, but no accompanying dream imagery [2, 31–33].

Epidemiology

Sleep terrors are more common in preschool children with 20–40% of children younger than 3 years experiencing an event and reduces to less than 14% of school aged children [37]. It is rare for adults, but prevalence has been reported to be around 2.7% [2].

Etiology/Pathophysiology

Sleep terrors occur from an incomplete arousal from SWS as with the other disorders of arousals above. The exact cause is unknown, but a strong genetic component is suspected based on strong family histories in patients and concordance twin studies. Patients have been shown to have more fragmented N3 sleep [2].

Diagnosis

The diagnosis can be made by clinical history. The key is related to the piercing scream at the beginning of the event. The ICSD-3 requires the following items to establish the diagnosis [1]:

1. The disorder must meet the general criteria for NREM disorders of arousal.
2. The events are characterized by episodes of abrupt terror, typically beginning with an alarming vocalization such as a frightening scream.
3. The events also have accompanying features of intense fear and signs of autonomic arousal, including mydriasis, tachycardia, tachypnea, and diaphoresis during an episode.

Sleep terrors can be distinguished from nightmares as night terrors tend occur in the first third of the night, when N3 is most prevalent, and there is lack of memory for the event and the patient is difficult to arouse. By contrast, nightmares occur from REM sleep, and the patient is not confused and is easily arousable. There is also story-like recall in the case of nightmares, whereas night terrors are only associated with vague, fragmented memory if any [2, 37].

Treatment

Sleep terrors are very dramatic and patients must first be protected from harming themselves or others. Typically the patients are trying to escape and may even fling themselves out of windows. The environment must be made safe from potential hazards, and windows need to be blocked. Other means are locks on doors or notification alarms to avoid the patient leaving the house. Treatment should be focused on addressing predisposing factors as mentioned above and examination for other sleep and medical disorders such as sleep apnea that need treatment. Some have recommended that anticipatory awakening therapy can be helpful in this population. For this therapy the patient is awakened roughly 10–30 minutes prior to the usual event time each night for 2 weeks, then allowed to sleep to see if the events resume. The process can be repeated; however this should only be performed once other disorders such as sleep apnea have been ruled out. In cases that are refractory to the nonpharmacologic interventions or there is risk of harm to self or others, clonazepam or tricyclic antidepressants have been used [2, 25, 33].

Sleep-Related Eating Disorder

Sleep-related eating disorder is characterized by patients having repeated bouts of eating while in a partial sleep state. Unlike the other NREM parasomnias, sleep-related eating disorder is not considered one of the disorders of arousal as discussed above. However, SRED has similar characteristics including occurring from NREM sleep and is also associated with incomplete arousal. The eating occurs after sleep onset has occurred and needs to be distinguished from nocturnal eating syndrome (NES) as discussed below.

Clinical Presentation

This condition is characterized by recurrent eating episodes that occur after an arousal from sleep. During these events patients may consume unusual to bizarre foods including raw meats, cake batter, and frozen foods to inedible non-foodstuffs like buttered cigarettes to toxins such as cleaning liquids. In addition to ingesting harmful foods or substances, there is risk of harm from improperly attempting to prepare foods [38–41]. The person with sleep-related eating disorder (SRED) has partial or total amnesia for the event. The events occur almost nightly. Occurring during NREM sleep they tend to occur in the first half of the night. SRED is, not surprisingly, associated with weight gain and morning anorexia, but also injury from eating toxic substances or inedible items. These types of events also raise several issues beyond being unusual stories, and a complete evaluation is vital for the patients' well being.

Epidemiology

The prevalence of SRED is estimated at 1–4.6% in the general population [38–40]. However Winkelman found up to 17% in patients with other eating disorders and that these symptoms are more common in those patients who have been hospitalized for eating disorders than the general population [42]. Sleep-related eating disorder appears to have a peak incidence in young adulthood and is more common in females than males. Santin, who examined a Chilean population, described a peak age of diagnosis around 39 years, but symptoms starting on average 8 years prior to diagnosis [43]. Concomitant sleep disorders are present in up to 80% of patients with SRED [38].

Etiology/Pathophysiology

A familial relationship has been shown in 5–26% of patients [38]. This may be in part related to the possible relationship to the DOA for some of these patients; however, other contributors such as eating disorders also appear to run in families. Thus the pathophysiology is not known, but it is surmised that arousals from NREM sleep may result in varying levels of consciousness resulting in SRED in susceptible individuals. The strongest association is with other eating disorders, and this may have a relationship to the underlying focus on food and eating. There is also an association with restless leg syndrome, suggesting a possible dopaminergic pathway involving the reward system of the mesolimbic region. Some medications such as zolpidem are associated with episodes of sleep-related eating, and there is also an association with many psychoactive drugs. Sedative hypnotics, antidepressants, and antipsychotics have all been associated with SRED [38, 40, 41].

There is a high rate of psychiatric comorbidity and SRED as well. In the original description of SRED over 40% of the patients had a coexisting mood disorder [41]. The rate of depression has been reported at 37% and 18% for anxiety disorder. The rate of substance abuse is also high at 24% [38]. Daytime eating disorders, i.e., anorexia and bulimia, also have a high association with SRED. The frequent co-occurrence of SRED and psychiatric illness suggests a similar underlying pathology [41].

Diagnosis

The diagnosis of SRED is typically based upon the clinical features presented at the initial history and physical examination. The key element is to have a reliable witness of the events describe the features of several events. The ICSD-3 sets four criteria for diagnosing SRED. These include:

1. Recurrent episodes of dysfunctional eating occurring after an arousal from sleep
2. The presence of one of the following: ingestion of odd or peculiar foodstuffs or combinations or inedible or toxic substances, injuries sustained by or potentially injurious behavior when getting food or in the preparation of food that is sleep related, and adverse health consequences, e.g., weight gain or diabetes
3. Partial or complete amnesia for the event
4. And finally that the above is not better explained by some other disorder, substance, or medication

Although the presence of SRED can usually be diagnosed based on the clinical history, the clinician needs to have a high suspicion for other sleep, neurological, or psychiatric disorders. If the episodes are stereotypic or other sleep disorders are considered in the differential, then the VPSG should be performed. During this study, the usual foods that the patient tends to eat during SRED should be available in the room during the overnight study [38].

Differential Diagnosis

– SRED needs to be distinguished from another form of abnormal nighttime eating disorder. Nocturnal eating syndrome (NES) is defined differently depending on the literature, but key distinctions are the level of consciousness, timing of eating, and frequency of comorbid sleep disorders [41]. Nocturnal eating syndrome has similar features of eating during the night, but, as opposed to SRED, these patients are fully conscious during the nocturnal eating. In addition, nighttime eating very often occurs prior to sleep onset as NES is actually a circadian phase delay in the eating schedule. Finally, SRED is more associated with other sleep disorders, e.g., sleep apnea, than patients with NES [38, 41]. There is, however, considerable overlap in other features of NES and SRED. NES can also be accompanied by an eating episode after arousal from sleep. In addition, affective disorders are also highly associated with NES as with SRED [38]. The astute clinician may be able to delineate the two disorders by careful history; however the diagnosis of NES should be on the differential with any sleep disturbance accompanied by eating. On PSG studies of NES eating was accompanied by full consciousness and no other sleep disorders were described, save for decreased total sleep time and sleep efficiency [38].

Treatment

In general most treatments of SRED are anecdotal reports. If a patient started the sleep-related eating events with the initiation of a medication such as a short-acting hypnotic, then the hypnotic should be discontinued. Similarly good sleep hygiene and avoidance of initiating or provoking factors are a foundation point for therapy. Pharmacologic treatment includes pramipexole which showed some modest effectiveness in a small placebo controlled trial [40]. Another trial has shown the antiepileptic medication topiramate to be effective as well. Case reports have shown the SSRIs fluvoxamine, paroxetine, and fluoxetine to be successful [38, 40]. Treatment should also be aimed at any sleep disruptors, including other sleep disorders that may arouse the patient from NREM.

REM-Related Parasomnias

REM sleep is characterized by relative atonia of the voluntary muscles, rapid eye movements, and vivid dream mentation. Portions of these characteristics are key in the description of REM-related parasomnias as a group of parasomnias that, obviously, arise out of REM sleep. These disorders share many of the characteristics of REM but represent a variety of underlying pathologies. The disorders can be an intrusion of REM sleep into wake, such as sleep paralysis, demonstrate a vulnerable neurocircuitry as in REM sleep behavior disorder, or an over expression of emotion into the state such as in nightmare disorder. Arising from REM sleep these parasomnias tend to occur in the second half of the night. They affect both children and adults, and in the case of REM behavior disorder can be a sign of or precursor to a neurodegenerative disorder.

REM Sleep Behavior Disorder

REM sleep behavior disorder (RBD) is characterized by the loss of the usual paralysis during REM sleep resulting in the patient acting out their dreams. These events are often violent resulting in injury of the patient as well as the bed partner. RBD has a high association with a group of neurodegenerative disorders and can precede the hallmark clinical characteristics by years.

Clinical Presentation

RBD is a parasomnia that is characterized by abnormal behaviors occurring during REM sleep. Due to the loss of the muscle atonia that normally accompanies REM sleep, the affected sleeper has motor responses correlating to dream imagery. In general RBD manifests as dream enactment, resulting in thrashing, slapping, or kicking of the extremities and even yelling [44–47]. Self-injury is a common occurrence and a little over 60% of patients injuring a bed partner [44]. The usual dream semiology involves predominantly defensive types of events in which the patient is being attacked or threatened by animals or intruders or has to defend in a sport. The resulting behaviors are the result of attempts at self-defense or the defense of others. The patient usually wakes at the end of the dream and can recall the dream content that parallels the observed behavior while asleep.

Epidemiology

The prevalence of RBD in the general population has been reported to be from 0.38 to roughly 2% [47]. However, the prevalence has been suggested to be as high as 5–13% of adults aged 60–99 [46]. The disorder is thought to be more common in men than women, yet some of this may be related to reporting bias. In younger onset patients, those under 50 years old, men and women are equal [46].

Etiology/Pathophysiology

The exact mechanisms underlying RBD appear to be related to impairment of the pathway that induces atonia during REM sleep. This syndrome can be created in animal models by lesions involving the REM atonia pathways, suggesting involvement of the REM sleep control centers located in the pons and medulla. The resulting dysfunction results in loss of the normal atonia associated with REM sleep [45]. Although several reports show that lesions in the pons, midbrain, and medulla can elicit RBD, in older adults there is a high association with RBD, and a group of neurodegenerative disorders called alpha-synucleinopathies. This group is named for the protein that can be found intracellularly in these disorders. The alpha-synucleinopathies include Parkinson's disease (PD), multiple system atrophy (MSA), and dementia with Lewy bodies (DLB). RBD is considered a predictor for future conversion to one of the above disorders. Indeed RBD may precede phenoconversion to one of the alpha-synucleinopathies by decades. The risk of conversion over 2–5 years is roughly 15–35% and after 25 years is over 90% [45]. Many medications have been associated with RBD as well. SSRIs and SNRIs are well known to cause REM sleep without atonia (RSWA) and are associated with RBD. Up to 15% of patients taking SSRIs have been shown to have RSWA [18]. In younger patients with the onset of RBD, narcolepsy may be a key driver. As with other partial induction of the REM sleep state in narcolepsy, RBD can occur with the same violent behaviors [48].

Diagnosis

The diagnosis of RBD requires two major features, the presence of dream enactment and the loss of REM sleep-related atonia. The ICSD-3 requires the following features to make the diagnosis of RBD:

A. A. Repeated episodes of sleep-related complex motor behaviors and/or vocalization.
B. The behaviors are documented on polysomnography to arise during REM sleep or, based on the description of the events including dream enactment, they are presumed to occur during REM sleep.
C. Polysomnographic recording demonstrates the loss of REM sleep atonia.
D. The disturbance is not better explained by another sleep or mental disorder, medication, or substance.

Thus unlike the NREM-related parasomnias, the diagnosis of RBD requires a polysomnogram to document the loss of atonia in REM sleep (Fig. 16.2). The loss of atonia is best demonstrated with recording EMG activity from all four extremities. Events do not need to be captured during the recording; however, the diagnosis can be made either with a clinical history consistent with RBD and the findings of REM sleep without atonia on polysomnogram. If there is no history of dream enactment, the diagnosis can be made by capturing an episode of complex behavior or vocalizations during REM on the study. RBD should be distinguished from other diseases that have vivid dreams with dream enactment, such as PTSD and obstructive sleep apnea [46].

Clinical Approach

For patients suspected of having RBD, historical features of dream enactment with clear description of the events are key. These events should vary in their content but may center around the theme of defending. For patients over 55 years, clinicians should ask about the other non-motor signs of alpha-synucleinopathies such as constipation, loss of smell, or orthostatic hypotension. These features may co-exist with the RBD events and precede other manifestations by years. Similarly, a detailed neurological exam is essential to evaluate for other neurological features. Since RBD can be related to other processes impairing the atonia pathways, patients should also be evaluated for possible underlying structural causes of RBD such as stroke, demyelinating lesions, or tumors and undergo brain imaging.

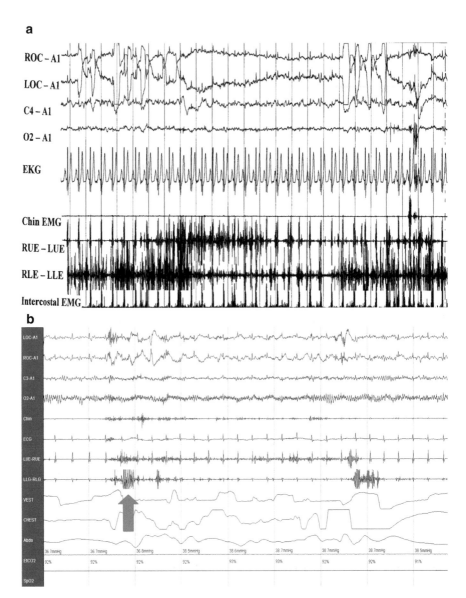

Fig. 16.2 This polysomnogram is a representative sample of loss of atonia during REM sleep. Note that the submental EMG does not have a high amount of AMG activity but the extremities are noted to demonstrate significant muscle activity. (**a**) This tracing is from a 76-year-old man with multiple system atrophy and history of violent dream enactment. (**b**) It is from a 65-year-old female who was not being evaluated for parasomnia and had incidental sudden movement of her arm and leg during REM sleep and noted dreaming she was shooing a cat off the bed. The patient later admitted to multiple events of dream enactment

Treatment

Patients should be counseled on bedroom safety to prevent injury. This includes removal of furniture near the bed, placing the mattress on the floor, and removal of weapons from the bedroom. The patient or the bed partner should be advised to sleep in another bed or another room to prevent injury to others. Any OSA, if present, should be treated as this may reduce incidence of events [45, 46]. The mainstay of pharmacologic treatment is melatonin and clonazepam. Melatonin of 3–15 mg dosed at bedtime has been shown in trials to reduce the incidence and severity of events. In addition, clonazepam 0.25–2.0 mg at bedtime can be used as well. However, the cautious use of clonazepam is advised in patients with dementia, gait difficulties, and OSA as the medication can worsen these conditions [44–47].

Recurrent Isolated Sleep Paralysis

Recurrent isolated sleep paralysis is the phenomenon of the inability to move any part of the body during the sleep-wake transition or vice versa. These events leave a lasting impression upon the subject that can be remembered for decades. The events typically occur upon awakening but may be related to going to sleep. Although events are fairly uncommon, the events are noted to be described across a variety of cultures and given sacred explanations.

Clinical Presentation

Sleep paralysis is the phenomenon of the inability to move the limbs, head, or trunk at the onset of sleep or upon awakening. The episodes only last a few seconds to minutes and resolve abruptly. Respiratory muscles are not affected, and the patient is usually fully conscious of their environment. The episodes are frequently accompanied by an overwhelming sense of impending doom or hallucinations of someone or thing in the room, a sense of pressure as if someone sitting on their chest, and a sense of fear or distress [3, 49–51]. Patients remember these events for decades with unusual clarity.

Epidemiology

Sleep paralysis is fairly uncommon in the full-blown events; however partial events may have a lifetime prevalence as high as 7.6% in the general population. Events appear to be more prevalent in students with history of sleep deprivation and circadian rhythm phase shifts ranging up to 28% in selected series, and almost 32% of patients with psychiatric illness [49]. Women are slightly more likely to experience sleep paralysis than men.

Etiology/Pathophysiology

Sleep paralysis is thought to be a mixture of states with elements of REM invading the waking state. Risk factors for experiencing sleep paralysis include sleep deprivation, sleep disruption, or shifts in circadian rhythm. Shift workers are noted to experience sleep paralysis more commonly. Sleep paralysis is also more likely to occur when sleeping in the supine position. Psychiatric illness has also been reported to be a risk factor for sleep paralysis [3, 49–51].

Diagnosis

Recurrent isolated sleep paralysis is diagnosed by the clinical history and requires that the episodes cause significant distress including fear of sleep and/or the bedtime/bedroom. The ICSD-3 requires the following criteria to establish the diagnosis:

1. Recurrent episodes of inability to move the trunk and all of the limbs at sleep onset or upon awakening from sleep.
2. Each of the individual episodes should last seconds to a few minutes.
3. The episodes cause significant distress which can include bedtime anxiety or fear.
4. The disturbance is not better explained by another sleep disorder (especially narcolepsy), mental or medical disorder, or medication, or substance use.

As noted in the criteria, recurrent isolated sleep paralysis should not be diagnosed in a patient with symptoms consistent with narcolepsy. The patient with sleep paralysis will not have daytime sleepiness nor cataplexy [1, 51]. VPSG does not need to be performed unless an underlying sleep disorder is suspected; however rarely an event can be captured during a recording (Fig. 16.3).

Treatment

For the most part, patients do not need to be treated for recurrent isolated sleep paralysis as the majority do not have significant distress associated with the events. The pharmacologic treatment is based on treatment for narcolepsy. SSRIs and tricyclic antidepressants have been used to effectively treat sleep paralysis, presumably for their REM suppressant effects [51].

Nightmare Disorder

Nightmare disorder involves recurrent frightening dreams that cause the patient anxiety or daytime distress. There is a high association with psychiatric illness, particularly PTSD. Nightmares are common and affect both children and adults. They are often associated with awakening and, unlike night terrors, are associated

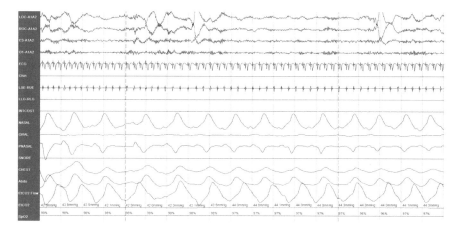

Fig. 16.3 This is the tracing of a 27-year-old male with recurrent episodes of sleep paralysis, who woke after this epoch, that he was having one of his events of paralysis. He noted a visual hallucination of a small older man sitting on his chest. The epoch shows typical features of REM sleep. (Reprinted with permission from Bradley Vaughn)

with complete recall and quick orientation to full consciousness. Nightmare disorder, however, results in daytime sequelae, which is what distinguishes it from the general occurrence of nightmares.

Clinical Presentation

Nightmare disorder consists of repeated episodes of nightmares that cause clinically significant impairment in social, occupational, or other important areas of functioning. When the patient wakes from the nightmare, they are immediately oriented and alert, and there is recall of the dream imagery. Nightmares are defined as dysphoric dreams and usually involve threat of harm to the person [1]. The nightmares are associated with negative emotions, most commonly fear. The nightmares can be idiopathic or post-traumatic. Idiopathic nightmares are more imaginative and do not have a traumatic content. Post-traumatic nightmares usually involve the direct replication of the traumatic event or contain material that is symbolically related to the trauma [52, 53].

Epidemiology

Occasional nightmares are relatively common in the general population, and approximately 3–8% of adults report recurrent nightmares. Although more common in childhood roughly 7–11%, the rate increases to 15 to as high as 67% of adult patients with psychiatric illness. Men and women appear to be equally affected, but the overall prevalence of nightmare disorder is unclear.

Etiology/Pathophysiology

Nightmares by themselves usually occur in relationship to either an experience of the day, such as a horror movie, or related to a substance consumed – such as alcohol. Nightmare disorder, however, is associated with psychopathologies, particularly PTSD, and personality characteristics. Some medications that affect serotonin, norepinephrine, GABA, histamine, acetylcholine, and dopamine are associated with nightmares. The withdrawal of REM suppressant medication is also associated with nightmares [1, 52]. Dream generation is thought to be a process of brain regions and mechanisms independent of REM generation. Nightmare disorder has been proposed to be due to a two-factor process of hyperarousal and impaired fear extinction. Hyperarousal is a hallmark of not only insomnia but PTSD in which 80% of patients report nightmares [53, 54].

Diagnosis

Diagnosis is usually established by clinical history. Nightmares should be distinguished from night terrors as discussed above. The ICSD-3 requires the following for the diagnosis:

1. Recurrent extremely dysphoric, distressing well-remembered dreams that usually involve threats to survival, security, or physical integrity.
2. Upon awakening from the nightmare, the person quickly becomes oriented and alert.
3. When awakening from the nightmare, the person has clinically significant distress or impairment in social, occupational, or other important areas of functioning as indicated by the report of at least one of the following:

   - Mood disturbance (e.g., persistence of nightmare affect, anxiety, dysphoria)
   - Sleep resistance (e.g., bedtime anxiety, fear of sleep/subsequent nightmares)
   - Cognitive impairments (e.g., intrusive nightmare imagery, impaired concentration, or memory)
   - Negative impact on caregiver or family functioning (e.g., nighttime disruption)
   - Behavioral problems (e.g., bedtime avoidance, fear of the dark)
   - Daytime sleepiness
   - Fatigue or low energy
   - Impaired occupational or educational function
   - Impaired Interpersonal/Social Function

When considering this diagnosis, the key is to have a clear description of the nightmare events, and also the key features of the sequelae during wake. The later part is what distinguishes nightmare disorder, from the occasional disturbing dream. Many times patients may not spontaneously disclose the impairment in social, occupational, or other important areas as they have not drawn the connection. Thus further questioning may be needed.

Treatment

Non-pharmacologic treatment consists of image rehearsal therapy (IRT), cognitive behavioral therapy (CBT), lucid dreaming therapy, and hypnosis, among others [52]. IRT is part of the recommended guidelines and appears to be successful in patients with history of trauma. IRT consists of changing dream content by recreating the dream with positive images and rehearsing the dream for 10–20 minutes daily while awake. Several RCTs have shown efficacy of IRT in the treatment of nightmare disorder with reduction in nightmare frequency [52, 53]. Pharmacologic treatment of nightmare disorder is based on studies of their efficacy in treating PTSD-associated nightmares. Prazosin was initially thought to reduce the recurrence of nightmares but has mixed results in larger trials [55]. Other commonly used medications in this instance include the atypical antipsychotics, clonidine, cyproheptadine, trazodone, tricyclic antidepressants, and clonazepam with mixed results [52].

Other Parasomnias

Other parasomnias include a collection of disorders that are either related to sleep-wake transitions, or have no clear tie to a particular sleep stage. Some of these are very specific phenomena, while others are more general catch-all disorders. Each has specific criteria to help the clinician distinguish the syndromes.

Exploding Head Syndrome

Exploding head syndrome is named due to the phenomenon of the sudden sensation of an explosion or loud noise going off in the head. This usually occurs at sleep onset, but can occur upon awakening. The person usually has an abrupt arousal immediately after the event, which is brief, and is accompanied by a sense of fright, but is not accompanied or associated with any significant pain [1, 56]. The prevalence is not well known due to the transient nature of the phenomenon and due to underreporting and under recognition. However, prevalence has been reported to be roughly 11% in the general population. Individuals may only have one episode in a lifetime or may have clusters of events over a night or more. The most common concern for a patient is bleeding or a tumor. Treatment is focused on reassurance as the condition is benign and usually self-limiting. In the instances that exploding head syndrome is recurrent or results in distress for the patient, medications may be tried. Several medications, such as clonazepam, clomipramine, and topiramate, have had varying success [57, 58].

Sleep-Related Hallucinations

Hypnic hallucinations are dreamlike imagery that occur during the wake-sleep transition or vice versa. Hypnopompic hallucinations occur on the transition from sleep to wake, and hypnogogic hallucinations occur at the onset of sleep and are thought to be the intrusion of REM into the wake state [59–61]. The hallucinations are most often visual, but can be auditory or tactile. Though hypnic hallucinations occur commonly in narcolepsy, they can occur independent of any other disorder and are common in the general population. Hypnogogic hallucinations are more common than hypnopompic, with a reported prevalence of 37% and 12.5%, respectively [62]. Sleep-related hallucinations are associated with sleep problems, such as insomnia or poor sleep/wake schedules. Treatment is not usually necessary as the episodes are short-lived and benign. Most individuals are aware that the images are not real, but they can be distressing [59–61]. Treatment with benzodiazepines and tricyclics has been unsuccessful, but there are reports of success with melatonin [59].

Sleep Enuresis or Nocturnal Enuresis

Sleep enuresis is the phenomenon of involuntary voiding during sleep in a patient that is older than 5, occurring at least 2 nights a week, for at least 3 months. Sleep enuresis or nocturnal bedwetting is delineated into primary and secondary nocturnal enuresis, wherein primary there has never been dry periods of at least 6 months and in secondary forms the patient had previously been dry. Though there is a common symptomatology of wetting the bed a night, the two have distinct etiologies [1]. The prevalence is between 6 and 10% by age 7, which then decreases to 2% and less than 2% in teenagers and adults, respectively. The pathophysiology of nocturnal enuresis is thought to involve nocturnal polyuria, decreased bladder storage ability, and poor arousal [63]. Primary nocturnal enuresis is usually considered a disorder of acquired developmental skills, and therefore there is a range of ages when these skills are acquired. However, in secondary nocturnal enuresis it can be caused by a number of problems, including diabetes, urinary tract infections, urinary tract malformations, and psychosocial factors [1, 64]. In addition, there is a high rate of sleep disordered breathing associated with nocturnal enuresis, being reported in 8–47% of cases. Diagnosis involves a careful history, and it is important to distinguish between primary and secondary enuresis as further workup is warranted in the latter. The mainstay of treatment in primary enuresis is bed alarms. In secondary enuresis the underlying cause should be investigated and treatment targeted based on the underlying pathology. In suspected cases of sleep apnea, a PSG may need to be performed [63–65].

Approach to Distinguishing Nocturnal Events

The goal of any evaluation of a patient with nocturnal events is to prevent harm to the patient or others. For this the clinician should focus the initial consultation upon answering the following questions: (1) Is the patient at risk potential for harm or causing harming to someone else? (2) What may be driving the appearance of these events? (3) Are these events indicating another underlying disorder?

In general, an astute clinician can differentiate parasomnias by looking for key distinguishing features (Table 16.2). The key for any evaluation of nocturnal events is a thorough history and excellent physical exam. Although these are foundational, the underpinning of the evaluation is based on a clear description of the events from witnesses who can give an accurate testimony of the behaviors. Key historical features such as time of night, duration, frequency of occurrence, behavioral characteristics with each event, eyes open or closed, memory recall, age of onset, and family history of nocturnal events may help differentiate these disorders [66]. The physician should also search for factors that precipitate parasomnias such as poor sleep environment, improper sleep hygiene, sleep deprivation, circadian rhythm abnormalities, other sleep disorders, medical issues, fever or other illnesses, emotional stress, medication use, and ingestion of alcohol or sedatives before sleep onset [22, 67–69]. Additional search for other neurological symptoms such as decrease sense of smell, constipation, or other autonomic issues may give clues to REM sleep behavior disorder [46]. Similarly, features suggesting cognitive decline in adult may provide the opening for further investigation of encephalopathic processes or dementia [69].

Further testing may be indicated for patients with parasomnia. Key features may elucidate the need for further study in the sleep lab (Table 16.4). Polysomnographic recording can also provide important information in determining the etiology of the nocturnal events, with the goal of capturing the physiology of each sleep state and to evaluate the possibility of other contributing sleep disorders. Overnight polysomnography is necessary if the history is atypical, sleepiness is significant, other sleep disorders are suspected, or the patient is at risk for harming themselves or others

Table 16.4   Indications for polysomnography in patients with nocturnal events. Reprinted with permission from Bradley Vaughn

Unusual or atypical presentation for a parasomnia (time of night, behavioral description)
Events injurious or with significant risk for injury
Significant disturbance to patient's home life
Unusual age of onset
Events stereotyped or repetitive
High frequency of the events
Patient has excessive daytime sleepiness or complaints of insomnia
Complaints suggestive of sleep apnea, periodic limb movements, or other sleep disorders

[70]. Studies should include complete respiratory monitoring, time-synchronized video monitoring, additional electromyographic recording from all four limbs, a complete set of cephalic electrodes, and ability to extensively review the electroencephalogram [5, 71, 72]. Incorporation of a full 10- to 20-electrode array and ability to view the tracing at 10 second windows is necessary in evaluating for seizures and the differentiation of the epileptiform discharges from potential normal variants or artifacts [73].

Parasomnias may be distinguished using key features. The challenge for the ardent clinician is to utilize historical and physical examination clues and appropriate diagnostic tools to distinguish the underlying causes and propose directed therapy to improve the patient's condition.

References

1. American Academy of Sleep Medicine. International classification of sleep disorders. 3rd ed. Darien, IL: American Academy of Sleep Medicine, 2014.
2. Provini F, Tinuper P, Bisulli F, Lugaresi E. Arousal disorders. Sleep Med. 2011;12(Suppl 2):S22–6. https://doi.org/10.1016/j.sleep.2011.10.007.
3. Denis D, French CC, Gregory AM. A systematic review of variables associated with sleep paralysis. Sleep Med Rev. 2018;38:141–57. PMID: 28735779. https://doi.org/10.1016/j.smrv.2017.05.005.
4. Stefani A, Holzknecht E, Högl B. Clinical neurophysiology of REM parasomnias. Handb Clin Neurol. 2019;161:381–96.
5. Gieselmann A, Ait Aoudia M, Carr M, Germain A, Gorzka R, Holzinger B, Kleim B, Krakow B, Kunze AE, Lancee J, Nadorff MR, Nielsen T, Riemann D, Sandahl H, Schlarb AA, Schmid C, Schredl M, Spoormaker VI, Steil R, van Schagen AM, Wittmann L, Zschoche M, Pietrowsky R. Aetiology and treatment of nightmare disorder: state of the art and future perspectives. J Sleep Res. 2019;28:e12820.
6. Gaudreau H, Joncas S, Zadra A, Montplaisir J. Dynamics of slow-wave activity during the NREM sleep of sleepwalkers and control subjects. Sleep. 2000;23:755–60.
7. Desjardins M, Carrier J, Lina J, et al. EEG functional connectivity prior to sleepwalking: evidence of interplay between sleep and wakefulness. Sleep. 2017;40:zsx024.
8. Heidbreder A, Stefani A, Brandauer E, et al. Gray matter abnormalities of the dorsal posterior cingulate in sleep walking. Sleep Med. 2017;36:152–5.
9. Gibbs SA, Proserpio P, Terzaghi M, et al. Sleep-related epileptic behaviors and non-REM-related parasomnias: insights from stereo-EEG. Sleep Med Rev. 2016;25:4–20.
10. Januszko P, Niemcewicz S, Gajda T, et al. Sleepwalking episodes are preceded by arousal-related activation in the cingulate motor area: EEG current density imaging. Clin Neurophysiol. 2016;127(1):530–6.
11. Bassetti C, Vella S, Donati F, et al. SPECT during sleepwalking. Lancet. 2000;356(9228):484–5.
12. Oliviero A, Della Marca G, Tonali PA, et al. Functional involvement of cerebral cortex in adult sleepwalking. J Neurol. 2007;254(8):1066–72.
13. Labelle MA, Dang-Vu TT, Petit D, Desautels A, Montplaisir J, Zadra A. Sleep deprivation impairs inhibitory control during wakefulness in adult sleepwalkers. J Sleep Res. 2015;24:658–65.
14. Di Gennaro G, Autret A, Mascia A, et al. Night terrors associated with thalamic lesion. Clin Neurophysiol. 2004;115(11):2489–92.

15. Daftary AS, Walker JM, Farney RJ. NREM sleep parasomnia associated with Chiari I malformation. J Clin Sleep Med. 2011;7(5):526–9.
16. Giuliano L, Fatuzzo D, Mainieri G, La Vignera S, Sofia V, Zappia M. Adult-onset sleepwalking secondary to hyperthyroidism: polygraphic evidence. J Clin Sleep Med. 2018;14(2):285–7.
17. Labelle M, Desautels A, Montplaisir J, Zadra A. Psychopathologic correlates of adult sleepwalking. Sleep Med. 2013;14:1348–55.
18. Ohayon MM, Guilleminault C, Priest RG. Night terrors, sleepwalking, and confusional arousals in the general population: their frequency and relationship to other sleep and mental disorders. J Clin Psychiatry. 1999;60:268–76.
19. Howell MJ. Parasomnias: an updated review. Neurotherapeutics. 2012;9(4):753–75.
20. Goodwin JL, Kaemingk KL, Fregosi RF, et al. Parasomnias and sleep disordered breathing in Caucasian and Hispanic children – the Tucson children's assessment of sleep apnea study. BMC Med. 2004;2:14.
21. Lundetræ RS, Saxvig IW, Pallesen S, Aurlien H, Lehmann S, Bjorvatn B. Prevalence of parasomnias in patients with obstructive sleep apnea. A registry-based cross-sectional study. Front Psychol. 2018;9:1140.
22. Stallman HM, Kohler M, White J. Medication induced sleepwalking: a systematic review. Sleep Med Rev. 2018;37:105–13. PMID: 28363449. https://doi.org/10.1016/j.smrv.2017.01.005.
23. Fois C, Wright MA, Sechi GP, et al. The utility of polysomnography for the diagnosis of NREM parasomnias: an observational study over 4 years of clinical practice. J Neurol. 2015;262(2):385–93.
24. Pilon M, Montplaisir J, Zadra A. Precipitating factors of somnambulism: impact of sleep deprivation and forced arousals. Neurology. 2008;70(24):2274–5.
25. Pressman MR. Factors that predispose, prime and precipitate NREM parasomnias in adults: clinical and forensic implications. Sleep Med Rev. 2007;11(1):5–30.
26. Attarian H. Treatment options for parasomnias. Neurol Clin. 2010;28(4):1089–106.
27. Schenck CH, Mahowald MW. Long-term, nightly benzodiazepine treatment of injurious parasomnias and other disorders of disrupted nocturnal sleep in 170 adults. Am J Med. 1996;100(3):333–7.
28. Cooper AJ. Treatment of coexistent night-terrors and somnambulism in adults with imipramine and diazepam. J Clin Psychiatry. 1987;48:209–10.
29. Balon R. Sleep terror disorder and insomnia treated with trazodone: a case report. Ann Clin Psychiatry. 1994;6:161–3.
30. Wilson SJ, Lillywhite AR, Potokar JP, et al. Adult night terrors and paroxetine. Lancet. 1997;350:185.
31. Ekambaram V, Maski K. Non-rapid eye movement arousal parasomnias in children. Pediatr Ann. 2017;46(9):e327–31. https://doi.org/10.3928/19382359-20170814-01.
32. Castelnovo A, Lopez R, Proserpio P, Nobili L, Dauvilliers Y. NREM sleep parasomnias as disorders of sleep-state dissociation. Nat Rev Neurol. 2018;14(8):470–81. https://doi.org/10.1038/s41582-018-0030-y.
33. Drakatos P, Leschziner G. Diagnosis and management of nonrapid eye movement-parasomnias. Curr Opin Pulm Med. 2019;25(6):629–35. https://doi.org/10.1097/MCP.0000000000000619.
34. Bargiotas P, Arnet I, Frei M, Baumann CR, Schindler K, Bassetti CL. Demographic, clinical and polysomnographic characteristics of childhood- and adult-onset sleepwalking in adults. Eur Neurol. 2017;78(5–6):307–11. https://doi.org/10.1159/000481685.
35. Stallman HM, Kohler M. Prevalence of sleepwalking: a systematic review and meta-analysis. PLoS One. 2016;11(11):e0164769. Published 2016 Nov 10. https://doi.org/10.1371/journal.pone.0164769.
36. Baldini T, Loddo G, Sessagesimi E, et al. Clinical features and pathophysiology of disorders of arousal in adults: a window into the sleeping brain. Front Neurol. 2019;10:526. Published 2019 May 17. https://doi.org/10.3389/fneur.2019.00526.
37. Ellington E. It's not a nightmare: understanding sleep terrors. J Psychosoc Nurs Ment Health Serv. 2018;56(8):11–4. https://doi.org/10.3928/02793695-20180723-03.

38. Auger RR. Sleep-related eating disorders. Psychiatry (Edgmont). 2006;3(11):64–70.
39. Komada Y, Takaesu Y, Matsui K, et al. Comparison of clinical features between primary and drug-induced sleep-related eating disorder. Neuropsychiatr Dis Treat. 2016;12:1275–80. Published 2016 May 26. https://doi.org/10.2147/NDT.S107462.
40. Chiaro G, Caletti MT, Provini F. Treatment of sleep-related eating disorder. Curr Treat Options Neurol. 2015;17(8):361. https://doi.org/10.1007/s11940-015-0361-6.
41. Inoue Y. Sleep-related eating disorder and its associated conditions. Psychiatry Clin Neurosci. 2015;69(6):309–20. https://doi.org/10.1111/pcn.12263.
42. Winkelman JW, Herzog DB, Fava M. The prevalence of sleep-related eating disorder in psychiatric and non-psychiatric populations. Psychol Med. 1999;29:1461–6.
43. Santin J, Mery V, Elso MJ, Retamal E, Torres C, Ivelic J, Godoy J. Sleep-related eating disorder: a descriptive study in Chilean patients. Sleep Med. 2014;15(2):163–7.
44. McGrane IR, Leung JG, St Louis EK, Boeve BF. Melatonin therapy for REM sleep behavior disorder: a critical review of evidence. Sleep Med. 2015;16(1):19–26. https://doi.org/10.1016/j.sleep.2014.09.011.
45. Barone DA, Henchcliffe C. Rapid eye movement sleep behavior disorder and the link to alpha-synucleinopathies. Clin Neurophysiol. 2018;129(8):1551–64. https://doi.org/10.1016/j.clinph.2018.05.003.
46. St Louis EK, Boeve BF. REM sleep behavior disorder: diagnosis, clinical implications, and future directions. Mayo Clin Proc. 2017;92(11):1723–36. https://doi.org/10.1016/j.mayocp.2017.09.007.
47. Porter VR, Avidan AY. Clinical overview of REM sleep behavior disorder. Semin Neurol. 2017;37(4):461–70. https://doi.org/10.1055/s-0037-1605595.
48. Zhou J, Zhang J, Du L, Li Z, Li Y, Lei F, Wing YK, Kushida CA, Zhou D, Tang X. Characteristics of early- and late-onset rapid eye movement sleep behavior disorder in China: a case-control study. Sleep Med. 2014;15(6):654–60.
49. Sharpless BA, Kliková M. Clinical features of isolated sleep paralysis. Sleep Med. 2019;58:102–6. https://doi.org/10.1016/j.sleep.2019.03.007.
50. Ramos DF, Magalhães J, Santos P, Vale J, Santos MI. Recurrent sleep paralysis – fear of sleeping. Rev Paul Pediatr. 2019;38:e2018226. Published 2019 Nov 25. https://doi.org/10.1590/1984-0462/2020/38/2018226.
51. Sharpless BA. A clinician's guide to recurrent isolated sleep paralysis. Neuropsychiatr Dis Treat. 2016;12:1761–7. Published 2016 Jul 19. https://doi.org/10.2147/NDT.S100307.
52. Morgenthaler TI, Auerbach S, Casey KR, et al. Position paper for the treatment of nightmare disorder in adults: an american academy of sleep medicine position paper. J Clin Sleep Med. 2018;14(6):1041–55. Published 2018 Jun 15. https://doi.org/10.5664/jcsm.7178.
53. Gieselmann A, Ait Aoudia M, Carr M, et al. Aetiology and treatment of nightmare disorder: state of the art and future perspectives. J Sleep Res. 2019;28(4):e12820. https://doi.org/10.1111/jsr.12820.
54. Simor P, Blaskovich B. The pathophysiology of nightmare disorder: signs of impaired sleep regulation and hyperarousal. J Sleep Res. 2019;28(6):e12867. https://doi.org/10.1111/jsr.12867.
55. Rubin ML, Copeland LA, Kroll-Desrosiers AR, Knittel AG. Demographic variation in the use of prazosin for treatment of sleep disturbance in combat veterans with PTSD. Psychopharmacol Bull. 2020;50:26–35.
56. Ceriani CEJ, Nahas SJ. Exploding head syndrome: a review. Curr Pain Headache Rep. 2018;22(10):63. Published 2018 Jul 30. https://doi.org/10.1007/s11916-018-0717-1.
57. Sharpless BA. Exploding head syndrome. Sleep Med Rev. 2014;18(6):489–93. https://doi.org/10.1016/j.smrv.2014.03.001.
58. Palikh GM, Vaughn BV. Topiramate responsive exploding head syndrome. J Clin Sleep Med. 2010;6:382–3.
59. Lysenko L, Bhat S. Melatonin-responsive complex nocturnal visual hallucinations. J Clin Sleep Med. 2018;14(4):687–91. Published 2018 Apr 15. https://doi.org/10.5664/jcsm.7074.

60. Silber MH, Hansen MR, Girish M. Complex nocturnal visual hallucinations. Sleep Med. 2005;6(4):363–6. https://doi.org/10.1016/j.sleep.2005.03.002.
61. Mishra BR, Sarkar S, Mishra S, Mishra A, Praharaj SK, Nizamie SH. Isolated nocturnal auditory hallucinations: a case report. Gen Hosp Psychiatry. 2011;33(5) https://doi.org/10.1016/j.genhosppsych.2011.04.008.
62. Ohayon MM, Priest RG, Caulet M, Guilleminault C. Hypnagogic and hypnopompic hallucinations: pathological phenomena? Br J Psychiatry. 1996;169(4):459–67. https://doi.org/10.1192/bjp.169.4.459.
63. Harari MD. Nocturnal enuresis. J Paediatr Child Health. 2013;49(4):264–71. https://doi.org/10.1111/j.1440-1754.2012.02506.x.
64. Graham KM, Levy JB. Enuresis [published correction appears in Pediatr Rev. 2009 Sep;30(9):369]. Pediatr Rev. 2009;30(5):165–73. https://doi.org/10.1542/pir.30-5-165.
65. Kuwertz-Bröking E, von Gontard A. Clinical management of nocturnal enuresis. Pediatr Nephrol. 2018;33(7):1145–54. https://doi.org/10.1007/s00467-017-3778-1.
66. Singh S, Kaur H, Singh S, Khawaja I. Parasomnias: a comprehensive review. Cureus. 2018;10:e3807. PMID: 30868021.
67. Pressman M, Mahowald M, Schenck C, et al. Alcohol-induced sleepwalking or confusional arousal as a defense to criminal behavior: a review of scientific evidence, methods and forensic considerations. J Sleep Rev. 2007;16:198–212.
68. Papadimitriou GN, Linkowski P. Sleep disturbance in anxiety disorders. Int Rev Psychiatry. 2005;17:229–36.
69. Khachiyants N, Trinkle D, Son SJ, Kim KY. Sundown syndrome in persons with dementia: an update. Psychiatry Investig. 2011;8:275–87.
70. Kushida CA, Littner MR, Morgenthaler T, et al. Practice parameters for the indications for polysomnography and related procedures: an update for 2005. Sleep. 2005;28:499–521.
71. Schenck CH, Boyd JL, Mahowald MW. A parasomnia overlap disorder involving sleepwalking, sleep terrors, and REM sleep behavior disorder in 33 polysomnographically confirmed cases. Sleep. 1997;20:972–81.
72. Proserpio P, Loddo G, Zubler F, Ferini-Strambi L, Licchetta L, Bisulli F, Tinuper P, Agostoni EC, Bassetti C, Tassi L, Menghi V, Provini F, Nobili L. Polysomnographic features differentiating disorder of arousals from sleep-related hypermotor epilepsy. Sleep. 2019;42(12):zsz166.
73. Foldvary N, Caruso AC, Mascha E, et al. Identifying montages that best detect electrographic seizure activity during polysomnography. Sleep. 2000;23:221–9.

Chapter 17
Rapid Eye Movement Parasomnias

Jordan Taylor Standlee and Margaret A. Kay-Stacey

Keywords REM parasomnias · REM sleep behavior disorder · Recurrent isolated sleep paralysis · Nightmare disorder

REM Sleep Behavior Disorder

Definition

REM Sleep Behavior Disorder (RBD) is clinically defined as having all of the following: (A) repeated sleep-related vocalizations and/or complex motor behaviors, (B) the episodes are documented to occur in REM sleep either based on PSG or clinical history, (C) PSG demonstrates REM sleep without atonia (RSWA), and (D) the episodes are not better explained by an alternative disorder [1– 3].

Clinical Features

The usual presentation of RBD is dramatic, aggressive physical activity during sleep. Patients may punch, kick, scream, curse, or even run or fall out of bed. It is not uncommon for these activities to be associated with injury to the individuals and bed partners, or to damage to objects around the bedroom. The movements tend to be brief and can appear purposeful to observers. Bruises, fractures, and even legal issues can result from these activities. In contrast to NREM parasomnias, it is

J. T. Standlee · M. A. Kay-Stacey (✉)
Northwestern University Feinberg School of Medicine, Department of Neurology,
Chicago, IL, USA
e-mail: Jordan.standlee@northwestern.edu; Margaret-stacey@northwestern.edu

© Springer Nature Switzerland AG 2022   381
M. S. Badr, J. L. Martin (eds.), *Essentials of Sleep Medicine*,
Respiratory Medicine, https://doi.org/10.1007/978-3-030-93739-3_17

uncommon for the behaviors to be elaborate or involve leaving the room, though relatively complex behaviors have occasionally been described in children and teen-agers, and in non-Western populations [4, 5]. When questioned afterward, patients report vivid dreams that commonly obtain life-threatening, action-filled content. As a distinction from a confusional arousal, the patient will rapidly reorient upon awak-ening and have clear recollection of dream content. There is usually no associated daytime somnolence. As is true with all REM-related conditions, they are much more common in the middle or latter third of the night, though this may not be the case in patients with narcolepsy, as those patients often have REM abnormally early within a sleep period. Frequency of events can be quiet variable, ranging from mul-tiple events per night to one every few months. The onset of symptoms tends to be gradual and slowly progressive, with usually a long lag between initial symptom onset and diagnosis. When asked in retrospect, patients often report a gradual pro-drome of limb jerking, teeth grinding, or sleep talking for years prior to RBD diag-nosis [3, 6–9].

As will be discussed below, there is a strong association between idiopathic RBD and alpha-synucleinopathies, and RBD is often one of the cardinal prodromal symp-toms portending later neurodegeneration. As such, at the point where patients are diagnosed with RBD, they often have other signs of early alpha-synucleinopathies: loss of olfaction, chronic constipation, autonomic dysfunction (particularly ortho-stasis), and impaired visuospatial abilities [2, 10–13].

Risk Factors

There is a clear association between RBD and neurodegenerative diseases, particu-larly alpha-synucleinopathies (idiopathic Parkinson disease, dementia with Lewy bodies, multiple system atrophy), though a huge range of other non-synuclein degenerative diseases have been implicated including tauopathies like Alzheimer disease, frontotemporal dementia, and progressive supranuclear palsy; Huntington disease; amyotrophic lateral sclerosis; myotonic dystrophy; paraneoplastic and autoimmune encephalitides; and spinal cerebellar ataxia [2, 3, 14–17]. Given the association of RBD with neurodegenerative disease, it is unsurprising that the stron-gest risk factor for RBD is older age, particularly age greater than 50 [3], and the median age of diagnosis is 60–70 years old [18]. However, the absence of a comor-bid neurodegenerative syndrome should not rule out clinical suspicion for RBD, since RBD tends to be part of the initial prodrome of the syndrome and can precede development of further symptoms by up to 50 years [19]. Often, the only comorbid symptoms are anosmia and constipation which, together with RBD, make up the classic prodrome for alpha-synucleinopathies. A 2019 meta-analysis found that among patients diagnosed with RBD, at 5-year follow-up, a third (33.5%) had developed a neurodegenerative disorder, whereas by 14-year follow-up, nearly everyone (96.6%) had developed one [20]. This finding speaks to both the robust association between RBD and neurodegenerative diseases, as well as the relatively long lag time that can separate the two.

Male sex is another very strong risk factor, though the mechanism for this is unknown [3]. Some case series report a male-female prevalence of 9:1, though this is likely inflated due to both the fact that women generally express less injurious dream enactment behaviors, which makes them less likely to seek medical attention, and that older women often outlive their spouses and therefore do not have a bed partner to report their symptoms [21]. Other risk factors include the presence of comorbid psychiatric conditions and antidepressant use, especially in cases where RBD has a relatively rapid onset [22–24]. Antidepressants of nearly all categories have been observed to acutely precipitate or exacerbate RBD episodes, including SSRIs, SNRIs, tricyclic acids (TCAs), monoamine oxidase inhibitors (MAOIs), and mirtazapine, though notably this has not been seen with bupropion [3, 23, 25, 26]. Further medications which have been implicated include beta-blockers and selegiline, and anticholinesterase inhibitors [3]. PTSD has an association with RBD, though it is more commonly associated with a different REM parasomnia, nightmare disorder, as discussed in section "Nightmare Disorder". There is also a clear association with narcolepsy, primarily narcolepsy type 1 [27]. Up to 50% of patients with narcolepsy type 1 may demonstrate RBD, though the mechanism for this is distinct from other causes of RBD, as discussed below. Unfortunately, treatments aimed at reducing cataplexy in narcolepsy patients, such as TCAs or SNRIs, may exacerbate RBD symptoms. While patients commonly report dreams with aggressive content, in waking life there is no clear association with aggressive personality traits; therefore, no particular personality traits are thought to impart risk [28–30]. Traumatic brain injury is a risk factor for all types of parasomnia (both NREM and REM), with one study estimating new onset of RBD in 8% of TBI patients [31]. Family history is also a risk factor, with one study showing that among patients with confirmed idiopathic RBD, 14% had a close family member with a history of dream enactment [32]. Tobacco smokers are also more likely to develop RBD, both among those with Parkinson disease and among the general population [33, 34].

Pathophysiology

While numerous distinct neurodegenerative diseases have all been associated with RBD, the underlying pathophysiology connecting them appears to be disruption of the dopaminergic and noradrenergic pathways through the pons, striatum, and frontal lobes, as demonstrated by functional neuroimaging [3, 20, 35–42]. These pathways are integral to normal sleep physiology, involving the usual paralysis of skeletal muscles during REM sleep. Alpha-synucleinopathies tend to target these pontine nuclei of sleep early-on, which explains their strong association with RBD. The exception to this physiology is in narcolepsy, where orexin deficiency from the hypothalamus is the culprit, leading to destabilization of sleep architecture.

Epidemiology

Prevalence of RBD in the general population is thought to range from 0.5% to 1%, though some studies estimate a higher prevalence in the elderly population, around 2% [3, 43, 44]. As discussed above, it is more common in elderly males, though it has been reported in women, children, and teenagers.

Diagnostic Workup

In-laboratory video polysomnography (PSG) demonstrating REM sleep without atonia (RSWA) is required for a diagnosis of RBD; this entails capturing REM sleep with simultaneous capturing of excessive EMG activity on chin or limb leads. When RSWA occurs in the setting of a clinical complaint of dream enactment, then the diagnosis of RBD can be made. Practically speaking, when setting up for an RSWA screen, EMG leads should be placed on upper and lower limbs as well as the chin in order to increase sensitivity for muscle activity. RSWA tends to occur in all REM periods throughout the night, though it is often most prominent in latter portions of the night, when REM sleep is more emphasized. Home sleep apnea testing is not a useful screen for this condition, as the lack of sleep stage identification prevents an evaluation of RSWA.

Though there is a strong association between RBD and neurodegenerative diseases, identification of such processes is not necessary for a diagnosis of RBD. As such, it is not required to send diagnostic tests such as a dopamine transport scan (DAT) or a neuropsychological battery to evaluate for neurodegeneration, though these tests could be considered as part of a patient's larger multidisciplinary care plan, and would generally be coordinated by a neurologist.

The presence of significant autonomic activation such as tachycardia during a behavioral episode should raise a diagnostic red flag because while this does not rule out RBD, it is uncommon in this condition whereas it is quite common in the NREM parasomnias associated with arousals. Also, in RBD, general sleep architecture is preserved between wake, NREM, and REM stages, which differentiates it from status dissociatus (as discussed in 17.1.9).

Differential Diagnosis

Other conditions that can manifest as dramatic sleep-related behaviors are NREM parasomnias such as sleepwalking and sleep terrors, sleep-related hypermotor epilepsy (SHE), rhythmic movement disorders, and OSA.

To distinguish REM from NREM parasomnias, PSG and clinical history can be used to elucidate the stage of sleep associated with the behavior. Often the dramatic behavior itself is not captured on a single night PSG, so clinical history is relied on to clarify how early in the sleep cycle the behavior emerges. Typically, NREM parasomnias occur within the first one-third of the night, and REM parasomnias occur in the latter two-thirds of the night [3]. Further, RBD is characterized by rapid alertness and orientation, whereas NREM parasomnias may have a prolonged period of confusion [45]. Individuals with RBD tend to report vivid dream content, whereas those with NREM parasomnias have at most a fragmentary, limited recall of dream content. Vocalizations can be seen in both RBD and NREM parasomnias, but those due to RBD are often loud and feature expletives or aggressive content, whereas NREM vocalizations more often resemble usual conversation, though this can be seen in REM as well [45]. NREM parasomnias tend to present in childhood or young adulthood, whereas REM parasomnias traditionally present in older age, though as discussed above, there are exceptions in both directions [3].

Sleep-related hypermotor epilepsy (SHE), formerly known as Nocturnal Frontal Lobe Epilepsy (NFLE), is characterized by recurrent motor behaviors arising from sleep which can sometimes by dramatic or injurious in nature, similar to RBD. A key feature to screen for, especially from bed partners who can better describe the specific motions being performed, is whether the behaviors are stereotyped, as RBD tends to involve a range of vocalizations and actions, whereas epilepsy-induced behaviors tend to be a very stereotyped action or set of actions which can occur more than a dozen times throughout the night [46, 47].

Rhythmic movement disorder tends to be seen in childhood and only rarely occurs in adults. It consists of rhythmic movement of large muscle groups, such as body rocking or head-banging during sleep. These movements often occur in developmentally normal children and do not cause harm or distress to the affected individuals. When seen in adults, it may be related to other underlying sleep disorders such as restless leg syndrome or obstructive sleep apnea.

Periodic limb movements of sleep (PLMS), while also consisting of movements during sleep, are differentiated from RBD in that they predominantly occur during NREM and often consist of a stereotyped triple flexion of a leg (hip flexion, knee flexion, ankle dorsiflexion) that can occur frequently through the night around once per minute [3]. These movements do not have an association with dream content.

Untreated obstructive sleep apnea (OSA) should be considered in any case of parasomnia, given that it is a common condition that causes fractured sleep, which can provoke parasomnias. Pseudo-RBD, as it is known, occurs when a patient with sleep apnea presents with symptoms of RBD. However, the RSWA and dream enactment are secondary to apneas and hypopneas disrupting REM sleep. Treatment of OSA with CPAP or other therapies leads to resolution of the RBD symptoms [2].

Treatment

The predominant goal of all treatment strategies is to prevent injury by reducing the burden of behavioral events.

First, clinicians should screen for any factors that may have provoked secondary RBD and address those triggers. For instance, in cases of OSA-provoked parasomnias, appropriately treating the OSA generally resolves the symptoms [48, 49]. Further, if a medication, such as an antidepressant, is thought to be contributing, then that medication should be discontinued if possible.

Second, if no provoking factor is identified, then the patient is considered to have idiopathic primary RBD and warrants symptomatic treatment. Pharmacotherapy is a mainstay of treatment, though optimizing the sleeping environment to minimize injuries and property damage should also be part of treatment. For example, walls should be padded, dangerous or breakable objects should be moved away from the bed, and bed partners may be counseled to sleep in a separate bed. The primary pharmacologic agents are melatonin and clonazepam [50, 51]. Both medications have shown efficacy in reducing or eliminating RBD. Many clinicians prefer melatonin as an initial agent given its favorable side effect profile, especially since clonazepam's sedating properties can predispose elderly patients to falls, particularly those with dementia or gait disorders, which is a large portion of the RBD population [51]. There has never been a head-to-head trial between these agents, but clonazepam may be more likely to eliminate symptoms than melatonin, so it is a reasonable second-line agent if patients do not respond to an adequate melatonin trial (3–15 mg of melatonin).

Other medications which have some evidence suggesting their efficacy toward RBD include "z-drugs" such as zopiclone, benzodiazepines other than clonazepam, acetylcholinesterase inhibitors such as donepezil and rivastigmine, carbamazepine, sodium oxybate, clozapine, pramipexole, levodopa, and paroxetine. Many of these drugs have only been studied in case reports or limited populations and are rarely used. However, they could be considered when both melatonin and clonazepam have been ineffective.

Subtypes

Status Dissociatus

Status dissociatus is a subtype of RBD where the individual expresses clinical behaviors suggestive of classic RBD (e.g., aggressive dream enactment), but on PSG, there is a lack of identifiable sleep stages. The PSG has a mixture of markers for wakefulness, NREM, and REM, without a clear delineation between these stages. Even more than in classical RBD, individuals with status dissociatus are often interpreted by observers to be awake when engaging in dream enactment behaviors, and these individuals may often be confused about whether they are awake or asleep [3]. If this condition is accompanied by generalized motor overactivity during wakefulness, loss of slow wave sleep, and sympathetic overactivation, then this would be consistent with a syndrome called "agrypnia excitata" and raises concern for an autoimmune/paraneoplastic encephalitis, delirium tremens, or fatal familial insomnia [3]. The prevalence of this subtype is unknown.

Parasomnia Overlap

Parasomnia overlap disorder refers to patients who meet clinical criteria for RBD and, in addition, have an NREM-related parasomnia or rhythmic movement disorder. Unlike isolated RBD, overlap syndrome is much more common in younger ages, often beginning during childhood and adolescence, though any age range could be affected. The associated pathophysiology is not as clear as with isolated RBD, and many diverse causes have been implicated, including pharmacotherapies, substance use, various psychiatric disorders, multiple sclerosis, narcolepsy, and traumatic brain injury [3]. As with status dissociatus, the prevalence is unknown. While this disorder may sound like status dissociatus in that REM and NREM conditions are blended, parasomnia overlap disorder does not feature involvement of the awake state, and affected individuals do not report confusion about whether they are awake, asleep, or dreaming.

Recurrent Isolated Sleep Paralysis

Definition

Recurrent isolated sleep paralysis is defined as (A) a recurrent inability to move the trunk and all limbs at onset or offset of sleep, (B) the episodes last seconds to minutes, (C) the episodes cause distress, and (D) the episodes are not better explained by a different medical condition [3].

Clinical Features

Recurrent isolated sleep paralysis is a recurrent distressing sensation of an inability to move one's body while transitioning to or from sleep [52, 53]. While it is benign, it can be associated with significant anxiety during and after an episode. Affected individuals are unable to speak or move, though they are fully conscious. Respiratory muscles are unaffected. These episodes tend to resolve spontaneously within a short period, usually seconds though it can last up to a few minutes, and sometimes an episode can be ended early if an observer speaks to or touches the patient. These episodes are not classified as a disease unless they are associated with significant distress to the patient, such as inducing bedtime anxiety or fear of sleep. Hallucinations often occur, including visual, auditory, or tactile hallucinations such as a sensation of a creature sitting on the individual's chest. The condition often presents in adolescence, with mean age of onset 14–17 years old, and most episodes occur in patient's teens and 20s [3].

Risk Factors

A familial form of sleep paralysis has been reported in two families, suggesting that underlying genetics may play a role; however, most cases do not have a clear familial component. Male and female sexes appear to have equal risk. As with all parasomnias, sleep deprivation and irregular sleep cycles are risk factors [54]. Patients who sleep supine appear to be at higher risk, though the mechanism for this is not understood. One case has been reported of isolated sleep paralysis induced by the abrupt withdrawal of bupropion [55]. As with all parasomnias, psychiatric disease is a risk factor [24].

Pathophysiology

Like narcolepsy, isolated sleep paralysis is thought to occur from a state dissociation, with the normal expected REM paralysis of skeletal muscles continuing abnormally into wakefulness. Brainstem systems that control serotonin, norepinephrine, and acetylcholine appear to be affected. Individuals who are sensitive to sleep disruptions may be particularly vulnerable, and abrupt awakenings from REM may produce an episode [3].

Epidemiology

There are limited global data on the prevalence of recurrent isolated sleep paralysis, partially due to the various definitions that have been used. When examining for single occurrences of isolated sleep paralysis, prevalence may range from 5% to 40% [3, 56].

Diagnostic Workup

A polysomnogram (PSG) is not required for diagnosis, and subjective history can be sufficient. A PSG may be supportive if it demonstrates REM atonia on EMG leads that persists into wakefulness.

Differential Diagnosis

The primary disease to consider is narcolepsy, which also often includes sleep paralysis episodes and hypnagogic and/or hypnopompic hallucinations. However, the prominent features of narcolepsy are extreme daytime somnolence and reduced mean sleep latency time, whereas these features are absent from recurrent isolated sleep paralysis. Another related phenomenon, cataplexy, also involves REM atonia invading the awake state, though it occurs during full wakefulness rather than at periods of transition to and from sleep; cataplexy also tends to be triggered by intense emotions, whereas sleep paralysis does not. Similar to cataplexy, atonic seizures can involve preserved consciousness with inability to move limbs, but atonic seizures occur during wakefulness rather than only at times of sleep transition.

Periodic paralysis syndromes may resemble isolated sleep paralysis in that the affected individual is conscious but unable to move the body. These episodes may occur during wakefulness or at periods of sleep transition; if the latter is the case, the primary way to differentiate these syndromes from isolated sleep paralysis is that periodic paralysis lasts for hours rather than seconds. Periodic paralysis is also less likely to affect bulbar muscles the way sleep paralysis can. These periodic paralysis syndromes include a hypokalemic, hyperkalemic, and thyrotoxic form, and involve mutations in skeletal muscle ions channels. Paralysis attacks can be precipitated by a large intake of carbohydrates, excessive exercise, or alcohol intake. Most cases of periodic paralysis are hereditary with an autosomal dominant inheritance [57].

Treatment

If sleep deprivation is thought to be a provoking factor, then that component can be addressed, such as avoiding shift work, addressing jet lag, or other general sleep hygiene components. Further pharmacotherapy options include tricyclic antidepressants (e.g., imipramine and clomipramine) or SSRIs (e.g., fluoxetine or escitalopram), all of which are thought to work by suppressing REM [58, 59].

Nightmare Disorder

Definition

Nightmare disorder is defined as (A) repeated, extended, well-remembered dreams associated with intensely unpleasant emotions, (B) rapid, full alertness on awakening, and (C) associated distress or impairment in functioning [3].

Clinical Features

Nightmares entail a realistic and vivid dream sequence that tends to become increasingly frightening, though other negative emotions can be predominant such as anger, disgust, guilt, or embarrassment. There is often a theme of imminent bodily harm, though this is not universally true. On awakening, affected individuals are quickly oriented, and can vividly recall dream content. There is often difficulty returning to sleep after an episode, and individuals may note signs of increased sympathetic activity such as rapid heart rate or piloerection. These episodes tend to occur in the latter third of a sleep session, as this is when REM sleep is most prominent. Nightmares associated with PTSD may be more variable in their timing within a sleep cycle, and can occur at sleep onset or from NREM sleep [3].

While occasional nightmares are quite common among the general population, a diagnosis of nightmare disorder is only made if these occurrences are persistent and affect a person's daily functioning. Distress can be manifested by any of the following: mood disturbances, sleep resistance, cognitive impairment such as concentration difficulties, negative impact on family functioning, behavioral disturbances, daytime somnolence, low energy, impairment in one's education or occupation, or impaired social function [3].

Risk Factors

The greatest risk factor for nightmare disorder is exposure to severe psychosocial stressors. This is particularly true in children, though in all age groups there is an association between physical or sexual abuse and nightmares. Trauma often precedes the onset of nightmares, though there may be a prolonged delay prior to nightmare onset. In acute stress disorder, symptoms occur immediately after a trauma, whereas in posttraumatic stress disorder, symptoms may arise more than a month after the event [3, 60].

Individuals who had recurrent nightmares as children are more likely to report recurrent nightmares as an adult, suggesting that predisposition to nightmares may be a component of one's personality traits. Twin studies also demonstrate that there are genetic predispositions to nightmares, analogous to the pattern seen with NREM parasomnias such as sleepwalking and sleep talking [61].

Nightmares can be induced by pharmaceuticals that affect neurotransmitter concentrations and function, particularly for serotonin, dopamine, and norepinephrine [62, 63]. Medications of interest include antidepressants of all classes; antihypertensive agents including beta-blockers and calcium channel blockers; dopaminergic drugs including levodopa and methylphenidate; atypical antipsychotics including risperidone and olanzapine; sedatives including alcohol and barbiturates (particularly withdrawal from these); acetylcholinesterase inhibitors, including donepezil and rivastigmine; and varenicline, which is a nicotinic acetylcholine receptor antagonist. Another class of implicated medications is antimicrobials (e.g., cipro-floxacin, ganciclovir, and mefloquine) which, in contrast to the above list, are thought to act via modulation of cytokines that are involved in sleep such as IL-1B and TNF-alpha. Implicated medical conditions include hypoglycemia induced by nocturnal insulin use [64], as well as all mood disorders including major depression, bipolar affective disorder, and schizoaffective disorder [24, 65]. As with all para-somnias, sleep deprivation and OSA can be a predisposing factor [66].

Pathophysiology

The pathophysiology of nightmares is not known.

Epidemiology

Occasional nightmares occur in 60–75% of children, and in most cases these night-mares are sporadic. Only in a small minority of children are nightmares frequent and extensive, occurring in 1–5% of children [3]. Among the general population, 2–8% report distress related to nightmares, and the age most likely to be affected is between 6 and 10 years old [67–69]. However, the incidence is increased among adults with psychopathology, most notable among those with PTSD where 80% report recurrent nightmares.

Diagnostic Workup

Patient history is sufficient for diagnosis of nightmare disorder, and further PSG evaluation is not required [70]. However, it may be considered if during the patients' nightmares they perform actions that either cause harm to self or others, or are highly stereotyped in nature, as this would raise clinical suspicion for other condi-tions, as described below.

Differential Diagnosis

The main conditions to distinguish from nightmare disorder are sleep terrors, noc-turnal panic attacks, seizures, RBD, and sleep paralysis.

Sleep terrors also involve an awakening from sleep with appearance of distress. However, with sleep terrors there is a prominent component of confusion and dis-orientation, which is not seen with nightmares. Further, in sleep terrors there is a lack of recall of dream content, whereas dream recall tends to be vivid with night-mares. Prominent autonomic activity (e.g., diaphoresis, pupillary dilatation) is more common with sleep terrors than nightmares. As sleep terrors arise from NREM sleep, they tend to occur earlier in the night, while nightmares occur later in the night. Similarly, nocturnal panic attacks tend to arise from NREM sleep, occurring earlier in the night and are not typically associated with vivid dream content.

Nocturnal seizures can, in rare cases, present only with recurrent nightmares [71]. These can be difficult to distinguish from true nightmares by history, though suspicion should be raised in patients with underlying cerebral disease or a history of epilepsy. Nightmares from epilepsy are more likely to resemble classic temporal lobe auras, such as déjà vu or intense panic without any associated dream content to induce the fear. These episodes come from NREM sleep rather than true REM sleep. A PSG, preferably with an extended EEG montage, is required to capture and prove that episodes are epileptic in nature.

REM sleep behavior disorder (RBD), as discussed in section "REM Sleep Behavior DisorderS30", involves involuntary acting out of dream content, much of which tends to involve frightening and life-threatening situations. While the dream content can be analogous between these two conditions, nightmare disorder does not involve any physical action, movement, or injury, so the presence of these would be strongly suggestive of RBD. RBD is most common in older age, whereas night-mare disorder is most common in childhood, though there are exceptions in both directions, as discussed above.

Sleep paralysis, whether occurring as part of isolated recurrent sleep paralysis (see section "Recurrent Isolated Sleep Paralysis") or narcolepsy, occurs at periods of transition to or from sleep and can often be associated with anxiety during the episode. Hallucinations commonly co-occur and can be disturbing in nature. While nightmares can occasionally involve an inability to move or speak, a recurrent experience of total paralysis with simultaneous wakefulness is much more suggestive of sleep paralysis.

Treatment

Nightmares on their own do not necessitate treatment, as they can often be self-limited. In particular, nightmares occurring in the context of recent bereavement tend to resolve over time [72]. For those patients who do require treatment, the next step is to address general sleep hygiene and any predisposing medications or medi-cal conditions. When this approach is insufficient, then a choice or combination between cognitive behavioral therapy (CBT) and pharmacotherapy can be employed [73].

CBT interventions for nightmare disorder emphasize stress management and repeated exposures [74]. As with other forms of CBT, it consists of a limited set of therapy sessions, aimed at addressing the maladaptive thoughts, emotions, and behaviors that disrupt patients' lives. One option is image rehearsal therapy, where patients recall the nightmare while awake, write down its details including emotional content, modify the story to have a more positive ending, and then rehearse the new narrative with the goal of replacing the nightmare if the dream recurs [73, 75, 76]. Another option is lucid dreaming treatment, where the patient is taught to identify that they are dreaming during a nightmare and then actively change the ending of the nightmare to a positive one [77]. Hypnosis has also been shown in small case studies to be effective in decreasing nightmare frequency [78]. Finally, systemic desensitization, where patients are gradually exposed to cues associated with their nightmares and taught stress management techniques, can be used [79].

The best-studied pharmacotherapy option is prazosin, which is a centrally active alpha1-adrenergic antagonist, and has been well-described to be effective in both PTSD and other nightmare disorders [73, 80–83]. It is thought to act via blunting of the sympathetic arousal state associated with nightmares. The only other medications recommended by the American Academy of Sleep Medicine (AASM) are triazepam and nitrazolam [84]. If these medications are ineffective or not tolerated, then there are many other options, which have primarily been studied in the context of PTSD nightmares: topiramate [85, 86], trazodone [87], risperidone [87], gabapentin [73, 88], olanzapine [89, 90], clonidine [73], aripiprazole [84], cyproheptadine [84], phenelzine [84], tricyclic antidepressants [84], and synthetic cannabinoids [91, 92]. Two medications which the AASM specifically recommends against using are venlafaxine and clonazepam, as the limited studies looking at these two have shown no efficacy [84]. Once a patient has attained prolonged relief from nightmares, pharmacotherapy can be tapered off.

References

1. Gagnon J-F, Postuma RB, Mazza S, Doyon J, Montplaisir J. Rapid-eye-movement sleep behaviour disorder and neurodegenerative diseases. Lancet Neurol. 2006;5(5):424–32.
2. Boeve B. Updated review of the core features, the REM sleep behavior disorder-neurodegenerative disease association, evolving concepts, controversies, and future directions. Ann N Y Acad Sci. 2010;1184:15–54.
3. Sateia MJ. International classification of sleep disorders. Chest. 2014;146(5):1387–94.
4. Stores G. Rapid eye movement sleep behaviour disorder in children and adolescents. Dev Med Child Neurol. 2008;50(10):728–32.
5. Lin FC, Lai CL, Huang P, Liu CK, Hsu CY. The rapid-eye-movement sleep behavior disorder in Chinese-Taiwanese patients. Psychiatry Clin Neurosci. 2009;63(4):557–62.
6. Tachibana N, Yamanaka K, Kaji R, Nagamine T, Watatani K, Kimura J, et al. Sleep bruxism as a manifestation of subclinical rapid eye movement sleep behavior disorder. Sleep. 1994;17(6):555–8.
7. Abe S, Gagnon J-F, Montplaisir JY, Postuma RB, Rompré PH, Huynh NT, et al. Sleep bruxism and oromandibular myoclonus in rapid eye movement sleep behavior disorder: a preliminary report. Sleep Med. 2013;14(10):1024–30.
8. Covassin N, Neikrug AB, Liu L, Corey-Bloom J, Loredo JS, Palmer BW, et al. Clinical correlates of periodic limb movements in sleep in Parkinson's disease. J Neurol Sci. 2012;316(1–2):131–6.

9. Fantini M, Michaud M, Gosselin N, Lavigne G, Montplaisir J. Periodic leg movements in REM sleep behavior disorder and related autonomic and EEG activation. Neurology. 2002;59(12):1889–94.

10. Postuma RB, Gagnon JF, Vendette M, Desjardins C, Montplaisir JY. Olfaction and color vision identify impending neurodegeneration in rapid eye movement sleep behavior disorder. Ann Neurol. 2011;69(5):811–8.

11. Fantini ML, Farini E, Ortelli P, Zucconi M, Manconi M, Cappa S, et al. Longitudinal study of cognitive function in idiopathic REM sleep behavior disorder. Sleep. 2011;34(5):619–25.

12. Kawamura M, Sugimoto A, Kobayakawa M, Tsuruya N. Neurological disease and facial recognition. Brain Nerve. 2012;64(7):799–813.

13. Génier Marchand D, Postuma RB, Escudier F, De Roy J, Pelletier A, Montplaisir J, et al. How does dementia with Lewy bodies start? prodromal cognitive changes in REM sleep behavior disorder. Ann Neurol. 2018;83(5):1016–26.

14. Coco DL, Cupidi C, Mattaliano A, Baiamonte V, Realmuto S, Cannizzaro E. REM sleep behavior disorder in a patient with frontotemporal dementia. Neurol Sci. 2012;33(2):371–3.

15. Chokroverty S, Bhat S, Rosen D, Farheen A. REM behavior disorder in myotonic dystrophy type 2. Neurology. 2012;78(24):2004.

16. Ebben MR, Shahbazi M, Lange DJ, Krieger AC. REM behavior disorder associated with familial amyotrophic lateral sclerosis. Amyotroph Lateral Scler. 2012;13(5):473–4.

17. Nomura T, Inoue Y, Takigawa H, Nakashima K. Comparison of REM sleep behaviour disorder variables between patients with progressive supranuclear palsy and those with Parkinson's disease. Parkinsonism Relat Disord. 2012;18(4):394–6.

18. Olson EJ, Boeve BF, Silber MH. Rapid eye movement sleep behaviour disorder: demographic, clinical and laboratory findings in 93 cases. Brain. 2000;123(2):331–9.

19. Claassen D, Josephs KA, Ahlskog J, Silber M, Tippmann-Peikert M, Boeve BF. REM sleep behavior disorder preceding other aspects of synucleinopathies by up to half a century. Neurology. 2010;75(6):494–9.

20. Galbiati A, Verga L, Giora E, Zucconi M, Ferini-Strambi L. The risk of neurodegeneration in REM sleep behavior disorder: a systematic review and meta-analysis of longitudinal studies. Sleep Med Rev. 2019;43:37–46.

21. Bodkin CL, Schenck CH. Rapid eye movement sleep behavior disorder in women: relevance to general and specialty medical practice. J Women's Health. 2009;18(12):1955–63.

22. Teman PT, Tippmann-Peikert M, Silber MH, Slocumb NL, Auger RR. Idiopathic rapid-eye-movement sleep disorder: associations with antidepressants, psychiatric diagnoses, and other factors, in relation to age of onset. Sleep Med. 2009;10(1):60–5.

23. Schenck CH, Mahowald MW, Kim SW, O'Connor KA, Hurwitz TD. Prominent eye movements during NREM sleep and REM sleep behavior disorder associated with fluoxetine treatment of depression and obsessive-compulsive disorder. Sleep. 1992;15(3):226–35.

24. Waters F, Moretto U, Dang-Vu TT. Psychiatric illness and parasomnias: a systematic review. Curr Psychiatry Rep. 2017;19(7):37.

25. Hoque R, Chesson AL Jr. Pharmacologically induced/exacerbated restless legs syndrome, periodic limb movements of sleep, and REM behavior disorder/REM sleep without atonia: literature review, qualitative scoring, and comparative analysis. J Clin Sleep Med. 2010;6(01):79–83.

26. Frauscher B, Jennum P, Ju Y-ES, Postuma RB, Arnulf I, De Cock VC, et al. Comorbidity and medication in REM sleep behavior disorder: a multicenter case-control study. Neurology. 2014;82(12):1076–9.

27. Nightingale S, Orgill J, Ebrahim I, De Lacy S, Agrawal S, Williams A. The association between narcolepsy and REM behavior disorder (RBD). Sleep Med. 2005;6(3):253–8.

28. Fantini ML, Corona A, Clerici S, Ferini-Strambi L. Aggressive dream content without daytime aggressiveness in REM sleep behavior disorder. Neurology. 2005;65(7):1010–5.

29. D'Agostino A, Manni R, Limosani I, Terzaghi M, Cavallotti S, Scarone S. Challenging the myth of REM sleep behavior disorder: no evidence of heightened aggressiveness in dreams. Sleep Med. 2012;13(6):714–9.

30. Sasai T, Inoue Y, Matsuura M. Do patients with rapid eye movement sleep behavior disorder have a disease-specific personality? Parkinsonism Relat Disord. 2012;18(5):616–8.
31. Verma A, Anand V, Verma NP. Sleep disorders in chronic traumatic brain injury. J Clin Sleep Med. 2007;3(04):357–62.
32. Dauvilliers Y, Postuma RB, Ferini-Strambi L, Arnulf I, Högl B, Manni R, et al. Family history of idiopathic REM behavior disorder: a multicenter case-control study. Neurology. 2013;80(24):2233–5.
33. Jacobs ML, Dauvilliers Y, St Louis EK, McCarter SJ, Romenets SR, Pelletier A, et al. Risk factor profile in Parkinson's disease subtype with REM sleep behavior disorder. J Parkinsons Dis. 2016;6(1):231–7.
34. Yao C, Fereshtehnejad S-M, Keezer MR, Wolfson C, Pelletier A, Postuma RB. Risk factors for possible REM sleep behavior disorder: a CLSA population-based cohort study. Neurology. 2019;92(5):e475–e85.
35. Postuma R, Gagnon J, Vendette M, Fantini M, Massicotte-Marquez J, Montplaisir J. Quantifying the risk of neurodegenerative disease in idiopathic REM sleep behavior disorder. Neurology. 2009;72(15):1296–300.
36. Iranzo A, Santamaria J, Tolosa E. The clinical and pathophysiological relevance of REM sleep behavior disorder in neurodegenerative diseases. Sleep Med Rev. 2009;13(6):385–401.
37. Iranzo A, Tolosa E, Gelpi E, Molinuevo JL, Valldeoriola F, Serradell M, et al. Neurodegenerative disease status and post-mortem pathology in idiopathic rapid-eye-movement sleep behaviour disorder: an observational cohort study. Lancet Neurol. 2013;12(5):443–53.
38. Heller J, Brcina N, Dogan I, Holtbernd F, Romanzetti S, Schulz JB, et al. Brain imaging findings in idiopathic REM sleep behavior disorder (RBD)–a systematic review on potential biomarkers for neurodegeneration. Sleep Med Rev. 2017;34:23–33.
39. Eisensehr I, Linke R, Tatsch K, Kharraz B, Gildehaus JF, Wetter CT, et al. Increased muscle activity during rapid eye movement sleep correlates with decrease of striatal presynaptic dopamine transporters. IPT and IBZM SPECT imaging in subclinical and clinically manifest idiopathic REM sleep behavior disorder, Parkinson's disease, and controls. Sleep. 2003;26(5):507–12.
40. Albin R, Koeppe R, Chervin R, Consens F, Wernette K, Frey K, et al. Decreased striatal dopaminergic innervation in REM sleep behavior disorder. Neurology. 2000;55(9):1410–2.
41. Gilman S, Koeppe R, Chervin R, Consens F, Little R, An H, et al. REM sleep behavior disorder is related to striatal monoaminergic deficit in MSA. Neurology. 2003;61(1):29–34.
42. Shirakawa SI, Takeuchi N, Uchimura N, Ohyama T, Maeda H, Abe T, et al. Study of image findings in rapid eye movement sleep behavioural disorder. Psychiatry Clin Neurosci. 2002;56(3):291–2.
43. Haba-Rubio J, Frauscher B, Marques-Vidal P, Toriel J, Tobback N, Andries D, et al. Prevalence and determinants of rapid eye movement sleep behavior disorder in the general population. Sleep. 2018;41(2):zsx197.
44. Kang S-H, Yoon I-Y, Lee SD, Han JW, Kim TH, Kim KW. REM sleep behavior disorder in the Korean elderly population: prevalence and clinical characteristics. Sleep. 2013;36(8):1147–52.
45. Howell MJ. Parasomnias: an updated review. Neurotherapeutics. 2012;9(4):753–75.
46. Tinuper P, Bisulli F. From nocturnal frontal lobe epilepsy to sleep-related hypermotor epilepsy: a 35-year diagnostic challenge. Seizure. 2017;44:87–92.
47. Provini F, Plazzi G, Tinuper P, Vandi S, Lugaresi E, Montagna P. Nocturnal frontal lobe epilepsy: a clinical and polygraphic overview of 100 consecutive cases. Brain. 1999;122(6):1017–31.
48. Henriques-Filho PSA, Pratesi R. Sleep apnea and REM sleep behavior disorder in patients with Chiari malformations. Arq Neuropsiquiatr. 2008;66(2B):344–9.
49. Iranzo A, Santamaría J. Severe obstructive sleep apnea/hypopnea mimicking REM sleep behavior disorder. Sleep. 2005;28(2):203–6.
50. Kunz D, Mahlberg R. A two-part, double-blind, placebo-controlled trial of exogenous melatonin in REM sleep behaviour disorder. J Sleep Res. 2010;19(4):591–6.

51. Zak RS, Maganti RK, Auerbach SH, Casey KR, Chowdhuri S, Karippot A, et al. Best practice guide for the treatment of REM sleep behavior disorder (RBD). J Clin Sleep Med. 2010;6(01):85–95.
52. Goode GB. Sleep paralysis. Arch Neurol. 1962;6(3):228–34.
53. Sharpless BA. A clinician's guide to recurrent isolated sleep paralysis. Neuropsychiatr Dis Treat. 2016;12:1761.
54. Takeuchi T, Miyasita A, Sasaki Y, Inugami M, Fukuda K. Isolated sleep paralysis elicited by sleep interruption. Sleep. 1992;15(3):217–25.
55. Bieber ED, Bieber DA, Romanowicz M, Voort JLV, Kolla BP, McKean AJ. Recurrent isolated sleep paralysis following bupropion cessation: a case report. J Clin Psychopharmacol. 2019;39(4):407–9.
56. Ohayon MM, Zulley J, Guilleminault C, Smirne S. Prevalence and pathologic associations of sleep paralysis in the general population. Neurology. 1999;52(6):1194.
57. Fontaine B, Lapie P, Plassart E, Tabti N, Nicole S, Reboul J, et al. Periodic paralysis and voltage-gated ion channels. Kidney Int. 1996;49(1):9–18.
58. Mitler MM, Hajdukovic R, Erman M, Koziol JA. Narcolepsy. J Clin Neurophysiol. 1990;7(1):93.
59. Hintze JP, Gault D. Escitalopram for recurrent isolated sleep paralysis. J Sleep Res. 2020;29:e13027.
60. Lavie P. Sleep disturbances in the wake of traumatic events. N Engl J Med. 2001;345(25): 1825–32.
61. Hublin C, Kaprio J, Partinen M, Koskenvuo M. Nightmares: familial aggregation and association with psychiatric disorders in a nationwide twin cohort. Am J Med Genet. 1999;88(4):329–36.
62. Pagel J, Helfter P. Drug induced nightmares—an etiology based review. Hum Psychopharmacol Clin Exp. 2003;18(1):59–67.
63. Foral P, Knezevich J, Dewan N, Malesker M. Medication-induced sleep disturbances. Consult Pharm. 2011;26(6):414–25.
64. Allen KV, Frier BM. Nocturnal hypoglycemia: clinical manifestations and therapeutic strategies toward prevention. Endocr Pract. 2003;9(6):530–43.
65. Beauchemin KM, Hays P. Dreaming away depression: the role of REM sleep and dreaming in affective disorders. J Affect Disord. 1996;41(2):125–33.
66. Schredl M, Schmitt J, Hein G, Schmoll T, Eller S, Haaf J. Nightmares and oxygen desaturations: is sleep apnea related to heightened nightmare frequency? Sleep Breath. 2006;10(4):203–9.
67. Levin R, Fireman G. Nightmare prevalence, nightmare distress, and self-reported psychological disturbance. Sleep. 2002;25(2):205–12.
68. Zadra A, Donderi D. Nightmares and bad dreams: their prevalence and relationship to well-being. J Abnorm Psychol. 2000;109(2):273.
69. Gauchat A, Seguin J, Zadra A. Prevalence and correlates of disturbed dreaming in children. Pathol Biol. 2014;62(5):311–8.
70. Boursoulian LJ, Schenck CH, Mahowald MW, Lagrange AH. Differentiating parasomnias from nocturnal seizures. J Clin Sleep Med. 2012;8(01):108–12.
71. Silvestri R, Bromfield E. Recurrent nightmares and disorders of arousal in temporal lobe epilepsy. Brain Res Bull. 2004;63(5):369–76.
72. Wright ST, Kerr CW, Doroszczuk NM, Kuszczak SM, Hang PC, Luczkiewicz DL. The impact of dreams of the deceased on bereavement: A survey of hospice caregivers. Am J Hosp Palliat Med. 2014;31(2):132–8.
73. Zak RS, Auerbach SH, Casey KR, Chowdhuri S, Karippot A, Maganti RK, et al. Best practice guide for the treatment of nightmare disorder in adults. J Clin Sleep Med. 2010;6(04):389–401.
74. Lancee J, Spoormaker VI, Krakow B, van den Bout J. A systematic review of cognitive-behavioral treatment for nightmares: toward a well-established treatment. J Clin Sleep Med. 2008;4(05):475–80.

75. Seda G, Sanchez-Ortuno MM, Welsh CH, Halbower AC, Edinger JD. Comparative meta-analysis of prazosin and imagery rehearsal therapy for nightmare frequency, sleep quality, and posttraumatic stress. J Clin Sleep Med. 2015;11(01):11–22.
76. Krakow B, Hollifield M, Johnston L, Koss M, Schrader R, Warner TD, et al. Imagery rehearsal therapy for chronic nightmares in sexual assault survivors with posttraumatic stress disorder: a randomized controlled trial. JAMA. 2001;286(5):537–45.
77. Spoormaker VI, Van Den Bout J. Lucid dreaming treatment for nightmares: a pilot study. Psychother Psychosom. 2006;75(6):389–94.
78. Committee SP, Aurora RN, Zak RS, Auerbach SH, Casey KR, Chowdhuri S, et al. Best practice guide for the treatment of nightmare disorder in adults. J Clin Sleep Med. 2010;6(4):389–401.
79. Grandi S, Fabbri S, Panattoni N, Gonnella E, Marks I. Self-exposure treatment of recurrent nightmares: waiting-list-controlled trial and 4-year follow-up. Psychother Psychosom. 2006;75(6):384–8.
80. Daly CM, Doyle ME, Radkind M, Raskind E, Daniels C. Clinical case series: the use of prazosin for combat-related recurrent nightmares among Operation Iraqi Freedom combat veterans. Mil Med. 2005;170(6):513–5.
81. Miller LJ. Prazosin for the treatment of posttraumatic stress disorder sleep disturbances. Pharmacotherapy. 2008;28(5):656–66.
82. Taylor F, Raskind MA. The α1-adrenergic antagonist prazosin improves sleep and nightmares in civilian trauma posttraumatic stress disorder. J Clin Psychopharmacol. 2002;22(1):82–5.
83. Taylor HR, Freeman MK, Cates ME. Prazosin for treatment of nightmares related to posttraumatic stress disorder. Am J Health Syst Pharm. 2008;65(8):716–22.
84. Morgenthaler TI, Auerbach S, Casey KR, Kristo D, Maganti R, Ramar K, et al. Position paper for the treatment of nightmare disorder in adults: an American Academy of Sleep Medicine position paper. J Clin Sleep Med. 2018;14(6):1041.
85. Nadorff MR, Lambdin KK, Germain A. Pharmacological and non-pharmacological treatments for nightmare disorder. Int Rev Psychiatry. 2014;26(2):225–36.
86. Aalbersberg C, Mulder J. Topiramate for the treatment of post traumatic stress disorder. A case study. Tijdschr Psychiatr. 2006;48(6):487–91.
87. Nielsen T, Levin R. Nightmares: a new neurocognitive model. Sleep Med Rev. 2007;11(4):295–310.
88. Hamner MB, Brodrick PS, Labbate LA. Gabapentin in PTSD: a retrospective, clinical series of adjunctive therapy. Ann Clin Psychiatry. 2001;13(3):141–6.
89. Detweiler MB, Pagadala B, Candelario J, Boyle JS, Detweiler JG, Lutgens BW. Treatment of post-traumatic stress disorder nightmares at a veterans affairs medical center. J Clin Med. 2016;5(12):117.
90. Jakovljević M, Šagud M, Mihaljević-Peleš A. Olanzapine in the treatment-resistant, combat-related PTSD–a series of case reports. Acta Psychiatr Scand. 2003;107(5):394–6.
91. Jetly R, Heber A, Fraser G, Boisvert D. The efficacy of nabilone, a synthetic cannabinoid, in the treatment of PTSD-associated nightmares: a preliminary randomized, double-blind, placebo-controlled cross-over design study. Psychoneuroendocrinology. 2015;51:585–8.
92. Fraser GA. The use of a synthetic cannabinoid in the management of treatment-resistant nightmares in posttraumatic stress disorder (PTSD). CNS Neurosci Ther. 2009;15(1):84–8.

Chapter 18
Movement Disorders

Salam Zeineddine and Nidhi S. Undevia

Keywords Sleep-related movement disorders · Restless legs syndrome · Periodic limb movement disorder · Sleep-related leg cramps · Sleep-related bruxism · Sleep-related rhythmic movement disorder

Introduction

Sleep-related movement disorders are conditions that are characterized by simple, usually stereotyped, movements that disturb sleep or its onset, such as RLS. The Third Edition of the *International Classification of Sleep Disorders* (ICSD-3) includes restless legs syndrome (RLS), periodic limb movement disorder (PLMD), sleep-related leg cramps, sleep-related bruxism and sleep-related rhythmic movement disorder (RMD). Propriospinal myoclonus at sleep onset, sleep-related movement disorder due to a medical disorder, and sleep-related movement disorder due to a medication or substance are also included under this heading [1] (Table 18.1). RLS is classified within this group of disorders due to its close association with PLMD. Movement alone is not sufficient for the diagnosis of a sleep-related movement disorder as an associated sleep disturbance or an impairment of daytime functioning is required. Daytime impairment can affect any important area of functioning

S. Zeineddine
Department of Medicine, John D. Dingell VA Medical Center and Wayne State University School of Medicine, Detroit, MI, USA

N. S. Undevia (✉)
Department of Medicine, Division of Pulmonary and Critical Care Medicine, Loyola Center for Sleep Disorders, Loyola University Medical Center, Maywood, IL, USA
e-mail: nundevia@lumc.edu

Table 18.1 Sleep-related movement disorders

Restless legs syndrome
Periodic limb movement disorder
Sleep-related leg cramps
Sleep-related bruxism
Sleep-related rhythmic movement disorder
Propriospinal myoclonus at sleep onset
Sleep-related movement disorder due to a medical disorder
Sleep-related movement disorder due to a medication or substance

such as mental, physical, social, behavioral, educational, or others. Each of these topics will be discussed in this chapter.

Restless Legs Syndrome

RLS is a sensorimotor disorder characterized by a distressing urge to move the legs and sometimes other parts of the body such as the arms. The British physician Sir Thomas Willis first described RLS in the seventeenth century by these very descriptive words "Wherefore to some, when being abed they betake themselves to sleep, presently in the arms and legs, leapings and contractions of the tendons, and so great a restlessness and tossings of their members ensue that the diseased are no more able to sleep than if they were in a place of the greatest torture" [2]. The first significant clinical review was carried out by the Swedish neurologist Karl-Axel Ekbom in the 1940s who also coined the term "restless legs" [3]. The severity of RLS can vary from mild with only occasional symptoms to daily severe symptoms that can have a profound effect on sleep and daytime functioning. The pathophysiology of RLS is incompletely understood, but probably results from derangements in iron and dopamine metabolism and has a genetic component [4–6].

Demographics

The prevalence of RLS varies from region to region; in Europe, South and North America, and the Indian subcontinent, it is estimated to be 4–10% of the adult population, while in Japan, Korea, and China, for example, it is 0.6, 0.9, and 1.6%, respectively [7–9]. In the United States, it is believed to affect more than ten million adults. The 2005 National Sleep Foundation Poll reported RLS symptoms in 8% of men and 11% of women [10]. Women and older adults appear to be at increased risk [11]. The prevalence of RLS in women is roughly twice that reported in men [12]. A population survey study reported that the prevalence of symptoms of RLS was

3% between the ages of 18 and 29 years, 10% between the ages of 30 and 79 years, and 19% in persons older than 80 years of age [13].

Diagnosis

RLS diagnosis is based on clinical grounds and no laboratory study reliably identifies RLS. It does not require a polysomnogram (PSG) unless an additional sleep disorder is thought to be present. The diagnosis of RLS in adults according to ICSD-3 requires the following: (a) The patient reports an urge to move the legs, usually accompanied or caused by uncomfortable and unpleasant sensation in the legs. (b) The urge to move or the unpleasant sensations begin or worsen during periods of rest or inactivity such as lying or sitting. (c) The urge to move or the unpleasant sensations are partially or totally relieved by movement, such as walking or stretching, at least as long as the activity continues. (d) The urge to move or the unpleasant sensations are worse, or only occur, in the evening or night. (e) The condition is not better explained by another current sleep disorder, medical or neurological disorder, mental disorder, medication use, or substance use disorder. (f) The symptoms cause concern, distress, sleep disturbance, or impairment in daytime functionning [1] (Table 18.2). Separate diagnostic criteria have been developed for cognitively impaired adults and young children (age 2–12 years) who have difficulty in reporting these symptoms.

Associated Features

There are several supportive clinical features which, while not required, may assist in diagnosis. These include a response to dopaminergic agents, the presence of periodic leg movements (PLMs) on diagnostic polysomnography (PSG), and a positive family history for RLS. PLMs may occur in sleep (PLMS) and resting wakefulness (PLMW). PLMS ≥5/hour is a highly sensitive marker for RLS, occurring in 80–90% of patients, but has low specificity as it is also frequently associated with narcolepsy, rapid eye movement behavioral disorder (RBD), and even healthy individuals, notably the elderly [14, 15]. PLMW may be noted during the wake time on standard

Table 18.2 Diagnostic criteria for restless legs syndrome (RLS)

Uncomfortable sensation in the legs associated with an urge to move
Symptoms are worse at rest
Symptoms are temporarily relieved by movement
Symptoms are worse or only occur at night
The condition is not better explained by another disorder
Symptoms cause concern, distress, sleep disturbance, or impairment in daytime functioning

PSG recorded 1 hour before the usual bedtime while the patient is upright in bed with stretched-out legs (Suggested Immobilization Test – SIT). A rate greater than 40 PLMW/hour supports the diagnosis of RLS [1]. RLS is associated with PLMW in ≈ 1/3 of patients [14]. The frequency of RLS among first-degree relatives of people with RLS is 3–5 times greater than in people without RLS [16]. There is a negative impact of RLS symptoms on sleep including reports of disrupted sleep, an inability to fall asleep, and insufficient hours of sleep [11]. Sleep disruption has also been associated with negative effects on cognitive function in patients with RLS [17]. Onset occurs at all ages from early childhood to late adult life with a mean age of onset between the third and fifth decade [18]. In children RLS may be misdiagnosed as "growing pains" or attention deficit hyperactivity disorder (ADHD). Two age-of-onset phenotypes for RLS have been described. Early-onset RLS usually starts before the age of 45 years with intermittent symptoms and progresses slowly. Late-onset RLS is usually either stable at onset or rapidly progresses over 5 years to a stable pattern. Patients may describe the symptoms as creeping, crawling, pulling, aching, prickling, or tingling. RLS can occur unilaterally or bilaterally in the lower extremities. About half (48.7%) of patients with RLS complain of restlessness in the arms as well. However, every patient who had arm restlessness also had leg restlessness. In most mild cases or RLS, symptoms are localized to the lower extremities, and only with increased severity do they also affect the arms and other parts of the body [19]. Peak intensity of RLS symptoms is on the falling phase of the core temperature cycle suggesting that RLS is related to the circadian rhythm [20].

Differential Diagnosis

The differential diagnosis of RLS includes neuropathic paresthesias, positional discomfort, akathisia, sleep starts (hypnic jerks), PLMD, sleep-related leg cramps, habitual foot tapping, and pain from other conditions. RLS can be distinguished from positional discomfort as the discomfort is resolved with change of body position without the need for continued movement and an urge to move the legs is not present. Akathisia involves a generalized need to move the body and often in association with neuroleptic medication. Akathisia sufferers frequently report an inner sense of restlessness rather than leg discomfort and lack the circadian pattern characteristic of RLS. Sleep starts produce brief body movements during the transition from wake to sleep, and an urge to move is not present. PLMD is a disorder that is only present during sleep without the essential diagnostic features of RLS. Sleep-related leg cramps are painful sensations caused by sudden and intense involuntary contractions of muscles and require stretching the legs to relieve symptoms rather than movement alone. Patients also describe hardening of the leg muscles that is not typical of RLS. Residual pain is also usually present with sleep-related leg cramps. Pain may be worse at rest but does not include an urge to move the legs. The presence of pain does not exclude a diagnosis or RLS as some patients report their RLS symptoms as pain; however, the additional characteristic features must also be present. Habitual foot tapping is easily differentiated from RLS but the absence of nocturnal predominance of symptoms except when exacerbated by alcohol or medications taken in the evening.

Primary Versus Secondary Factors

RLS can be classified as primary or secondary. The majority of cases of primary RLS are hereditary (autosomal dominant) with possible loci on chromosomes 12, 14, and 9. Onset of symptoms before the age of 40 years indicates an increased risk of RLS occurrence in the family. Physical and neurologic examinations are normal in the majority of primary RLS cases [21]. A number of secondary causes can contribute to RLS and can be expected to improve when the other disorders are treated. Iron deficiency has been associated with RLS. Pathologic studies suggest decreased iron and ferritin in the substantia nigra of RLS patients [22]. Low serum ferritin levels (< 45 µg/l) correlate significantly with increased RLS symptoms and with decreased sleep efficiency. A significant correlation to serum iron levels has not been found [23, 24]. Studies suggest disordered transport of iron from the periphery to the central nervous system [25]. The most commonly reported neurologic cause of secondary RLS is peripheral neuropathy [21]. Uremia associated with renal failure has also been identified as a cause of RLS. A 2008 study found that as many as 58.3% of dialysis patients have RLS [26]. Renal transplantation, unlike dialysis, causes significant or complete resolution of RLS symptoms [27]. Ekbom made the first observation that there is a high prevalence of RLS in pregnancy. In a study of 642 pregnant women, 26% were found to be affected by RLS during pregnancy. RLS was strongly associated with the third trimester [12]. A recent study in a French population of women in their third trimester of pregnancy found that 32% were affected by RLS. RLS disappeared after delivery in 64.8% of the women [28]. In a study of 184 narcolepsy with cataplexy patients, RLS was found to be significantly more prevalent compared to controls (14.7% vs. 3%). In this population, RLS symptoms occurred more than 10 years after narcolepsy onset and were less familial and, in contrast to idiopathic RLS, not more prevalent in women [29]. Transient RLS has been described in those undergoing spinal anesthesia [30]. Other secondary causes of RLS include myelopathy, Parkinson's disease, and diabetes. Medications may also precipitate RLS symptoms. Common medications which can precipitate RLS include those with dopamine receptor-blocking properties (sedating antihistamines, antipsychotics, and antinausea drugs) and those with serotonin-promoting activity (most antidepressants with the exception of bupropion, with its dopamine-promoting properties). There is limited or contradictory evidence for caffeine, tobacco, and alcohol as aggravating factors for RLS [31–33]. Multimorbidity was shown to be a strong risk factor for RLS in two independent German cohort studies indicating that the severity of underlying morbidity is a stronger risk factor for RLS than any specific single disease. Furthermore, the association was stronger with incident than with preexisting RLS, suggesting that RLS developed subsequently to preexisting comorbid diseases [34].

Management

The first step in managing RLS is performing a medication review. Medications that can precipitate or worsen RLS should be discontinued if possible. Secondary causes should undergo evaluation and treatment as this may resolve or improve symptoms. Patients with iron deficiency will benefit from iron replacement therapy to target ferritin levels ≥75 µg/l [35]. Intravenous (IV) iron may be considered when oral iron is not appropriate provided ferritin ≤100 µg/l. IV iron, unlike oral iron whose absorption in the gastrointestinal tract is highly variable, helps to achieve higher levels of peripheral iron required to increase cerebral iron levels. Vitamin C may enhance oral iron absorption. Non-pharmacologic treatments include improving sleep hygiene, warm baths, leg massage, and acupuncture. Only one study assessed the effect of a 12-week moderate-intensity aerobic and resistance exercise program and found 39% improvement in symptoms with a ceiling effect after 6 weeks [36]. Two studies, to date, have investigated the effectiveness of sequential compression devices for the treatment of RLS [37, 38]. In a prospective, randomized, double-blinded, sham-controlled trial, there was significant improvement in RLS severity and quality of life measures in those using the sequential compression device compared to the sham devices. Complete relief occurred in one-third of the therapeutic group in this study [38]. There has been one case reporting the improvement in RLS symptoms with a 4-week near-infrared light therapy [39]. A subsequent study by the same group, with 34 volunteers, reported significant improvement in RLS symptoms in the near-infrared light treatment group compared to the control group [40]. More research is necessary to investigate these and other potential non-pharmacologic therapies.

Pharmacologic treatment of RLS consists of four classes of medications which include dopaminergic agents, anticonvulsants, benzodiazepines, and opioids though other agents have been used (Table 18.3). An evidence-based review produced by a task force commissioned by the Movement Disorder Society concluded that levodopa, ropinirole, pramipexole, cabergoline, pergolide, and gabapentin were efficacious for the treatment of RLS, while rotigotine, bromocriptine, oxycodone, carbamazepine, valproic acid, and clonidine were likely efficacious [41]. Levodopa/benserazide or levodopa/carbidopa at dosages of 100/25 to 200/50 mg is considered efficacious for the treatment of RLS. The side-effect profile of levodopa is favorable; however treatment carries the highest incidence of augmentation among all dopamine agonists; hence levodopa is used mainly to treat intermittent RLS [42]. The dopamine agonists ropinirole and pramipexole are FDA approved for the treatment of RLS. Ropinirole (0.25–4 mg, mean 2 mg) and pramipexole (0.75 mg) are efficacious for treating RLS in patients with moderate to severe symptoms. Several studies have demonstrated the effectiveness of the rotigotine transdermal patch for

Table 18.3 Treatment for RLS

Non-pharmacological treatments
Improved sleep hygiene
Exercise
Massage
Acupuncture
Sequential compression devices
Near-infrared light
Pharmacological treatments
Dopaminergic agents
Antiepileptics
Benzodiazepines
Opioids
Iron

treatment of RLS including a randomized, double-blinded, placebo-controlled trial including 505 participants with moderate to severe RLS [43–47]. Ergot-derived dopamine agonists, including bromocriptine, pergolide, and cabergoline, require special monitoring due to increased incidence of cardiac valvular fibrosis and other fibrotic side effects. While efficacious, these agents are rarely used currently. Augmentation is the main side effect of long-term dopaminergic treatment of RLS and is characterized by an earlier onset of symptoms (≥ 4 hours) or a shorter time advance (2–4 hours) along with other required features such as an overall increase in severity of symptoms, a faster onset of symptoms at rest, and extension of the symptoms to other body parts, notably the upper extremities. A paradoxical response to dopaminergic agonists (worsening of symptoms with dosage increase and vice versa) constitutes an alternative diagnostic criterion [48, 49]. Mild cases may be followed with either a trial of judicious dose increase or dividing the dose and earlier dose administration, while in more severe cases, a complete change in treatment is indicated [49]. Ferritin may play a role as a biomarker for patients likely to develop augmentation [50], and treatment with oral/intravenous iron should be strongly considered in combination with other measures if ferritin levels <50–75 μg/l. Side effects of dopaminergic agents include excessive daytime sleepiness, nausea, vomiting, hallucinations, and insomnia. Dopaminergic therapy for RLS has also been associated with impulse control behaviors such as compulsive gambling and shopping. Antiepileptics used in the treatment of RLS include carbamazepine, gabapentin, pregabalin, and lamotrigine. Antiepileptics may be considered first-line therapy in those with concomitant neuropathy or painful leg symptoms. Gabapentin has been reported to be as effective as ropinirole in improving the sensorimotor symptoms in idiopathic RLS [51]. Pregabalin also has been demonstrated to improve RLS symptoms in double-blinded, placebo-controlled trial [52, 53]. Of the benzodiazepines, clonazepam is the best documented for treatment of RLS. Side effects of these agents include sleepiness and tolerance. Opioids are used in the treatment of RLS; however at sufficient analgesic doses, they cause a series of minor and major adverse effects including sedation, fatigue, and constipation. Short-acting agents including hydrocodone, oxycodone, and codeine may be used for intermittent or nightly symptoms. Tramadol has also been used. For more severe symptoms, low dose of longer-acting opioids such as oxycodone and methadone is usually very effective and safe in appropriate patients.

Periodic Limb Movement Disorder

Initially termed "nocturnal myoclonus" by the English neurologist Charles P Symonds in 1953, the term periodic movements in sleep was suggested by Coleman in 1980 [54, 55]. PLMD is characterized by periodic episodes of repetitive, highly stereotyped, limb movements that occur during sleep (PLMS) and by clinical sleep disturbance that cannot be accounted for by another primary sleep disorder. PLMS typically involve the extension of the big toe, often in combination with partial flexion of the ankle, the knee, and sometimes the hip. Similar movements can occur in the upper limb. They can occur individually in association with arousals or awakenings from sleep. PLMS may occur unilaterally, alternate between legs, or occur simultaneously in both legs. Significant night-to-night variability may be present.

Demographics

In a study of randomly selected community-dwelling persons 65 years and older, the prevalence rate of PLMS was 45% [56]. Considerable clinical evidence suggests that although PLMS are common, the diagnosis of PLMD is extremely rare in adults and is best thought of as a diagnosis of elimination.

Diagnosis

The diagnosis of PLMD in adults according to the ICSD-3 requires the following: (a) Polysomnography demonstrates repetitive, highly stereotyped, limb movements that are 0.5–5 seconds in duration, of amplitude greater than or equal to 25% of toe dorsiflexion during calibration, in a sequence of four or more movements, and separated by an interval of more than 5 seconds and less than 90 seconds. (b) The PLMS index exceeds 5/hour in children and 15/hour in most adult cases. (c) There is clinical sleep disturbance or a complaint of daytime fatigue. (d) The PLMS are not better explained by another current sleep disorder, medical or neurological disorder, mental disorder, medication use, or substance use disorder [1] (Table 18.4).

Table 18.4 Diagnostic criteria for periodic limb movement disorder (PLMD)

Polysomnography demonstrates repetitive, highly stereotyped, limb movements
The periodic limb movement index exceeds 15/hour in most adult cases
Clinical sleep disturbance or daytime fatigue
Limb movements during sleep are not better explained by another disorder

Associated Features

Patients often report history of sleep onset or maintenance problems, unrefreshing sleep, or excessive daytime hypersomnolence or fatigue. However, the presence of insomnia or hypersomnia with PLMS is insufficient to diagnose PLMD, as in most cases, the sleep disturbance is better explained by another underlying sleep disorder. In that case, PLMS are solely noted as polysomnographic findings. PLMS have been associated with a number of sleep disorders including narcolepsy, RBD, and sleep apnea as well as with a number of neurologic disorders. PSG is necessary to exclude sleep-related breathing disorders as the cause of the PLMS. Bed partner observations of leg movements may help in the clinical evaluation of PLMS. PLMD cannot be diagnosed if sleep disruption of the bed partner is the only complaint. PLMS should also be distinguished from other movements such as change in body position, stretching, or leg cramps. Movements are reported as an index of the number of leg movements per hour of sleep called the PLM index. PLMS may produce no change in the EEG or associated arousal or may be associated with K complexes, K alpha complexes, alpha activity, or other evidence of arousal. In a study of 23 patients with PLMs and/or RLS, 60% of PLMS were associated with microarousals, 4% were associated with slow-wave activity, and 36% showed no electroencephalographic changes. There was a prevalence of leg movements with microarousals in stage N1 and N2 sleep, while PLMS without microarousals were prevalent in slow-wave sleep [57].

PLMS are usually absent during rapid eye movement (REM) sleep. Two types of PLMS have been described. Type I has a peak frequency between midnight and 3 a.m. followed by a decrease in late morning hours and is seen in those with RLS and idiopathic PLMS. In Type II, leg movements are more evenly distributed throughout the night and are associated with sleep-related breathing disorders, RBD, and narcolepsy.

Differential Diagnosis

The differential diagnosis includes sleep starts, normal phasic REM activity, and fragmentary myoclonus. Sleep starts are limited to the transition from wakefulness to sleep and are shorter than PLMS. Normal phasic REM activity is usually associated with bursts of rapid eye movements and does not have the periodicity of

PLMS. Fragmentary myoclonus activity is briefer and is primarily an EMG diagnosis with little or no visible movement.

Management

Similar to management of RLS, an investigation to identify secondary causes of PLMD is recommended. Consideration should be given to discontinuing medications that may contribute to PLMD. The decision to treat PLMD should be based on signs of EEG arousal, disturbed nocturnal sleep, or associated daytime mental or functional impairment. Medication treatment is similar to that of RLS and includes dopaminergic agents, anticonvulsants, benzodiazepines, and opioids. Given that many patients may not be aware of PLMS, assessment of response to therapy is dependent on improvement in sleep quality and daytime symptoms, including fatigue. In some instances, PSG performed on treatment is required to assess response to therapy.

Sleep-Related Leg Cramps

Sleep-related leg cramps are painful sensations caused by sudden and intense involuntary contractions of muscles or muscle groups, usually in the calf or small muscles of the foot and occurring during the sleep period. The lay term is "Charley horse." These episodes may last up to a few minutes, awaken the patient, and interrupt sleep.

Diagnosis

The diagnosis of sleep-related leg cramps according to ICSD-3 requires the following: (a) A painful sensation in the leg or foot is associated with sudden muscle hardness or tightness indicating a strong muscle contraction. (b) The painful muscle contraction in the legs or feet occurs during the sleep period, although they may arise from either wakefulness or sleep. (c) The pain is relieved by forceful stretching of the affected muscles, releasing the contraction [1] (Table 18.5).

Table 18.5 Diagnostic criteria for sleep-related leg cramps

Painful sensation in the leg or foot associated with strong muscle contraction
Painful muscle contraction occurs during the sleep period
Pain is relieved by forceful stretching of the affected muscles

Demographics

Sleep-related leg cramps appear to occur at any age but are more common and frequent in the elderly. In an epidemiologic study in children, an overall incidence of 7.3% was reported [58]. In a general practice-based study of 233 people older than age 60, almost one-third had cramps during the previous 2 months, and this increased to one-half in those older than 80. In addition, 40% had cramps more than 3 times a week and 6% reported daily cramps [59]. A study of outpatient veterans found that 56% reported leg cramps [60]. Sleep-related leg cramps may appear or worsen during pregnancy and were reported in 75% of women in their third trimester in a study of 12 women [61].

Differential Diagnosis

The differential diagnosis of sleep-related leg cramps includes muscle strain, dystonia, claudication, RLS, PLMS, and nocturnal myoclonus. The pain associated with muscle strain is often associated with overuse or injury and does not usually occur only at night. The pain associated with claudication is usually relieved by rest. RLS involves an urge to move the legs with temporary relief with movement and does not require stretching of the muscle. PLMS occur during sleep and are not associated with pain or muscle hardening. Muscle cramps may also be a feature of a number of other neurologic conditions; however these cramps are not usually restricted to nighttime or the legs alone.

Associated Features

During the cramp the muscles are firm and tender. Tenderness and discomfort in the muscle may persist for several hours after the cramping. Delayed sleep onset and awakenings from sleep are often present with persistent discomfort delaying return to sleep. Patients may need to get out of bed to stand and stretch to alleviate symptoms. Sleep-related leg cramps are not sleep-stage specific as they may occur in any sleep stage. Although sleep-related leg cramps are idiopathic in most individuals, a large number of potential contributing factors have been reported. Medications that have been reported to cause leg cramps include diuretics, nifedipine, statins, β-agonists, steroids, morphine, cimetidine, penicillamine, and lithium. Medical conditions associated with sleep-related leg cramps include uremia, diabetes, thyroid disease, hypoparathyroidism, hypomagnesemia, hypocalcemia, hyponatremia, and hypokalemia. Additional predisposing factors include vigorous exercise during the day, oral contraceptive use, peripheral vascular disease, and dehydration. PSG is not routinely recommended for the evaluation of sleep-related leg cramps, but may show bursts of increased electromyographic activity over the affected area.

Treatment

A careful history to identify and treat any precipitating factors is important in patients with sleep-related leg cramps. Patients should be reassured regarding the benign nature of the disease. Adjustment of possible contributing medications should be considered. Cramps, once present, can be aborted by forcible dorsiflexion of the foot with the knee extended. This is often discovered by patients while dealing with cramps acutely at night and may be all that is required when sleep-related leg cramps are infrequent. Passive massage or stretching may also help. However, research data on the efficacy of stretching exercises are contradictory. A randomized controlled trial of 80 adults above 55 years found that stretching of the calves and hamstrings before sleep effectively reduced the frequency and severity of leg cramps, while a previous trial found this treatment to be ineffective [62]. Pharmacological treatment of leg cramps may be necessary when symptoms are severe and frequent. A number of treatments have been investigated. Quinine, an alkaloid agent, reduces the excitability of the motor end plate to nerve stimulation and increases the refractory period of skeletal muscle contraction. It has been used with great efficacy to treat leg cramps since 1940 though there were significant concerns regarding the risk/benefit ratio with this drug [63, 64]. In 1995, the FDA concluded that the risks of quinine outweighed any possible benefit and ordered a stop to the marketing of quinine for off-label use for prevention or treatment of sleep-related leg cramps. Quinine-induced thrombocytopenia and hypersensitivity reactions are among the most serious complications of quinine. Naftidrofuryl oxalate, a vasodilator, significantly reduced the frequency of cramps and increased the number of cram-free days by a third in a double-blind, placebo-controlled trial in 14 patients [65]. Orphenadrine citrate, an anticholinergic, reduced the frequency of leg cramps by a third in the majority of patients in a double-blind crossover trial [66]. Verapamil at 120 mg given at bedtime for 8 weeks resulted in an improvement in cramp symptoms in seven out of eight patients during an uncontrolled study [67]. Magnesium was effective in treating sleep-related leg cramps in pregnant women in several double-blind, randomized, placebo-controlled studies [68–70]; however, no significant effect was seen in the study of nonpregnant adults [71–73]. It was suggested that possible underlying pregnancy-induced magnesium deficiency may have led to positive results in pregnant patients and measurements of baseline and posttreatment serum magnesium in all patients should be conducted to highlight that finding. Vitamin E use yielded conflicting results among two randomized blinded studies [74, 75]. In the only randomized, double-blind, placebo-controlled study evaluating the efficacy of vitamin B complex capsules, 86% of the patients had prominent remission of leg cramps at 3 months compared to placebo [76]. Several studies have demonstrated the effectiveness of gabapentin in the treatment of leg cramps in those with neurologic conditions though its usefulness in idiopathic leg cramps remains unclear [77, 78]. The effectiveness of lidocaine injection at the gastrocnemius trigger point and botulinum injection into calf muscles for treatment of sleep-related leg cramps has also been reported [79, 80]. Finally, continuous positive airway pressure (CPAP) cured leg cramps in patients in a report of four patients with comorbid obstructive sleep apnea (OSA) [81]. More research in this area is needed.

Sleep-Related Bruxism

One of the first reports of bruxism was from Black in 1886; however, the term bruxism was introduced by Miller in 1938 [82, 83]. Sleep-related bruxism is an oral activity characterized by grinding or clenching of the teeth during sleep usually associated with sleep arousals. Jaw activity during sleep includes tonic contractions and rhythmic masticatory muscle activity (RMMA) that occurs at about 1 Hz. Teeth-grinding sounds occur when these contractions are strong during sleep and are present in about 20% of episodes [84].

Demographics

Bruxism has the highest prevalence in childhood which decreases with increasing age. One study reported an overall prevalence of 8% with a frequency of 13% in those 18–29 years of age and only 3% in older individuals [85]. No gender differences have been found [86]. A familial pattern is seen in approximately 20–35% of patients [87]. Moderate to severe tooth wear and jaw discomfort is seen in about 5–10% of the population [84].

Diagnosis

The diagnosis of sleep-related bruxism according to the ICSD-3 requires the following: (a) The patient reports or is aware of tooth-grinding sounds or tooth clenching during sleep. (b) One or more of the following are present: abnormal wear of the teeth, transient morning jaw muscle discomfort, fatigue or pain, and/or jaw locking [1] (Table 18.6). Although PSG is not required for diagnosis, bruxism is ideally recorded via the masseter EMG showing characteristic RMMA either a phasic pattern of activity at 1 Hz frequency lasting 0.25–2 s, sustained tonic activity lasting longer than 2 s, or a mixed pattern. Simultaneous audiovisual recording increases diagnostic reliability distinguishing between RMMA episodes and orofacial and other muscular activities that occur during sleep (swallowing, sleep talking, etc.). The RMMA episodes are associated with sleep arousal and are preceded by signs of increased autonomic activity (such as increased heart rate). PSG will also assess comorbid sleep disorders that may worsen bruxism such as OSA or RBD [88].

Differential Diagnosis

Sleep-related bruxism must be distinguished from other nocturnal faciomandibular activities including idiopathic myoclonus, RBD, parasomnias such as night terrors and confusional arousals, and dyskinetic jaw movements persisting in sleep. Very rarely, nocturnal partial or complex seizures may present as isolated bruxism.

Associated Features

Sleep-related bruxism can lead to abnormal wear of the teeth, tooth pain, jaw muscle pain, or temporal headache. Fractured teeth and buccal lacerations and temporomandibular joint pain can also occur as a consequence. Sleep disruption is also prevalent. Over time, hypertrophy of the masseter and other facial muscles can develop. Sleep bruxism has been attributed to several etiologies though the theory that malocclusion was the cause has fallen out of favor. Presumed mechanisms include sleep arousal, autonomic sympathetic cardiac activation, genetic predisposition, psychological components, and comorbidities such as sleep-disordered breathing and acid reflux. Medications such as selective serotonin reuptake inhibitors (SSRI) and amphetamines have been associated with bruxism. Bruxism is frequently associated with Down's syndrome, autism, and ADHD [89, 90]. Although bruxism can occur during any sleep stage, including REM sleep, it is most often seen during arousals from stage N1 and N2 sleep.

Management

Therapies for sleep-related bruxism can be divided into orthodontic, behavioral, and pharmacologic. Non-pharmacological treatments include occlusal bite splints that are extensively used in clinical practice to provide protection against tooth damage, although there is a lack of evidence to support their role in halting bruxism [88]. Furthermore, side effects of such treatment include changes in dental occlusion, dental hypersensitiveness, and worsening of orofacial pain and SDB by reducing the intraoral cavity space [91]. Patients should be followed by a dentist who can

Table 18.6 Diagnostic criteria for sleep-related bruxism

Tooth-grinding sounds or tooth clenching during sleep
One or more of the following are present: abnormal wear of the teeth, jaw muscle discomfort, fatigue or pain, and jaw lock upon awakening

monitor dental wear. Excessively worn teeth may need to be crowned. OSA is a risk factor for sleep-related bruxism, and successful treatment of sleep-disordered breathing may eliminate bruxism during sleep [92]. Psychological counseling may be helpful in stress-related cases of bruxism. Albeit, there is little evidence to support the use of antidepressants to treat bruxism. Amitriptyline (a tricyclic antidepressant) was found to be ineffective, and SSRI worsened bruxism in some reports [93, 94]. Benzodiazepines and muscle relaxants may be necessary in more severe cases though they may contribute to daytime sleepiness. Randomized, controlled, and double-blinded studies investigating the pharmacologic therapies for sleep-related bruxism are lacking. Other medications that have been reported to be used for bruxism include propranolol, L-dopa, pergolide, bromocriptine, clonidine, and gabapentin [95–99]. A recent systematic review of four randomized controlled trials assessing the effect of botulinum toxin in the treatment of bruxism concluded that botulinum toxin injection in the masseter muscles resulted in a significant reduction of the frequency and severity of bruxism episodes, as well as pain intensity and improved patients' quality of life. In addition, doses <100 IU are safe and effective treatment with a low risk of adverse side effects. Therefore the authors recommended botulinum toxin in patients with severe bruxism who did not respond to conventional therapy [100].

Sleep-Related Rhythmic Movement Disorder

Described in 1905 by Zappert as "jactatio capitis nocturna" and independently by Cruchet as "rhythmie du sommeil," the term "rhythmic movement disorder" was adopted by the ICSD in 1990. RMD is characterized by repetitive, stereotyped, and rhythmic motor behaviors that occur predominantly during drowsiness or sleep and involve large muscle groups. Initially classified as a sleep-wake transition disorder, the revised ICSD reclassified RMD under the heading of sleep-related movement disorders. Sleep-related rhythmic movements are normal in children, and a disorder should be diagnosed when significant consequences are present. RMD is typically seen in infants and children. Body rocking, head banging, and head rolling are subtypes of RMD. Combined types may also be observed.

Demographics

RMD is most commonly observed in children. The incidence of RMD is 66% in 9-month-old infants and decreases to 8% in 4-year-olds [101]. In one study, head banging persisted beyond the age of 4 in 30% of patients but usually ended by age 10

Table 18.7 Diagnostic criteria for sleep-related rhythmic movement disorder (RMD)

Repetitive, stereotyped, and rhythmic motor behaviors
Involving large muscle groups
Movements are predominantly sleep related or occur near nap or bedtime
A significant complaint such as interference with sleep, significant impairment in daytime function, or self-inflicted bodily injury is present
Rhythmic movements are not better explained by another disorder

[102]. Though most common in children, RMD has also been reported in adolescents and adults. When observed in older children and adults, there have been conflicting reports regarding persistent RMD and its association with neurodevelopmental and psychiatric disorders as cases in adults of normal intelligence have been reported [103–105]. Therefore, there is insufficient evidence to fully understand the true natural history of the condition. No sex differences have been found in patients with RMD.

Diagnosis

RMD can be recognized by its characteristic clinical features. However, in some instances PSG may be useful. The diagnosis of RMD according to the ICSD-3 requires the following: (a) The patient exhibits repetitive, stereotyped, and rhythmic motor behaviors involving large muscle groups. (b) The movements are predominantly sleep related, occurring near nap or bedtime or when the individual appears drowsy or asleep. (c) The behaviors result in a significant complaint as manifest by at least one of the following: interference with normal sleep, significant impairment in daytime function, or self-inflicted bodily injury or likelihood of injury if preventive measures are not used. (d) The rhythmic movements are not better explained by another movement disorder or epilepsy [1] (Table 18.7).

Associated Features

While PSG have shown rhythmic movements to occur most often in stage N1 and N2 sleep, there have been reports of RMD in REM (24%) [104, 106, 107]. In the case of RMD occurring in REM sleep, concurrent RBD has not been reported [104, 107, 108]. Exclusively REM-RMD occurs more frequently in adults. The most common subtypes of RMD are body rocking (19.1%), head banging (5.1%), and head rolling (6.3%). Body rolling, head rolling, and leg banging subtypes have also been described. As noted previously patients may also have combinations of the noted subtypes. Sleep is not fragmented by RMD and sleep stages do not usually change as a result of movement. RMD does not usually interrupt sleep and patients have minimal recall. A review of ten subjects with RMD persisting beyond 5 years of age found a strong association with ADHD [104]. Several studies have reported RMD in adults with OSA with RMD initiated by arousals at the termination of the apneas. Improvement in RMD was noted with treatment of OSA with CPAP [109–111]. PSG is useful to uncover RMD aggravated by another sleep disorder, such as OSA, RBD, and RLS. On PSG the frequency of movements ranges from 0.5 to 2 Hz.

Differential Diagnosis

The clinical history of RMD is usually clear though the differential diagnosis of RMD includes RLS and sleep-related epilepsy. In contrast to RLS, the movements of RMD are continuous for short periods of time rather than periodic jerking. Electroencephalographic studies are normal between RMD episodes in most individuals. Polysomnographic findings of RMD may be confused with bruxism, thumb sucking, and rhythmic sucking of the lips or a pacifier. RMD should also be distinguished from akathisia which is not sleep related and involves a feeling of generalized restlessness.

Treatment

For the majority of RMD patients, no treatment other than reassurance is required. Parents should be advised that neurologic damage is unlikely and that the child will outgrow the problem. RMD has rarely been associated with head injury, carotid artery dissection, and ocular injury [112–114]. In cases where there is concern regarding serious injury, treatment is warranted. There is a lack of systematic studies assessing the risk of injury or daytime consequences of RMD and clinical trials evaluating its treatment. Contemporary management of RMD is guided by clinical experience and reports of case studies. Hypnosis was reported as an effective treatment in a 26-year-old woman with body rocking since infancy [115]. Other treatments that have been used include behavioral interventions [116]. Almost complete resolution of rhythmic movements was noted in six children with 3 weeks of controlled sleep restriction with hypnotic administration in the first week [117]. Tricyclic antidepressants have also been used to treat RMD. One study documented failure of doxepin, amitriptyline, and imipramine, while another reported success with imipramine [118, 119] . In one report citalopram at a dose of 20 mg was effective in eliminating head banging in a 5-year-old with ADHD [120]. Several studies have demonstrated the utility of low-dose clonazepam. Clonazepam at a starting dose of 0.5 mg was not sufficient to decrease the intensity or frequency of events, but 1 mg was found to be effective [121, 122]. The use of the dopamine antagonists haloperidol and pimozide decreased the intensity and duration of head punching in a 17-year-old boy [123].

Propriospinal Myoclonus at Sleep Onset

Propriospinal myoclonus at sleep onset (PSM) was first described in 1997 in three patients with jerks occurring only during relaxed wakefulness preceding sleep and at the sleep-wake transition (N1 sleep) and quickly disappears when N2 sets in [124–126]. Few reports showed persistence of jerks during sleep [127, 128]. Myoclonus is termed "propriospinal" when it doesn't remain restricted to its segmental origin and it propagates along the spinal cord with a slow conduction velocity. PSM usually originates from the thoracoabdominal myelomere and less often from cervical ones. It provokes spontaneous and repetitive flexion of the trunk and neck. Less frequently an extension pattern has been reported.

Finally, a striking shift came with the first description of a case of functional (psychogenic) PSM and with the paper by Kang and Shon reporting that the typical pattern of PSM may be mimicked voluntary by healthy volunteers [129, 130]. Afterward, a number of cohorts with functional PSM have been described and so far, and more than 50% of all the reported cases of PSM appear to be functional [131]. Hence, our current knowledge of PSM presents heterogeneous features that are difficult to disentangle.

Diagnosis

PSM was previously classified among the "isolated symptoms, apparently normal variants and unresolved issues." ICSD-3 reclassified PSM at sleep onset among the "sleep-related movement disorders" since it is very rarely associated with spinal injury or disease and most patients with this disorder have a normal spinal MRI. Its diagnosis compromises a combination of all the following criteria: (a) A complaint of sudden jerks, mainly of the abdomen, trunk, and neck. (b) The jerks appear during relaxed wakefulness and during sleep-wake transition. (c) The jerks disappear upon mental activation and with onset of stable sleep. (d) The jerks are so bothersome, and they preclude sleep onset. (e) The disorder is not better explained by another sleep, mental, medical, or neurological disorder, as well as by a medication or substance use disorder [1] (Table 18.8).

Table 18.8 Diagnostic criteria for propriospinal myoclonus at sleep onset

Sudden jerks, mainly of the abdomen, trunk, and neck
The jerks appear during relaxed wakefulness and during sleep-wake transition
The jerks disappear upon mental activation and with onset of stable sleep
The jerks are so bothersome, and they preclude sleep onset
The disorder is not better explained by another sleep, mental, medical, or neurological disorder, as well as by a medication or substance use disorder

Demographics

Epidemiologic data are lacking. PSM appears to be typical of middle-aged subjects and extremely rare in children [131]. PSM is considered position dependent, with worsening in the supine position in >50% of the cases. In at least one-third of the cases, the movements are stimulus-sensitive.

Associated Features

PSM appears to be idiopathic in around 80% of cases. Etiology is postulated to involve a functional abnormality of the spinal generator with afferent stimuli from the distal part of the spinal cord triggering hyperexcitability of the myoclonic volleys [131]. The remainder consists of "symptomatic forms" that include a wide range of organic lesions of the spine or other central nervous system levels and medical conditions such as herpes zoster, Lyme disease, hepatitis C, myasthenia gravis, breast cancer, and *Escherichia coli* infection. Isolated reports associated the development of PSM with use of certain drugs such as interferon-alpha, intrathecal bupivacaine, ciprofloxacin, and cannabis; however, causality remains to be proven [132–136]. Sleep-onset insomnia is a common and peculiar feature of PSM. The movements disappear once stable sleep is reached but may reappear during arousals or awakenings with similar features. Patients may develop a fear of falling asleep, anxiety, and depression. PSM has also been described in association with RLS [137]. Remarkably, in those patients PSM coexisted with prominent PLM during relaxed wakefulness and significant restlessness and leg discomfort, typical of RLS.

Differential Diagnosis

The sleep-wake transition stage appears to act as a pacemaker for many sleep-related movement disorders besides PSM, such as hypnic jerks and restless legs syndrome (RLS). Hypnic jerks similarity to PSM might be the caudal propagation from facial and cervical muscles but is easily differentiated given the absence of periodicity and slow propagation velocity. Hypnic jerks do not typically cause sleep-onset insomnia, a hallmark feature of PSM. PLMS generally spare the trunk and abdomen and are longer in duration. RLS is differentiated from PSM given associated prominent leg discomfort. Functional (psychogenic) PSM mimics a typical PSM presentation in healthy adults; however the muscle recruitment pattern and the spread velocity differ [130]. Associated psychological disturbances as well as intraindividual variability over time are also common features on functional PSM. Differentiating PSM and tic disorders should also be taken into account. The "tic-like" myoclonus with jerks, involving the trunk and arms, if present, lacks the positional triggering (supine position) and is not usually limited to the trunk. Finally, epileptic myoclonus is not confined to relaxed wakefulness, and electroencephalography may show epileptic discharges.

Treatment

There are no current guidelines for idiopathic PSM treatment. Treatment of underlying condition is mainstay of symptomatic PSM management, even if this doesn't lead to a complete PSM resolution in most cases [131]. For example, almost complete resolution of PSM anterior cervical discectomy with fusion significantly improved PSM in a patient with cord compression in the absence of myelopathy [138]. Clonazepam at doses 0.5–2 mg given at bedtime to 65 patients was an effective treatment in 52% of patients [139]. Anecdotal use of other medical treatments that were sporadically effective in some cases include valproate, SSRI, zonisamide, and intrathecal infusion of baclofen [131, 140–142]. A case study of a 62-year-old male patient with comorbid PSM at sleep onset and OSA reported that CPAP decreased the frequency of the events [143].

Sleep-Related Movement Disorder Due to a Medical Disorder

The ICSD-3 intends this diagnosis for sleep-related movement disorders due to an underlying medical or neurological condition that does not meet criteria for another specific movement disorder. Often, this is a transient diagnosis until the underlying medical or neurological condition is fully diagnosed, and therefore the latter will take precedence in terms of the final diagnosis.

Diagnosis

According to ICSD-3, all the three following criteria must be met for diagnosis: (a) The patient manifests sleep-related movements that disturb sleep or its onset. (b) The movement disorder occurs as a consequence of a significant underlying medical or neurological condition. (c) The symptoms are not better explained by another sleep-related movement disorder, other sleep or mental disorder, or substance use [1] (Table 18.9).

Sleep-Related Movement Disorder Due to a Medication or Substance

The ICSD-3 intends this diagnosis for sleep-related movement disorder due to a medication or substance that does not meet criteria for another specific movement disorder. Since movement abnormalities during sleep or wake is a common and often anticipated complication of multiple medications or substances, the clinician must not resort to this diagnosis unless the sleep-related aspects of the abnormal movements are the focus of independent clinical attention.

Diagnosis

According to ICSD-3, all the three following criteria must be met for diagnosis: (a) The patient manifests sleep-related movements that disturb sleep or its onset. (b) The movement disorder occurs as a consequence of a current medication or substance use or withdrawal from a wake-promoting medication or substance. (c) The symptoms are not better explained by another sleep-related movement disorder and other untreated sleep, medical, neurological, or mental disorder [1] (Table 18.10).

Table 18.9 Diagnostic criteria for sleep-related movement disorder due to a medical disorder

The patient manifests sleep-related movements that disturb sleep or its onset
The movement disorder occurs as a consequence of a significant underlying medical or neurological condition
The symptoms are not better explained by another sleep-related movement disorder, other sleep or mental disorder, or substance use

Table 18.10 Diagnostic criteria for sleep-related movement disorder due to a medication or substance

The patient manifests sleep-related movements that disturb sleep or its onset
The movement disorder occurs as a consequence of a current medication or substance use or withdrawal from a wake-promoting medication or substance
The symptoms are not better explained by another sleep-related movement disorder and other untreated sleep, medical, neurological, or mental disorder

Conclusion

Sleep-related movement disorders include a varied group of diseases which are quite prevalent and can cause significant sleep disturbance and impairment in daytime functioning and compromise quality of life. These disorders are frequently encountered yet may be confused or misdiagnosed by healthcare professionals. Increasing awareness of these conditions is necessary to allow for prompt identification and management as this can significantly improve quality of life.

Summary of Keypoints
- Restless legs syndrome (RLS) is a common sensorimotor disorder characterized by a distressing urge to move the legs and sometimes other parts of the body such as the arms. RLS affects approximately 10% of US adults. Difficulty falling asleep may frequently be associated with moderate to severe RLS.
- The diagnosis of RLS is based on clinical criteria and does not require a polysomnogram unless an additional sleep disorder is suspected.
- The majority of cases of primary RLS are hereditary (autosomal dominant). Causes of secondary RLS include iron deficiency, peripheral neuropathy, uremia associated with renal failure, and pregnancy. Common medications which can precipitate RLS include tricyclic antidepressants, SSRI, lithium, antihistamines, and dopamine antagonists. RLS affects approximately 10% of US adults.
- RLS diagnostic criteria:

  1. Uncomfortable sensation in the legs associated with an urge to move.
  2. Symptoms are worse at rest.
  3. Symptoms are temporarily relieved by movement.
  4. Symptoms are worse or only occur at night.

- Medications that can worsen RLS should be discontinued, and secondary causes should be evaluated and treated.
- Management strategy consists of discontinuation of medications that can worsen RLS, treatment of secondary causes of RLS such as iron deficiency, conservative treatment, and pharmacologic treatment. Four classes of medications have been used for the treatment of RLS, including dopaminergic agents, anticonvulsants, benzodiazepines, and opioids.
- Periodic limb movement disorder (PLMD) is a sleep disorder characterized by rhythmic movements of the limbs during sleep, involving the legs, but upper extremity movements may also occur. Movements tend to cluster in episodes that last anywhere from a few minutes to several hours.
- The causes of PLMD are unknown. However, people with a variety of medical problems, including Parkinson's disease and narcolepsy, may

have frequent periodic limb movements in sleep. PLMD may be caused by medications, most notably antidepressants. Periodic leg movements (PLMs) occur in at least 85% of people with RLS. PLMS are not usually seen in REM sleep.

- Rhythmic movement disorder (RMD) occurs mainly in infants and children, and it is usually a benign condition that does not require intervention.
- Propriospinal myoclonus at sleep onset (PSM) is a rare disorder, mostly idiopathic, that causes severe sleep-onset insomnia. There are no current guidelines for treatment of PSM.

References

1. American Academy of Sleep Medicine. International classification of sleep disorders. 3rd edition. Darien, IL.: American Academy of Sleep Medicine; 2014.
2. Willis T. The London practice of physick: or the whole practical part of physick contained in the works of Dr. Willis. Faithfully made English, and printed together for the publick good. 1685.
3. Ekbom K-A FH. Restless legs, a clinical study of a hitherto overlooked disease in the legs characterized by peculiar paresthesia ("anxietas tibiarum"), pain and weakness and occurring in two main forms, asthenia crurum paraesthetica and asthenia crurum dolorosa. A short review of paresthesias in general. Stockholm. 1945.
4. Allen RP, Barker PB, Wehrl FW, Song HK, Earley CJ. MRI measurement of brain iron in patients with restless legs syndrome. Neurology. 2001;56(2):263–5.
5. Turjanski N, Lees AJ, Brooks DJ. Striatal dopaminergic function in restless legs syndrome: 18F-dopa and 11C-raclopride PET studies. Neurology. 1999;52(5):932–7.
6. Winkelmann J, Wetter TC, Collado-Seidel V, et al. Clinical characteristics and frequency of the hereditary restless legs syndrome in a population of 300 patients. Sleep. 2000;23(5):597–602.
7. Chen NH, Chuang LP, Yang CT, et al. The prevalence of restless legs syndrome in Taiwanese adults. Psychiatry Clin Neurosci. 2010;64(2):170–8.
8. Cho SJ, Hong JP, Hahm BJ, et al. Restless legs syndrome in a community sample of Korean adults: prevalence, impact on quality of life, and association with DSM-IV psychiatric disorders. Sleep. 2009;32(8):1069–76.
9. Zucconi M, Ferini-Strambi L. Epidemiology and clinical findings of restless legs syndrome. Sleep Med. 2004;5(3):293–9.
10. Phillips B, Hening W, Britz P, Mannino D. Prevalence and correlates of restless legs syndrome: results from the 2005 National Sleep Foundation Poll. Chest. 2006;129(1):76–80.
11. Allen RP, Walters AS, Montplaisir J, et al. Restless legs syndrome prevalence and impact: REST general population study. Arch Intern Med. 2005;165(11):1286–92.
12. Manconi M, Ulfberg J, Berger K, et al. When gender matters: restless legs syndrome. Report of the "RLS and woman" workshop endorsed by the European RLS Study Group. Sleep Med Rev. 2012;16(4):297–307.
13. Phillips B, Young T, Finn L, Asher K, Hening WA, Purvis C. Epidemiology of restless legs symptoms in adults. Arch Intern Med. 2000;160(14):2137–41.
14. Ferri R, Manconi M, Plazzi G, et al. Leg movements during wakefulness in restless legs syndrome: time structure and relationships with periodic leg movements during sleep. Sleep Med. 2012;13(5):529–35.
15. Montplaisir J, Lapierre O, Warnes H, Pelletier G. The treatment of the restless leg syndrome with or without periodic leg movements in sleep. Sleep. 1992;15(5):391–5.

16. Allen RP, Picchietti D, Hening WA, et al. Restless legs syndrome: diagnostic criteria, special considerations, and epidemiology. A report from the restless legs syndrome diagnosis and epidemiology workshop at the National Institutes of Health. Sleep Med. 2003;4(2):101–19.

17. Pearson VE, Allen RP, Dean T, Gamaldo CE, Lesage SR, Earley CJ. Cognitive deficits associated with restless legs syndrome (RLS). Sleep Med. 2006;7(1):25–30.

18. Gonzalez-Latapi P, Malkani R. Update on restless legs syndrome: from mechanisms to treatment. Curr Neurol Neurosci Rep. 2019;19(8):54.

19. Michaud M, Chabli A, Lavigne G, Montplaisir J. Arm restlessness in patients with restless legs syndrome. Mov Disord. 2000;15(2):289–93.

20. Trenkwalder C, Hening WA, Walters AS, Campbell SS, Rahman K, Chokroverty S. Circadian rhythm of periodic limb movements and sensory symptoms of restless legs syndrome. Mov Disord. 1999;14(1):102–10.

21. Ondo W, Jankovic J. Restless legs syndrome: clinicoetiologic correlates. Neurology. 1996;47(6):1435–41.

22. Connor JR, Boyer PJ, Menzies SL, et al. Neuropathological examination suggests impaired brain iron acquisition in restless legs syndrome. Neurology. 2003;61(3):304–9.

23. O'Keeffe ST, Gavin K, Lavan JN. Iron status and restless legs syndrome in the elderly. Age Ageing. 1994;23(3):200–3.

24. Sun ER, Chen CA, Ho G, Earley CJ, Allen RP. Iron and the restless legs syndrome. Sleep. 1998;21(4):371–7.

25. Mizuno S, Mihara T, Miyaoka T, Inagaki T, Horiguchi J. CSF iron, ferritin and transferrin levels in restless legs syndrome. J Sleep Res. 2005;14(1):43–7.

26. Enomoto M, Inoue Y, Namba K, Munezawa T, Matsuura M. Clinical characteristics of restless legs syndrome in end-stage renal failure and idiopathic RLS patients. Mov Disord. 2008;23(6):811–6; quiz 926

27. Chrastina M, Martinkova J, Minar M, Zilinska Z, Valkovic P, Breza J. Impact of kidney transplantation on restless legs syndrome. Bratisl Lek Listy. 2015;116(7):404–7.

28. Neau JP, Marion P, Mathis S, et al. Restless legs syndrome and pregnancy: follow-up of pregnant women before and after delivery. Eur Neurol. 2010;64(6):361–6.

29. Plazzi G, Ferri R, Antelmi E, et al. Restless legs syndrome is frequent in narcolepsy with cataplexy patients. Sleep. 2010;33(5):689–94.

30. Hogl B, Frauscher B, Seppi K, Ulmer H, Poewe W. Transient restless legs syndrome after spinal anesthesia: a prospective study. Neurology. 2002;59(11):1705–7.

31. Duz OA, Yilmaz NH, Olmuscelik O. Restless legs syndrome in aircrew. Aerosp Med Hum Perform. 2019;90(11):934–7.

32. Hadjigeorgiou GM, Stefanidis I, Dardiotis E, et al. Low RLS prevalence and awareness in Central Greece: an epidemiological survey. Eur J Neurol. 2007;14(11):1275–80.

33. Oksenberg A. Alleviation of severe restless legs syndrome (RLS) symptoms by cigarette smoking. J Clin Sleep Med. 2010;6(5):489–90.

34. Szentkiralyi A, Volzke H, Hoffmann W, Trenkwalder C, Berger K. Multimorbidity and the risk of restless legs syndrome in 2 prospective cohort studies. Neurology. 2014;82(22):2026–33.

35. Allen RP, Picchietti DL, Auerbach M, et al. Evidence-based and consensus clinical practice guidelines for the iron treatment of restless legs syndrome/Willis-Ekbom disease in adults and children: an IRLSSG task force report. Sleep Med. 2018;41:27–44.

36. Aukerman MM, Aukerman D, Bayard M, Tudiver F, Thorp L, Bailey B. Exercise and restless legs syndrome: a randomized controlled trial. J Am Board Fam Med. 2006;19(5):487–93.

37. Eliasson AH, Lettieri CJ. Sequential compression devices for treatment of restless legs syndrome. Medicine (Baltimore). 2007;86(6):317–23.

38. Lettieri CJ, Eliasson AH. Pneumatic compression devices are an effective therapy for restless legs syndrome: a prospective, randomized, double-blinded, sham-controlled trial. Chest. 2009;135(1):74–80.

39. Mitchell UH. Use of near-infrared light to reduce symptoms associated with restless legs syndrome in a woman: a case report. J Med Case Rep. 2010;4:286.

40. Mitchell UH, Myrer JW, Johnson AW, Hilton SC. Restless legs syndrome and near-infrared light: an alternative treatment option. Physiother Theory Pract. 2011;27(5):345–51.
41. Trenkwalder C, Hening WA, Montagna P, et al. Treatment of restless legs syndrome: an evidence-based review and implications for clinical practice. Mov Disord. 2008;23(16):2267–302.
42. Allen RP, Earley CJ. Augmentation of the restless legs syndrome with carbidopa/levodopa. Sleep. 1996;19(3):205–13.
43. Hening WA, Allen RP, Ondo WG, et al. Rotigotine improves restless legs syndrome: a 6-month randomized, double-blind, placebo-controlled trial in the United States. Mov Disord. 2010;25(11):1675–83.
44. Oertel WH, Benes H, Garcia-Borreguero D, et al. Efficacy of rotigotine transdermal system in severe restless legs syndrome: a randomized, double-blind, placebo-controlled, six-week dose-finding trial in Europe. Sleep Med. 2008;9(3):228–39.
45. Oertel WH, Benes H, Garcia-Borreguero D, et al. One year open-label safety and efficacy trial with rotigotine transdermal patch in moderate to severe idiopathic restless legs syndrome. Sleep Med. 2008;9(8):865–73.
46. Stiasny-Kolster K, Kohnen R, Schollmayer E, Moller JC, Oertel WH, Rotigotine Sp 666 Study G. Patch application of the dopamine agonist rotigotine to patients with moderate to advanced stages of restless legs syndrome: a double-blind, placebo-controlled pilot study. 2004;19(12):1432–8.
47. Trenkwalder C, Benes H, Poewe W, et al. Efficacy of rotigotine for treatment of moderate-to-severe restless legs syndrome: a randomised, double-blind, placebo-controlled trial. Lancet Neurol. 2008;7(7):595–604.
48. Garcia-Borreguero D, Allen RP, Kohnen R, et al. Diagnostic standards for dopaminergic augmentation of restless legs syndrome: report from a World Association of Sleep Medicine-International Restless Legs Syndrome Study Group consensus conference at the Max Planck Institute. Sleep Med. 2007;8(5):520–30.
49. Garcia-Borreguero D, Silber MH, Winkelman JW, et al. Guidelines for the first-line treatment of restless legs syndrome/Willis-Ekbom disease, prevention and treatment of dopaminergic augmentation: a combined task force of the IRLSSG, EURLSSG, and the RLS-foundation. Sleep Med. 2016;21:1–11.
50. Trenkwalder C, Hogl B, Benes H, Kohnen R. Augmentation in restless legs syndrome is associated with low ferritin. Sleep Med. 2008;9(5):572–4.
51. Happe S, Sauter C, Klosch G, Saletu B, Zeitlhofer J. Gabapentin versus ropinirole in the treatment of idiopathic restless legs syndrome. Neuropsychobiology. 2003;48(2):82–6.
52. Allen R, Chen C, Soaita A, et al. A randomized, double-blind, 6-week, dose-ranging study of pregabalin in patients with restless legs syndrome. Sleep Med. 2010;11(6):512–9.
53. Garcia-Borreguero D, Larrosa O, Williams AM, et al. Treatment of restless legs syndrome with pregabalin: a double-blind, placebo-controlled study. Neurology. 2010;74(23):1897–904.
54. Coleman RM, Pollak CP, Weitzman ED. Periodic movements in sleep (nocturnal myoclonus): relation to sleep disorders. Ann Neurol. 1980;8(4):416–21.
55. Symonds CP. Nocturnal myoclonus. J Neurol Neurosurg Psychiatry. 1953;16(3):166–71.
56. Ancoli-Israel S, Kripke DF, Klauber MR, Mason WJ, Fell R, Kaplan O. Periodic limb movements in sleep in community-dwelling elderly. Sleep. 1991;14(6):496–500.
57. Sforza E, Jouny C, Ibanez V. Time course of arousal response during periodic leg movements in patients with periodic leg movements and restless legs syndrome. Clin Neurophysiol. 2003;114(6):1116–24.
58. Leung AK, Wong BE, Chan PY, Cho HY. Nocturnal leg cramps in children: incidence and clinical characteristics. J Natl Med Assoc. 1999;91(6):329–32.
59. Naylor JR, Young JB. A general population survey of rest cramps. Age Ageing. 1994;23(5):418–20.
60. Haskell SG, Fiebach NH. Clinical epidemiology of nocturnal leg cramps in male veterans. Am J Med Sci. 1997;313(4):210–4.

61. Hertz G, Fast A, Feinsilver SH, Albertario CL, Schulman H, Fein AM. Sleep in normal late pregnancy. Sleep. 1992;15(3):246–51.
62. Hallegraeff JM, van der Schans CP, de Ruiter R, de Greef MH. Stretching before sleep reduces the frequency and severity of nocturnal leg cramps in older adults: a randomised trial. J Physiother. 2012;58(1):17–22.
63. Jansen PH, Veenhuizen KC, Wesseling AI, de Boo T, Verbeek AL. Randomised controlled trial of hydroquinine in muscle cramps. Lancet. 1997;349(9051):528–32.
64. Moss HK, Herrmann LG. Night cramps in human extremities; a clinical study of the physiologic action of quinine and prostigmine upon the spontaneous contractions of resting muscles. Am Heart J. 1948;35(3):403–8.
65. Young JB, Connolly MJ. Naftidrofuryl treatment for rest cramp. Postgrad Med J. 1993;69(814):624–6.
66. Popkin RJ. Orphenadrine citrate (Norflex) for the treatment of "restless legs" and related syndromes. J Am Geriatr Soc. 1971;19(1):76–9.
67. Baltodano N, Gallo BV, Weidler DJ. Verapamil vs quinine in recumbent nocturnal leg cramps in the elderly. Arch Intern Med. 1988;148(9):1969–70.
68. Dahle LO, Berg G, Hammar M, Hurtig M, Larsson L. The effect of oral magnesium substitution on pregnancy-induced leg cramps. Am J Obstet Gynecol. 1995;173(1):175–80.
69. Nygaard IH, Valbo A, Pethick SV, Bohmer T. Does oral magnesium substitution relieve pregnancy-induced leg cramps? Eur J Obstet Gynecol Reprod Biol. 2008;141(1):23–6.
70. Supakatisant C, Phupong V. Oral magnesium for relief in pregnancy-induced leg cramps: a randomised controlled trial. Matern Child Nutr. 2015;11(2):139–45.
71. Frusso R, Zarate M, Augustovski F, Rubinstein A. Magnesium for the treatment of nocturnal leg cramps: a crossover randomized trial. J Fam Pract. 1999;48(11):868–71.
72. Garrison SR, Birmingham CL, Koehler BE, McCollom RA, Khan KM. The effect of magnesium infusion on rest cramps: randomized controlled trial. J Gerontol A Biol Sci Med Sci. 2011;66(6):661–6.
73. Roffe C, Sills S, Crome P, Jones P. Randomised, cross-over, placebo controlled trial of magnesium citrate in the treatment of chronic persistent leg cramps. Med Sci Monit. 2002;8(5):CR326–30.
74. Connolly PS, Shirley EA, Wasson JH, Nierenberg DW. Treatment of nocturnal leg cramps. A crossover trial of quinine vs vitamin E. Arch Intern Med. 1992;152(9):1877–80.
75. Roca AO, Jarjoura D, Blend D, et al. Dialysis leg cramps. Efficacy of quinine versus vitamin E. ASAIO J. 1992;38(3):M481–5.
76. Chan P, Huang TY, Chen YJ, Huang WP, Liu YC. Randomized, double-blind, placebo-controlled study of the safety and efficacy of vitamin B complex in the treatment of nocturnal leg cramps in elderly patients with hypertension. J Clin Pharmacol. 1998;38(12):1151–4.
77. Mueller ME, Gruenthal M, Olson WL, Olson WH. Gabapentin for relief of upper motor neuron symptoms in multiple sclerosis. Arch Phys Med Rehabil. 1997;78(5):521–4.
78. Serrao M, Rossi P, Cardinali P, Valente G, Parisi L, Pierelli F. Gabapentin treatment for muscle cramps: an open-label trial. Clin Neuropharmacol. 2000;23(1):45–9.
79. Bertolasi L, Priori A, Tomelleri G, et al. Botulinum toxin treatment of muscle cramps: a clinical and neurophysiological study. Ann Neurol. 1997;41(2):181–6.
80. Prateepavanich P, Kupniratsaikul V, Charoensak T. The relationship between myofascial trigger points of gastrocnemius muscle and nocturnal calf cramps. J Med Assoc Thail. 1999;82(5):451–9.
81. Westwood AJ, Spector AR, Auerbach SH. CPAP treats muscle cramps in patients with obstructive sleep apnea. J Clin Sleep Med. 2014;10(6):691–2.
82. SC M. Textbook of periodontia (oral medicine). Philadelphia: P. Blakiston's Son; 1938.
83. WF L. The American system of dentistry, in treatises by various authors. Philadelphia: Lea Brothers; 1886.
84. Rugh JD, Harlan J. Nocturnal bruxism and temporomandibular disorders. Adv Neurol. 1988;49:329–41.

85. Lavigne GJ, Montplaisir JY. Restless legs syndrome and sleep bruxism: prevalence and association among Canadians. Sleep. 1994;17(8):739–43.

86. Bader G, Lavigne G. Sleep bruxism; an overview of an oromandibular sleep movement disorder. REVIEW ARTICLE. Sleep Med Rev. 2000;4(1):27–43.

87. Abe K, Shimakawa M. Genetic and developmental aspects of sleeptalking and teeth-grinding. Acta Paedopsychiatr. 1966;33(11):339–44.

88. Carra MC, Huynh N, Lavigne G. Sleep bruxism: a comprehensive overview for the dental clinician interested in sleep medicine. Dent Clin N Am. 2012;56(2):387–413.

89. DeMattei R, Cuvo A, Maurizio S. Oral assessment of children with an autism spectrum disorder. J Dent Hyg. 2007;81(3):65.

90. Ghanizadeh A. ADHD, bruxism and psychiatric disorders: does bruxism increase the chance of a comorbid psychiatric disorder in children with ADHD and their parents? Sleep Breath. 2008;12(4):375–80.

91. Gagnon Y, Mayer P, Morisson F, Rompre PH, Lavigne GJ. Aggravation of respiratory disturbances by the use of an occlusal splint in apneic patients: a pilot study. Int J Prosthodont. 2004;17(4):447–53.

92. Oksenberg A, Arons E. Sleep bruxism related to obstructive sleep apnea: the effect of continuous positive airway pressure. Sleep Med. 2002;3(6):513–5.

93. Ellison JM, Stanziani P. SSRI-associated nocturnal bruxism in four patients. J Clin Psychiatry. 1993;54(11):432–4.

94. Raigrodski AJ, Christensen LV, Mohamed SE, Gardiner DM. The effect of four-week administration of amitriptyline on sleep bruxism. A double-blind crossover clinical study. Cranio. 2001;19(1):21–5.

95. Amir I, Hermesh H, Gavish A. Bruxism secondary to antipsychotic drug exposure: a positive response to propranolol. Clin Neuropharmacol. 1997;20(1):86–9.

96. Lobbezoo F, Lavigne GJ, Tanguay R, Montplaisir JY. The effect of catecholamine precursor L-dopa on sleep bruxism: a controlled clinical trial. Mov Disord. 1997;12(1):73–8.

97. Sjoholm TT, Lehtinen I, Piha SJ. The effect of propranolol on sleep bruxism: hypothetical considerations based on a case study. Clin Auton Res. 1996;6(1):37–40.

98. Van der Zaag J, Lobbezoo F, Van der Avoort PG, Wicks DJ, Hamburger HL, Naeije M. Effects of pergolide on severe sleep bruxism in a patient experiencing oral implant failure. J Oral Rehabil. 2007;34(5):317–22.

99. Huynh N, Lavigne GJ, Lanfranchi PA, Montplaisir JY, de Champlain J. The effect of 2 sympatholytic medications--propranolol and clonidine--on sleep bruxism: experimental randomized controlled studies. Sleep. 2006;29(3):307–16.

100. Fernandez-Nunez T, Amghar-Maach S, Gay-Escoda C. Efficacy of botulinum toxin in the treatment of bruxism: systematic review. Med Oral Patol Oral Cir Bucal. 2019;24(4):e416–24.

101. Klackenberg G. A prospective longitudinal study of children. Data on psychic health and development up to 8 years of age. Acta Paediatr Scand Suppl. 1971;224:1–239.

102. Kravitz H, Rosenthal V, Teplitz Z, Murphy JB, Lesser RE. A study of head-banging in infants and children. Dis Nerv Syst. 1960;21:203–8.

103. Happe S, Ludemann P, Ringelstein EB. Persistence of rhythmic movement disorder beyond childhood: a videotape demonstration. Mov Disord. 2000;15(6):1296–8.

104. Stepanova I, Nevsimalova S, Hanusova J. Rhythmic movement disorder in sleep persisting into childhood and adulthood. Sleep. 2005;28(7):851–7.

105. Gwyther ARM, Walters AS, Hill CM. Rhythmic movement disorder in childhood: an integrative review. Sleep Med Rev. 2017;35:62–75.

106. Kaneda R, Furuta H, Kazuto K, Arayama K, Sano J, Koshino Y. An unusual case of rhythmic movement disorder. Psychiatry Clin Neurosci. 2000;54(3):348–9.

107. Kohyama J, Matsukura F, Kimura K, Tachibana N. Rhythmic movement disorder: polysomnographic study and summary of reported cases. Brain and Development. 2002;24(1):33–8.

108. Kempenaers C, Bouillon E, Mendlewicz J. A rhythmic movement disorder in REM sleep: a case report. Sleep. 1994;17(3):274–9.

109. Chirakalwasan N, Hassan F, Kaplish N, Fetterolf J, Chervin RD. Near resolution of sleep related rhythmic movement disorder after CPAP for OSA. Sleep Med. 2009;10(4):497–500.

110. Gharagozlou P, Seyffert M, Santos R, Chokroverty S. Rhythmic movement disorder associated with respiratory arousals and improved by CPAP titration in a patient with restless legs syndrome and sleep apnea. Sleep Med. 2009;10(4):501–3.

111. Mayer G, Wilde-Frenz J, Kurella B. Sleep related rhythmic movement disorder revisited. J Sleep Res. 2007;16(1):110–6.

112. Jackson MA, Hughes RC, Ward SP, McInnes EG. "Headbanging" and carotid dissection. Br Med J (Clin Res Ed). 1983;287(6401):1262.

113. Mackenzie JM. "Headbanging" and fatal subdural haemorrhage. Lancet. 1991;338(8780):1457–8.

114. Noel LP, Clarke WN. Self-inflicted ocular injuries in children. Am J Ophthalmol. 1982;94(5):630–3.

115. Rosenberg C. Elimination of a rhythmic movement disorder with hypnosis--a case report. Sleep. 1995;18(7):608–9.

116. Ross RR. Treatment of nocturnal headbanging by behavior modification techniques: a case report. Behav Res Ther. 1971;9(2):151–4.

117. Etzioni T, Katz N, Hering E, Ravid S, Pillar G. Controlled sleep restriction for rhythmic movement disorder. J Pediatr. 2005;147(3):393–5.

118. Drake ME Jr. Jactatio nocturna after head injury. Neurology. 1986;36(6):867–8.

119. Regestein QR, Hartmann E, Reich P. Single case study. A head movement disorder occurring in dreaming sleep. J Nerv Ment Dis. 1977;164(6):432–6.

120. Vogel W, Stein DJ. Citalopram for head-banging. J Am Acad Child Adolesc Psychiatry. 2000;39(5):544–5.

121. Chisholm T, Morehouse RL. Adult headbanging: sleep studies and treatment. Sleep. 1996;19(4):343–6.

122. Manni R, Tartara A. Clonazepam treatment of rhythmic movement disorders. Sleep. 1997;20(9):812.

123. Lee SK. A case with dopamine-antagonist responsive repetitive head punching as rhythmic movement disorder during sleep. J Epilepsy Res. 2013;3(2):74–5.

124. Khoo SM, Tan JH, Shi DX, Jamil HK, Rajendran N, Lim TK. Propriospinal myoclonus at sleep onset causing severe insomnia: a polysomnographic and electromyographic analysis. Sleep Med. 2009;10(6):686–8.

125. Montagna P, Provini F, Plazzi G, Liguori R, Lugaresi E. Propriospinal myoclonus upon relaxation and drowsiness: a cause of severe insomnia. Mov Disord. 1997;12(1):66–72.

126. Oguri T, Hisatomi K, Kawashima S, Ueki Y, Tachibana N, Matsukawa N. Postsurgical propriospinal myoclonus emerging at wake to sleep transition. Sleep Med. 2014;15(1):152–4.

127. Brown P, Thompson PD, Rothwell JC, Day BL, Marsden CD. Axial myoclonus of propriospinal origin. Brain. 1991;114(Pt 1A):197–214.

128. Manconi M, Sferrazza B, Iannaccone S, Massimo A, Zucconi M, Ferini-Strambi L. Case of symptomatic propriospinal myoclonus evolving toward acute "myoclonic status". Mov Disord. 2005;20(12):1646–50.

129. Kang SY, Sohn YH. Electromyography patterns of propriospinal myoclonus can be mimicked voluntarily. Mov Disord. 2006;21(8):1241–4.

130. Williams DR, Cowey M, Tuck K, Day B. Psychogenic propriospinal myoclonus. Mov Disord. 2008;23(9):1312–3.

131. Antelmi E, Provini F. Propriospinal myoclonus: the spectrum of clinical and neurophysiological phenotypes. Sleep Med Rev. 2015;22:54–63.

132. Abrao J, Bianco Mde P, Roma W, Krippa JE, Hallak JE. Spinal myoclonus after subarachnoid anesthesia with bupivacaine. Rev Bras Anestesiol. 2011;61(5):619–23, 339-640

133. Benatru I, Thobois S, Andre-Obadia N, et al. Atypical propriospinal myoclonus with possible relationship to alpha interferon therapy. Mov Disord. 2003;18(12):1564–8.

134. Lozsadi DA, Forster A, Fletcher NA. Cannabis-induced propriospinal myoclonus. Mov Disord. 2004;19(6):708–9.
135. Post B, Koelman JH, Tijssen MA. Propriospinal myoclonus after treatment with ciprofloxacin. Mov Disord. 2004;19(5):595–7.
136. Zamidei L, Bandini M, Michelagnoli G, Campostrini R, Consales G. Propriospinal myoclonus following intrathecal bupivacaine in hip surgery: a case report. Minerva Anestesiol. 2010;76(4):290–3.
137. Vetrugno R, Provini F, Plazzi G, Cortelli P, Montagna P. Propriospinal myoclonus: a motor phenomenon found in restless legs syndrome different from periodic limb movements during sleep. Mov Disord. 2005;20(10):1323–9.
138. Shprecher D, Silberstein H, Kurlan R. Propriospinal myoclonus due to cord compression in the absence of myelopathy. Mov Disord. 2010;25(8):1100–1.
139. van der Salm SM, Erro R, Cordivari C, et al. Propriospinal myoclonus: clinical reappraisal and review of literature. Neurology. 2014;83(20):1862–70.
140. Fouillet N, Wiart L, Arne P, Alaoui P, Petit H, Barat M. Propriospinal myoclonus in tetraplegic patients: clinical, electrophysiological and therapeutic aspects. Paraplegia. 1995;33(11):678–81.
141. Roze E, Bounolleau P, Ducreux D, et al. Propriospinal myoclonus revisited: clinical, neurophysiologic, and neuroradiologic findings. Neurology. 2009;72(15):1301–9.
142. Wong SH, Selvan A, White RP. Propriospinal myoclonus associated with fragile-X-premutation and response to selective serotonin reuptake inhibitor. Parkinsonism Relat Disord. 2011;17(7):573–4.
143. Okura M, Tanaka M, Sugita H, Taniguchi M, Ohi M. Obstructive sleep apnea syndrome aggravated propriospinal myoclonus at sleep onset. Sleep Med. 2012;13(1):111–4.

Part IV
Sleep in Special Conditions

Chapter 19
Sleep in Critical Illness

Michael T. Y. Lam, Atul Malhotra, Jamie Nicole LaBuzetta, and Biren B. Kamdar

Keywords Critical illness · Sleep · Circadian rhythms · Delirium
Sleep fragmentation · Sleep disruption · Sleep deprivation · Intensive care unit

The importance of sleep to overall wellness and physiological homeostasis has been increasingly appreciated. For critically ill patients in the intensive care unit (ICU) setting, physiological disruptions are common, highlighting sleep as an important factor in this vulnerable population. In this chapter, we review existing literature on sleep in the ICU and provide ideas for future research. After providing an overview of sleep in healthy and critically ill patients, we review tools to measure sleep and causes of sleep disruption in the ICU. We also highlight the impact of sleep disruption on two systems that are essential to recovery: the immune system and brain.

M. T. Y. Lam · A. Malhotra
Department of Medicine, Division of Pulmonary, Critical Care, Sleep Medicine
and Physiology, University of California San Diego Health, La Jolla, CA, USA

J. N. LaBuzetta
Department of Neurosciences, Division of Neurocritical Care, University of California San Diego Health, La Jolla, CA, USA

B. B. Kamdar (✉)
Department of Medicine, Division of Pulmonary, Critical Care and Sleep Medicine, University of California San Diego Health, La Jolla, CA, USA
e-mail: kamdar@ucsd.edu

© Springer Nature Switzerland AG 2022
M. S. Badr, J. L. Martin (eds.), *Essentials of Sleep Medicine*,
Respiratory Medicine, https://doi.org/10.1007/978-3-030-93739-3_19

Sleep Patterns in the ICU

Sleep in Healthy Adults

An understanding of sleep in healthy adults (summarized in greater detail in other chapters of this book) is necessary to appreciate the sleep experienced by critically ill patients. In healthy adults, sleep architecture—as measured using polysomnography (PSG)—is divided into non-rapid eye movement (NREM) sleep, comprised of N1 (2–5% of total sleep time), N2 (45–55%), and N3 (3–15%), and REM (20–25%). Sleep onset usually occurs within 10–20 minutes, and the first REM period usually begins 90–120 minutes into sleep. In healthy adults, total consolidated nightly sleep time is usually 7–9 hours. Arousals occur roughly ten times per hour (even in normal individuals), although higher figures have been reported [1–3].

The drive to sleep is primarily governed by two factors: homeostatic and circadian. The homeostatic drive refers to the impact of antecedent sleep deprivation on the urge to sleep, i.e., the longer an individual is awake, the more tired they get and more pressure to sleep. The circadian drive is based on an endogenous body clock, which increases or decreases the propensity to sleep during the 24-hour day.

The importance of circadian rhythms has been well established in health and in disease, as the circadian system—consisting of a central oscillator and peripheral "clocks"—can affect cells in nearly every vital organ system [4]. The clinical relevance of the circadian system is represented by the disproportionate number of myocardial infarctions and ischemic strokes that occur in the morning and asthma flares that occur at night [5–7]. Sleep-wake coordination, rest-activity maintenance, light-dark exposure, feeding timing, and social interactions follow a circadian pattern and are modifiable factors for circadian rhythm alignment [8, 9].

Sleep in Critically Ill Patients

In contrast to healthy adults, sleep in critically ill patients is characterized by low total sleep time (~5 hr) and interruption of the normal diurnal pattern, with approximately 50% of sleep occurring during daytime hours [10–14]. Critically ill patients undergoing polysomnography (PSG) have been shown to experience mostly N1 and N2 sleep, with notably reduced or absent slow-wave sleep (N3) and REM (Fig. 19.1) [10–14]. Sleep in the ICU is also severely fragmented, with frequent interruptions and arousals resulting in discrete and frequent sleep episodes [10–14]. This sleep fragmentation was highlighted in a landmark study demonstrating that critically ill patients undergoing PSG experienced 41 ± 28 sleep episodes each day, with each episode averaging 15 ± 9 minutes [15].

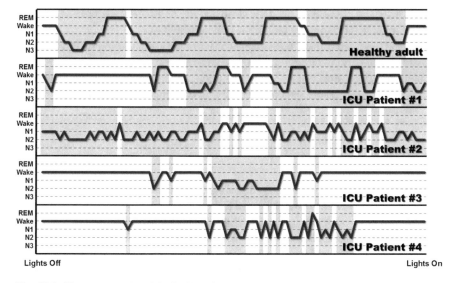

Fig. 19.1 Sleep patterns in critically ill patients, as recorded using polysomnography, as compared to a healthy adult. Gray areas represent sleep and white areas represent wakefulness; notable in critically ill patients is the lack of consolidated sleep, N3 and REM. ICU intensive care unit, REM rapid eye movement. (From Knauert, with permission [14])

Sleep Measurement in the ICU

Large-scale, accurate measurement of sleep in the ICU setting is challenging and represents a key barrier to efforts aimed at building knowledge in this area. Nevertheless, sleep measurement in the ICU is a topic of great interest motivating many prior and ongoing investigations.

Polysomnography

In the ICU setting, PSG is cumbersome and expensive; furthermore, it is not feasible to perform for longer than 24 hours [13]. Additionally, interpretation of the PSG differs substantially when comparing prototypical critically ill patients with community-dwelling adults [16]. For example, while N2 sleep is characterized by sleep spindles, benzodiazepines—sedative medications commonly used in the ICU—can produce spindles on EEG that are qualitatively similar but functionally different than those occurring during natural sleep. Thus, the N2 designation in the ICU can be problematic due to its inability to discriminate between natural and benzodiazepine-induced N2. Similarly, N3 (slow-wave) sleep is characterized by delta activity, a brain wave pattern also resembling that seen in ICU patients experiencing encephalopathy, i.e., diffuse slowing [14, 17, 18]. Finally, submentalis electromyography

(EMG), which is commonly used for sleep staging (e.g., REM vs. NREM), can be affected in the ICU setting by paralytics or comorbidities.

While ICU-based efforts to define new criteria for sleep staging of PSG recordings are ongoing, no major consensus has been reached [16]. As a result, efforts to evaluate the effectiveness of sleep interventions remain hampered by difficulties in assessing sleep, e.g., scoring sleep according to conventional methods.

Actigraphy

Actigraphy involves accelerometry, often via a wristwatch-like device, to evaluate cycles of rest and activity. A decades-old technology, actigraphy has received recent attention for large-scale use in the ICU since it is inexpensive and well tolerated and can wirelessly capture continuous rest-activity data across daytime and nighttime periods [19–21]. Moreover, as demonstrated in nursing home and ICU survivor populations, actigraphic rest-activity data can be used to approximate circadian rhythm alignment [22, 23]. Despite these strengths, actigraphy is challenging in the ICU as critically ill patients are mostly inactive, resulting in overestimation of sleep using traditional scoring algorithms [19, 20, 24]. Moreover, actigraphy-based activity monitoring can be confounded by common ICU factors such as sedating medications, delirium, and staff interventions such as turning and bathing. Nevertheless, actigraphy is a promising method for capturing rest-activity rhythms in critically ill patients, especially if ICU-specific scoring algorithms are developed.

Subjective Measures

Subjective measurement of sleep is a practical, low-cost option for evaluating sleep at a large scale in the ICU. Currently, the Richards-Campbell Sleep Questionnaire (RCSQ), which involves a 5-item visual analogue scale (VAS), and the Verran/Snyder-Halpern Sleep Scale [25, 26]—which involves a 14-item VAS—represent the most commonly used sleep questionnaires in the ICU [27–32]. The RCSQ is the only instrument validated against PSG [26, 33]. While easy to collect and inexpensive to use in the ICU setting, subjective instruments have inherent limitations, including recall bias and fatigue across repeated assessments. Notably, ICU staff may complete subjective instruments for patients with altered cognition and/or consciousness [28, 34, 35]; however these ratings tend to be overestimated [36]. Whether by observation or validated instruments, subjective sleep measurement in the ICU must be performed with caution.

Causes of Sleep Disruption in the ICU

The nature of the ICU environment could be described as a "constant routine" in which noise, light, and biological stress occur 24/7. As such, critically ill patients are felt to experience substantial circadian rhythm disruption, but data are sparse to support the presence of circadian misalignment or the therapeutic benefits of circadian rhythm entrainment in the ICU [4, 8, 9, 37, 38]. Several factors can contribute to disrupted sleep in critically ill patients, many of which are modifiable (Fig. 19.2). In theory, modulation of ambient light and noise, timing of food and medication administration (e.g., melatonin, ramelteon), as well as adjusting mechanical ventilation could influence sleep-wake rhythms highlighting these factors as potential targets for ICU-based interventions aimed at improving clinical outcomes [18, 39].

Noise

Noise, defined as an unpleasant, unwanted, and/or disruptive sound, is common in the ICU setting [40, 41]. Noises produced by people (e.g., staff, visitors), machines (e.g., ventilator alarms, IV pumps), or objects (e.g., doors, squeaky shoes) can

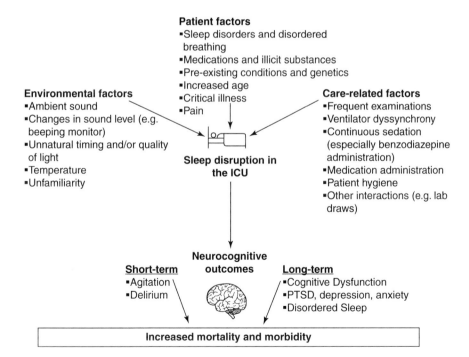

Fig. 19.2 Causes and consequences of sleep disruption in the ICU

disrupt sleep [42, 43]. In the ICU, noise levels range from 55 to 65 dB [15, 44–46] but often exceed 80 dB, a level sufficient for sleep arousal [47]. In comparison, the Environmental Protection Agency recommends hospital noise levels average less than 35–45 dB during the day and 30–35 dB at night [48]. Some data suggest that absolute noise levels are less critical than sound-level changes [49]. Abrupt changes in noise level—for example, an IV pump alarming in an otherwise quiet room—are common in the ICU and may disrupt sleep more than constant background sounds. Additionally, recent studies have shown that the majority of noise in the ICU originates from sources near the ears of the patient and is often due to staff conversations and nonessential alarms [42, 43]. As patients and survivors consistently report noise as a disruptive factor needing improvement [18, 50], efforts are needed to identify and minimize noise in the ICU.

Light

Despite suboptimal day-night light exposure in the ICU setting, critically ill patients generally report light to be less disruptive than other factors such as noise and care-based interactions [28, 51]. Nevertheless, mistimed, excessive, or inadequate environmental light exposure can affect sleep-wake rhythms. As described above and in other chapters, sleep-wake rhythms follow a circadian pattern, with the suprachiasmatic nucleus (SCN) acting as a central 24-hour pacemaker. Light represents the strongest zeitgeber (environmental cues that entrain the central clock) for sleep-wake rhythms by regulating melatonin secretion from the SCN. Typically, retinal receptors receive early morning light, which signal the SCN to suppress melatonin secretion from the pineal gland. Melatonin levels accumulate in the early evening to promote sleep.

When compared to indoor light (~1000 lux), subjects exposed to natural light (>4000 lux) over longer durations have been shown to exhibit improved melatonin and sleep-wake rhythms [52]. Unfortunately, in the ICU setting, light levels range from 30 to 165 lux during the day, below the level needed to inhibit melatonin, and can rise as high as 1445 lux at night, above the level needed to suppress melatonin release [49, 53–57]. Light levels during bedside procedures have been shown to reach 10,000 lux [56]. Interestingly, independent of light exposure, impaired melatonin secretion has been observed in patients with sepsis [58] and delirium [59, 60], highlighting bright light exposure as a potentially important intervention in critically ill patients [56]. Additionally, melatonin and melatonin-receptor agonists are receiving attention as part of ICU-based sleep-wake improvement efforts [61–66].

Care-Related Interactions

While vigilant monitoring is required in the ICU setting, in some circumstances excessive or poorly timed staff interactions can be deleterious. For example, hourly assessments may capture signs of deterioration early in an ICU course, but may disrupt sleep once a patient achieves clinical stability. When surveyed, ICU patients report blood draws, vital signs, and nurse visits among the most disruptive factors, along with radiographs, baths, wound care, and suctioning and non-care-related interactions from family and visitors.

When quantified, ICU patients can experience up to 8 care-related interactions per hour while sleeping [67] and 50 across the night shift [68, 69]. When evaluated against PSG in one study, one out of every five interactions resulted in a sleep arousal or awakening [12]. Hence, efforts to improve sleep should involve individualization of bedside interactions, consideration of nondisruptive technologies (e.g., devices with outside-of-the-room alarms and controls), and bundling of care [70, 71]. Vital to such efforts is multidisciplinary and staff engagement to develop interventions to minimize interactions and to evaluate their feasibility [72].

Medications

Via mechanisms including sympathetic activation, deliriogenicity, and drug-drug interactions, nearly every medication administered in the ICU can disrupt patient sleep (Table 19.1). Notably, chronotherapy—treatments provided in the context of the body clock—is gaining interest, as data suggest that the timing of treatment may impact the safety and efficacy of various treatments [73]. For example, inhaled steroid use at 3 pm has been shown to have similar efficacy to more frequent dosing [74]. Additionally, chemotherapy may be safer and more effective when administered at specific times [75]. Understanding and optimizing the timing of medications in critically ill patients represents a compelling area of research, along with other common ICU practices such as enteral feeding and mechanical ventilation.

Mechanical Ventilation

While mechanical ventilation (MV) is a cornerstone of critical care, inappropriate patient-ventilator interactions can result in profound sleep disruption. In general, patients receiving mechanical ventilation report worse sleep quality compared to those not receiving MV, for various reasons including patient-ventilator dyssynchrony, endotracheal tube discomfort, alarms, and ventilator-related care interactions (i.e., suctioning) [51, 76, 77]. Additionally, small studies in patients receiving MV suggest that spontaneous modes such as pressure support (PSV) may inhibit sleep by inducing central apneas from intermittent bursts of excessive support [78]. Controlled modes of ventilation, such as volume control (VC), pressure control (PC), and proportional assist ventilation (PAV), may be better for sleep, in particular PAV via matching of driving pressure with patient effort [79]. However, one study involving clinician-adjusted PSV [80] and another involving addition of dead space to the ventilator circuit in patients receiving PSV [81] demonstrated improvement in central apneas and associated sleep disruption as compared to PSV alone, suggesting that individualized instead of "one size fits all" approaches are vital for

Table 19.1 Commonly used ICU medications and their effect on sleep

Medication class	Mechanism of action	Effect on sleep
Sedative		
Benzodiazepines	GABA receptor agonist	↓W, ↑TST, ↓N3, ↓REM, ↓SL
Dexmedetomidine	α_2-Agonist	↑N3, ↓SL, ↓REM, ↑N2 with spindles, ↑SE
Propofol	GABA receptor agonist	↑TST, ↓SL, ↓W, ↓REM
Nonbenzodiazepine hypnotics	GABA receptor agonist	↓N2, ↑TST, ↓N3, ↑↓REM, ↓SL, ↓W
Analgesic		
Opioids	μ-Receptor agonist	↓TST, ↓N3, ↓REM, ↑W
Antipsychotic		
Haloperidol	Dopamine-receptor antagonist	↑TST, ↑N3, ↑SE, ↓SL, ↓W
Olanzapine	$5HT_2$-, D_2-receptor antagonist	↑TST, ↑N3, ↑SE, ↓SL, ↓W
Trazodone	SSRI, $5HT_{1a/1c/2}$-receptor antagonist, H_1-receptor antagonist	↑N3, ↑↓REM,? ↑SE, ↓SL
Antihistamine		
Diphenhydramine	H1-receptor antagonist	?↑N3, ↓REM,? ↑SE, ↓SL
Melatonin and melatonin-receptor agonist		
Ramelteon	Melatonin 1 and 2 receptor agonist	↑TST, ↓SL, ↑SE
Immunosuppressant		
Corticosteroids	Decreased melatonin secretion	↑W, ↓N3, ↓REM, insomnia
Tacrolimus	Calcineurin inhibitor	Insomnia
Cyclosporine	Inhibits production and release of IL-2	Insomnia
Cardiovascular		
Norepinephrine/epinephrine	α- and β-receptor agonist	↓N3, ↓REM, insomnia
Dopamine	D_2-, β_1-, α_1-receptor agonist	↓N3, ↓REM, insomnia
Phenylephrine	α_1-Receptor agonist	↓N3, ↓REM
β-Blockers	CNS β-receptor antagonist	↑W, ↓REM, nightmares, insomnia
Amiodarone	Various pathways	Nightmares
Clonidine	α_2-Agonist	↓REM
Antimicrobial		
Fluoroquinolones	GABA type A receptor inhibition	Insomnia

Abbreviations: *ICU* intensive care unit, *GABA* gamma-aminobutyric acid, *W* wake, *TST* total sleep time, *N2* deeper sleep, *N3* restorative/slow-wave sleep, *REM* rapid eye movement sleep, *SL* sleep latency, *SE* sleep efficiency, *SSRI* selective serotonin reuptake inhibitor, *CNS* central nervous system, *W* wake

optimizing sleep quality. Other strategies to improve sleep quality could include adjusting positive end-expiratory pressure (PEEP) to lessen respiratory effort for patients with auto-PEEP, increasing the inspiratory flow rate in the setting of air hunger, shortening inspiratory time to prevent double triggering, and minimizing sleep-disrupting sedative medications. Additionally, modes such as neurally adjusted ventilator assist (NAVA), which involves neuromechanical coupling to promote patient-ventilator synchrony, may also be considered [82]. While the 2018 Clinical Practice Guidelines for Pain, Agitation/Sedation, Delirium, Immobility, and Sleep Disruption (PADIS) conditionally recommend controlled ventilation modes for sleep at night, large multi-site studies are needed to fill substantial knowledge gaps [83].

Sleep, Immunity, and Cognition in Critically Ill Patients

Sleep disruption can have a profound effect on nearly every major organ system, thus impeding recovery for critically ill patients (Fig. 19.3). The SARS-CoV-2 (COVID-19) pandemic has increased attention toward critical care, specifically highlighting the poor sleep patients experience in the ICU setting [84] and its possible association with immune dysfunction [85] and—in the context of delirium and dementia—cognitive dysfunction [86, 87]. As a summary of the multi-organ effects of sleep disruption would be beyond the scope of this chapter, this section instead will focus specifically on the role of sleep disruption on immune and cognition function in critically ill patients.

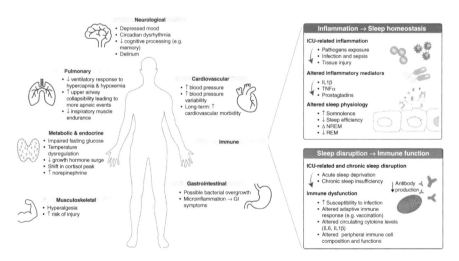

Fig. 19.3 The effect of disrupted sleep on major organ systems, with a focus on the relationship of poor sleep, immunity, and inflammation. (Adapted from Chang et al. [146])

Sleep and Immunity

Adequate sleep is critical to immune function (Fig. 19.3). Outside of the ICU, clinicians and researchers observed the development of respiratory infections as a consequence of sleep deprivation, which has more recently been supported by high-quality studies. First, a rhinovirus inoculation study in healthy human volunteers observed a higher rate of infection in subjects obtaining 7 hours or less of sleep, as compared to rested controls [88]. Second, in large epidemiological cohorts, reported sleep duration of 5 hours—as compared to matched controls obtaining 7–8 hours of sleep—has been associated with an increased incidence of pneumonia [89] and upper respiratory tract infections [90]. Third, in response to influenza [91, 92] and hepatitis vaccination [93, 94], a slowed peak in antibody levels has been noted in those who are sleep deprived as compared to those obtaining adequate sleep. The findings may suggest an adequate but delayed antigenic response due to sleep deprivation. Lastly, acute sleep deprivation in healthy individuals alters circulating cytokine levels [95] and the transcriptome relevant to immune function in blood cells [96, 97]. While these studies suggest that sleep disruption may alter humoral and cellular immunity, other studies suggest that chronic sleep disruption may exacerbate inflammatory states such as atherosclerosis [98–100], metabolic syndrome [101–105], stroke [106, 107], and tumor immunity [108, 109] (Fig. 19.3).

Reciprocally, infection also has an important relationship with sleep. Somnolence is a cardinal symptom of infection, and sleep is therefore considered an acute-phase compensatory response. In animal models, viral and bacterial infections, as well as the inoculation of pathogenic components (e.g., muramyl peptide, lipopolysaccharide), are sufficient to alter sleep [110]. In a series of studies in healthy volunteers, low doses of systemic endotoxin resulted in changes in sleep patterns on PSG, prolonging NREM sleep while suppressing REM sleep [111]. Moreover, sleep is altered differentially depending on the timing and dosing of a septic challenge [112], highlighting the complex relationship between acute inflammation and sleep. Indeed, the effect of sepsis on sleep architecture is likely influenced by a complex combination of factors, including cytokines IL (interleukin)-1β, TNF (tumor necrosis factor)-α, and prostaglandins [95].

In the ICU setting, the relationship between sleep disruption and immune function is unclear and complicated by the ubiquity of sleep disruption and infection in critically ill patients. Research in animals has contributed valuable knowledge in this area. Sleep-deprived mice have a higher mortality after a septic challenge as compared to non-sleep-deprived controls [113–115], an observation that could be attributed to impaired pathogen clearance [114]. Furthermore, as the somnogenic effect of sepsis depends on a neuronal-specific isoform of IL1 receptor accessory protein, mice deficient of this gene lacked the sleep response when given a septic challenge with influenza and experienced higher mortality than controls [116]. Moreover, animals invariably died after 6–8 weeks of chronic total sleep deprivation [117] and showed signs of bacterial infection before death [118]. While these studies support the notion of compromised microbial defense as a consequence of sleep deprivation, the levels of sleep deprivation and stress imposed by these models may not generalize to critically ill patients. Last, it is unclear whether acute-on-chronic sleep disruption predisposes critically ill patients to a hyper-inflammatory state.

Overall, the collective body of research provides a biological plausibility for the sleep-immunity association, particularly in critically ill patients who experience sepsis as a common cause of mortality [119–121]. Sepsis survivors have poor long-term prognosis, with infection as the most common reason for rehospitalization [122]. For critically ill patients, an intact immune system may play a vital role in noninfectious processes such as wound healing and tissue repair (e.g., after trauma, surgery, or acute myocardial infarction). Understanding the sleep-immune axis in the critically ill is of paramount importance. The awareness to improve sleep may have an immediate implication in immune-related ICU outcomes (e.g., enhanced pathogen clearance and improved recovery from sepsis) as well as long-term consequences (e.g., mounting an adequate adaptive immune response for a robust acquired immunity).

Sleep Disruption and Cognition

A comprehensive pathophysiological review of the relationship between sleep, delirium, and cognition is outside the scope of this chapter, but briefly is believed to include common pathophysiologic pathways, mechanisms, and neurotransmitters [34, 123]. Sleep disruption likely plays a role in the development of delirium, and vice versa, though a causal relationship has not been established [124, 125]. Approximately one-third of critically ill patients experience delirium, including up to 80% of those receiving mechanical ventilation [123]. Patients experiencing delirium are at high risk of devastating outcomes, including longer duration of mechanical ventilation and prolonged ICU and hospital length of stay [126]. Over the past decade, increased attention has been paid to the long-term sequelae of ICU delirium, in particular its association with severe and disabling long-term neurocognitive impairments [127–129]. Another study observed an eightfold increase in developing dementia for elderly (>85-year-old) patients who developed delirium during their hospital stay [130].

Risk factors for delirium in the ICU include critical illness, older age, preexisting cognitive impairments, and genetic predisposition [123]. Disrupted sleep has received particular attention as a modifiable risk factor for delirium in the ICU and is supported by observational studies demonstrating increased mental status change frequency among critically ill patients experiencing more sleep interruptions [131] and higher delirium incidence after thoracic surgery in patients reporting sleep deprivation [132]. More objectively, a study involving PSG in mechanically ventilated patients demonstrated a higher rate of incident delirium in patients with REM suppression [133].

The interaction between pharmacological agents and delirium has been studied extensively, with benzodiazepine infusions being identified consistently as a risk factor for delirium development [125, 134–138]. Several studies have examined strategies to prevent or treat delirium, with inconclusive results [83]. Antipsychotics are traditionally administered off-label for delirium, but have not been shown to be effective in large studies [139, 140]. Dexmedetomidine has been a subject of interest as it has a favorable deliriogenicity profile [141, 142] and may act via the ventrolateral preoptic nucleus of the hypothalamus [143], thus promoting biological sleep rather than sedation seen with benzodiazepines and propofol. However, a large, randomized control trial did not show any major benefits of dexmedetomidine when compared with usual care [144]. Thus, strategies to address delirium have largely focused on non-pharmacological strategies such as sleep promotion and early mobility and, from a pharmacological perspective, avoidance of deliriogenic medications such as benzodiazepines (Table 19.2) [72, 83]. As sleep-focused improvement efforts have been shown to reduce delirium in ICU settings [28, 29], design and implementation of larger interventions is a high priority [145], in large part due to heightened awareness of delirium and its associated short- and long-term consequences [83].

Future Directions

This chapter highlights the important intersection between sleep and critical illness and reviews some of the short- and long-term consequences when sleep is disrupted during critical illness. However, a dearth of data highlights the vast array of research opportunities in the area. Further research is needed to evaluate the role of ICU-related sleep disruption on clinically important patient outcomes, in particular on immunity and cognition. Circadian rhythms are also gaining attention in the ICU, in particular in the context of balancing the provision of potentially lifesaving treatments while minimizing the short- and long-term impairments imposed by critical illness itself. While multicomponent bundled interventions are recommended for all critically ill patients, the ideal strategy to optimize sleep and associated outcomes remains unknown and represents a complex and fascinating topic of future investigation.

Table 19.2 Interventions to promote sleep in the ICU setting

Study	Behav. Mod: ↓ Average peak sound	Behav. Mod: ↑ Sleep quality	Behav. Mod: ↓ Delirium	Behav. Mod: ↓ Ambient light and/or noise	Ear Plugs: ↑ Sleep quality	Eye Mask: ↑ Sleep quality	Music: ↓ Anxiety	Music: ↓ Sedative use	Music: ↑ Subjective sleep	White Noise: ↑ Subjective sleep	Massage: ↑ Sleep quality	Massage: ↑ Sleep efficiency (men)	Aromatherapy: ↑ Sleep quality	Acupressure: ↓ Waking	Acupressure: ↑ Sleep quality	Foot reflexology: ↑ Subjective sleep	Guided Imagery: No improvement
Kahn et al [n= all ICU staff] (147)	✓																
Olson et al [n=239] (148)	✓																
Monsen and Edell-Gustafsson [n=23] (149)	✓																
Dennis et al [n=50] (55)	✓																
Li et al [n=55] (30)	✓																
Faraklas et al [n=130] (150)	✓																
Maidl et al [n=129] (151)	✓																
Foster and Kelly [n=32] (152)	✓		✓														
Hansen et al [n=37] (153)	✓		✓														
Walder et al [n=17] (154)	✓				✓	✓	✓										
Kamdar et al [n=300] (28)	✓				✓	✓	✓		✓								
Patel et al [n=338] (29)	✓				✓	✓	✓										
Boyko et al [n=17] (155)	✓				✓	✓	✓										
Haddock [n=18] (156)					✓												
Scotto et al [n=88] (31)					✓												
Neyse et al [n=60] (157)					✓												
Van Rompaey et al [n=136] (158)					✓												
Richardson at al [n=64] (159)					✓	✓											
Ryu et al [n=58] (160)					✓	✓											
Jones and Dawson [n=100] (161)					✓	✓											
Le Guen et al [n=41] (162)					✓	✓											
Yazdannik et al [n=50] (32)					✓	✓											
Dave et al [n=50] (163)					✓	✓											
Mashayekhi et al [n=90] (164)					✓	✓	✓										
Bajwa et al [n=100] (165)					✓	✓											
Hu et al [n=45] (166)					✓	✓											
Babaii [n=60] (167)						✓											
Mashayekhi et al [n=60] (168)						✓											
Daneshmandi et al [n=60] (169)						✓											✓
Richardson [n=36] (170)									✓								
Chlan et al [n=373] (171)									✓								
Su et al [n=28] (172)									✓								
Gragert [n=40] (173)																	
Williamson [n=60] (174)										✓							
Afshar et al [n=60] (175)										✓							
Richards [n=69] (27)									✓	✓							✓
Nerbass et al [n=57] (176)											✓						
Oshvandi et al [n=60] (177)											✓						
Shinde and Anjum [n=60] (178)											✓						
Hsu et al [n=60] (179)											✓						
Moeini et al [n=64] (180)													✓				
Cho et al [n=56] (181)													✓				
Hajibagheri et al [60] (182)													✓				
Karadag e a [n=60] (183)													✓				
Cho et al [n=60] (184)													✓				
Chen et al [85] (185)														✓			
Bagheri-Nesami et al [n=90] (186)													✓	✓			
Rahmani et al [n=140] (187)																✓	

Acknowledgments Dr. Malhotra is funded by the NIH. He reports income related to medical education from LivaNova and Equillium and serves on a DSMB for Corvus. ResMed provided a philanthropic donation to UC San Diego. Dr. Kamdar is supported by a Paul B. Beeson Career Development Award through the National Institutes of Health/National Institute on Aging (K76 AG059936).

Dr. Lam is supported by the Academic Sleep Pulmonary Integrated Research/Clinical Fellowship through the American Thoracic Society and by the NIH (5T32HL134632-04).

References

1. Mathur R, Douglas NJ. Frequency of EEG arousals from nocturnal sleep in normal subjects. Sleep. 1995;18(5):330–3.
2. Boselli M, Parrino L, Smerieri A, Terzano MG. Effect of age on EEG arousals in normal sleep. Sleep. 1998;21(4):351–7.
3. Bonnet MH, Arand DL. EEG arousal norms by age. J Clin Sleep Med. 2007;3(3):271–4.
4. Oldham MA, Lee HB, Desan PH. Circadian rhythm disruption in the critically ill: an opportunity for improving outcomes. Crit Care Med. 2016;44(1):207–17.
5. Elliott WJ. Circadian variation in the timing of stroke onset: a meta-analysis. Stroke. 1998;29(5):992–6.
6. Martin RJ. Nocturnal asthma: circadian rhythms and therapeutic interventions. Am Rev Respir Dis. 1993;147(6 Pt 2):S25–8.
7. Muller JE, Stone PH, Turi ZG, Rutherford JD, Czeisler CA, Parker C, et al. Circadian variation in the frequency of onset of acute myocardial infarction. N Engl J Med. 1985;313(21):1315–22.
8. Brainard J, Gobel M, Bartels K, Scott B, Koeppen M, Eckle T. Circadian rhythms in anesthesia and critical care medicine: potential importance of circadian disruptions. Semin Cardiothorac Vasc Anesth. 2015;19(1):49–60.
9. McKenna H, Reiss I, Martin D. The significance of circadian rhythms and dysrhythmias in critical illness. J Intensive Care Soc. 2017;18(2):121–9.
10. Hilton BA. Quantity and quality of patients' sleep and sleep-disturbing factors in a respiratory intensive care unit. J Adv Nurs. 1976;1(6):453–68.
11. Aurell J, Elmqvist D. Sleep in the surgical intensive care unit: continuous polygraphic recording of sleep in nine patients receiving postoperative care. Br Med J. 1985;290(6474):1029–32.
12. Gabor JY, Cooper AB, Crombach SA, Lee B, Kadikar N, Bettger HE, et al. Contribution of the intensive care unit environment to sleep disruption in mechanically ventilated patients and healthy subjects. Am J Respir Crit Care Med. 2003;167(5):708–15.
13. Knauert MP, Yaggi HK, Redeker NS, Murphy TE, Araujo KL, Pisani MA. Feasibility study of unattended polysomnography in medical intensive care unit patients. Heart Lung. 2014;43(5):445–52.
14. Knauert MP, Malik V, Kamdar BB. Sleep and sleep disordered breathing in hospitalized patients. Semin Respir Crit Care Med. 2014;35(5):582–92.
15. Freedman NS, Gazendam J, Levan L, Pack AI, Schwab RJ. Abnormal sleep/wake cycles and the effect of environmental noise on sleep disruption in the intensive care unit. Am J Respir Crit Care Med. 2001;163(2):451–7.
16. Watson PL, Pandharipande P, Gehlbach BK, Thompson JL, Shintani AK, Dittus BS, et al. Atypical sleep in ventilated patients: empirical electroencephalography findings and the path toward revised ICU sleep scoring criteria. Crit Care Med. 2013;41(8):1958–67.
17. King LM, Bailey KB, Kamdar BB. Promoting sleep in critically ill patients. Nurs Crit Care. 2015;10(3):37–43.
18. Kamdar BB, Needham DM, Collop NA. Sleep deprivation in critical illness: its role in physical and psychological recovery. J Intensive Care Med. 2012;27(2):97–111.

19. Schwab KE, To AQ, Chang J, Ronish B, Needham DM, Martin JL, et al. Actigraphy to measure physical activity in the intensive care unit: a systematic review. J Intensive Care Med. 2019;35(11):1323–31. https://doi.org/10.1177/0885066619863654.
20. Schwab KE, Ronish B, Needham DM, To AQ, Martin JL, Kamdar BB. Actigraphy to evaluate sleep in the intensive care unit. A systematic review. Ann Am Thorac Soc. 2018;15(9):1075–82.
21. Kamdar BB, Kadden DJ, Vangala S, Elashoff DA, Ong MK, Martin JL, et al. Feasibility of continuous actigraphy in patients in a medical intensive care unit. Am J Crit Care. 2017;26(4):329–35.
22. Martin J, Marler M, Shochat T, Ancoli-Israel S. Circadian rhythms of agitation in institutionalized patients with Alzheimer's disease. Chronobiol Int. 2000;17(3):405–18.
23. Yang P-L, Ward TM, Burr RL, Kapur VK, McCurry SM, Vitiello MV, et al. Sleep and circadian rhythms in survivors of acute respiratory failure. Front Neurol. 2020;11:94.
24. Gupta P, Martin JL, Needham DM, Vangala S, Colantuoni E, Kamdar BB. Use of actigraphy to characterize inactivity and activity in patients in a medical ICU. Heart Lung. 2020;49(4):398–406.
25. Snyder-Halpern R, Verran JA. Instrumentation to describe subjective sleep characteristics in healthy subjects. Res Nurs Health. 1987;10(3):155–63.
26. Shahid A, Wilkinson K, Marcu S, Shapiro C. Verran and Snyder-Halpern sleep scale (VSH). In: Shahid A, Wilkinson K, Marcu S, Shapiro CM, editors. STOP, THAT and one hundred other sleep scales. New York: Springer; 2012. p. 397–8.
27. Richards KC. Effect of a back massage and relaxation intervention on sleep in critically ill patients. Am J Crit Care. 1998;7(4):288–99.
28. Kamdar BB, King LM, Collop NA, Sakamuri S, Colantuoni E, Neufeld KJ, et al. The effect of a quality improvement intervention on perceived sleep quality and cognition in a medical ICU. Crit Care Med. 2013;41(3):800–9.
29. Patel J, Baldwin J, Bunting P, Laha S. The effect of a multicomponent multidisciplinary bundle of interventions on sleep and delirium in medical and surgical intensive care patients. Anaesthesia. 2014;69(6):540–9.
30. Li SY, Wang TJ, Vivienne Wu SF, Liang SY, Tung HH. Efficacy of controlling night-time noise and activities to improve patients' sleep quality in a surgical intensive care unit. J Clin Nurs. 2011;20(3–4):396–407.
31. Scotto CJ, McClusky C, Spillan S, Kimmel J. Earplugs improve patients' subjective experience of sleep in critical care. Nurs Crit Care. 2009;14(4):180–4.
32. Yazdannik AR, Zareie A, Hasanpour M, Kashefi P. The effect of earplugs and eye mask on patients' perceived sleep quality in intensive care unit. Iran J Nurs Midwifery Res. 2014;19(6):673–8.
33. Shahid A, Wilkinson K, Marcu S, Shapiro C. Richards–Campbell sleep questionnaire (RCSQ). In: Shahid A, Wilkinson K, Marcu S, Shapiro CM, editors. STOP, THAT and one hundred other sleep scales. New York: Springer; 2012. p. 299–302.
34. Figueroa-Ramos MI, Arroyo-Novoa CM, Lee KA, Padilla G, Puntillo KA. Sleep and delirium in ICU patients: a review of mechanisms and manifestations. Intensive Care Med. 2009;35(5):781–95.
35. Nicolas A, Aizpitarte E, Iruarrizaga A, Vazquez M, Margall A, Asiain C. Perception of night-time sleep by surgical patients in an intensive care unit. Nurs Crit Care. 2008;13(1):25–33.
36. Kamdar BB, Shah PA, King LM, Kho ME, Zhou X, Colantuoni E, et al. Patient-nurse inter-rater reliability and agreement of the Richards-Campbell sleep questionnaire. Am J Crit Care. 2012;21(4):261–9.
37. Engwall M, Fridh I, Johansson L, Bergbom I, Lindahl B. Lighting, sleep and circadian rhythm: an intervention study in the intensive care unit. Intensive Crit Care Nurs. 2015;31(6):325–35.
38. Simons KS, Laheij RJ, van den Boogaard M, Moviat MA, Paling AJ, Polderman FN, et al. Dynamic light application therapy to reduce the incidence and duration of delirium in intensive-care patients: a randomised controlled trial. Lancet Respir Med. 2016;4(3):194–202.
39. Dorsch JJ, Martin JL, Malhotra A, Owens RL, Kamdar BB. Sleep in the intensive care unit: strategies for improvement. Semin Respir Crit Care Med. 2019;40(5):614–28.

40. Kamdar BB, Simons KS, Spronk PE. Can ICUs create more sleep by creating less noise? Intensive Care Med. 2020;46(3):498–500.
41. Kamdar BB, Martin JL, Needham DM. Noise and light pollution in the hospital: a call for action. J Hosp Med. 2017;12(10):861–2.
42. Darbyshire JL, Muller-Trapet M, Cheer J, Fazi FM, Young JD. Mapping sources of noise in an intensive care unit. Anaesthesia. 2019;74(8):1018–25.
43. Park M, Kohlrausch A, de Bruijn W, de Jager P, Simons K. Analysis of the soundscape in an intensive care unit based on the annotation of an audio recording. J Acoust Soc Am. 2014;135(4):1875–86.
44. Elbaz M, Leger D, Sauvet F, Champigneulle B, Rio S, Strauss M, et al. Sound level intensity severely disrupts sleep in ventilated ICU patients throughout a 24-h period: a preliminary 24-h study of sleep stages and associated sound levels. Ann Intensive Care. 2017;7(1):25.
45. Tainter CR, Levine AR, Quraishi SA, Butterly AD, Stahl DL, Eikermann M, et al. Noise levels in surgical ICUs are consistently above recommended standards. Crit Care Med. 2016;44(1):147–52.
46. Darbyshire JL, Young JD. An investigation of sound levels on intensive care units with reference to the WHO guidelines. Crit Care. 2013;17(5):R187.
47. Gardner G, Collins C, Osborne S, Henderson A, Eastwood M. Creating a therapeutic environment: a non-randomised controlled trial of a quiet time intervention for patients in acute care. Int J Nurs Stud. 2009;46(6):778–86.
48. Horsten S, Reinke L, Absalom AR, Tulleken JE. Systematic review of the effects of intensive-care-unit noise on sleep of healthy subjects and the critically ill. Br J Anaesth. 2018;120(3):443–52.
49. Jaiswal SJ, Garcia S, Owens RL. Sound and light levels are similarly disruptive in ICU and non-ICU wards. J Hosp Med. 2017;12(10):798–804.
50. Jha AK, Orav EJ, Zheng J, Epstein AM. Patients' perception of hospital care in the United States. N Engl J Med. 2008;359(18):1921–31.
51. Freedman NS, Kotzer N, Schwab RJ. Patient perception of sleep quality and etiology of sleep disruption in the intensive care unit. Am J Respir Crit Care Med. 1999;159(4 Pt 1):1155–62.
52. Wright KP Jr, McHill AW, Birks BR, Griffin BR, Rusterholz T, Chinoy ED. Entrainment of the human circadian clock to the natural light-dark cycle. Curr Biol. 2013;23(16):1554–8.
53. Voigt LP, Reynolds K, Mehryar M, Chan WS, Kostelecky N, Pastores SM, et al. Monitoring sound and light continuously in an intensive care unit patient room: a pilot study. J Crit Care. 2017;39:36–9.
54. Fan EP, Abbott SM, Reid KJ, Zee PC, Maas MB. Abnormal environmental light exposure in the intensive care environment. J Crit Care. 2017;40:11–4.
55. Dennis CM, Lee R, Woodard EK, Szalaj JJ, Walker CA. Benefits of quiet time for neuro-intensive care patients. J Neurosci Nurs. 2010;42(4):217–24.
56. Verceles AC, Liu X, Terrin ML, Scharf SM, Shanholtz C, Harris A, et al. Ambient light levels and critical care outcomes. J Crit Care. 2013;28(1):110.e1–8.
57. Meyer TJ, Eveloff SE, Bauer MS, Schwartz WA, Hill NS, Millman RP. Adverse environmental conditions in the respiratory and medical ICU settings. Chest. 1994;105(4):1211–6.
58. Mundigler G, Delle-Karth G, Koreny M, Zehetgruber M, Steindl-Munda P, Marktl W, et al. Impaired circadian rhythm of melatonin secretion in sedated critically ill patients with severe sepsis. Crit Care Med. 2002;30(3):536.
59. Yoshitaka S, Egi M, Morimatsu H, Kanazawa T, Toda Y, Morita K. Perioperative plasma melatonin concentration in postoperative critically ill patients: its association with delirium. J Crit Care. 2013;28(3):236–42.
60. Miyazaki T, Kuwano H, Kato H, Ando H, Kimura H, Inose T, et al. Correlation between serum melatonin circadian rhythm and intensive care unit psychosis after thoracic esophagectomy. Surgery. 2003;133(0039-6060; 0039-6060; 6):662.
61. Mo Y, Scheer CE, Abdallah GT. Emerging role of melatonin and melatonin receptor agonists in sleep and delirium in intensive care unit patients. J Intensive Care Med. 2016;31(7):451–5.

62. Shilo L, Dagan Y, Smorjik Y, Weinberg U, Dolev S, Komptel B, et al. Effect of melatonin on sleep quality of COPD intensive care patients: a pilot study. Chronobiol Int. 2000;17(1):71–6.
63. Bourne RS, Mills GH, Minelli C. Melatonin therapy to improve nocturnal sleep in critically ill patients: encouraging results from a small randomised controlled trial. Crit Care. 2008;12(2):R52.
64. Ibrahim MG, Bellomo R, Hart GK, Norman TR, Goldsmith D, Bates S, et al. A double-blind placebo-controlled randomised pilot study of nocturnal melatonin in tracheostomised patients. Crit Care Resusc. 2006;8(3):187–91.
65. Jaiswal SJ, Vyas AD, Heisel AJ, Ackula H, Aggarwal A, Kim NH, et al. Ramelteon for prevention of postoperative delirium: a randomized controlled trial in patients undergoing elective pulmonary thromboendarterectomy. Crit Care Med. 2019;47(12):1751–8.
66. Hatta K, Kishi Y, Wada K, Takeuchi T, Odawara T, Usui C, et al. Preventive effects of ramelteon on delirium: a randomized placebo-controlled trial. JAMA Psychiat. 2014;71(4):397–403.
67. Malik V, Parthasarathy S. Sleep in intensive care units. Curr Resp Care Rep. 2014;3(2):35–41.
68. Tamburri LM, DiBrienza R, Zozula R, Redeker NS. Nocturnal care interactions with patients in critical care units. Am J Crit Care. 2004;13(2):102–12; quiz 14–5.
69. Celik S, Oztekin D, Akyolcu N, Issever H. Sleep disturbance: the patient care activities applied at the night shift in the intensive care unit. J Clin Nurs. 2005;14(1):102.
70. Kamdar BB, Kamdar BB, Needham DM. Bundling sleep promotion with delirium prevention: ready for prime time? Anaesthesia. 2014;69(6):527–31.
71. Kamdar BB, Yang J, King LM, Neufeld KJ, Bienvenu OJ, Rowden AM, et al. Developing, implementing, and evaluating a multifaceted quality improvement intervention to promote sleep in an ICU. Am J Med Qual. 2014;29(6):546–54.
72. Kamdar BB, Martin JL, Needham DM, Ong MK. Promoting sleep to improve delirium in the ICU. Crit Care Med. 2016;44(12):2290–1.
73. Smolensky MH, Hermida RC, Reinberg A, Sackett-Lundeen L, Portaluppi F. Circadian disruption: new clinical perspective of disease pathology and basis for chronotherapeutic intervention. Chronobiol Int. 2016;33(8):1101–19.
74. Song J-U, Park HK, Lee J. Impact of dosage timing of once-daily inhaled corticosteroids in asthma: a systematic review and meta-analysis. Ann Allergy Asthma Immunol. 2018;120(5):512–9.
75. Ozturk N, Ozturk D, Kavakli IH, Okyar A. Molecular aspects of circadian pharmacology and relevance for cancer chronotherapy. Int J Mol Sci. 2017;18(10):2168.
76. Cooper AB, Thornley KS, Young GB, Slutsky AS, Stewart TE, Hanly PJ. Sleep in critically ill patients requiring mechanical ventilation. Chest. 2000;117(3):809–18.
77. Hardin KA, Seyal M, Stewart T, Bonekat HW. Sleep in critically ill chemically paralyzed patients requiring mechanical ventilation. Chest. 2006;129(0012-3692; 0012-3692; 6):1468.
78. Poongkunran C, John SG, Kannan AS, Shetty S, Bime C, Parthasarathy S. A meta-analysis of sleep-promoting interventions during critical illness. Am J Med. 2015;128(10):1126–37.
79. Bosma K, Ferreyra G, Ambrogio C, Pasero D, Mirabella L, Braghiroli A, et al. Patient-ventilator interaction and sleep in mechanically ventilated patients: pressure support versus proportional assist ventilation. Crit Care Med. 2007;35(4):1048.
80. Cabello B, Thille AW, Drouot X, Galia F, Mancebo J, d'Ortho MP, et al. Sleep quality in mechanically ventilated patients: comparison of three ventilatory modes. Crit Care Med. 2008;36(6):1749.
81. Parthasarathy S, Tobin MJ. Effect of ventilator mode on sleep quality in critically ill patients. Am J Respir Crit Care Med. 2002;166(1073-449; 1073-449; 11):1423.
82. Delisle S, Ouellet P, Bellemare P, Tetrault JP, Arsenault P. Sleep quality in mechanically ventilated patients: comparison between NAVA and PSV modes. Ann Intensive Care. 2011;1(1):42.
83. Devlin JW, Skrobik Y, Gelinas C, Needham DM, Slooter AJC, Pandharipande PP, et al. Clinical practice guidelines for the prevention and management of pain, agitation/sedation, delirium, immobility, and sleep disruption in adult patients in the ICU. Crit Care Med. 2018;46(9):e825–e73.

84. Cardinali DP, Brown GM, Reiter RJ, Pandi-Perumal SR. Elderly as a high-risk group during COVID-19 pandemic: effect of circadian misalignment, sleep dysregulation and melatonin administration. Sleep Vigil. 2020;4:81–7.
85. Zhang J, Xu D, Xie B, Zhang Y, Huang H, Liu H, et al. Poor-sleep is associated with slow recovery from lymphopenia and an increased need for ICU care in hospitalized patients with COVID-19: a retrospective cohort study. Brain Behav Immun. 2020;88:50–8.
86. Zambrelli E, Canevini M, Gambini O, D'Agostino A. Delirium and sleep disturbances in COVID–19: a possible role for melatonin in hospitalized patients? Sleep Med. 2020;70:111.
87. LaHue SC, Douglas VC, Miller BL. The one-two punch of delirium and dementia during the COVID-19 pandemic and beyond. Front Neurol. 2020;11:1409.
88. Cohen S, Doyle WJ, Alper CM, Janicki-Deverts D, Turner RB. Sleep habits and susceptibility to the common cold. Arch Intern Med. 2009;169(1):62–7.
89. Patel SR, Malhotra A, Gao X, Hu FB, Neuman MI, Fawzi WW. A prospective study of sleep duration and pneumonia risk in women. Sleep. 2012;35(1):97–101.
90. Prather AA, Leung CW. Association of insufficient sleep with respiratory infection among adults in the United States. JAMA Intern Med. 2016;176(6):850–2.
91. Spiegel K, Sheridan JF, Van Cauter E. Effect of sleep deprivation on response to immunization. JAMA. 2002;288(12):1471–2.
92. Benedict C, Brytting M, Markstrom A, Broman JE, Schioth HB. Acute sleep deprivation has no lasting effects on the human antibody titer response following a novel influenza A H1N1 virus vaccination. BMC Immunol. 2012;13:1.
93. Lange T, Perras B, Fehm HL, Born J. Sleep enhances the human antibody response to hepatitis A vaccination. Psychosom Med. 2003;65(5):831–5.
94. Lange T, Dimitrov S, Bollinger T, Diekelmann S, Born J. Sleep after vaccination boosts immunological memory. J Immunol. 2011;187(1):283–90.
95. Besedovsky L, Lange T, Haack M. The sleep-immune crosstalk in health and disease. Physiol Rev. 2019;99(3):1325–80.
96. Möller-Levet CS, Archer SN, Bucca G, Laing EE, Slak A, Kabiljo R, et al. Effects of insufficient sleep on circadian rhythmicity and expression amplitude of the human blood transcriptome. Proc Natl Acad Sci U S A. 2013;110(12):E1132–41.
97. Foo JC, Trautmann N, Sticht C, Treutlein J, Frank J, Streit F, et al. Longitudinal transcriptome-wide gene expression analysis of sleep deprivation treatment shows involvement of circadian genes and immune pathways. Transl Psychiatry. 2019;9(1):343.
98. Aggarwal B, Makarem N, Shah R, Emin M, Wei Y, St-Onge MP, et al. Effects of inadequate sleep on blood pressure and endothelial inflammation in women: findings from the American Heart Association go red for women strategically focused research network. J Am Heart Assoc. 2018;7(12):e008590.
99. Dominguez F, Fuster V, Fernandez-Alvira JM, Fernandez-Friera L, Lopez-Melgar B, Blanco-Rojo R, et al. Association of sleep duration and quality with subclinical atherosclerosis. J Am Coll Cardiol. 2019;73(2):134–44.
100. McAlpine CS, Kiss MG, Rattik S, He S, Vassalli A, Valet C, et al. Sleep modulates haematopoiesis and protects against atherosclerosis. Nature. 2019;566(7744):383–7.
101. Bakker JP, Weng J, Wang R, Redline S, Punjabi NM, Patel SR. Associations between obstructive sleep apnea, sleep duration, and abnormal fasting glucose. The multi-ethnic study of atherosclerosis. Am J Respir Crit Care Med. 2015;192(6):745–53.
102. Tanno S, Tanigawa T, Saito I, Nishida W, Maruyama K, Eguchi E, et al. Sleep-related intermittent hypoxemia and glucose intolerance: a community-based study. Sleep Med. 2014;15(10):1212–8.
103. Stamatakis KA, Punjabi NM. Effects of sleep fragmentation on glucose metabolism in normal subjects. Chest. 2010;137(1):95–101.
104. Wang Y, Carreras A, Lee S, Hakim F, Zhang SX, Nair D, et al. Chronic sleep fragmentation promotes obesity in young adult mice. Obesity. 2013;22(3):758–62.
105. Poroyko VA, Carreras A, Khalyfa A, Khalyfa AA, Leone V, Peris E, et al. Chronic sleep disruption alters gut microbiota, induces systemic and adipose tissue inflammation and insulin resistance in mice. Sci Rep. 2016;6(1):35405.

106. Redline S, Yenokyan G, Gottlieb DJ, Shahar E, O'Connor GT, Resnick HE, et al. Obstructive sleep apnea-hypopnea and incident stroke: the sleep heart health study. Am J Respir Crit Care Med. 2010;182(2):269–77.
107. Yaggi HK, Concato J, Kernan WN, Lichtman JH, Brass LM, Mohsenin V. Obstructive sleep apnea as a risk factor for stroke and death. N Engl J Med. 2005;353(19):2034–41.
108. Hakim F, Wang Y, Zhang SXL, Zheng J, Yolcu ES, Carreras A, et al. Fragmented sleep accelerates tumor growth and progression through recruitment of tumor-associated macrophages and TLR4 signaling. Cancer Res. 2014;74(5):1329–37.
109. Nieto FJ, Peppard PE, Young T, Finn L, Hla KM, Farré R. Sleep-disordered breathing and cancer mortality. Am J Respir Crit Care Med. 2012;186(2):190–4.
110. Majde JA, Krueger JM. Links between the innate immune system and sleep. J Allergy Clin Immunol. 2005;116(6):1188–98.
111. Pollmächer T, Schreiber W, Gudewill S, Vedder H, Fassbender K, Wiedemann K, et al. Influence of endotoxin on nocturnal sleep in humans. Am J Phys. 1993;264(6 Pt 2):R1077–83.
112. Mullington J, Korth C, Hermann DM, Orth A, Galanos C, Holsboer F, et al. Dose-dependent effects of endotoxin on human sleep. Am J Phys Regul Integr Comp Phys. 2000;278(4):R947–55.
113. Friese RS, Bruns B, Sinton CM. Sleep deprivation after septic insult increases mortality independent of age. J Trauma. 2009;66(1):50–4.
114. Lungato L, Gazarini ML, Paredes-Gamero EJ, Tufik S, D'Almeida V. Paradoxical sleep deprivation impairs mouse survival after infection with malaria parasites. Malar J. 2015;14:183.
115. Chou KT, Cheng SC, Huang SF, Perng DW, Chang SC, Chen YM, et al. Impact of intermittent hypoxia on sepsis outcomes in a murine model. Sci Rep. 2019;9(1):12900.
116. Davis CJ, Dunbrasky D, Oonk M, Taishi P, Opp MR, Krueger JM. The neuron-specific interleukin-1 receptor accessory protein is required for homeostatic sleep and sleep responses to influenza viral challenge in mice. Brain Behav Immun. 2015;47(C):35–43.
117. Rechtschaffen A, Bergmann BM. Sleep deprivation in the rat: an update of the 1989 paper. Sleep. 2002;25(1):18–24.
118. Everson CA, Toth LA. Systemic bacterial invasion induced by sleep deprivation. Am J Physiol Regul Integr Comp Physiol. 2000;278(4):R905–16.
119. Liu V, Escobar GJ, Greene JD, Soule J, Whippy A, Angus DC, et al. Hospital deaths in patients with sepsis from 2 independent cohorts. JAMA. 2014;312(1):90–2.
120. Fleischmann C, Scherag A, Adhikari NKJ, Hartog CS, Tsaganos T, Schlattmann P, et al. Assessment of global incidence and mortality of hospital-treated sepsis. Current estimates and limitations. Am J Respir Crit Care Med. 2016;193(3):259–72.
121. Rudd KE, Johnson SC, Agesa KM, Shackelford KA, Tsoi D, Kievlan DR, et al. Global, regional, and national sepsis incidence and mortality, 1990-2017: analysis for the Global Burden of Disease Study. Lancet (London, England). 2020;395(10219):200–11.
122. Shankar-Hari M, Rubenfeld GD. Understanding long-term outcomes following sepsis: implications and challenges. Curr Infect Dis Rep. 2016;18(11):37.
123. Wilson JE, Mart MF, Cunningham C, Shehabi Y, Girard TD, MacLullich AMJ, et al. Delirium. Nat Rev Dis Primers. 2020;6(1):90.
124. Kamdar BB, Knauert MP, Jones SF, Parsons EC, Parthasarathy S, Pisani MA, et al. Perceptions and practices regarding sleep in the intensive care unit. A survey of 1,223 critical care providers. Ann Am Thorac Soc. 2016;13(8):1370–7.
125. Kamdar BB, Niessen T, Colantuoni E, King LM, Neufeld KJ, Bienvenu OJ, et al. Delirium transitions in the medical ICU: exploring the role of sleep quality and other factors. Crit Care Med. 2015;43(1):135–41.
126. Salluh JIF, Wang H, Schneider EB, Nagaraja N, Yenokyan G, Damluji A, et al. Outcome of delirium in critically ill patients: systematic review and meta-analysis. BMJ. 2015;350:h2538.
127. Gunther ML, Morandi A, Krauskopf E, Pandharipande P, Girard TD, Jackson JC, et al. The association between brain volumes, delirium duration, and cognitive outcomes in intensive care unit survivors: the VISIONS cohort magnetic resonance imaging study*. Crit Care Med. 2012;40(7):2022–32.

128. Morandi A, Rogers BP, Gunther ML, Merkle K, Pandharipande P, Girard TD, et al. The relationship between delirium duration, white matter integrity, and cognitive impairment in intensive care unit survivors as determined by diffusion tensor imaging: the VISIONS prospective cohort magnetic resonance imaging study*. Crit Care Med. 2012;40(7):2182–9.

129. Pandharipande PP, Girard TD, Jackson JC, Morandi A, Thompson JL, Pun BT, et al. Long-term cognitive impairment after critical illness. N Engl J Med. 2013;369(14):1306–16.

130. Davis DH, Muniz Terrera G, Keage H, Rahkonen T, Oinas M, Matthews FE, et al. Delirium is a strong risk factor for dementia in the oldest-old: a population-based cohort study. Brain. 2012;135(Pt 9):2809–16.

131. Helton MC, Gordon SH, Nunnery SL. The correlation between sleep deprivation and the intensive care unit syndrome. Heart Lung. 1980;9(3):464.

132. Yildizeli B, Ozyurtkan MO, Batirel HF, Kuscu K, Bekiroglu N, Yuksel M. Factors associated with postoperative delirium after thoracic surgery. Ann Thorac Surg. 2005;79(3):1004.

133. Trompeo AC, Vidi Y, Locane MD, Braghiroli A, Mascia L, Bosma K, et al. Sleep disturbances in the critically ill patients: role of delirium and sedative agents. Minerva Anestesiol. 2011;77(6):604–12.

134. Lonardo NW, Mone MC, Nirula R, Kimball EJ, Ludwig K, Zhou X, et al. Propofol is associated with favorable outcomes compared with benzodiazepines in ventilated intensive care unit patients. Am J Respir Crit Care Med. 2014;189(11):1383–94.

135. Pandharipande P, Shintani A, Peterson J, Pun BT, Wilkinson GR, Dittus RS, et al. Lorazepam is an independent risk factor for transitioning to delirium in intensive care unit patients. Anesthesiology. 2006;104(1):21–6.

136. Maldonado JR. Pathoetiological model of delirium: a comprehensive understanding of the neurobiology of delirium and an evidence-based approach to prevention and treatment. Crit Care Clin. 2008;24(4):789–856, ix.

137. Pandharipande P, Cotton BA, Shintani A, Thompson J, Pun BT, Morris JA Jr, et al. Prevalence and risk factors for development of delirium in surgical and trauma intensive care unit patients. J Trauma. 2008;65(1):34.

138. McPherson JA, Wagner CE, Boehm LM, Hall JD, Johnson DC, Miller LR, et al. Delirium in the cardiovascular ICU: exploring modifiable risk factors. Crit Care Med. 2013;41(2):405–13.

139. Girard TD, Exline MC, Carson SS, Hough CL, Rock P, Gong MN, et al. Haloperidol and ziprasidone for treatment of delirium in critical illness. N Engl J Med. 2018;379(26):2506–16.

140. Van Den Boogaard M, Slooter AJ, Brüggemann RJ, Schoonhoven L, Beishuizen A, Vermeijden JW, et al. Effect of haloperidol on survival among critically ill adults with a high risk of delirium: the REDUCE randomized clinical trial. JAMA. 2018;319(7):680–90.

141. Pandharipande PP, Pun BT, Herr DL, Maze M, Girard TD, Miller RR, et al. Effect of sedation with dexmedetomidine vs lorazepam on acute brain dysfunction in mechanically ventilated patients: the MENDS randomized controlled trial. JAMA. 2007;298(22):2644.

142. Riker RR, Shehabi Y, Bokesch PM, Ceraso D, Wisemandle W, Koura F, et al. Dexmedetomidine vs midazolam for sedation of critically ill patients: a randomized trial. JAMA. 2009;301(5):489.

143. Nelson Laura E, Lu J, Guo T, Saper Clifford B, Franks Nicholas P, Maze M. The α2-adrenoceptor agonist dexmedetomidine converges on an endogenous sleep-promoting pathway to exert its sedative effects. Anesthesiology. 2003;98(2):428–36.

144. Shehabi Y, Howe BD, Bellomo R, Arabi YM, Bailey M, Bass FE, et al. Early sedation with dexmedetomidine in critically ill patients. N Engl J Med. 2019;380(26):2506–17.

145. Pandharipande PP, Ely EW, Arora RC, Balas MC, Boustani MA, La Calle GH, et al. The intensive care delirium research agenda: a multinational, interprofessional perspective. Intensive Care Med. 2017;43(9):1329–39.

146. Chang VA, Owens RL, LaBuzetta JN. Impact of sleep deprivation in the neurological intensive care unit: a narrative review. Neurocrit Care. 2020;32(2):596–608.

147. Kahn DM, Cook TE, Carlisle CC, Nelson DL, Kramer NR, Millman RP. Identification and modification of environmental noise in an ICU setting. Chest. 1998;114(0012-3692; 0012-3692; 2):535.

148. Olson DM, Borel CO, Laskowitz DT, Moore DT, McConnell ES. Quiet time: a nursing intervention to promote sleep in neurocritical care units. Am J Crit Care. 2001;10(2):74–8.

149. Monsen MG, Edell-Gustafsson UM. Noise and sleep disturbance factors before and after implementation of a behavioural modification programme. Intensive Crit Care Nurs. 2005;21(4):208.

150. Faraklas I, Holt B, Tran S, Lin H, Saffle J, Cochran A. Impact of a nursing-driven sleep hygiene protocol on sleep quality. J Burn Care Res. 2013;34(2):249–54.

151. Maidl CA, Leske JS, Garcia AE. The influence of "quiet time" for patients in critical care. Clin Nurs Res. 2014;23(5):544–59.

152. Foster J, Kelly M. A pilot study to test the feasibility of a nonpharmacologic intervention for the prevention of delirium in the medical intensive care unit. Clin Nurse Spec. 2013;27(5):231–8.

153. Hansen IP, Langhorn L, Dreyer P. Effects of music during daytime rest in the intensive care unit. Nurs Crit Care. 2018;23(4):207–13.

154. Walder B, Francioli D, Meyer JJ, Lancon M, Romand JA. Effects of guidelines implementation in a surgical intensive care unit to control nighttime light and noise levels. Crit Care Med. 2000;28(7):2242–7.

155. Boyko Y, Jennum P, Nikolic M, Holst R, Oerding H, Toft P. Sleep in intensive care unit: the role of environment. J Crit Care. 2017;37:99–105.

156. Haddock J. Reducing the effects of noise in hospital. Nurs Stand. 1994;8(43):25–8.

157. Neyse F, Daneshmandi M, Sadeghi Sharme M, Ebadi A. The effect of earplugs on sleep quality in patients with acute coronary syndrome. Iran J Crit Care Nurs. 2011;4(3):127–34.

158. Van Rompaey B, Elseviers MM, Van Drom W, Fromont V, Jorens PG. The effect of earplugs during the night on the onset of delirium and sleep perception: a randomized controlled trial in intensive care patients. Crit Care. 2012;16(3):R73.

159. Richardson A, Allsop M, Coghill E, Turnock C. Earplugs and eye masks: do they improve critical care patients' sleep? Nurs Crit Care. 2007;12(6):278.

160. Ryu MJ, Park JS, Park H. Effect of sleep-inducing music on sleep in persons with percutaneous transluminal coronary angiography in the cardiac care unit. J Clin Nurs. 2012;21(5–6):728–35.

161. Jones C, Dawson D. Eye masks and earplugs improve patient's perception of sleep. Nurs Crit Care. 2012;17(5):247–54.

162. Le Guen M, Nicolas-Robin A, Lebard C, Arnulf I, Langeron O. Earplugs and eye masks vs routine care prevent sleep impairment in post-anaesthesia care unit: a randomized study. Br J Anaesth. 2014;112(1):89–95.

163. Dave K, Qureshi A, Gopichandran L. Effects of earplugs and eye masks on perceived quality of sleep during night among patients in intensive care units. Int J Sci Res (Ahmedabad). 2015;5(3):319–22.

164. Mashayekhi F, Rafiei H, Arab M, Abazari F, Ranjbar HJ. The effect of sleep quality on patients in a coronary care unit. Br J Cardiac Nurs. 2013;8(9):443–7.

165. Bajwa N, Saini P, Kaur H, Kalra S, Kaur J. Effect of ear plugs and eye mask on sleep among ICU patients: a randomized control trial. Int J Curr Res. 2015;7(12):23741–5.

166. Hu RF, Jiang XY, Hegadoren KM, Zhang YH. Effects of earplugs and eye masks combined with relaxing music on sleep, melatonin and cortisol levels in ICU patients: a randomized controlled trial. Crit Care. 2015;19:115.

167. Babaii A, Adib-Hajbaghery M, Hajibagheri A. Effect of using eye mask on sleep quality in cardiac patients: a randomized controlled trial. Nurs Midwifery Stud. 2015;4(4):e28332.

168. Mashayekhi F, Pilevarzadeh M, Amiri M, Rafiei H. The effect of eye mask on sleep quality in patients of coronary care unit o efeito da mascara de olhos na qualidade de sono em pacientes em uma unidade coronariana. Sleep Sci. 2013;6(3):108–11.

169. Daneshmandi M, Neiseh F, SadeghiShermeh M, Ebadi A. Effect of eye mask on sleep quality in patients with acute coronary syndrome. J Caring Sci. 2012;1(3):135–43.

170. Richardson S. Effects of relaxation and imagery on the sleep of critically ill adults. Dimens Crit Care Nurs. 2003;22(4):182–90.

171. Chlan LL, Weinert CR, Heiderscheit A, Tracy MF, Skaar DJ, Guttormson JL, et al. Effects of patient-directed music intervention on anxiety and sedative exposure in critically ill patients receiving mechanical ventilatory support: a randomized clinical trial. JAMA. 2013;309(22):2335–44.

172. Su CP, Lai HL, Chang ET, Yiin LM, Perng SJ, Chen PW. A randomized controlled trial of the effects of listening to non-commercial music on quality of nocturnal sleep and relaxation indices in patients in medical intensive care unit. J Adv Nurs. 2013;69(6):1377–89.

173. Gragert MD. The use of a masking signal to enhance the sleep of men and women 65 years of age and older in the critical care environment: University of Texas at Austin; 1991.

174. Williamson JW. The effects of ocean sounds on sleep after coronary artery bypass graft surgery. Am J Crit Care. 1992;1(1):91.

175. Farokhnezhad Afshar P, Bahramnezhad F, Asgari P, Shiri M. Effect of white noise on sleep in patients admitted to a coronary care. J Caring Sci. 2016;5(2):103–9.

176. Nerbass FB, Feltrim MI, Souza SA, Ykeda DS, Lorenzi-Filho G. Effects of massage therapy on sleep quality after coronary artery bypass graft surgery. Clinics (Sao Paulo). 2010;65(11):1105–10.

177. Oshvandi K, ABDI S, Karampourian A, Moghimbaghi A, Homayounfar S. The effect of foot massage on quality of sleep in ischemic heart disease patients hospitalized in CCU. 2014.

178. Shinde MB, Anjum S. Effectiveness of slow back massage on quality of sleep among ICU patent's. Int J Sci Res. 2014;3(3):292–8.

179. Hsu WC, Guo SE, Chang CH. Back massage intervention for improving health and sleep quality among intensive care unit patients. Nurs Crit Care. 2019;24(5):313–9.

180. Moeini M, Khadibi M, Bekhradi R, Mahmoudian SA, Nazari F. Effect of aromatherapy on the quality of sleep in ischemic heart disease patients hospitalized in intensive care units of heart hospitals of the Isfahan University of Medical Sciences. Iran J Nurs Midwifery Res. 2010;15(4):234–9.

181. Cho M-Y, Min ES, Hur M-H, Lee MS. Effects of aromatherapy on the anxiety, vital signs, and sleep quality of percutaneous coronary intervention patients in intensive care units. Evid Based Complement Alternat Med. 2013;2013:381381.

182. Hajibagheri A, Babaii A, Adib-Hajbaghery M. Effect of Rosa damascene aromatherapy on sleep quality in cardiac patients: a randomized controlled trial. Complement Ther Clin Pract. 2014;20(3):159–63.

183. Karadag E, Samancioglu S, Ozden D, Bakir E. Effects of aromatherapy on sleep quality and anxiety of patients. Nurs Crit Care. 2017;22(2):105–12.

184. Cho EH, Lee MY, Hur MH. The effects of aromatherapy on intensive care unit patients' stress and sleep quality: a nonrandomised controlled trial. Evid Based Complement Alternat Med. 2017;2017:2856592.

185. Chen JH, Chao YH, Lu SF, Shiung TF, Chao YF. The effectiveness of valerian acupressure on the sleep of ICU patients: a randomized clinical trial. Int J Nurs Stud. 2012;49(8):913–20.

186. Bagheri-Nesami M, Gorji MA, Rezaie S, Pouresmail Z, Cherati JY. Effect of acupressure with valerian oil 2.5% on the quality and quantity of sleep in patients with acute coronary syndrome in a cardiac intensive care unit. J Tradit Complement Med. 2015;5(4):241–7.

187. Rahmani A, Naseri M, Salaree MM, Nehrir B. Comparing the effect of foot reflexology massage, foot bath and their combination on quality of sleep in patients with acute coronary syndrome. J Caring Sci. 2016;5(4):299–306.

Chapter 20
Sleep in Hospitalized Patients

Nancy H. Stewart and Vineet M. Arora

Keywords Sleep · Hospital · ICU · Medical care

Abbreviations

ACOVE-3	Assessing Care of Vulnerable Elders-3
AGS	American Geriatrics Society
CABG	Coronary artery bypass graft
CPAP	Continuous positive airway pressure
EEG	Electroencephalogram
HELP	Hospital Elder Life Program
ICU	Intensive care unit
NICU	Neuro-intensive care unit
OSA	Obstructive sleep apnea
RCT	Randomized controlled trial
REM	Rapid eye movement
SIESTA	Sleep for Inpatients: Empowering Staff to Act

Sleep Loss in Adults

Over 70 million Americans suffer from a chronic disorder of sleep, which adversely affects their health [1]. It is estimated by the National Academy of Medicine that hundreds of billions of dollars per year are spent caring for patients with sleep disorders [1]. Regardless of this, a staggering number of patients suffering from sleep

N. H. Stewart
Department of Medicine, University of Kansas Medical Center, Kansas City, KS, USA

V. M. Arora (✉)
Department of Medicine, University of Chicago Medical Center, Chicago, IL, USA
e-mail: varora@uchicago.edu

© Springer Nature Switzerland AG 2022   453
M. S. Badr, J. L. Martin (eds.), *Essentials of Sleep Medicine*,
Respiratory Medicine, https://doi.org/10.1007/978-3-030-93739-3_20

disorders remain undiagnosed. Nearly half of the general population (30–48%) report difficulty initiating or maintaining sleep [2]. Awareness of diagnoses and treatment of sleep disorders among healthcare professionals and the public remain very low. The lack of awareness among the general public results from the absence of sleep awareness in public health education programs [1]. This in turn causes patients to be hesitant to discuss sleep issues with their healthcare providers.

Sleep is considered a protector of the normal brain activity and strikes a balance between the various functions of the central nervous system [3]. Shortened sleep duration is characterized on polysomnography with decreased stage N3 sleep, and chronic sleep loss can demonstrate a greater percentage of rapid eye movement sleep [4]. Interestingly, effects of health conditions can also be noted on polysomnography [5].

Sleep Loss in Older Adults

Although sleep architecture changes as one ages, there is not a decreased need for sleep, and sleep disturbance is not an inherent aspect of the aging process [6]. Sleep disturbance is common in aging adults, not due to aging, in fact due to comorbidities and psychosocial and polypharmacy factors that elderly often face [6]. A multidisciplinary approach to care is encouraged with these patients [6]. Sleep disturbances in older adults are reported more frequently later in life, among females, among those with physical disabilities, among those experiencing psychiatric health concerns [7].

Health Effects of Sleep Loss in Hospitalized Patients

Unfortunately, the patients most at risk for poor, non-restorative sleep are often also acutely ill and hospitalized, when they need sleep to recover from their acute illness. Predictors of poor inpatient sleep quality include decreased sleep duration, increased nighttime awakenings, younger age, and female [8]. Acute sleep loss in the hospital has been associated with poor patient outcomes, including cardiometabolic effects such as high blood pressure, hyperglycemia, as well as delirium [9–11]. In-hospital acute sleep loss is implicated by Krumholz as a factor in "post-hospital syndrome" development, an acquired condition of vulnerability and increased risk of hospital readmission for diseases unrelated to their index admission [12]. Although studies of long-term consequences of acute sleep loss are lacking, in-hospital sleep loss was implicated as a potential mediator of post-hospital syndrome.

Prior research has demonstrated in-hospital sleep loss is associated with worse psychological and cardiometabolic outcomes [11]. Up to 40 percent of hospitalized medical patients without a diagnosed sleep disorder are at high risk for sleep apnea [13]. Although patients experience acute in-hospital sleep loss, one would expect sleep to improve on discharge, yet sleep loss does not recover in the week following discharge [14]. The time spent in-hospital provides an opportunity not only to optimize the sleep environment for patients but also to screen patients for undiagnosed sleep disorders and reduce unnecessary admissions [15].

Barriers to Healthy Sleep in Hospitalized Patients

Despite a paucity of literature regarding sleep loss in hospitalized patients, multiple factors have been noted to affect the sleep of patients while they are hospitalized. To understand factors affecting sleep while hospitalized, it is imperative to first understand the effects that hospitalization has upon sleep. Several laboratory and epidemiological studies suggest sleep deprivation in itself can lead to a variety of intrinsic physiologic health consequences (i.e., delirium development and metabolic derangements in blood sugar and blood pressure) [16–19]. Interestingly, these health consequences are also known complications of hospitalization in patients. [20, 21] In addition to the health consequences linked to sleep deprivation during hospitalization (delirium, hyperglycemia, and hypertension), these health conditions are often associated with administration of medications and increased dosages of medications to ameliorate or control the condition: antipsychotics for delirium, insulin for hyperglycemia, and antihypertensives to enable blood pressure control. As such, a significant number of these medications may be continued on after patient discharge, which subsequently can result in downstream patient harm (i.e., polypharmacy, hypoglycemia, and hypotension) [22]. Sleep loss can also impair recovery during hospitalization due to daytime fatigue and excessive daytime sleepiness, hindering participation in recovery activities such as physical or occupational therapy, as well as participation in important healthcare discussions (i.e., informed consent, understanding medication changes, discussion discharge/follow-up plans) [23, 24]. Decreased daytime physical activity is a known contributor to functional decline, an unfortunate consequence of hospitalization for older adults. In addition, adults who are less empowered and informed regarding their hospital care are more likely to experience readmission [25].

Medical Care Interruptions

Obtaining a good night of sleep is not an easy task during hospitalization. Many factors can lead to sleep disruptions, including environmental factors (e.g., noise), medical care factors (e.g., medication distribution, vital sign checks, phlebotomy), and patient factors (e.g., pain, anxiety). Hospitalized patients report difficulty with sleep initiation and sleep maintenance, decreased sleep quality, and increased daytime sleepiness [26]. Frequent awakenings by members of the care team represent a significant barrier to sleep in the hospital setting. One study on patients in the neuro-intensive care unit (NICU) demonstrated that although hourly neurological exams may be beneficial in the acute phase of a neurological injury, surprisingly, prolonged use of these exams was associated with a 75% increase in development of delirium [27]. Patients awakened often may be unable to complete an entire sleep cycle and may struggle with falling back to sleep, leading to deprivation of slow-wave sleep, e.g., stage 3 sleep, and rapid eye movement (REM) sleep (e.g., "dream" sleep). Routine night awakenings by care team members are often to complete day-time tasks requested by clinicians, such as vital signs or blood draws [28, 29].

Environmental Factors Disrupting Sleep

Sounds within the walls of the hospital are more than an irritation [32]. The auditory environment in the hospital should complement high standards of compassionate patient care. Failure to provide patients with quiet hospital rooms affects clinical patient outcomes through multiple mechanisms. Increased noise within the hospital affects clinical outcomes through increased physiological and stress responses, medical errors, sleep disturbances, and interference with privacy practices [33, 34]. While the United States Environmental Protection Agency recommends a maximum noise level of 45 decibels (dB) throughout the day and 35 dB at night, most hospitals have noise levels ranging from 50 to 70 dB during the daytime and averaging just under 70 dB (67 dB) at nighttime [35]. Regrettably, this data demonstrates only 62% of Americans report their hospital rooms "always quiet" at night, which is one of the worst performing patient experience measures in the entire Hospital Consumer Assessment of Healthcare Providers and Systems Survey. Moreover, patients staying in the loudest rooms reportedly get significantly less sleep [36]. In addition, the elimination of diurnal light-dark cycles in hospital environments can result in disruption of circadian rhythm and entrainment of sleep [12].

Patient Factors Influencing Sleep

Conditions such as multiple comorbidities, anxiety, and depression often associated with acute and chronic illness and repeated hospitalizations and contribute to diminished sleep among hospitalized inpatients [30]. Studies show poor self-rated health and presence of chronic conditions (cardiovascular disease, lung disease, gastro-esophageal reflux disease, and arthritis) are all associated with increased complaints of poor sleep [7]. Pain is also a frequently reported factor causing sleep disruptions and nighttime awakenings [31].

Prevalence of Sleep Disorders Among Hospitalized Patients

Hospitalization represents a "missed opportunity" to screen patients for sleep disorders. The high prevalence of untreated sleep disorders may often complicate or worsen patients' underlying conditions. For instance, two in every five patients older than age 50 screened at high risk for having obstructive sleep apnea (OSA) and were also found to have worse in-hospital sleep quality and quantity [37]. In addition, in a small single-center study of hospitalized patients, up to 80% screened high risk for OSA using the STOP-BANG questionnaire [38]. Despite a high prevalence, few had been evaluated with a sleep study, diagnosed with OSA, or were receiving treatment with continuous positive airway pressure (CPAP) therapy, which is known to improve quality of life and reduce complications [39, 40]. The prevalence of insomnia is also increased, with several studies finding nearly two out of every five patients screen positive for insomnia [41, 42]. Another study of hospitalized patients noted half of inpatients reported chronic sleep complaints, and nearly one-third of patients screened positive for insomnia, yet *no mention* of sleep complaints was found in the hospital admission documentation [43]. Additionally, even if sleep disorders are suspected or recognized during hospitalization, therapy is frequently unavailable or suboptimal. For example, in a nationally representative sample of nearly 300,000 discharges of patients with OSA from nonfederal acute care hospitals in the United States, only 5.8% of patients were documented to have received CPAP therapy [44]. Given that sleep disorders can exacerbate cardiopulmonary health conditions and may actually result in heart failure or chronic obstructive pulmonary disease (COPD) exacerbations, it is crucial to recognize sleep disorders as an underlying health condition [45–48]. Certain inpatient diagnoses, such as acute stroke and heart failure, are associated with a higher prevalence of sleep-disordered breathing, poor outcomes, and even death [49–56]. Moreover, treatment of OSA with CPAP therapy in patients with acute stroke, systolic heart failure, or COPD improves outcomes and decreases readmission rates [40, 57–60]. The presence of a highly treatable disease and a very prevalent disorder such as sleep-disordered breathing warrants early recognition and treatment.

Perhaps most concerning is that acute sleep loss in the hospital may precipitate insomnia, leading to chronic insomnia after discharge. [61] This is particularly concerning given the association of chronic insomnia and poor long-term health consequences [62]. Early recognition of insomnia is imperative [62]. Lastly, poor self-reported sleep quality predicts 1-year mortality among adults who received inpatient rehabilitation [63]. In a similar study among geriatric hospitalized patients, observed sleep disturbances determined by hourly observations were associated with higher mortality at 2 years [64].

Interventions to Improve Sleep in Hospitalized Patients

Interventions to improve sleep in hospitalized patients can be categorized in two categories: pharmacologic and nonpharmacologic. While hospitalized patients often request pharmacological sleep aids, they are generally not recommended for first-line therapy [65]. It determined that a pharmacologic sleep aid would be of benefit to the patient; general consensus is that the choice of sleep aid should be customized based on patient needs and comorbidity profile to minimize any potential drug side effect and ultimate polypharmacy.

Pharmacologic

Melatonin

If a pharmacologic sleep aid is deemed necessary, melatonin may be an appropriate first-line treatment due to its minimal side effect profile and low likelihood of potential drug-drug interactions, as well as its ability to improve circadian rhythm disturbances [66, 67]. Small randomized studies done in simulated sleep environments, hospitalized patients, and intensive care unit (ICU) patients note improved sleep duration (by polysomnography) and improved sleep quality (by actigraphy) when initiating 1 mg to 5 mg of melatonin at nighttime [68–70]. Although rates of melatonin usage in hospitalized patients have increased, no dosing standard exists [71]. The typical dose used during initiation of melatonin for a hospitalized patient is 1 mg to 5 mg at night, usually dispensed between 2100 and 2200, depending on patient sleep habits, and should be given 30 minutes prior to the desired bedtime. Notably, melatonin given nightly to hospitalized patients over age 65 did not prevent delirium.

Sleep Initiation and Sleep Maintenance Aids

Sleep aids are generally not recommended. In a single-center retrospective study in 2014 determined over a 2-month period, 26.2% of patients received a sleep aid, with trazodone being the most commonly prescribed sleep aid medication 30.4% of the time [72]. In a 2005 meta-analysis by Glass et al., risks and benefits of sedative hypnotic utilization in patients over age 60 found a statistically significant improvement in sleep quality and sleep quantity with sedative use compared to use of placebo, although the magnitude of the effect was small and the patient risk was great (e.g., falls and cognitive impairment) [73]. Notably, while four classes of medications for insomnia have been FDA approved (benzodiazepines, non-benzodiazepines, melatonin receptor agonists, and benzodiazepine receptor agonist hypnotics ("Z drugs")), three of these are also found on the Beers Criteria list from the American Geriatrics

Society (AGS) of medications to avoid in the elderly population (benzodiazepines, non-benzodiazepines, benzodiazepine receptor agonist hypnotics) [74, 75].

Nonpharmacologic Interventions

Nonpharmacologic therapies are the first line of therapy for sleep disturbances in the hospital setting. There is great interest in evidence-based interventions that demonstrate improvement in sleep and related outcomes among hospitalized patients, yet data are limited. To this end, two relevant symptomatic reviews have summarized extant evidence. A Cochrane review in 2015 on improving sleep in the ICU setting evaluated multiple points of potential interventions including type of ventilator used, eye masks used in collaboration with ear plugs, relaxation therapy, sleep-inducing music, aromatherapy, foot baths, acupressure, and visit times for family members of the hospitalized patient, yet the evidence was low [76]. In 2014 the *Journal of General Internal Medicine* found only 13 intervention studies, 4 of which were randomized controlled trials [77]. Despite the limited evidence, some data existed for improving sleep quality, interventions to improve sleep hygiene, interventions to reduce nighttime interruptions, and daytime bright light exposure [77]. These nonpharmacologic interventions are discussed in more detail below.

Relaxation Techniques

Despite the low level of evidence and limited data, several methods of relaxation techniques have been suggested. A systematic review in 2014 by Tamrat et al. in the *Journal of General Internal Medicine* evaluated four randomized controlled trials (RCT) on relaxation techniques and found a 0–28% improvement of overall sleep quality [77].

Soden et al. evaluated the use of aromatherapy, aromatherapy and massage, or usual care and found no difference between groups [78]. In a pilot study by Toth et al. on the effect of guided imagery for 20 minutes daily compared to solitary activity of choice, no difference was noted between groups [79]. Finally, a study randomizing patients postcoronary artery bypass graft (CABG) to a music intervention involving a soothing music video, 30 minutes of rest, or 30 minutes of music via headphones demonstrated a 28% improvement in self-reported sleep quality in those patients that received the soothing music video when compared to the control group [80].

Bright Light Therapy

Several small studies have been performed evaluating the impact of bright light therapy on sleep. Three studies investigated bright light therapy (3000–5000 lux) use during daytime hours. Wakmurua et al. exposed seven older (mean age 67) hospitalized patients to 5 hours of bright light therapy during daytime hours (1000 to 1500) and noted a 7% increase in total sleep duration in the intervention arm [81]. This study also noted increased "immobile minutes" via wrist Actiwatch, suggesting illuminating conditions for elder hospitalized patients may improve nocturnal sleep [81]. A study by Mishima et al. in hospitalized dementia patients exposed to bright light therapy between 0900 and 1100 for 4 weeks found an improvement in average sleep time in the patients in the intervention arm [82]. Twenty-seven patients with Alzheimer-type dementia were treated with bright light therapy in the morning for 4 consecutive weeks and noted to have an increase in total nighttime sleep time [83]. In a 2018 systematic review of the effects of bright light therapy on sleep, mood, and cognition in Alzheimer's patients, 32 studies were evaluated based on the United States Preventive Services Task Force Guidelines, and although the results were mixed, a trend toward benefit was noted [84].

Noise Reduction

Uncontrolled in-hospital noise can have a negative physiological and psychological effect on patients and care staff. A quality improvement study in 2018 by McGough et al. described the implementation and improvement in noise perception using a "Quiet Time Bundle" on four different progressive care units [85]. Another study performed on a medical-surgical unit demonstrated an overwhelmingly favorable response from staff and patients following the implementation of a "Quiet Time Noise Reduction" program [86]. Due to the increased number of monitors and acuity, modalities for noise reduction in the intensive care unit have been evaluated. These approaches include the use of eye masks in conjunction with ear plugs [87], the use of "white noise" also known as sound masking [88, 89],and the installation of soundproof ceiling materials [90]. Sound absorbing modalities are relatively effective at noise reduction, whereas sound masking modalities appear to be the most effective at actually improving sleep [91].

Sleep Hygiene

Promoting good sleep hygiene during hospitalization can be challenging. Gathecha et al. described a nurse-delivered sleep-promoting intervention augmented by sleep hygiene education in the *Journal of Hospital Medicine* as an opportunity for improvement [92]. A randomized controlled trial by Lareau et al. in geriatric hospitalized patients evaluated a nighttime intervention of minimizing patient contact, clustering nursing care, as well as decreasing sounds and lights, as compared to usual care. The group found that intervention was associated with a decrease in the use of sleep aid medications and a 7% improvement in sleep quality [93]. Another study evaluated a sleep hygiene program in hospitalized psychiatric patients. The intervention in this study by Edinger et al. included the standardization of wake and sleep times and the removal of the opportunity for daytime napping [94]. This intervention was associated with an increase of 18 minutes in total sleep time; however neither sleep quality nor significant testing was discussed [94].

Reduction of Nighttime Interruptions

The goal of reducing nighttime interruptions of patient sleep during hospitalized patient sleep may seem ambitious, yet as the most cited nighttime disruption, action is warranted [95]. For example, many nighttime disruptions in the intensive care unit could be safely omitted or clustered, noted Le et al. [96] A recent study evaluating nearly 3500 patients determined that passive vital sign monitoring and reduction in nighttime noise ultimately led to a decreased hospital length of stay and an increase in patient self-reported emotional and mental health [97]. Future studies are needed to best determine methods to implement reductions in nighttime interactions, which in turn improves hospital sleep, enhancing quality and safety.

Sleep Education and Empowerment

Improving patient knowledge and education on health and disease is essential. In a recent randomized controlled trial, non-ICU patients who received sleep-enhancing tools (a white noise machine, ear plugs, and an eye mask) along with sleep education reported decreased sleep impairment and less fatigue than those who received only the sleep-enhancing tool kit [98].

Multifaceted Protocols

The "Somerville" multifaceted protocol implemented several components for sleep improvement. These components included an 8-hour quiet time, "lights off" lullaby, staff-monitored noise control, and avoidance of staff disruptions for routine vitals and medications. The study investigators reported fewer patients reporting nighttime disruptions and fewer patients requesting sleep aid/sedatives [99]. Another multifaceted protocol program of electronic health record reminders and nursing "nudges," "Sleep for Inpatients: Empowering Staff to Act (SIESTA)," demonstrated that a unit-based nursing empowerment approach was associated with fewer nighttime hospital room entries and overall improved patient experiences [28]. Finally, the Hospital Elder Life Program (HELP) designed in 1999 by SK Inouye was successfully implemented across 200 German hospitals [100]. This protocol consisted of multiple strategies to aid in delirium prevention in hospitalized elderly including (re)orientation, cognitive activation, mobilization, meal companionship, and non-pharmacological sleep promotion [100].

Pain and Sleep

Pain should be evaluated frequently on every patient during hospitalization. It is not only a barrier to hospital discharge, but its management is a quality of care issue [101]. Optimal treatment of pain is recommended, as pain can interfere with falling asleep and with the ability to participate in recovery activities during hospitalization [102, 103]. Pharmacologic and nonpharmacologic management options should be evaluated for treatment of pain [103].

Sleep in Hospitalized Patients with Underlying Disorders of Mental Health

Associations between sleep health and mental health are many, yet knowledge of this association is lacking [104]. Among patients hospitalized with depressive disorder, 25–40% report almost always having daytime sleepiness, and a more individualized sleep-wake schedule should be applied in these patients [105]. In a small study of inpatients hospitalized with moderate-to-severe depression undergoing chronotherapy, a significant number of patients (>40%) reported a significant improvement in their depressive symptoms [106].

Hospitalized Older Adults

Predisposing factors and precipitating factors play a role in delirium development in hospitalized older patients [20]. Sleep loss in hospitalized older adults can slow recovery during hospitalization due to fatigue and excessive daytime sleepiness, which leads to decreased participation in recovery activities such as participation with therapy and in important healthcare discussions and decisions with social work and case management [22, 23]. Coaching and empowerment of hospitalized older adults and their caregivers to confirm their needs are met during transitions of care may reduce rates of rehospitalization [24].

Moreover, sleep deprivation has been associated with a variety of significant outcomes of relevance to hospitalized older adults as they recover from acute illness. In addition to delirium, sleep loss has been associated with other health conditions often seen in the elderly population, such as falls. For example, one study by Stone et al. noted women with shorter sleep duration (< 7 hours) or lower sleep efficiency (<70%), as determined by wrist actigraphy, were more likely to suffer from falls in the subsequent year compared to women with normal sleep duration and sleep efficiency [107]. Additionally, sleep deprivation has also been associated with impaired immune function in healthy humans as well as animals, which most certainly has implications for hospitalized older adults [108]. Scientists have also noted genes in *Drosophila* flies – which promote increased sleep – in turn promote survival following infection [109, 110]. Sleep disturbances in hospitalized elderly patients are associated with increased mortality at 2 years [63]. As previously noted, the AGS has recommended against certain medications to aid in sleep initiation and maintenance in the hospitalized elderly due to increased risk of falls and cognitive impairment, specifically benzodiazepines and non-benzodiazepines. Melatonin remains the sleep aid of choice in this patient population. The Assessing Care of Vulnerable Elders-3 (ACOVE-3) program utilizes quality metrics to assess and promote best practices of elder care [111]. Medications such as anticholinergics (including antihistamines) should be avoided [75]. Other medications frequently utilized to aid in sleep, but not recommended, in the elderly population such as antihistamines, oral decongestants (pseudoephedrine and ephedrine), and stimulants (amphetamine and methylphenidate) make insomnia worse, are associated with anticholinergic side effects, and are *not* recommended in the elder population [75, 103].

Sleep in the Intensive Care Unit (ICU)

A study in the ICU found that 51% of noise was modifiable, while patients report staff conversations as well as television noise as the most irritating disturbances [112]. In addition, this noise was notable and found to interfere with sleep as seen on electroencephalogram (EEG) recordings [112]. Light disruptions of the circadian rhythm are particularly problematic in the ICU setting. Due to continued exposure of differing levels of light in the ICU, melatonin secretion patterns are atypical, and in turn the circadian rhythms of these patients are markedly abnormal [113, 114]. Modifiable factors in the ICU which lead to sleep disturbances are best dealt with from a multidisciplinary approach involving multiple ICU stakeholders [115].

Assess and Treat Underlying Sleep Disorders

Several studies have shown that early recognition and treatment of sleep disorders in hospitalized patients is associated with improved outcomes. To illustrate, in a small study by Konikkara, patients hospitalized with a COPD exacerbation were screened for sleep apnea, and if positive, CPAP therapy was initiated. Patients with COPD and OSA overlap disease that were adherent to CPAP therapy were noted to demonstrate a reduction in 6-month hospital readmission rates and emergency room visits [46]. In another study of hospitalized patients with congestive heart failure, those patients compliant with CPAP for a minimum of 4 hours for 70% of the nights in the month (Medicare PAP compliance guidelines) had fewer hospital readmissions when compared to those patients who were not compliant with their CPAP therapy following hospital discharge [116]. To that end, in another study involving early diagnosis of sleep-disordered breathing utilizing portable sleep study equipment, patients hospitalized with cardiac disease demonstrated significantly lower hospital readmission rates and decreased emergency department visits in those adherent with PAP therapy [117]. Initiation of CPAP therapy for patients with OSA is associated with decreased hospital readmissions [116].

Conclusions

Hospitalization is a period of acute illness and multifactorial acute sleep deprivation. Sleep deprivation in hospitalized patients can be related to patient factors, environmental factors, as well as medical interventions. Sleep loss in the hospital is also associated with poor health outcomes, including an increased risk of delirium and cardiometabolic derangements. Both pharmacologic and nonpharmacologic interventions have shown promise in improving sleep loss in patients while hospitalized. Awareness and consideration of implicit sleep loss in hospitalization is warranted, and implementation of treatment measures is justified.

References

1. Institute of Medicine (US) Committee on Sleep Medicine and Research. In: Colten HR, Altevogt BM, editors. Sleep disorders and sleep deprivation: an unmet public health problem. Washington DC: National Academies Press (US); 2006. Accessed 13 June 2020. http://www.ncbi.nlm.nih.gov/books/NBK19960/.
2. Ohayon MM. Epidemiological overview of sleep disorders in the general population. Published online 2011. Accessed 13 June 2020. https://doi.org/10.17241/smr.2011.2.1.1
3. Guyton AC, Hall JE. States of brain activity-sleep, brain waves, epilepsy, psychoses. In: Textbook of medical physiology. 13th ed. Mississippi: Elsevier Saunders; 2011. p. 763–72.
4. Åkerstedt T, Lekander M, Nilsonne G, et al. Effects of late-night short-sleep on in-home polysomnography: relation to adult age and sex. J Sleep Res. 2018;27(4):e12626. https://doi.org/10.1111/jsr.12626.
5. Miner B, Kryger MH. Sleep in the aging population. Sleep Med Clin. 2017;12(1):31–8. https://doi.org/10.1016/j.jsmc.2016.10.008.
6. Blazer DG, Hays JC, Foley DJ. Sleep complaints in older adults: a racial comparison. J Gerontol A Biol Sci Med Sci. 1995;50(5):M280–4. https://doi.org/10.1093/gerona/50a.5.m280.
7. Sorensen, RT, Bergholt, MD, Herning, M, Noiesen, E, Szots K, Harboe, G, Troosborg, I, Konradsen, H. To sleep or not to sleep during hospitalisation - a mixed-method study of patient reported sleep quality and the experience of sleeping poorly during hospitalisation. Published online 2018.

8. Pilkington S. Causes and consequences of sleep deprivation in hospitalised patients. Nurs Stand. 2013;27(49):35–42. https://doi.org/10.7748/ns2013.08.27.49.35.e7649.

9. DePietro RH, Knutson KL, Spampinato L, et al. Association between inpatient sleep loss and hyperglycemia of hospitalization. Diabetes Care. 2017;40(2):188–93. https://doi.org/10.2337/dc16-1683.

10. Arora VM, Chang KL, Fazal AZ, et al. Objective sleep duration and quality in hospitalized older adults: associations with blood pressure and mood. J Am Geriatr Soc. 2011;59(11):2185–6. https://doi.org/10.1111/j.1532-5415.2011.03644.x.

11. Krumholz HM. Post-hospital syndrome--an acquired, transient condition of generalized risk. N Engl J Med. 2013;368(2):100–2. https://doi.org/10.1056/NEJMp1212324.

12. Shear TC, Balachandran JS, Mokhlesi B, et al. Risk of sleep apnea in hospitalized older patients. J Clin Sleep Med. 2014;10(10):1061–6. https://doi.org/10.5664/jcsm.4098.

13. Shah MS, Spampinato LM, Beveridge C, Meltzer DO, Arora VM. Quantifying post hospital syndrome: sleeping longer and physically stronger?. Abstracted presented at the Society of Hospital Medicine Annual Meeting, 2016, March 6–9, San Diego, Calif. Abstract 340. J Hosp Med. 11(1). https://shmabstracts.org/abstract/quantifying-post-hospital-syndrome-sleeping-longer-and-physically-stronger/. June 13th 2020.

14. Sharma S. Hospital sleep medicine: the elephant in the room? J Clin Sleep Med. 2014;10(10):1067–8. https://doi.org/10.5664/jcsm.4100.

15. Knutson KL, Spiegel K, Penev P, Van Cauter E. The metabolic consequences of sleep deprivation. Sleep Med Rev. 2007;11(3):163–78. https://doi.org/10.1016/j.smrv.2007.01.002.

16. Spiegel K, Leproult R, Van Cauter E. Impact of sleep debt on metabolic and endocrine function. Lancet. 1999;354(9188):1435–9. https://doi.org/10.1016/S0140-6736(99)01376-8.

17. Meisinger C, Heier M, Loewel H, MONICA/KORA Augsburg Cohort Study. Sleep disturbance as a predictor of type 2 diabetes mellitus in men and women from the general population. Diabetologia. 2005;48(2):235–41. https://doi.org/10.1007/s00125-004-1634-x.

18. Yaggi HK, Araujo AB, McKinlay JB. Sleep duration as a risk factor for the development of type 2 diabetes. Diabetes Care. 2006;29(3):657–61. https://doi.org/10.2337/diacare.29.03.06.dc05-0879.

19. Inzucchi SE. Clinical practice. Management of hyperglycemia in the hospital setting. N Engl J Med. 2006;355(18):1903–11. https://doi.org/10.1056/NEJMcp060094.

20. Inouye SK. Prevention of delirium in hospitalized older patients: risk factors and targeted intervention strategies. Ann Med. 2000;32(4):257–63. https://doi.org/10.3109/07853890009011770.

21. Bell CM, Fischer HD, Gill SS, et al. Initiation of benzodiazepines in the elderly after hospitalization. J Gen Intern Med. 2007;22(7):1024–9. https://doi.org/10.1007/s11606-007-0194-4.

22. Ancoli-Israel S, Cooke JR. Prevalence and comorbidity of insomnia and effect on functioning in elderly populations. J Am Geriatr Soc. 2005;53(7 Suppl):S264–71. https://doi.org/10.1111/j.1532-5415.2005.53392.x.

23. Gooneratne NS, Weaver TE, Cater JR, et al. Functional outcomes of excessive daytime sleepiness in older adults. J Am Geriatr Soc. 2003;51(5):642–9. https://doi.org/10.1034/j.1600-0579.2003.00208.x.

24. Coleman EA, Parry C, Chalmers S, Min S-J. The care transitions intervention: results of a randomized controlled trial. Arch Intern Med. 2006;166(17):1822–8. https://doi.org/10.1001/archinte.166.17.1822.

25. Redeker NS. Sleep in acute care settings: an integrative review. J Nurs Scholarsh. 2000;32(1):31–8. https://doi.org/10.1111/j.1547-5069.2000.00031.x.

26. McLaughlin DC, Hartjes TM, Freeman WD. Sleep deprivation in neurointensive care unit patients from serial neurological checks: how much is too much? J Neurosci Nurs. 2018;50(4):205–10. https://doi.org/10.1097/JNN.0000000000000378.

27. Grossman MN, Anderson SL, Worku A, et al. Awakenings? patient and hospital staff perceptions of nighttime disruptions and their effect on patient sleep. J Clin Sleep Med. 2017;13(2):301–6. https://doi.org/10.5664/jcsm.6468.

28. Arora VM, Machado N, Anderson SL, et al. Effectiveness of SIESTA on Objective and Subjective Metrics of Nighttime Hospital Sleep Disruptors. J Hosp Med. 2019;14(1):38–41. https://doi.org/10.12788/jhm.3091.
29. Hoffman S. Sleep in the older adult: implications for nurses (CE). Geriatr Nurs. 2003;24(4):210–4; quiz 215-216. https://doi.org/10.1016/s0197-4572(03)00213-1.
30. Ersser S, Wiles A, Taylor H, Wade S, Walsh R, Bentley T. The sleep of older people in hospital and nursing homes. J Clin Nurs. 1999;8(4):360–8. https://doi.org/10.1046/j.1365-2702.1999.00267.x.
31. Hospital Compare. U.S. Department of Health and Human Services. Available at: https://www.medicare.gov/hospitalcompare/search.html.
32. Buxton OM, Ellenbogen JM, Wang W, et al. Sleep disruption due to hospital noises: a prospective evaluation. Ann Intern Med. 2012;157(3):170–9. https://doi.org/10.7326/0003-4819-157-3-201208070-00472.
33. Pope DS, Miller-Klein ET. Acoustic assessment of speech privacy curtains in two nursing units. Noise Health. 2016;18(80):26–35. https://doi.org/10.4103/1463-1741.174377.
34. Tullmann DF, Dracup K. Creating a healing environment for elders. AACN Clin Issues. 2000;11(1):34–50; quiz 153-154. https://doi.org/10.1097/00044067-200002000-00006.
35. Yoder JC, Staisiunas PG, Meltzer DO, Knutson KL, Arora VM. Noise and sleep among adult medical inpatients: far from a quiet night. Arch Intern Med. 2012;172(1):68–70. https://doi.org/10.1001/archinternmed.2011.603.
36. Monk TH, Buysse DJ, Billy BD, Kennedy KS, Kupfer DJ. The effects on human sleep and circadian rhythms of 17 days of continuous bedrest in the absence of daylight. Sleep. 1997;20(10):858–64. https://doi.org/10.1093/sleep/20.10.858.
37. Kumar S, McElligott D, Goyal A, Baugh M, Ionita RN. Risk of obstructive sleep apnea (OSA) in hospitalized patients. Chest. 2010;138(4):supp 779A. Available at: https://journal.chestnet.org/article/S0012-3692(16)42455-4/abstract. Presented at the:
38. Javaheri S, Caref EB, Chen E, Tong KB, Abraham WT. Sleep apnea testing and outcomes in a large cohort of Medicare beneficiaries with newly diagnosed heart failure. Am J Respir Crit Care Med. 2011;183(4):539–46. https://doi.org/10.1164/rccm.201003-0406OC.
39. Kaneko Y, Floras JS, Usui K, et al. Cardiovascular effects of continuous positive airway pressure in patients with heart failure and obstructive sleep apnea. N Engl J Med. 2003;348(13):1233–41. https://doi.org/10.1056/NEJMoa022479.
40. Kokras N, Kouzoupis AV, Paparrigopoulos T, et al. Predicting insomnia in medical wards: the effect of anxiety, depression and admission diagnosis. Gen Hosp Psychiatry. 2011;33(1):78–81. https://doi.org/10.1016/j.genhosppsych.2010.12.003.
41. Isaia G, Corsinovi L, Bo M, et al. Insomnia among hospitalized elderly patients: prevalence, clinical characteristics and risk factors. Arch Gerontol Geriatr. 2011;52(2):133–7. https://doi.org/10.1016/j.archger.2010.03.001.
42. Meissner HH, Riemer A, Santiago SM, Stein M, Goldman MD, Williams AJ. Failure of physician documentation of sleep complaints in hospitalized patients. West J Med. 1998;169(3):146–9.
43. Spurr KF, Graven MA, Gilbert RW. Prevalence of unspecified sleep apnea and the use of continuous positive airway pressure in hospitalized patients, 2004 National Hospital Discharge Survey. Sleep Breath. 2008;12(3):229–34. https://doi.org/10.1007/s11325-007-0166-2.
44. Gay PC. Sleep and sleep-disordered breathing in the hospitalized patient. Respir Care. 2010;55(9):1240–54.
45. Shorofsky M, Bourbeau J, Kimoff J, et al. Impaired sleep quality in COPD is associated with exacerbations: The CanCOLD Cohort Study. Chest. Published online 28 May 2019. https://doi.org/10.1016/j.chest.2019.04.132.
46. Konikkara J, Tavella R, Willes L, Kavuru M, Sharma S. Early recognition of obstructive sleep apnea in patients hospitalized with COPD exacerbation is associated with reduced readmission. Hosp Pract. 2016;44(1):41–7. https://doi.org/10.1080/21548331.2016.1134268.

47. Kendzerska T, Leung RS, Aaron SD, Ayas N, Sandoz JS, Gershon AS. Cardiovascular outcomes and all-cause mortality in patients with obstructive sleep apnea and chronic obstructive pulmonary disease (overlap syndrome). Ann Am Thorac Soc. 2019;16(1):71–81. https://doi.org/10.1513/AnnalsATS.201802-136OC.
48. Mohsenin V, Valor R. Sleep apnea in patients with hemispheric stroke. Arch Phys Med Rehabil. 1995;76(1):71–6. https://doi.org/10.1016/s0003-9993(95)80046-8.
49. Harbison J, Ford GA, James OFW, Gibson GJ. Sleep-disordered breathing following acute stroke. QJM. 2002;95(11):741–7. https://doi.org/10.1093/qjmed/95.11.741.
50. Brown DL, Shafie-Khorassani F, Kim S, et al. Sleep-disordered breathing is associated with recurrent ischemic stroke. Stroke. 2019;50(3):571–6. https://doi.org/10.1161/STROKEAHA.118.023807.
51. Bassetti C, Aldrich MS. Sleep apnea in acute cerebrovascular diseases: final report on 128 patients. Sleep. 1999;22(2):217–23. https://doi.org/10.1093/sleep/22.2.217.
52. Wu Z, Chen F, Yu F, Wang Y, Guo Z. A meta-analysis of obstructive sleep apnea in patients with cerebrovascular disease. Sleep Breath. 2018;22(3):729–42. https://doi.org/10.1007/s11325-017-1604-4.
53. Yaggi HK, Concato J, Kernan WN, Lichtman JH, Brass LM, Mohsenin V. Obstructive sleep apnea as a risk factor for stroke and death. N Engl J Med. 2005;353(19):2034–41. https://doi.org/10.1056/NEJMoa043104.
54. Good DC, Henkle JQ, Gelber D, Welsh J, Verhulst S. Sleep-disordered breathing and poor functional outcome after stroke. Stroke. 1996;27(2):252–9. https://doi.org/10.1161/01.str.27.2.252.
55. Oldenburg O, Lamp B, Faber L, Teschler H, Horstkotte D, Töpfer V. Sleep-disordered breathing in patients with symptomatic heart failure: a contemporary study of prevalence in and characteristics of 700 patients. Eur J Heart Fail. 2007;9(3):251–7. https://doi.org/10.1016/j.ejheart.2006.08.003.
56. Bravata DM, Concato J, Fried T, et al. Continuous positive airway pressure: evaluation of a novel therapy for patients with acute ischemic stroke. Sleep. 2011;34(9):1271–7. https://doi.org/10.5665/SLEEP.1254.
57. Mansfield DR, Gollogly NC, Kaye DM, Richardson M, Bergin P, Naughton MT. Controlled trial of continuous positive airway pressure in obstructive sleep apnea and heart failure. Am J Respir Crit Care Med. 2004;169(3):361–6. https://doi.org/10.1164/rccm.200306-752OC.
58. Truong KK, De Jardin R, Massoudi N, Hashemzadeh M, Jafari B. Nonadherence to CPAP associated with increased 30-day hospital readmissions. J Clin Sleep Med. 2018;14(2):183–9. https://doi.org/10.5664/jcsm.6928.
59. Scalzitti NJ, O'Connor PD, Nielsen SW, et al. Obstructive sleep apnea is an independent risk factor for hospital readmission. J Clin Sleep Med. 2018;14(5):753–8. https://doi.org/10.5664/jcsm.7098.
60. Griffiths MF, Peerson A. Risk factors for chronic insomnia following hospitalization. J Adv Nurs. 2005;49(3):245–53. https://doi.org/10.1111/j.1365-2648.2004.03283.x.
61. Morin CM, Benca R. Chronic insomnia. Lancet. 2012;379(9821):1129–41. https://doi.org/10.1016/S0140-6736(11)60750-2.
62. Martin JL, Fiorentino L, Jouldjian S, Mitchell M, Josephson KR, Alessi CA. Poor self-reported sleep quality predicts mortality within one year of inpatient post-acute rehabilitation among older adults. Sleep. 2011;34(12):1715–21. https://doi.org/10.5665/sleep.1444.
63. Manabe K, Matsui T, Yamaya M, et al. Sleep patterns and mortality among elderly patients in a geriatric hospital. Gerontology. 2000;46(6):318–22. https://doi.org/10.1159/000022184.
64. Lenhart SE, Buysse DJ. Treatment of insomnia in hospitalized patients. Ann Pharmacother. 2001;35(11):1449–57. https://doi.org/10.1345/aph.1A040.
65. Brzezinski A, Vangel MG, Wurtman RJ, et al. Effects of exogenous melatonin on sleep: a meta-analysis. Sleep Med Rev. 2005;9(1):41–50. https://doi.org/10.1016/j.smrv.2004.06.004.

66. Zhdanova IV, Wurtman RJ, Regan MM, Taylor JA, Shi JP, Leclair OU. Melatonin treatment for age-related insomnia. J Clin Endocrinol Metab. 2001;86(10):4727–30. https://doi.org/10.1210/jcem.86.10.7901.
67. Andrade C, Srihari BS, Reddy KP, Chandramma L. Melatonin in medically ill patients with insomnia: a double-blind, placebo-controlled study. J Clin Psychiatry. 2001;62(1):41–5. https://doi.org/10.4088/jcp.v62n0109.
68. Shilo L, Dagan Y, Smorjik Y, et al. Effect of melatonin on sleep quality of COPD intensive care patients: a pilot study. Chronobiol Int. 2000;17(1):71–6. https://doi.org/10.1081/cbi-100101033.
69. Huang H-W, Zheng B-L, Jiang L, et al. Effect of oral melatonin and wearing earplugs and eye masks on nocturnal sleep in healthy subjects in a simulated intensive care unit environment: which might be a more promising strategy for ICU sleep deprivation? Crit Care. 2015;19:124. https://doi.org/10.1186/s13054-015-0842-8.
70. MacMillan TE, Lui P, Wu RC, Cavalcanti RB. Melatonin Increasingly Used in Hospitalized Patients. J Hosp Med. 2020;15(6):349–51. https://doi.org/10.12788/jhm.3408.
71. Jaiswal SJ, McCarthy TJ, Wineinger NE, et al. Melatonin and Sleep in Preventing Hospitalized Delirium: A Randomized Clinical Trial. Am J Med. 2018;131(9):1110–1117.e4. https://doi.org/10.1016/j.amjmed.2018.04.009.
72. Gillis CM, Poyant JO, Degrado JR, Ye L, Anger KE, Owens RL. Inpatient pharmacological sleep aid utilization is common at a tertiary medical center. J Hosp Med. 2014;9(10):652–7. https://doi.org/10.1002/jhm.2246.
73. Glass J, Lanctôt KL, Herrmann N, Sproule BA, Busto UE. Sedative hypnotics in older people with insomnia: meta-analysis of risks and benefits. BMJ. 2005;331(7526):1169. https://doi.org/10.1136/bmj.38623.768588.47.
74. Young JS, Bourgeois JA, Hilty DM, Hardin KA. Sleep in hospitalized medical patients, part 2: behavioral and pharmacological management of sleep disturbances. J Hosp Med. 2009;4(1):50–9. https://doi.org/10.1002/jhm.397.
75. By the 2019 American Geriatrics Society Beers Criteria® Update Expert Panel. American Geriatrics Society 2019 Updated AGS Beers Criteria® for Potentially Inappropriate Medication Use in Older Adults. J Am Geriatr Soc. 2019;67(4):674–94. https://doi.org/10.1111/jgs.15767.
76. Hu R-F, Jiang X-Y, Chen J, et al. Non-pharmacological interventions for sleep promotion in the intensive care unit. Cochrane Database Syst Rev. 2015;10:CD008808. https://doi.org/10.1002/14651858.CD008808.pub2.
77. Tamrat R, Huynh-Le M-P, Goyal M. Non-pharmacologic interventions to improve the sleep of hospitalized patients: a systematic review. J Gen Intern Med. 2014;29(5):788–95. https://doi.org/10.1007/s11606-013-2640-9.
78. Soden K, Vincent K, Craske S, Lucas C, Ashley S. A randomized controlled trial of aromatherapy massage in a hospice setting. Palliat Med. 2004;18(2):87–92. https://doi.org/10.1191/0269216304pm874oa.
79. Toth M, Wolsko PM, Foreman J, et al. A pilot study for a randomized, controlled trial on the effect of guided imagery in hospitalized medical patients. J Altern Complement Med. 2007;13(2):194–7. https://doi.org/10.1089/acm.2006.6117.
80. Zimmerman L, Nieveen J, Barnason S, Schmaderer M. The effects of music interventions on postoperative pain and sleep in coronary artery bypass graft (CABG) patients. Sch Inq Nurs Pract. 1996;10(2):153–70; discussion 171-174.
81. Wakamura T, Tokura H. Influence of bright light during daytime on sleep parameters in hospitalized elderly patients. J Physiol Anthropol Appl Hum Sci. 2001;20(6):345–51. https://doi.org/10.2114/jpa.20.345.
82. Mishima K, Okawa M, Hishikawa Y, Hozumi S, Hori H, Takahashi K. Morning bright light therapy for sleep and behavior disorders in elderly patients with dementia. Acta Psychiatr Scand. 1994;89(1):1–7. https://doi.org/10.1111/j.1600-0447.1994.tb01477.x.

83. Yamadera H, Ito T, Suzuki H, Asayama K, Ito R, Endo S. Effects of bright light on cognitive and sleep-wake (circadian) rhythm disturbances in Alzheimer-type dementia. Psychiatry Clin Neurosci. 2000;54(3):352–3. https://doi.org/10.1046/j.1440-1819.2000.00711.x.

84. Mitolo M, Tonon C, La Morgia C, Testa C, Carelli V, Lodi R. Effects of light treatment on sleep, cognition, mood, and behavior in Alzheimer's disease: a systematic review. Dement Geriatr Cogn Disord. 2018;46(5–6):371–84. https://doi.org/10.1159/000494921.

85. McGough NNH, Keane T, Uppal A, et al. Noise reduction in progressive care units. J Nurs Care Qual. 2018;33(2):166–72. https://doi.org/10.1097/NCQ.0000000000000275.

86. Applebaum D, Calo O, Neville K. Implementation of quiet time for noise reduction on a medical-surgical unit. J Nurs Adm. 2016;46(12):669–74. https://doi.org/10.1097/NNA.0000000000000424.

87. Richardson A, Allsop M, Coghill E, Turnock C. Earplugs and eye masks: do they improve critical care patients' sleep? Nurs Crit Care. 2007;12(6):278–86. https://doi.org/10.1111/j.1478-5153.2007.00243.x.

88. Gragert MD. The Use of Masking Signal to Enhance Sleep of Men and Women 65 Years of Age and Older in the Critical Care Environment. Austin: The University of Texas; 1990.

89. Stanchina ML, Abu-Hijleh M, Chaudhry BK, Carlisle CC, Millman RP. The influence of white noise on sleep in subjects exposed to ICU noise. Sleep Med. 2005;6(5):423–8. https://doi.org/10.1016/j.sleep.2004.12.004.

90. Blomkvist V, Eriksen CA, Theorell T, Ulrich R, Rasmanis G. Acoustics and psychosocial environment in intensive coronary care. Occup Environ Med. 2005;62(3):e1. https://doi.org/10.1136/oem.2004.017632.

91. Xie H, Kang J, Mills GH. Clinical review: the impact of noise on patients' sleep and the effectiveness of noise reduction strategies in intensive care units. Crit Care. 2009;13(2):208. https://doi.org/10.1186/cc7154.

92. Gathecha E, Rios R, Buenaver LF, Landis R, Howell E, Wright S. Pilot study aiming to support sleep quality and duration during hospitalizations. J Hosp Med. 2016;11(7):467–72. https://doi.org/10.1002/jhm.2578.

93. Lareau R, Benson L, Watcharotone K, Manguba G. Examining the feasibility of implementing specific nursing interventions to promote sleep in hospitalized elderly patients. Geriatr Nurs. 2008;29(3):197–206. https://doi.org/10.1016/j.gerinurse.2007.10.020.

94. Edinger JD, Lipper S, Wheeler B. Hospital ward policy and patients' sleep patterns: A multiple baseline study. Rehabil Psychol. 34(1):43. Published online 1989.

95. Freedman NS, Kotzer N, Schwab RJ. Patient perception of sleep quality and etiology of sleep disruption in the intensive care unit. Am J Respir Crit Care Med. 1999;159(4 Pt 1):1155–62. https://doi.org/10.1164/ajrccm.159.4.9806141.

96. Le A, Friese RS, Hsu C-H, Wynne JL, Rhee P, O'Keeffe T. Sleep disruptions and nocturnal nursing interactions in the intensive care unit. J Surg Res. 2012;177(2):310–4. https://doi.org/10.1016/j.jss.2012.05.038.

97. Milani RV, Bober RM, Lavie CJ, Wilt JK, Milani AR, White CJ. Reducing hospital toxicity: impact on patient outcomes. Am J Med. 2018;131(8):961–6. https://doi.org/10.1016/j.amjmed.2018.04.013.

98. Farrehi PM, Clore KR, Scott JR, Vanini G, Clauw DJ. Efficacy of Sleep Tool Education During Hospitalization: A Randomized Controlled Trial. Am J Med. 2016;129(12):1329.e9–1329.e17. https://doi.org/10.1016/j.amjmed.2016.08.001.

99. Bartick MC, Thai X, Schmidt T, Altaye A, Solet JM. Decrease in as-needed sedative use by limiting nighttime sleep disruptions from hospital staff. J Hosp Med. 2010;5(3):E20–4. https://doi.org/10.1002/jhm.549.

100. Singler K, Thomas C. HELP - Hospital Elder Life Program - multimodal delirium prevention in elderly patients. Internist (Berl). 2017;58(2):125–31. https://doi.org/10.1007/s00108-016-0181-0.

101. Carr ECJ, Meredith P, Chumbley G, Killen R, Prytherch DR, Smith GB. Pain: a quality of care issue during patients' admission to hospital. J Adv Nurs. 2014;70(6):1391–403. https://doi.org/10.1111/jan.12301.

102. Li JMW. Pain management in the hospitalized patient. Med Clin North Am. 2008; 92(2):371–85, ix. https://doi.org/10.1016/j.mcna.2007.11.003.

103. Martin JL, Fung CH. Quality indicators for the care of sleep disorders in vulnerable elders. J Am Geriatr Soc. 2007;55(Suppl 2):S424–30. https://doi.org/10.1111/j.1532-5415.2007. 01351.x.

104. Kragh M, Møller DN, Wihlborg CS, et al. Experiences of wake and light therapy in patients with depression: a qualitative study. Int J Ment Health Nurs. 2017;26(2):170–80. https://doi. org/10.1111/inm.12264.

105. Müller MJ, Olschinski C, Kundermann B, Cabanel N. Sleep duration of inpatients with a depressive disorder: associations with age, subjective sleep quality, and cognitive complaints. Arch Psychiatr Nurs. 2017;31(1):77–82. https://doi.org/10.1016/j.apnu.2016.08.008.

106. Kragh M, Larsen ER, Martiny K, et al. Predictors of response to combined wake and light therapy in treatment-resistant inpatients with depression. Chronobiol Int. 2018;35(9):1209–20. https://doi.org/10.1080/07420528.2018.1468341.

107. Stone KL, Ancoli-Israel S, Blackwell T, et al. Actigraphy-measured sleep characteristics and risk of falls in older women. Arch Intern Med. 2008;168(16):1768–75. https://doi. org/10.1001/archinte.168.16.1768.

108. Spiegel K, Sheridan JF, Van Cauter E. Effect of sleep deprivation on response to immunization. JAMA. 2002;288(12):1471–2. https://doi.org/10.1001/jama.288.12.1471-a.

109. Toda H, Williams JA, Gulledge M, Sehgal A. A sleep-inducing gene, nemuri, links sleep and immune function in drosophila. Science. 2019;363(6426):509–15. https://doi.org/10.1126/ science.aat1650.

110. Kuo T-H, Williams JA. Increased sleep promotes survival during a bacterial infection in drosophila. Sleep. 2014;37(6):1077–86, 1086A-1086D. https://doi.org/10.5665/sleep.3764.

111. Sinvani L, Kozikowski A, Smilios C, et al. Implementing ACOVE Quality Indicators as an Intervention Checklist to Improve Care for Hospitalized Older Adults. J Hosp Med. 2017;12(7):517–22. https://doi.org/10.12788/jhm.2765.

112. Kahn DM, Cook TE, Carlisle CC, Nelson DL, Kramer NR, Millman RP. Identification and modification of environmental noise in an ICU setting. Chest. 1998;114(2):535–40. https://doi.org/10.1378/chest.114.2.535.

113. Shilo L, Dagan Y, Smorjik Y, et al. Patients in the intensive care unit suffer from severe lack of sleep associated with loss of normal melatonin secretion pattern. Am J Med Sci. 1999;317(5):278–81. https://doi.org/10.1097/00000441-199905000-00002.

114. Pisani MA, Friese RS, Gehlbach BK, Schwab RJ, Weinhouse GL, Jones SF. Sleep in the intensive care unit. Am J Respir Crit Care Med. 2015;191(7):731–8. https://doi.org/10.1164/ rccm.201411-2099CI.

115. Knauert MP, Haspel JA, Pisani MA. Sleep loss and circadian rhythm disruption in the intensive care unit. Clin Chest Med. 2015;36(3):419–29. https://doi.org/10.1016/j.ccm.2015.05.008.

116. Sharma S, Mather P, Gupta A, et al. Effect of early intervention with positive airway pressure therapy for sleep disordered breathing on six-month readmission rates in hospitalized patients with heart failure. Am J Cardiol. 2016;117(6):940–5. https://doi.org/10.1016/j. amjcard.2015.12.032.

117. Kauta SR, Keenan BT, Goldberg L, Schwab RJ. Diagnosis and treatment of sleep disordered breathing in hospitalized cardiac patients: a reduction in 30-day hospital readmission rates. J Clin Sleep Med. 2014;10(10):1051–9. https://doi.org/10.5664/jcsm.4096.

Chapter 21
Sleep in Pregnancy

Keywords Pittsburgh Sleep Quality Index (PSQI) · Unrefreshed sleep · Sleep in mid-pregnancy · Sleep-disordered breathing (SDB) · RLS during pregnancy · Insufficient Sleep

Introduction

During pregnancy, a life stage during which there are significant hormonal, anatomic, physiological, and psychological changes, women experience unique challenges with sleep. Pregnancy can exacerbate preexisting sleep problems as well as cause the emergence of new ones. The impact of sleep deficiency – which includes insufficient sleep, poorly timed sleep, and clinical sleep disorders – is observed not only on the individual but also on the offspring, with potentially long-lasting implications.

Sleep in Normal Pregnancy

Due to physiological and hormonal changes related to pregnancy, most women experience changes in sleep [1]. In the first trimester, common complaints include daytime sleepiness and fatigue with many women reporting daytime naps. Sleep quality and slow-wave sleep (SWS) typically decrease compared to prepregnancy

L. M. O'Brien (✉)
Division of Sleep Medicine, Department of Neurology, Michigan Medicine, Ann Arbor, MI, USA

Department of Obstetrics & Gynecology, Michigan Medicine, Ann Arbor, MI, USA
e-mail: louiseo@med.umich.edu

© Springer Nature Switzerland AG 2022
M. S. Badr, J. L. Martin (eds.), *Essentials of Sleep Medicine*,
Respiratory Medicine, https://doi.org/10.1007/978-3-030-93739-3_21

or the nonpregnant state [1, 2] but improve in the second trimester, along with improvements in daytime sleepiness and fatigue [2–5]. Toward the end of the second trimester and into the third trimester, snoring is common along with restless legs and increased awakenings [6]. Indeed, in the third trimester, the vast majority of women endorse sleep deficiencies with insomnia symptoms, sleep-disordered breathing (SDB), frequent awakenings [2, 5, 7, 8], and increased napping [5, 7–9], with consequentially more light sleep [10, 11].

Insufficient Sleep

Although there are no guidelines specific to pregnant women, the National Sleep Foundation (www.sleepfoundation.org) recommends that adults obtain 7–9 hours of sleep per night, with <6 hours per night considered insufficient [12]. Nonetheless, definition of short sleep is likely dependent on the method of assessment, and short sleep in pregnancy has been suggested as being <7 hours if reported subjectively and <6 hours if data are collected objectively [13]. Individual studies differ in the definition of short sleep, which can range anywhere from 5 to 8 hours depending on the study and thus makes comparisons challenging. Regardless, insufficient sleep has been linked with poor cardiometabolic health in nonpregnant populations [14], and accumulating evidence, as discussed below, suggests that these findings are similar in pregnancy.

With regard to maternal health, few studies have specifically investigated the relationships between sleep duration and blood pressure in pregnancy. In a self-report study, Williams et al. found that both maternally reported short sleep duration (defined as ≤6 hours) and long sleep duration (defined as at least 9 hours) in early pregnancy were both associated with increases in systolic and diastolic blood pressure in the third trimester [15]. In particular, a report of <5 hours' sleep was found to have a particularly high odds of preeclampsia (aOR 9.5, 95%CI 1.8–49.4), although sleeping more than 10 hours did not show an increase in preeclampsia: aOR 2.5 (95%CI 0.7–8.2) [15]. Conversely, results from an actigraphy-based study in over 700 women found no relationship between short sleep duration (defined as <7 hours) and a diagnosis of hypertension [16]. Recently, Tang et al. have demonstrated that in the first trimester, both systolic and diastolic blood pressure was lower in women who slept longer; in longitudinal analyses across pregnancy, women with longer sleep durations had lower systolic blood pressure [17].

Associations between sleep duration and gestational diabetes (GDM) have been studied more than maternal blood pressure. A large study of >1200 women found that GDM risk was increased among those who slept ≤4 hours per night when compared to those sleeping at least 9 hours per night, with a relative risk (RR) of 5.6 (95%CI 1.3–23.7) [18]. Sleep duration has been reported to have a "J"-shaped association with GDM; in over 900 women, with sleep durations of ≥9 hours and <7 hours, the odds for GDM were 1.2 (95%CI 1.0–1.4) and 1.4 (95%CI 0.9–2.1), respectively, although the proportion of women in the short sleep category was small [19]. In a cohort of over 600 multiethnic Asian women, those who reported sleeping less than 6 hours per night had the highest frequency of GDM compared to those who slept 7–8 hours per night (27.3% vs. 16.8%), and fasting glucose levels were observed to decrease linearly with increasing sleep duration [20]. However, after accounting for other covariates, no relationship with sleep duration and glucose levels was evident. Associations between sleep duration and GDM have been reported to differ by prepregnancy obesity status. Findings from the multi-site Fetal Growth Study of approximately 2500 women [21] found that the association between maternal sleep duration and GDM was only significant among nonobese women, with a twofold higher increased risk of GDM in women who reported more or less than 8–9 hours. The highest adjusted relative risk for GDM (aRR 2.5, 95%CI 1.27–5.0) was observed among nonobese women who slept 5–6 hours in the second trimester. Specifically, in women who slept <7 hours, the risk for GDM was more than twice that of women who slept 8–9 (aRR 2.5, 95%CI 1.2–5.1), with long sleepers (at least 10 hours) who rarely or never napped having the highest risk of GDM (aRR 3.1, 95%CI 1.0–9.2) [21]. Napping appears to modify the sleep-GDM association with a significant association among women who rarely or never napped in the second trimester. Recent work in Chinese pregnant women supports these findings; the influence of shorter nighttime sleep duration on GDM was found to be weaker in women with more napping, and midday napping reduced the risk of GDM among women with insufficient sleep [22].

Objective data from 782 women with actigraphy also supports that sleep duration <7 hours per night is associated with an increased risk of GDM (aOR 2.2, 95%CI 1.1–4.5) [16]. Furthermore, an individual patient data (IPD) meta-analysis has demonstrated that pregnant women who slept <6–7 hours were at higher odds of GDM compared to those without short sleep: aOR 1.7 (95%CI, 1.2–2.3) [23]. In addition, compared to sleeping >6.25 hours, women who slept ≤6.25 hours had higher 1-hour glucose levels and an increased odds of GDM, aOR 2.8 (95%CI 1.3–6.4) [23]. Taken together, both subjective and objective data suggest that sleeping less than 7 hours in early-mid-pregnancy is associated with an approximate twofold increased risk for the development of GDM, with extremes of sleep (e.g., less than 4 hours or greater than 10 hours) possibly associated with even higher risks.

While short sleep duration in pregnancy has been linked with poor maternal outcomes, fewer studies have focused on fetal outcomes. Similar to the studies described above, those focused on sleep duration and fetal outcomes have inconsistent definitions of short sleep, ranging from between <4 hours and <8 hours per night. Fetal growth has been investigated in a few studies of maternal sleep duration. In a study of almost 1100 women, no differences in birth weight or being born small for gestational age (SGA; <10th percentile) were found in women who self-reported less than 5 hours of sleep per night [24]. Similarly, Howe et al. [25] found no differences in birth weight or percentile in infants born to women reporting sleep <6 hours per night. However, both SGA <5th percentile and low birth weight have been linked with sleeping less than 8 hours per night, with odds ratios of 2.2 and 2.8, respectively [26, 27]. In a prospective study of 32 depressed and 136 nondepressed pregnant women, it was only the depressed women who reported fewer than 7 hours of sleep at 30 weeks' gestation that had smaller babies than women who reported more than 9 hours' sleep [13].

Nonetheless, it should be noted that cross-sectional studies have limitations when measuring fetal outcomes. Insults in early pregnancy may influence subsequent fetal growth, which is not captured with cross-sectional designs. Longitudinal studies are therefore critical to investigate the impacts of maternal sleep on fetal health. For example, in 1500 women who were assessed at several times across pregnancy, those sleeping at least 9 hours per night hours before the 17- and 28-week assessments had mean birth weights 74 g and 60 g higher, respectively, compared to other women, and a linear trend was evident at 17 weeks [28]. In contrast, cross-sectional studies of those sleeping more than 9 hours per night find no association with a single measure of birth weight [25]. In a large cohort of over 3500 women, those who slept <7 hours in early pregnancy, compared to those who slept 8–9 hours, had a shorter birth length by 2.4 mm and a 42.7 g reduction in birth weight. The risk of low birth weight increased 83% and the risk of SGA increased 56% in women sleeping <7 hours [29]. More recently, a Brazilian study reported first-trimester 24-hour sleep duration and its change throughout pregnancy were inversely associated with birth weight such that women with greater decreases in sleep duration gave birth to infants with lower birth weight z-scores [30]. These findings were only in nulliparous women and no associations were detected in multiparous women. In a large study of women who had delivered at full term, no association between sleep durations in the second trimester was found with SGA [31]. A recent study in which subjective and objective sleep measures were collected in 166 low-risk women found that shorter self-reported sleep duration (but not actigraphy-assessed duration) was associated with shorter gestational age [32]. The authors posited that in otherwise healthy women, there appears to be minimal evidence that sleep measures in early gestation impact pregnancy outcomes. Despite this, findings of recent meta-analyses suggest that women with the shortest sleep duration have an increased relative risk of preterm birth compared to women with the longest sleep durations (RR1.23, 95%CI 1.01–1.50) [33] although findings are unclear in regard to whether short – or long – sleep duration impacts fetal growth as the adjusted odds ratios for SGA and large for gestational age (LGA) were found to be 1.3 "(95%CI 0.9–2.0) and 1.5 (95%CI 0.7–2.8) [34]. However, it should be noted that both of the latter meta-analyses included cross-sectional studies as well as longitudinal ones.

Sleep Quality

The National Women's Sleep Poll (www.sleepfoundation.org) found that 30% of pregnant women rarely/never get a good night's sleep, which is twice as many as nonpregnant women who endorsed the same question. Reasons for this include increased need to urinate, difficulty finding comfortable sleeping positions, and body aches [35]. Prevalence estimates of poor sleep quality in pregnancy, as measured by the Pittsburgh Sleep Quality Index (PSQI) [36] with a score of at least 5, range from 29% to 76% [5, 37], with a recent meta-analysis from over 11,000 pregnant women suggesting that the frequency of poor sleep quality is approximately 45% [38]. Indeed, waking up feeling unrefreshed is a very common complaint in pregnancy with most women endorsing unrefreshing sleep [5]. Parity and gestational age appear to play a role in reported sleep quality, with nulliparous women reporting worse sleep quality compared to multiparous women [39] and better sleep quality in early pregnancy compared to late pregnancy [38]. Unsurprisingly, poor sleep quality is also common in depressed women [13].

Several studies have suggested that poor sleep quality may impact blood pressure. In a study of 161 pregnant women that utilized sleep diaries and actigraphy, latency to sleep onset and wake after sleep onset – which are two measures of sleep continuity – were associated with higher blood pressures, despite accounting for covariates including BMI [40]. In a Japanese cohort, an increase in morning systolic blood pressure from the first to the third trimester was larger in women with poor sleep quality than in those with good sleep quality (7.1 ± 7.0 mmHg vs. 3.0 ± 5.6 mmHg, $p < 0.01$), suggesting that sleep quality early in pregnancy may contribute to a rise in systolic blood pressure in late pregnancy [41]. Similarly, a mixed model analysis of over 900 pregnant women in Singapore demonstrated an overall positive association between sleep quality, as measured by the PSQI score, and diastolic blood pressure [17]. In the latter study, overall poor sleep during pregnancy was also found to be associated with a higher uterine artery pulsatility index (an increased resistance to blood flow and thus increased risk for hypertension). However, it is possible that the influence of poor sleep and hypertension may be bidirectional. In a small cross-sectional study of 56 women with gestational hypertension and GDM, higher PSQI scores continued to worsen throughout pregnancy, and the authors suggested that the presence of hypertension may increase maternal stress and subsequently affect sleep [42].

In a multiethnic cohort of Asian women, Cai et al. reported that poor sleep quality – again measured by the PSQI – was independently associated with an increased risk of GDM with an adjusted odds ratio of 1.75 (95%CI 1.11–2.76) [20], similar to the findings in Chinese women [19]. However, other studies using the same measure of sleep quality have not supported these findings [43, 44]. In addition to the PSQI, sleep quality has also been investigated via a single self-reported question item although findings are inconsistent. Some studies have not found associations with GDM [45, 46], while two very large studies (over 4000 and 12,000 women, respectively) did find that poor sleep quality increased the odds of GDM 60–70% even after adjusting for other covariates [19, 47]. Indeed, a recent systematic review of sleep quality and GDM risk reported that subjectively measured poor sleep quality was associated with a higher risk for GDM (pooled OR 1.43; 95%CI, 1.16–1.77), but little evidence was found for associations when using objective measures [48]. It should be noted that the latter objectively measured studies were quite small and measure different aspects of sleep such as continuity or efficiency as opposed to self-report of perceived sleep quality, which is what is captured subjectively.

In recent years, data on poor sleep quality and fetal outcomes have begun to emerge. There appears to be little impact for maternal poor sleep quality on fetal growth [25, 43, 49] although one study reported lower birth weight in babies born to women with very high PSQI scores (greater than 18) compared to those with lower PSQI scores [50]. Women with "unrefreshed sleep" have been reported to be more likely to deliver babies with a birth weight of at least 3.5 kg compared to those who report refreshed sleep: 26% vs. 14%, $p < 0.03$ [51]. Nonetheless, a recent systematic review found that current evidence does not support differences in birth weight or fetal growth with poor maternal sleep quality [34]. It should be noted however that most studies have relatively small sample sizes which is particularly challenging when the exposure is a subjective measure.

Several studies have investigated associations between poor sleep quality and preterm birth; some have found no relationship [49, 52], while others have reported higher frequencies of preterm birth in women with poor sleep quality [53–55]. Interestingly, Blair et al. demonstrated that the odds of preterm birth were tenfold higher in African American women with poor sleep quality compared to those without, a finding that was not replicated in European women [54]. While data suggest a potential association between poor sleep quality and preterm birth, there is wide variability in sample sizes, differing study designs (such as preterm birth as an exposure in some studies and an outcome in others), and differing definitions of poor sleep quality which make it difficult to draw firm conclusions [34]. However, in studies that have measured sleep in mid-pregnancy, poor sleep quality was demonstrated to increase the odds for preterm birth in several studies in the United States, China, and Japan [53–57], with risk estimates being two-to fivefold higher for preterm birth. In a very recent meta-analysis, the pooled relative risk for preterm birth was 1.54 (95%CI 1.18–2.01) [33]. It is thus plausible that the impact of disturbed sleep on fetal outcome may begin in early pregnancy and that longitudinal studies are necessary for fully delineate any associations. Indeed, it has been suggested that disturbed sleep during early pregnancy may contribute to an increased inflammatory response or decreased uterine blood flow that could disrupt the normal remodeling of maternal blood vessels that perfuse the placenta and thus could subsequently result in poor pregnancy outcomes [58].

Insomnia

Insomnia, defined as difficulty falling asleep, staying asleep, or poor sleep quality, is one of the most common sleep complaints in pregnancy. The prevalence of insomnia disorder and clinically significant insomnia symptoms are much greater in pregnant women relative to the general population of women of childbearing age with 60% of pregnant women meeting criteria compared to only 11% of nonpregnant women [59]. The prevalence of insomnia symptoms also increases across pregnancy from 6.1% pregestation, 44.2% in the first trimester, and 46.3% in the second trimester to a peak of 63.7% in the third trimester [60]. Physiological and psychosocial changes that occur during the perinatal period contribute to the development and maintenance of insomnia within the framework of the diathesis-stress model of chronic insomnia, which identifies predisposing factors, precipitating events, and perpetuating factors (i.e., Spielman's "Three P Model" [61]) as critical to the evolution of insomnia into chronicity across time. Pregnant women experience more cognitive hyperarousal [62] than nonpregnant women who appear more likely to engage in nocturnal rumination (i.e., repetitive negative thinking at night) [63], possibly related to hormonal influences [64]. Insomnia symptoms are highly associated with PSQI scores, and the increased prevalence of poor sleep quality during pregnancy may indicate an increase in insomnia symptoms [38].

While insomnia in pregnancy is well-known to have strong associations with depressive symptomatology [65] and has been associated with higher blood pressures in the nonpregnant population [66], there is a dearth of data regarding its relationship with maternal and fetal outcomes. A study of 370 women found that presence of insomnia was associated with abnormalities of maternal body composition (increased weight and arm circumference) [67]. In pregnant women who were screened for insomnia as well as habitual snoring, only those with comorbid insomnia and habitual snoring had an increased odds for gestational hypertension (OR 3.6, 95%CI 1.1–11.7), but isolated insomnia had no association [68]. The same study also demonstrated that isolated insomnia increased the odds for babies being born large for gestational age even after adjustment for confounders. An observational study of approximately three million women reported that a diagnosis of insomnia was associated with a 30% in the odds of preterm birth [69]. Furthermore, women with a recorded insomnia diagnosis were almost twice as likely to deliver before 34 weeks' gestation (OR 1.7, 95% CI 1.1–2.6) compared to women without a sleep disorder diagnosis, and the risk was highest for preterm premature rupture of membranes at less than 34 weeks (OR 4.1, 95% CI 2.0–8.3). It should be noted insomnia is often discussed in the context of poor sleep quality and insufficient sleep, both of which have been associated with poor pregnancy outcomes [9], but studies focused on insomnia and pregnancy outcomes are lacking.

Sleep-Disordered Breathing

Sleep-disordered breathing (SDB) is common in pregnancy with up to 35% of women reporting habitual snoring by the third trimester [70]. However, the frequency of objectively measured SDB is somewhat less common, with approximately 3% of women in early pregnancy and 8% by mid-pregnancy having an apnea-hypopnea index of at least 5 [71]. Unsurprisingly, women with higher BMIs are more likely to have SDB [72, 73]. Furthermore, in women with hypertensive disorders of pregnancy, both symptoms of SDB and objectively defined SDB are much more common, with as many as 85% of hypertensive women endorsing habitual snoring and approximately 50% having underlying SDB [74–76].

A robust literature demonstrates strong associations between maternal SDB and gestational hypertension/preeclampsia, regardless of whether SDB is symptom-based or objectively measured [70, 71, 77, 78]. Furthermore, the timing of SDB onset is important; it has been shown that pregnancy-onset SDB may drive the relationship with maternal hypertension [70]. In a systematic review and meta-analysis, SDB during pregnancy has been related to a twofold increased risk of gestational hypertension/preeclampsia [77]. The NuMoM2b study, a large cohort of women who underwent home sleep testing during pregnancy, found that the presence of SDB (defined as an AHI ≥5) was associated with a twofold increase in odds for the development of preeclampsia [71]. Of note, in the latter study, the adjusted odds ratio for hypertensive disorders with early pregnancy SDB did not reach statistical significance, but SDB in mid-pregnancy was statistically significant: aOR 1.7 (95% CI 1.2–2.5). This supports prior reports using subjective symptoms of SDB that timing of SDB is important [70]. While obesity is common in pregnant women, it does not completely explain the higher odds of hypertension in women with SDB; application of causal mediation has demonstrated that the presence of new-onset maternal SDB accounts for 15% of the relationship between BMI and hypertension [79].

In addition to gestational hypertension/preeclampsia, there is an increasing literature that demonstrates associations between SDB and GDM. Several cohort studies utilizing retrospective and prospective data all found increased odds (approximately two- to fivefold) for GDM or impaired glucose tolerance in women with SDB symptoms [18, 56, 78, 80, 81]. Similar findings were reported when using a population-based study of ICD-9 codes to identify SDB up to a year prior to delivery [82], as did a national cohort of over 1.5 million women [83]. Moreover, in the NuMoM2b study of over 3000 women with objective sleep measures, women with an AHI ≥5 in early pregnancy had an aOR of 3.45 (95%CI 2.0–6.2) for the development of GDM [71]. Meta-analyses also support these findings [84, 85]. One study compared lean women (BMI < 25 kg/m^2) to overweight women (BMI ≥ 25 kg/m^2) and found that lean women who snored had double the odds for GDM compared to lean non-snorers, with overweight snoring women having the highest odds, at 5.0 (95%CU 2.7–9.3) [81].

While robust associations between SDB and maternal outcomes have been reported as described above, associations with fetal outcomes are not as strong. Although associations between maternal SDB and fetal well-being were first reported in 1978 [86], it was not until recently that work became focused in this area. In 2000 the first study of pregnant women with SDB suggested that habitual snoring was associated with infants born SGA [87]. However, data are conflicting, and several studies fail to find associations between SDB symptoms and birth weight or birth centile [25, 88–92]. In those studies that do find a relationship, SDB appears to be associated with both SGA and LGA. Some have reported SGA/growth restriction with odds ratios or relative risks of between 1.7 and 3.5 [24, 87, 93], while others have reported LGA with very similar relative risks of 1.7–2.6 [94–96]. Timing of onset of maternal SDB symptoms may also be relevant to fetal outcomes as only chronic habitual snoring but not pregnancy-onset snoring appears associated with SGA <10th percentile (aOR 1.7, 95% CI 1.0–2.7) [93]. Of note, studies that found an approximate twofold increase in LGA used the Berlin Questionnaire [94–98], which performs poorly in pregnancy [99], likely because it includes obesity in the scoring paradigm which may drive the relationship with poor outcomes [100].

In support of this, a study stratified by BMI found that the association with high birth weight in snoring women was only present in those with a BMI >30 kg/m^2 [96]. Further, when prepregnancy BMI is accounted for, the apparent association with abnormal glucose levels disappears [70]. Further research is needed to tease out the contributions of SDB and obesity to fetal growth.

Symptom-based studies are also conflicting with regard to associations with preterm birth. Several cross-sectional and cohort studies find no associations between snoring and preterm birth [24, 89, 95, 101, 102], although gasping has been associated with preterm birth with an odds of 1.8 (95% CI 1.1–3.2) [78] and witnessed apnea has demonstrated more than double an increased risk of preterm birth (aRR 2.6, 95%CI 1.2–5.2) [95]. Maternal snoring may also play a role in gestational length; deliveries before 38 weeks' gestation occurred among 25% of women with chronic, frequent-loud snoring, and women with the latter symptom had an increased hazard ratio for delivery of 1.60 (95% CI 1.04, 2.45) as well as a higher frequency of delivery prior to both 37 and 39 weeks' gestation compared with non-snorers (45% vs. 33% and 19% vs. 9%, respectively) [103].

Similar to the data for subjective SDB measures, most objective SDB assessments do not demonstrate differences in birth weight or percentile [104–107]. However, in 230 women who underwent polysomnography, a two- to threefold increase in SGA has been reported, with higher odds for SGA in those with more severe sleep disturbance [108]. Conversely, in 155 healthy Israeli women without comorbidities, SDB has been associated with LGA (aOR 5.1, 95%CI 1.3–20.1) [109]. Population-based studies of diagnostic codes have yielded inconsistent results with reports of SDB being associated with SGA [82], LGA [110], or no difference [73]. Large population-based studies are challenging to interpret because the true prevalence of SDB is not known nor is the proportion of women who receive and appropriately use treatment interventions. One further consideration in studies of fetal growth is that a single measure after delivery may not reflect the true pattern of fetal growth. Fetuses of women with SDB have been reported to demonstrate a fall in growth percentile between 32 weeks and delivery [106], while a causal relationship between maternal SDB and fetal growth is suggested by a study which showed a fall in fetal growth percentiles across the third trimester in women with untreated SDB, with no such slowing in growth in women treated with positive airway pressure [111]. A recent meta-analysis has demonstrated that both SDB symptoms and objective measures of SDB are independently associated with growth abnormalities, both SGA and LGA with similar pooled odds ratios of approximately 1.3–1.6 [34]. While these findings may appear counterintuitive, it is plausible that the underlying mechanisms of SDB may differentially affect fetal growth such that hypertension and its associated sympathetic activation may be associated with fetal growth restriction, while a poor metabolic environment may be more likely to be related to macrosomia.

In studies using clinical diagnoses of SDB, an increase in early preterm birth (<32 weeks) as well as an increase in delivery prior to 37 weeks has been reported in women with SDB compared to both obese women and to normal-weight women [112], with the presence of SDB doubling the odds for preterm birth. Small prospective studies, however, have generally found no differences in preterm birth whether that be defined as <32 weeks [72], <34 weeks [105], or <37 weeks [72, 108]. Nonetheless, rather than preterm birth as a dichotomous outcome, some studies have reported gestational length as a continuous variable although findings are mixed. Some do not support a difference in gestational length [104, 113], while others suggest a slightly shorter gestation in women with OSA [106]. Data from large population-based data sets do however appear to support a link [73, 82, 110, 114] with about a twofold increase in odds in earlier delivery.

Restless Leg Syndrome

Symptoms of restless leg syndrome (RLS) increase as pregnancy progresses, peaking in third trimester and resolving a few days before delivery [115–118]. A recent meta-analysis [119] reported that the frequency of RLS increases across the first, second, and third trimesters of pregnancy, with 8%, 16%, and 22% of women, respectively, reporting RLS symptoms, with a large decrease in frequency to 4% after delivery. RLS symptoms are associated with shorter total sleep time, more difficulty initiating and maintaining sleep, and more daytime sleepiness compared to pregnant women without RLS [115, 116, 118, 120]. In extreme cases, symptoms are so disturbing that evening relaxation and falling asleep is almost impossible and creates a high risk for depression [120, 121]. The prevalence of RLS is approximately two- to threefold higher in pregnant women compared to nonpregnant women [116], at about 3–36% [115, 116, 122]. In a prospective study of 1428 women, prepregnancy RLS was found to be a risk factor for both prenatal and postnatal depression, while no added risk was seen in those with new-onset RLS during pregnancy [121]. Moreover, RLS has been linked with poor sleep quality, poor daytime function, and excessive daytime sleepiness although it should be noted that despite the high frequency of RLS in pregnancy, there is little evidence to suggest an association with birth outcomes [122–124]. However, in a study that used a surrogate measure of RLS ("jumpy or jerky leg movements"), having such movements "always" was associated with an increased incidence of preterm birth and a lower birth weight [125].

Mechanisms for Cardiovascular Morbidity

The mechanisms of sleep disruption – especially SDB – that affect cardiovascular morbidity in nonpregnant adults are remarkably similar to the biological pathways for preeclampsia and include sympathetic activation, oxidative stress, inflammation, and endothelial dysfunction [126, 127]. In SDB, increased sympathetic activation is propagated by frequent arousals and repetitive apneas; the surges in sympathetic activity ultimately result in elevated nocturnal and daytime blood pressures, a key factor in the pathogenesis of cardiovascular morbidity [128]. In pregnancy, sympathetic overactivity is one of the hallmarks of preeclampsia [129]. Furthermore, episodes of intermittent hypoxia and reoxygenation are involved in the generation of reactive oxygen species and reduction in the levels of circulating antioxidants. The subsequent imbalance leads to oxidative stress which plays a central role in endothelial damage and ultimately hypertension [130]. It has been postulated that conditions of chronic sleep loss in pregnancy, such as insufficient sleep, insomnia, and poor sleep quality, could lead to sustained overload of the stress system, which may in turn impair the HPA axis and the proinflammatory system, leading to poor pregnancy outcomes [9, 127].

Treatment Interventions

Treatment intervention trials for sleep disturbance in pregnancy are limited. For pregnant women with SDB, small studies and case reports show that use of positive airway pressure is safe and appears to improve maternal blood pressure and insulin secretion, extend time in utero, and improve markers of maternal and fetal well-being [131–136]. For insomnia, cognitive behavioral therapy (CBTI) is efficacious during pregnancy [137, 138]. A 5-week CBTI program for pregnant women demonstrated significant reductions in insomnia symptoms and increases in subjective sleep quality as well as less time in bed, shorter sleep-onset latency, increased sleep efficiency, and increased subjective total sleep time. Importantly, symptoms of depression, pregnancy-specific anxiety, and fatigue all decreased over the course of treatment [138]. Moreover, since access to trained clinicians can be challenging to many women, delivery of digital CBTI online has also been shown to improve sleep onset and maintenance symptoms as well as sleep duration [139]. Importantly, CBTI during pregnancy appears to protect against sleep loss after childbirth. Support for other therapies to improve sleep quality such as yoga/mindfulness, relaxation, herbal therapies, and acupuncture has also been reported (see Bacaro [140] for a review). However, whether these interventions translate to improvements in fetal outcomes is yet to be tested. Effective treatments, either via therapies such as positive airway pressure for SDB or behavioral strategies to promote good hygiene, should be aggressively pursued in order to reduce the short- and long-term burden of the consequences of sleep deficiency during pregnancy.

Circadian Rhythm Disruption

The majority of studies of circadian rhythms focus on nonpregnant individuals with shift work and find associations with poor health outcomes, especially obesity and type 2 diabetes mellitus [141, 142]. Although an emerging area of investigation in pregnant women, circadian rhythm disruption has been associated with poorer fertility and early pregnancy loss via alterations in circadian rhythm-regulating gene expression [143]. Indeed, shift work has been reported to increase the risk of miscarriage [144–146]. However, data on circadian disruption and its relationship with pregnancy outcomes is scarce. Recently, a large multicenter study of over 7000 women found that those who self-reported a late sleep midpoint (>5 am) in early pregnancy – as a marker of circadian misalignment – had an aOR of 1.67 (95% CI 1.17–2.38) for GDM [147] and an aOR of 1.39 (95%CI 1.08–1.80) for preterm birth [148]. Similar findings were reported by the same group using a sub-cohort of women with actigraphic measures, with a later sleep midpoint being associated with an increased odds for GDM (aOR 2.58, 95%CI 1.24–5.36) [16] although the associations between later sleep midpoint and preterm birth were not quite significant in this smaller sample (aOR 1.68, 95%CI 0.88–3.20) [148].

Analysis of 24-hour rest-activity and saliva cortisol rhythms across the second and third trimester of gestation has shown that more robust activity rhythms are associated with more robust cortisol rhythms and suggest that more irregular sleep-activity rhythms may be associated with earlier gestational age [149]. Furthermore, women diagnosed with gestational-related disease (hypertension, gestational diabetes mellitus, and/or preeclampsia) showed a trend for higher cortisol levels [149], which is consistent with the relationship of hypercortisolism with gestational diabetes [150]. In light of these emerging findings, there is an urgent need to explore the impact of disrupted circadian rhythms among the pregnant women and their offspring. To that end, a large study in Malaysia is underway to investigate the role of circadian rhythms, activity, and nutrition during pregnancy on birth outcomes and infant growth [151].

Maternal Sleep Position

In recent years, data from several countries have shown that self-reported maternal supine going-to-sleep position is a significant risk factor for late-gestation stillbirth (stillbirth at 28 weeks' gestation or more). Report of supine sleep position is three- to eightfold higher in women who experience a late stillbirth [101, 152–155] with an individual patient data analysis showing a 2.6-fold increased odds [156]. While it has long been recognized that posture in pregnancy – particularly during labor – has a profound impact on maternal hemodynamics, few people have extrapolated these practices to how a pregnant woman sleeps. In the supine position, the inferior vena cava is compressed, with subsequent reduced blood flow and a reduction in cardiac output [157]. Even in healthy late-gestation pregnancies, maternal position results in an approximate 6% reduction in oxygen delivery to the fetus and 11% reduction in fetal umbilical venous blood flow [158]. Maternal supine position has been demonstrated to induce fetal quiescence [159], an oxygen conserving state observed during periods of fetal hypoxia, and a small cross-sectional study has suggested that maternal supine sleep was linked to a fivefold increase in low birth weight [101], a finding that was confirmed in a large individual patient data analysis of 1760 women and which found a threefold increase in small for gestational age [160]. Taken together, these findings provide evidence of biological plausibility in the relationship of supine sleep to late-gestation stillbirth. Unlike the studies that have used self-report of going-to-sleep position mentioned above, a study of home sleep testing found no association between sleep position prior to 30 weeks' gestation and stillbirth [161]. However, the latter study was conducted at a much earlier gestational age than other studies [101, 152–156], and this suggests that the heavier gravid uterus later in the third trimester likely conveys the risk. Other sleep behaviors such as long sleep duration, non-restless sleep, and not waking in the night have also been associated with late stillbirth [162], which raises the question of whether long periods of undisturbed sleep increase the risk of late fetal demise. Data are lacking on how the neuroendocrine and autonomic system pathways are regulated in pregnant women during sleep, and this is a fertile area for investigation.

Since most pregnant women spend at least some time in the supine position [163], supine sleep is a potentially modifiable risk factor which could prevent up to 10% of late stillbirths [154, 164]. While there is no intervention study adequately powered to investigate whether reduction in supine sleep translates to fewer stillbirths, several recent studies have shown promise in the ability to reduce time spent in the supine position without impacting sleep quality or duration [165–167] and even suggest that fetal heart rate decelerations can be reduced and infant birth weight may be increased [165, 167]. Work is ongoing in this area.

Summary

In summary, pregnancy is a vulnerable period for sleep disturbance and confers significant impact to both maternal and fetal health. Clinicians caring for pregnant women should be mindful of the accumulating evidence, and identification of sleep disturbance and clinical sleep disorders should be prioritized. Effective therapies to reduce the public health burden of sleep deficiencies are urgently needed since pregnancy offers a window of opportunity to improve long-term health outcomes for both mothers and their babies.

References

1. Lee KA, Zaffke ME, McEnany G. Parity and sleep patterns during and after pregnancy. Obstet Gynecol. 2000;95(1):14–8. PubMed PMID: 10636494.
2. Hedman C, Pohjasvaara T, Tolonen U, Suhonen-Malm AS, Myllyla VV. Effects of pregnancy on mothers' sleep. Sleep Med. 2002;3(1):37–42. PubMed PMID: 14592252.
3. Facco FL, Kramer J, Ho KH, Zee PC, Grobman WA. Sleep disturbances in pregnancy. Obstet Gynecol. 2010;115(1):77–83. PubMed PMID: 20027038. Epub 2009/12/23.
4. Lee KA, Zaffke ME. Longitudinal changes in fatigue and energy during pregnancy and the postpartum period. J Obstet Gynecol Neonatal Nurs. 1999;28(2):183–91.

5. Mindell JA, Cook RA, Nikolovski J. Sleep patterns and sleep disturbances across pregnancy. Sleep Med. 2015;16(4):483–8. PubMed PMID: 25666847. Epub 2015/02/11.

6. Izci-Balserak B, Pien GW. The relationship and potential mechanistic pathways between sleep disturbances and maternal hyperglycemia. Curr Diab Rep. 2014;14:459.

7. National Sleep Foundation. Women and sleep in America poll. Available at https://www.sleepfoundation.org/professionals/sleep-america-polls/2007-women-and-sleep. Accessed 30 Oct 2019. Washington, DC, 2007.

8. Beebe KR, Gay CL, Richoux SE, Lee KA. Symptom experience in late pregnancy. J Obstet Gynecol Neonatal Nurs. 2017;46(4):508–20. PubMed PMID: 28549613. Epub 2017/05/28.

9. Palagini L, Gemignani A, Banti S, Manconi M, Mauri M, Riemann D. Chronic sleep loss during pregnancy as a determinant of stress: impact on pregnancy outcome. Sleep Med. 2014;15(8):853–9. PubMed PMID: 24994566. Epub 2014/07/06.

10. Izci-Balserak B, Keenan BT, Corbitt C, Staley B, Perlis M, Pien GW. Changes in sleep characteristics and breathing parameters during sleep in early and late pregnancy. J Clin Sleep Med. 2018;14(7):1161–8. PubMed PMID: 23354511. PMCID: PMC3696035.

11. Brunner DP, Munch M, Biedermann K, Huch R, Huch A, Borbely AA. Changes in sleep and sleep electroencephalogram during pregnancy. Sleep. 1994;17(7):576–82.

12. Hirshkowitz M, Whiton K, Albert SM, Alessi C, Bruni O, DonCarlos L, et al. National Sleep Foundation's sleep time duration recommendations: methodology and results summary. Sleep Health. 2015;1(1):40–3. PubMed PMID: 29073412.

13. Okun ML, Kline CE, Roberts JM, Wettlaufer B, Glover K, Hall M. Prevalence of sleep deficiency in early gestation and its associations with stress and depressive symptoms. J Womens Health (Larchmt). 2013;22(12):1028–37. PubMed PMID: 24117003. PMCID: PMC3852611. Epub 2013/10/15.

14. Cappuccio FP, Miller MA. Sleep and cardio-metabolic disease. Curr Cardiol Rep. 2017;19(11):110. PubMed PMID: 28929340. PMCID: PMC5605599. Epub 2017/09/21.

15. Williams MA, Miller RS, Qiu C, Cripe SM, Gelaye B, Enquobahrie D. Associations of early pregnancy sleep duration with trimester-specific blood pressures and hypertensive disorders in pregnancy. Sleep. 2010;33(10):1363–71. PubMed PMID: 21061859. PMCID: PMC2941423. Epub 2010/11/11.

16. Facco FL, Grobman WA, Reid KJ, Parker CB, Hunter SM, Silver RM, et al. Objectively measured short sleep duration and later sleep midpoint in pregnancy are associated with a higher risk of gestational diabetes. Am J Obstet Gynecol. 2017;217(4):447 e1–e13. PubMed PMID: 28599896. PMCID: PMC5783638. Epub 2017/06/11.

17. Tang Y, Zhang J, Dai F, Razali NS, Tagore S, Chern B, et al. Poor sleep is associated with higher blood pressure and uterine artery pulsatility index in pregnancy: a prospective cohort study. BJOG. 2020. PubMed PMID: 33145901. Epub 2020/11/05.

18. Qiu C, Enquobahrie D, Frederick IO, Abetew D, Williams MA. Glucose intolerance and gestational diabetes risk in relation to sleep duration and snoring during pregnancy: a pilot study. BMC Womens Health. 2010;10:17. PubMed PMID: 20470416. PMCID: PMC2885310. Epub 2010/05/18.

19. Wang H, Leng J, Li W, Wang L, Zhang C, Li W, et al. Sleep duration and quality, and risk of gestational diabetes mellitus in pregnant Chinese women. Diabet Med. 2017;34(1):44–50. PubMed PMID: 27154471. Epub 2016/05/08.

20. Cai S, Tan S, Gluckman PD, Godfrey KM, Saw SM, Teoh OH, et al. Sleep quality and nocturnal sleep duration in pregnancy and risk of gestational diabetes mellitus. Sleep. 2017;40(2). PubMed PMID: 28364489. Epub 2017/04/02.

21. Buck Louis GM, Grewal J, Albert PS, Sciscione A, Wing DA, Grobman WA, et al. Racial/ethnic standards for fetal growth: the NICHD Fetal Growth Studies. Am J Obstet Gynecol. 2015;213(4):449 e1–e41. PubMed PMID: 26410205. PMCID: PMC4584427.

22. Wang W, Li M, Huang T, Fu Q, Zou L, Song B, et al. Effect of nighttime sleep duration and midday napping in early pregnancy on gestational diabetes mellitus. Sleep Breath. 2020. PubMed PMID: 32266661. Epub 2020/04/09.

23. Reutrakul S, Anothaisintawee T, Herring SJ, Balserak BI, Marc I, Thakkinstian A. Short sleep duration and hyperglycemia in pregnancy: aggregate and individual patient data meta-analysis. Sleep Med Rev. 2017. PubMed PMID: 29103944.

24. Micheli K, Komninos I, Bagkeris E, Roumeliotaki T, Koutis A, Kogevinas M, et al. Sleep patterns in late pregnancy and risk of preterm birth and fetal growth restriction. Epidemiology. 2011;22(5):738–44. PubMed PMID: 21734587. Epub 2011/07/08.

25. Howe LD, Signal TL, Paine SJ, Sweeney B, Priston M, Muller D, et al. Self-reported sleep in late pregnancy in relation to birth size and fetal distress: the E Moe, Mama prospective cohort study. BMJ Open. 2015;5(10):e008910. PubMed PMID: 26438138. PMCID: PMC4606387. Epub 2015/10/07.

26. Abeysena C, Jayawardana P, DE A Seneviratne R. Maternal sleep deprivation is a risk factor for small for gestational age: a cohort study. Aust N Z J Obstet Gynaecol. 2009;49(4):382–7. PubMed PMID: 19694692. Epub 2009/08/22.

27. Abeysena C, Jayawardana P, Seneviratne RA. Effect of psychosocial stress and physical activity on low birthweight: a cohort study. J Obstet Gynaecol Res. 2010;36(2):296–303. PubMed PMID: 20492380. Epub 2010/05/25.

28. Rabkin CS, Anderson HR, Bland JM, Brooke OG, Chamberlain G, Peacock JL. Maternal activity and birth weight: a prospective, population-based study. Am J Epidemiol. 1990;131(3):522–31. PubMed PMID: 2301361. Epub 1990/03/01.

29. Wang W, Zhong C, Zhang Y, Huang L, Chen X, Zhou X, et al. Shorter sleep duration in early pregnancy is associated with birth length: a prospective cohort study in Wuhan, China. Sleep Med. 2017;34:99–104. PubMed PMID: 28522106. Epub 2017/05/20.

30. Franco-Sena AB, Kahn LG, Farias DR, Ferreira AA, Eshriqui I, Figueiredo ACC, et al. Sleep duration of 24 h is associated with birth weight in nulli- but not multiparous women. Nutrition. 2018;55–56:91–8. PubMed PMID: 29980093. Epub 2018/07/07.

31. Morokuma S, Shimokawa M, Kato K, Sanefuji M, Shibata E, Tsuji M, et al. Maternal sleep and small for gestational age infants in the Japan Environment and Children's Study: a cohort study. BMC Res Notes. 2017;10(1):394. PubMed PMID: 28800769. PMCID: PMC5553583. Epub 2017/08/13.

32. Okun ML, Obetz V, Feliciano L. Sleep disturbance in early pregnancy, but not inflammatory cytokines, may increase risk for adverse pregnancy outcomes. Int J Behav Med. 2020. PubMed PMID: 32372169. Epub 2020/05/07.

33. Wang L, Jin F. Association between maternal sleep duration and quality, and the risk of preterm birth: a systematic review and meta-analysis of observational studies. BMC Pregnancy Childbirth. 2020;20(1):125. PubMed PMID: 32093626. PMCID: PMC7041242. Epub 2020/02/26.

34. Warland J, Dorrian J, Morrison JL, O'Brien LM. Maternal sleep during pregnancy and poor fetal outcomes: a scoping review of the literature with meta-analysis. Sleep Med Rev. 2018;41:197–219. PubMed PMID: 29910107. Epub 2018/06/19.

35. Mindell JA, Jacobson BJ. Sleep disturbances during pregnancy. J Obstet Gynecol Neonatal Nurs. 2000;29(6):590–7. PubMed PMID: 11110329. Epub 2000/12/08.

36. Buysse DJ, Reynolds CF 3rd, Monk TH, Berman SR, Kupfer DJ. The Pittsburgh Sleep Quality Index: a new instrument for psychiatric practice and research. Psychiatry Res. 1989;28(2):193–213. PubMed PMID: 2748771. Epub 1989/05/01.

37. Gelaye B, Barrios YV, Zhong QY, Rondon MB, Borba CP, Sanchez SE, et al. Association of poor subjective sleep quality with suicidal ideation among pregnant Peruvian women. Gen Hosp Psychiatry. 2015;37(5):441–7. PubMed PMID: 25983188. PMCID: PMC4558240. Epub 2015/05/20.

38. Sedov ID, Cameron EE, Madigan S, Tomfohr-Madsen LM. Sleep quality during pregnancy: a meta-analysis. Sleep Med Rev. 2018;38:168–76. PubMed PMID: 28866020. Epub 2017/09/04.

39. Signal TL, Gander PH, Sangalli MR, Travier N, Firestone RT, Tuohy JF. Sleep duration and quality in healthy nulliparous and multiparous women across pregnancy and post-

partum. Aust N Z J Obstet Gynaecol. 2007;47(1):16–22. PubMed PMID: 17261094. Epub 2007/01/31.

40. Haney A, Buysse DJ, Rosario BL, Chen YF, Okun ML. Sleep disturbance and cardiometabolic risk factors in early pregnancy: a preliminary study. Sleep Med. 2014;15(4):444–50. PubMed PMID: 24657205. PMCID: PMC4084505. Epub 2014/03/25.

41. Okada K, Saito I, Katada C, Tsujino T. Influence of quality of sleep in the first trimester on blood pressure in the third trimester in primipara women. Blood Press. 2019;28(5):345–55. PubMed PMID: 31266373. Epub 2019/07/04.

42. Hayase M, Shimada M, Seki H. Sleep quality and stress in women with pregnancy-induced hypertension and gestational diabetes mellitus. Women. Birth. 2014;27(3):190–5. PubMed PMID: 24881523. Epub 2014/06/03.

43. Sharma SK, Nehra A, Sinha S, Soneja M, Sunesh K, Sreenivas V, et al. Sleep disorders in pregnancy and their association with pregnancy outcomes: a prospective observational study. Sleep Breath. 2016;20(1):87–93. PubMed PMID: 25957617. Epub 2015/05/11.

44. Bisson M, Series F, Giguere Y, Pamidi S, Kimoff J, Weisnagel SJ, et al. Gestational diabetes mellitus and sleep-disordered breathing. Obstet Gynecol. 2014;123(3):634–41. PubMed PMID: 24499765. Epub 2014/02/07.

45. Xu X, Liu Y, Liu D, Li X, Rao Y, Sharma M, et al. Prevalence and determinants of gestational diabetes mellitus: a cross-sectional study in China. Int J Environ Res Public Health. 2017;14(12). PubMed PMID: 29292753. PMCID: PMC5750950. Epub 2018/01/03.

46. Ahmed AH, Hui S, Crodian J, Plaut K, Haas D, Zhang L, et al. Relationship between sleep quality, depression symptoms, and blood glucose in pregnant women. West J Nurs Res. 2019;41(9):1222–40. PubMed PMID: 30406728. Epub 2018/11/09.

47. Zhong C, Chen R, Zhou X, Xu S, Li Q, Cui W, et al. Poor sleep during early pregnancy increases subsequent risk of gestational diabetes mellitus. Sleep Med. 2018;46:20–5. PubMed PMID: 29773207. Epub 2018/05/19.

48. Zhu B, Shi C, Park CG, Reutrakul S. Sleep quality and gestational diabetes in pregnant women: a systematic review and meta-analysis. Sleep Med. 2020;67:47–55. PubMed PMID: 31911280. Epub 2020/01/09.

49. Hung HM, Ko SH, Chen CH. The association between prenatal sleep quality and obstetric outcome. J Nurs Res. 2014;22(3):147–54. PubMed PMID: 25111108. Epub 2014/08/12.

50. Rajendiran S, Swetha Kumari A, Nimesh A, Soundararaghavan S, Ananthanarayanan PH, Dhiman P. Markers of oxidative stress in pregnant women with sleep disturbances. Oman Med J. 2015;30(4):264–9. PubMed PMID: 26366260. PMCID: PMC4561639. Epub 2015/09/15.

51. Zafarghandi N, Hadavand S, Davati A, Mohseni SM, Kimiaiimoghadam F, Torkestani F. The effects of sleep quality and duration in late pregnancy on labor and fetal outcome. J Matern Fetal Neonatal Med. 2012;25(5):535–7. PubMed PMID: 21827377. Epub 2011/08/11.

52. Strange LB, Parker KP, Moore ML, Strickland OL, Bliwise DL. Disturbed sleep and preterm birth: a potential relationship? Clin Exp Obstet Gynecol. 2009;36(3):166–8. PubMed PMID: 19860360. Epub 2009/10/29.

53. Li R, Zhang J, Zhou R, Liu J, Dai Z, Liu D, et al. Sleep disturbances during pregnancy are associated with cesarean delivery and preterm birth. J Matern Fetal Neonatal Med. 2017;30(6):733–8. PubMed PMID: 27125889. Epub 2016/04/30.

54. Blair LM, Porter K, Leblebicioglu B, Christian LM. Poor sleep quality and associated inflammation predict preterm birth: heightened risk among African Americans. Sleep. 2015;38(8):1259–67. PubMed PMID: 25845693. PMCID: PMC4507731. Epub 2015/04/08.

55. Okun ML, Schetter CD, Glynn LM. Poor sleep quality is associated with preterm birth. Sleep. 2011;34(11):1493–8. PubMed PMID: 22043120. PMCID: PMC3198204. Epub 2011/11/02.

56. Reutrakul S, Zaidi N, Wroblewski K, Kay HH, Ismail M, Ehrmann DA, et al. Sleep disturbances and their relationship to glucose tolerance in pregnancy. Diabetes Care. 2011;34(11):2454–7. PubMed PMID: 21926292. PMCID: PMC3198297. Epub 2011/09/20.

57. Ota H, Hasegawa J, Sekizawa A. Effect of sleep disorders on threatened premature delivery. J Perinat Med. 2017;45(1):57–61. PubMed PMID: 27219094. Epub 2016/05/25.

58. Okun ML, Roberts JM, Marsland AL, Hall M. How disturbed sleep may be a risk factor for adverse pregnancy outcomes. Obstet Gynecol Surv. 2009;64(4):273–80. PubMed PMID: 19296861. PMCID: PMC2880322. Epub 2009/03/20.

59. Sivertsen B, Hysing M, Dorheim SK, Eberhard-Gran M. Trajectories of maternal sleep problems before and after childbirth: a longitudinal population-based study. BMC Pregnancy Childbirth. 2015;15:129. PubMed PMID: 26031504. PMCID: PMC4458335. Epub 2015/06/03.

60. Roman-Galvez RM, Amezcua-Prieto C, Salcedo-Bellido I, Martinez-Galiano JM, Khan KS, Bueno-Cavanillas A. Factors associated with insomnia in pregnancy: a prospective cohort study. Eur J Obstet Gynecol Reprod Biol. 2018;221:70–5. PubMed PMID: 29304393. Epub 2018/01/06.

61. Spielman AJ, Caruso LS, Glovinsky PB. A behavioral perspective on insomnia treatment. Psychiatr Clin North Am. 1987;10(4):541–53. PubMed PMID: 3332317.

62. Michopoulos V, Rothbaum AO, Corwin E, Bradley B, Ressler KJ, Jovanovic T. Psychophysiology and posttraumatic stress disorder symptom profile in pregnant African-American women with trauma exposure. Arch Womens Ment Health. 2015;18(4):639–48. PubMed PMID: 25278341. Epub 10/03. eng.

63. Kalmbach DA, Cheng P, Ong JC, Ciesla JA, Kingsberg SA, Sangha R, et al. Depression and suicidal ideation in pregnancy: exploring relationships with insomnia, short sleep, and nocturnal rumination. Sleep Med. 2020;65:62–73. PubMed PMID: 31710876. PMCID: PMC6980654. Epub 2019/11/12. eng.

64. Soldin OP, Guo T, Weiderpass E, Tractenberg RE, Hilakivi-Clarke L, Soldin SJ. Steroid hormone levels in pregnancy and 1 year postpartum using isotope dilution tandem mass spectrometry. Fertil Steril. 2005;84(3):701–10. PubMed PMID: 16169406. PMCID: PMC3640374. Epub 2005/09/20. eng.

65. Pauley AM, Moore GA, Mama SK, Molenaar P, Symons DD. Associations between prenatal sleep and psychological health: a systematic review. J Clin Sleep Med. 2020;16(4):619–30. PubMed PMID: 32003734. PMCID: PMC7161464. Epub 2020/02/01.

66. Bathgate CJ, Fernandez-Mendoza J. Insomnia, short sleep duration, and high blood pressure: recent evidence and future directions for the prevention and management of hypertension. Curr Hypertens Rep. 2018;20(6):52. PubMed PMID: 29779139. Epub 2018/05/21.

67. Fernandez-Alonso AM, Trabalon-Pastor M, Chedraui P, Perez-Lopez FR. Factors related to insomnia and sleepiness in the late third trimester of pregnancy. Arch Gynecol Obstet. 2012;286(1):55–61. PubMed PMID: 22331224. Epub 2012/02/15.

68. Okun ML, O'Brien LM. Concurrent insomnia and habitual snoring are associated with adverse pregnancy outcomes. Sleep Med. 2018;46:12–9. PubMed PMID: 29773206. Epub 2018/05/19.

69. Felder JN, Baer RJ, Rand L, Jelliffe-Pawlowski LL, Prather AA. Sleep disorder diagnosis during pregnancy and risk of preterm birth. Obstet Gynecol. 2017;130(3):573–81. PubMed PMID: 28796676. Epub 2017/08/11.

70. O'Brien LM, Bullough AS, Owusu JT, Tremblay KA, Brincat CA, Chames MC, et al. Pregnancy-onset habitual snoring, gestational hypertension, and preeclampsia: prospective cohort study. Am J Obstet Gynecol. 2012;207(6):487 e1–9. PubMed PMID: 22999158. PMCID: PMC3505221. Epub 2012/09/25.

71. Facco FL, Parker CB, Reddy UM, Silver RM, Koch MA, Louis JM, et al. Association between sleep-disordered breathing and hypertensive disorders of pregnancy and gestational diabetes mellitus. Obstet Gynecol. 2017;129(1):31–41. PubMed PMID: 27926645. PMCID: PMC5512455. Epub 2016/12/08.

72. Louis J, Auckley D, Miladinovic B, Shepherd A, Mencin P, Kumar D, et al. Perinatal outcomes associated with obstructive sleep apnea in obese pregnant women. Obstet Gynecol. 2012;120(5):1085–92. PubMed PMID: 23090526. PMCID: PMC3552141. Epub 2012/10/24.

73. Louis JM, Mogos MF, Salemi JL, Redline S, Salihu HM. Obstructive sleep apnea and severe maternal-infant morbidity/mortality in the United States, 1998-2009. Sleep. 2014;37(5):843–9. PubMed PMID: 24790262. PMCID: PMC3985102.

74. Izci B, Martin SE, Dundas KC, Liston WA, Calder AA, Douglas NJ. Sleep complaints: snoring and daytime sleepiness in pregnant and pre-eclamptic women. Sleep Med. 2005;6(2):163–9. PubMed PMID: 15716220. Epub 2005/02/18.

75. O'Brien LM, Bullough AS, Chames MC, Shelgikar AV, Armitage R, Guilleminualt C, et al. Hypertension, snoring, and obstructive sleep apnoea during pregnancy: a cohort study. BJOG. 2014;121(13):1685–93. PubMed PMID: 24888772. PMCID: PMC4241143. Epub 2014/06/04.

76. Reid J, Skomro R, Cotton D, Ward H, Olatunbosun F, Gjevre J, et al. Pregnant women with gestational hypertension may have a high frequency of sleep disordered breathing. Sleep. 2011;34(8):1033–8. PubMed PMID: 21804665. PMCID: PMC3138158. Epub 2011/08/02.

77. Pamidi S, Pinto LM, Marc I, Benedetti A, Schwartzman K, Kimoff RJ. Maternal sleep-disordered breathing and adverse pregnancy outcomes: a systematic review and metaanalysis. Am J Obstet Gynecol. 2014;210(1):52 e1–e14. PubMed PMID: 23911687. Epub 2013/08/06.

78. Bourjeily G, Raker CA, Chalhoub M, Miller MA. Pregnancy and fetal outcomes of symptoms of sleep-disordered breathing. Eur Respir J. 2010;36(4):849–55. PubMed PMID: 20525714. Epub 2010/06/08.

79. Dunietz GL, Shedden K, Lisabeth LD, Treadwell MC, O'Brien LM. Maternal weight, snoring, and hypertension: potential pathways of associations. Am J Hypertens. 2018;31(10):1133–8. PubMed PMID: 29788196. PMCID: PMC6132116. Epub 2018/05/23.

80. Facco FL, Grobman WA, Kramer J, Ho KH, Zee PC. Self-reported short sleep duration and frequent snoring in pregnancy: impact on glucose metabolism. Am J Obstet Gynecol. 2010;203(2):142 e1–5. PubMed PMID: 20510182. PMCID: PMC3178265. Epub 2010/06/01.

81. Qiu C, Lawrence W, Gelaye B, Stoner L, Frederick IO, Enquobahrie DA, et al. Risk of glucose intolerance and gestational diabetes mellitus in relation to maternal habitual snoring during early pregnancy. PLoS One. 2017;12(9):e0184966. PubMed PMID: 28926639. PMCID: PMC5605003. Epub 2017/09/20.

82. Chen YH, Kang JH, Lin CC, Wang IT, Keller JJ, Lin HC. Obstructive sleep apnea and the risk of adverse pregnancy outcomes. Am J Obstet Gynecol. 2012;206(2):136 e1–5. PubMed PMID: 22000892. Epub 2011/10/18.

83. Bourjeily G, Danilack VA, Bublitz MH, Lipkind H, Muri J, Caldwell D, et al. Obstructive sleep apnea in pregnancy is associated with adverse maternal outcomes: a national cohort. Sleep Med. 2017;38:50–7. PubMed PMID: 29031756. PMCID: PMC5677512. Epub 2017/10/17.

84. Luque-Fernandez MA, Bain PA, Gelaye B, Redline S, Williams MA. Sleep-disordered breathing and gestational diabetes mellitus: a meta-analysis of 9,795 participants enrolled in epidemiological observational studies. Diabetes Care. 2013;36(10):3353–60. PubMed PMID: 24065843. PMCID: PMC3781575. Epub 2013/09/26.

85. Li L, Zhao K, Hua J, Li S. Association between sleep-disordered breathing during pregnancy and maternal and fetal outcomes: an updated systematic review and meta-analysis. Front Neurol. 2018;9:91. PubMed PMID: 29892255. PMCID: PMC5985400. Epub 2018/06/13.

86. Joel-Cohen SJ, Schoenfeld A. Fetal response to periodic sleep apnea: a new syndrome in obstetrics. Eur J Obstet Gynecol Reprod Biol. 1978;8(2):77–81. PubMed PMID: 45501.

87. Franklin KA, Holmgren PA, Jonsson F, Poromaa N, Stenlund H, Svanborg E. Snoring, pregnancy-induced hypertension, and growth retardation of the fetus. Chest. 2000;117(1):137–41. PubMed PMID: 10631211. Epub 2000/01/13.

88. Ayrim A, Keskin EA, Ozol D, Onaran Y, Yiidirim Z, Kafali H. Influence of self-reported snoring and witnessed sleep apnea on gestational hypertension and fetal outcome in pregnancy. Arch Gynecol Obstet. 2011;283(2):195–9. PubMed PMID: 20033421. Epub 2009/12/25.

89. Koken G, Sahin FK, Cosar E, Saylan F, Yilmaz N, Altuntas I, et al. Oxidative stress markers in pregnant women who snore and fetal outcome: a case control study. Acta Obstet Gynecol Scand. 2007;86(11):1317–21. PubMed PMID: 17963059. Epub 2007/10/27.

90. Loube DI, Poceta JS, Morales MC, Peacock MD, Mitler MM. Self-reported snoring in pregnancy. Association with fetal outcome. Chest. 1996;109(4):885–9. PubMed PMID: 8635365.

91. Perez-Chada D, Videla AJ, O'Flaherty ME, Majul C, Catalini AM, Caballer CA, et al. Snoring, witnessed sleep apnoeas and pregnancy-induced hypertension. Acta Obstet Gynecol Scand. 2007;86(7):788–92. PubMed PMID: 17611822. Epub 2007/07/06.

92. Tauman R, Sivan Y, Katsav S, Greenfeld M, Many A. Maternal snoring during pregnancy is not associated with fetal growth restriction. J Matern Fetal Neonatal Med. 2012;25(8):1283–6. PubMed PMID: 21999115.

93. O'Brien LM, Bullough AS, Owusu JT, Tremblay KA, Brincat CA, Chames MC, et al. Snoring during pregnancy and delivery outcomes: a cohort study. Sleep. 2013;36(11):1625–32. PubMed PMID: 24179294. PMCID: PMC3792378. Epub 2013/11/02.

94. Antony KM, Agrawal A, Arndt ME, Murphy AM, Alapat PM, Guntupalli KK, et al. Association of adverse perinatal outcomes with screening measures of obstructive sleep apnea. J Perinatol. 2014;34(6):441–8. PubMed PMID: 24603455. Epub 2014/03/08.

95. Ge X, Tao F, Huang K, Mao L, Huang S, Niu Y, et al. Maternal snoring may predict adverse pregnancy outcomes: a cohort study in China. PLoS One. 2016;11(2):e0148732. PubMed PMID: 26871434. PMCID: PMC4752474.

96. Olivarez SA, Ferres M, Antony K, Mattewal A, Maheshwari B, Sangi-Haghpeykar H, et al. Obstructive sleep apnea screening in pregnancy, perinatal outcomes, and impact of maternal obesity. Am J Perinatol. 2011;28(8):651–8. PubMed PMID: 21480159. PMCID: PMC3966067. Epub 2011/04/12.

97. Higgins N, Leong E, Park CS, Facco FL, McCarthy RJ, Wong CA. The Berlin questionnaire for assessment of sleep disordered breathing risk in parturients and non-pregnant women. Int J Obstet Anesth. 2011;20(1):22–5. PubMed PMID: 21123046. Epub 2010/12/03.

98. Ko HS, Kim MY, Kim YH, Lee J, Park YG, Moon HB, et al. Obstructive sleep apnea screening and perinatal outcomes in Korean pregnant women. Arch Gynecol Obstet. 2013;287(3):429–33. PubMed PMID: 23086136. Epub 2012/10/23.

99. Tantrakul V, Numthavaj P, Guilleminault C, McEvoy M, Panburana P, Khaing W, et al. Performance of screening questionnaires for obstructive sleep apnea during pregnancy: a systematic review and meta-analysis. Sleep Med Rev. 2017;36:96–106. PubMed PMID: 28007402.

100. O'Brien LR, Dunietz GL. The Berlin questionnaire in pregnancy predominantly identifies obesity. J Clin Sleep Med. 2021;17(8):1553–61.

101. Owusu JT, Anderson FJ, Coleman J, Oppong S, Seffah JD, Aikins A, et al. Association of maternal sleep practices with pre-eclampsia, low birth weight, and stillbirth among Ghanaian women. Int J Gynaecol Obstet. 2013;121(3):261–5. PubMed PMID: 23507553. PMCID: PMC3662549. Epub 2013/03/20.

102. Leung PL, Hui DS, Leung TN, Yuen PM, Lau TK. Sleep disturbances in Chinese pregnant women. BJOG. 2005;112(11):1568–71. PubMed PMID: 16225581. Epub 2005/10/18.

103. Dunietz GL, Shedden K, Schisterman EF, Lisabeth LD, Treadwell MC, O'Brien LM. Associations of snoring frequency and intensity in pregnancy with time-to-delivery. Paediatr Perinat Epidemiol. 2018. PubMed PMID: 30266041.

104. Bassan H, Uliel-Sibony S, Katsav S, Farber M, Tauman R. Maternal sleep disordered breathing and neonatal outcome. Isr Med Assoc J. 2016;18(1):45–8. PubMed PMID: 26964280. Epub 2016/03/12.

105. Facco FL, Ouyang DW, Zee PC, Strohl AE, Gonzalez AB, Lim C, et al. Implications of sleep-disordered breathing in pregnancy. Am J Obstet Gynecol. 2014;210(6):559 e1–6. PubMed PMID: 24373947. PMCID: PMC4511595. Epub 2014/01/01.

106. Fung AM, Wilson DL, Lappas M, Howard M, Barnes M, O'Donoghue F, et al. Effects of maternal obstructive sleep apnoea on fetal growth: a prospective cohort study. PLoS One. 2013;8(7):e68057. PubMed PMID: 23894293. PMCID: PMC3722214. Epub 2013/07/31.

107. Sahin FK, Koken G, Cosar E, Saylan F, Fidan F, Yilmazer M, et al. Obstructive sleep apnea in pregnancy and fetal outcome. Int J Gynaecol Obstet. 2008;100(2):141–6. PubMed PMID: 17976624. Epub 2007/11/03.

108. Pamidi S, Marc I, Simoneau G, Lavigne L, Olha A, Benedetti A, et al. Maternal sleep-disordered breathing and the risk of delivering small for gestational age infants: a prospective cohort study. Thorax. 2016;71(8):719–25. PubMed PMID: 27084956. Epub 2016/04/17.

109. Telerant A, Dunietz GL, Many A, Tauman R. Mild maternal obstructive sleep apnea in non-obese pregnant women and accelerated fetal growth. Sci Rep. 2018;8(1):10768. PubMed PMID: 30018451. PMCID: PMC6050232. Epub 2018/07/19.

110. Bin YS, Cistulli PA, Ford JB. Population-based study of sleep apnea in pregnancy and maternal and infant outcomes. J Clin Sleep Med. 2016;12(6):871–7. PubMed PMID: 27070246. PMCID: PMC4877320. Epub 2016/04/14.

111. Kneitel AW, Treadwell MC, O'Brien LM. Effects of maternal obstructive sleep apnea on fetal growth: a case-control study. J Perinatol. 2018;38(8):982–8. PubMed PMID: 29785058. PMCID: PMC6092194. Epub 2018/05/23.

112. Louis JM, Auckley D, Sokol RJ, Mercer BM. Maternal and neonatal morbidities associated with obstructive sleep apnea complicating pregnancy. Am J Obstet Gynecol. 2010;202(3):261 e1–5. PubMed PMID: 20005507.

113. Olivarez SA, Maheshwari B, McCarthy M, Zacharias N, van den Veyver I, Casturi L, et al. Prospective trial on obstructive sleep apnea in pregnancy and fetal heart rate monitoring. Am J Obstet Gynecol. 2010;202(6):552 e1–7. PubMed PMID: 20171603. Epub 2010/02/23.

114. Spence DL, Allen RC, Lutgendorf MA, Gary VR, Richard JD, Gonzalez SC. Association of obstructive sleep apnea with adverse pregnancy-related outcomes in military hospitals. Eur J Obstet Gynecol Reprod Biol. 2017;210:166–72. PubMed PMID: 28040612. Epub 2017/01/04.

115. Manconi M, Ulfberg J, Berger K, Ghorayeb I, Wesstrom J, Fulda S, et al. When gender matters: restless legs syndrome. Report of the "RLS and woman" workshop endorsed by the European RLS Study Group. Sleep Med Rev. 2012;16(4):297–307. PubMed PMID: 22075215. Epub 2011/11/15.

116. Srivanitchapoom P, Pandey S, Hallett M. Restless legs syndrome and pregnancy: a review. Parkinsonism Relat Disord. 2014. PubMed PMID: 24768121. Epub 2014/04/29. Eng.

117. Hubner A, Krafft A, Gadient S. Characteristics and determinants of restless legs syndrome in pregnancy: a prospective study. Neurology. 2013;80:738–42.

118. Lee KA, Zaffke ME, Baratte-Beebe K. Restless legs syndrome and sleep disturbance during pregnancy: the role of folate and iron. J Womens Health Gend Based Med. 2001;10(4):335–41. PubMed PMID: 11445024. Epub 2001/07/11.

119. Chen SJ, Shi L, Bao YP, Sun YK, Lin X, Que JY, et al. Prevalence of restless legs syndrome during pregnancy: a systematic review and meta-analysis. Sleep Med Rev. 2018;40:43–54. PubMed PMID: 29169861. Epub 2017/11/25.

120. Manconi M, Govoni V, De Vito A, Economou NT, Cesnik E, Casetta I, et al. Restless legs syndrome and pregnancy. Neurology. 2004;63(6):1065–9.

121. Wesstrom J, Skalkidou A, Manconi M, Fulda S, Sundstrom-Poromaa I. Pre-pregnancy restless legs syndrome (Willis-Ekbom disease) is associated with perinatal depression. J Clin Sleep Med. 2014;10(5):527–33. PubMed PMID: 24812538. PMCID: PMC4013381. Epub 2014/05/09.

122. Dunietz GL, Lisabeth LD, Shedden K, Shamim-Uzzaman QA, Bullough AS, Chames MC, et al. Restless legs syndrome and sleep-wake disturbances in pregnancy. J Clin Sleep Med. 2017;13(7):863–70. PubMed PMID: 28633715. PMCID: PMC5482577. Epub 2017/06/22.

123. Minar M, Habanova H, Rusnak I, Planck K, Valkovic P. Prevalence and impact of restless legs syndrome in pregnancy. Neuro Endocrinol Lett. 2013;34(5):366–71. PubMed PMID: 23922045. Epub 2013/08/08.

124. Vahdat M, Sariri E, Miri S, Rohani M, Kashanian M, Sabet A, et al. Prevalence and associated features of restless legs syndrome in a population of Iranian women during pregnancy. Int J Gynaecol Obstet. 2013;123(1):46–9. PubMed PMID: 23886452. Epub 2013/07/28.

125. Oyieng'o DO, Kirwa K, Tong I, Martin S, Antonio Rojas-Suarez J, Bourjeily G. Restless legs symptoms and pregnancy and neonatal outcomes. Clin Ther. 2016;38(2):256–64. PubMed PMID: 26740290. PMCID: PMC6581560. Epub 2016/01/08.

126. Izci-Balserak B, Pien GW. Sleep-disordered breathing and pregnancy: potential mechanisms and evidence for maternal and fetal morbidity. Curr Opin Pulm Med. 2010;16(6):574–82. PubMed PMID: 20859210. PMCID: PMC3603138. Epub 2010/09/23.

127. Chang JJ, Pien GW, Duntley SP, Macones GA. Sleep deprivation during pregnancy and maternal and fetal outcomes: is there a relationship? Sleep Med Rev. 2010;14(2):107–14. PubMed PMID: 19625199. PMCID: PMC2824023. Epub 2009/07/25.

128. Nieto FJ, Young TB, Lind BK, Shahar E, Samet JM, Redline S, et al. Association of sleep-disordered breathing, sleep apnea, and hypertension in a large community-based study. Sleep Heart Health Study. JAMA. 2000;283(14):1829–36. PubMed PMID: 10770144. Epub 2000/04/19.

129. Schobel HP, Fischer T, Heuszer K, Geiger H, Schmieder RE. Preeclampsia -- a state of sympathetic overactivity. N Engl J Med. 1996;335(20):1480–5. PubMed PMID: 8890098. Epub 1996/11/14.

130. Lavie L. Oxidative stress--a unifying paradigm in obstructive sleep apnea and comorbidities. Prog Cardiovasc Dis. 2009;51(4):303–12. PubMed PMID: 19110132. Epub 2008/12/27.

131. Edwards N, Blyton DM, Kirjavainen T, Kesby GJ, Sullivan CE. Nasal continuous positive airway pressure reduces sleep-induced blood pressure increments in preeclampsia. Am J Respir Crit Care Med. 2000;162(1):252–7. PubMed PMID: 10903250. Epub 2000/07/21.

132. Guilleminault C, Palombini L, Poyares D, Takaoka S, Huynh NT, El-Sayed Y. Pre-eclampsia and nasal CPAP: part 1. Early intervention with nasal CPAP in pregnant women with risk-factors for pre-eclampsia: preliminary findings. Sleep Med. 2007;9(1):9–14. PubMed PMID: 17644420. Epub 2007/07/24.

133. Poyares D, Guilleminault C, Hachul H, Fujita L, Takaoka S, Tufik S, et al. Pre-eclampsia and nasal CPAP: part 2. Hypertension during pregnancy, chronic snoring, and early nasal CPAP intervention. Sleep Med. 2007;9(1):15–21. PubMed PMID: 17644475. Epub 2007/07/24.

134. Chirakalwasan N, Amnakkittikul S, Wanitcharoenkul E, Charoensri S, Saetung S, Chanprasertyothin S, et al. Continuous positive airway pressure therapy in gestational diabetes with obstructive sleep apnea: a randomized controlled trial. J Clin Sleep Med. 2018;14(3):327–36. PubMed PMID: 29458699. PMCID: PMC5837834. Epub 2018/02/21.

135. Blyton DM, Skilton MR, Edwards N, Hennessy A, Celermajer DS, Sullivan CE. Treatment of sleep disordered breathing reverses low fetal activity levels in preeclampsia. Sleep. 2013;36(1):15–21. PubMed PMID: 23288967. PMCID: PMC3524539. Epub 2013/01/05.

136. Whitehead C, Tong S, Wilson D, Howard M, Walker SP. Treatment of early-onset preeclampsia with continuous positive airway pressure. Obstet Gynecol. 2015;125(5):1106–9. PubMed PMID: 25774926. Epub 2015/03/17.

137. Manber R, Bei B, Simpson N, Asarnow L, Rangel E, Sit A, et al. Cognitive behavioral therapy for prenatal insomnia: a randomized controlled trial. Obstet Gynecol. 2019;133(5):911–9. PubMed PMID: 30969203. PMCID: PMC6485299. Epub 2019/04/11.

138. Tomfohr-Madsen LM, Clayborne ZM, Rouleau CR, Campbell TS. Sleeping for two: an open-pilot study of cognitive behavioral therapy for insomnia in pregnancy. Behav Sleep Med. 2017;15(5):377–93. PubMed PMID: 27124405. Epub 2016/04/29.

139. Kalmbach DA, Cheng P, O'Brien LM, Swanson LM, Sangha R, Sen S, et al. A randomized controlled trial of digital cognitive behavioral therapy for insomnia in pregnant women. Sleep Med. 2020;72:82–92. PubMed PMID: 32559716. Epub 2020/06/20.

140. Bacaro V, Benz F, Pappaccogli A, De Bartolo P, Johann AF, Palagini L, et al. Interventions for sleep problems during pregnancy: a systematic review. Sleep Med Rev. 2020;50:101234. PubMed PMID: 31801099. Epub 2019/12/05.

141. Hansen AB, Stayner L, Hansen J, Andersen ZJ. Night shift work and incidence of diabetes in the Danish Nurse Cohort. Occup Environ Med. 2016;73(4):262–8. PubMed PMID: 26889020. Epub 2016/02/19.

142. Rosa D, Terzoni S, Dellafiore F, Destrebecq A. Systematic review of shift work and nurses' health. Occup Med (Lond). 2019;69(4):237–43. PubMed PMID: 31132107. Epub 2019/05/28.

143. Mills J, Kuohung W. Impact of circadian rhythms on female reproduction and infertility treatment success. Curr Opin Endocrinol Diabetes Obes. 2019. PubMed PMID: 31644470. Epub 2019/10/24.

144. Grajewski B, Whelan EA, Lawson CC, Hein MJ, Waters MA, Anderson JL, et al. Miscarriage among flight attendants. Epidemiology. 2015;26(2):192–203. PubMed PMID: 25563432. PMCID: PMC4510952. Epub 2015/01/08.

145. Begtrup LM, Specht IO, Hammer PEC, Flachs EM, Garde AH, Hansen J, et al. Night work and miscarriage: a Danish nationwide register-based cohort study. Occup Environ Med. 2019;76(5):302–8. PubMed PMID: 30910992. Epub 2019/03/27.

146. Lawson CC, Rocheleau CM, Whelan EA, Lividoti Hibert EN, Grajewski B, Spiegelman D, et al. Occupational exposures among nurses and risk of spontaneous abortion. Am J Obstet Gynecol. 2012;206(4):327 e1–8. PubMed PMID: 22304790. PMCID: PMC4572732. Epub 2012/02/07.

147. Facco FL, Parker CB, Hunter S, Reid KJ, Zee PC, Silver RM, et al. Association of adverse pregnancy outcomes with self-reported measures of sleep duration and timing in women who are nulliparous. J Clin Sleep Med. 2018;14(12):2047–56. PubMed PMID: 30518449. PMCID: PMC6287730. Epub 2018/12/07.

148. Facco FL, Parker CB, Hunter S, Reid KJ, Zee PP, Silver RM, et al. Later sleep timing is associated with an increased risk of preterm birth in nulliparous women. Am J Obstet Gynecol MFM. 2019;1(4):100040. PubMed PMID: 33345835. PMCID: PMC7757682. Epub 2020/12/22.

149. Casey T, Sun H, Suarez-Trujillo A, Crodian J, Zhang L, Plaut K, et al. Pregnancy rest-activity patterns are related to salivary cortisol rhythms and maternal-fetal health indicators in women from a disadvantaged population. PLoS One. 2020;15(3):e0229567. PubMed PMID: 32126104. PMCID: PMC7053712. Epub 2020/03/04.

150. Ahmed SA, Shalayel MH. Role of cortisol in the deterioration of glucose tolerance in Sudanese pregnant women. East Afr Med J. 1999;76(8):465–7. PubMed PMID: 10520355. Epub 1999/10/16.

151. Kaur S, Teoh AN, Shukri NHM, Shafie SR, Bustami NA, Takahashi M, et al. Circadian rhythm and its association with birth and infant outcomes: research protocol of a prospective cohort study. BMC Pregnancy Childbirth. 2020;20(1):96. PubMed PMID: 32046676. PMCID: PMC7014629. Epub 2020/02/13.

152. Gordon A, Raynes-Greenow C, Bond D, Morris J, Rawlinson W, Jeffery H. Sleep position, fetal growth restriction, and late-pregnancy stillbirth: the Sydney stillbirth study. Obstet Gynecol. 2015;125(2):347–55. PubMed PMID: 25568999. Epub 2015/01/09.

153. Heazell A, Li M, Budd J, Thompson J, Stacey T, Cronin RS, et al. Association between maternal sleep practices and late stillbirth - findings from a stillbirth case-control study. BJOG. 2018;125(2):254–62. PubMed PMID: 29152887. PMCID: PMC5765411. Epub 2017/11/21.

154. McCowan LME, Thompson JMD, Cronin RS, Li M, Stacey T, Stone PR, et al. Going to sleep in the supine position is a modifiable risk factor for late pregnancy stillbirth; findings from the New Zealand multicentre stillbirth case-control study. PLoS One. 2017;12(6):e0179396. PubMed PMID: 28609468. PMCID: PMC5469491. Epub 2017/06/14.

155. Stacey T, Thompson JM, Mitchell EA, Ekeroma AJ, Zuccollo JM, McCowan LM. Association between maternal sleep practices and risk of late stillbirth: a case-control study. BMJ. 2011;342:d3403. PubMed PMID: 21673002. PMCID: PMC3114953. Epub 2011/06/16.

156. Cronin RS, Li M, Thompson JMD, Gordon A, Raynes-Greenow CH, Heazell AEP, et al. An individual participant data meta-analysis of maternal going-to-sleep position, interactions with fetal vulnerability, and the risk of late stillbirth. EClinicalMedicine. 2019;10:49–57. PubMed PMID: 31193832. PMCID: PMC6543252. Epub 2019/06/14.

157. Humphries A, Mirjalili SA, Tarr GP, Thompson JMD, Stone P. The effect of supine positioning on maternal hemodynamics during late pregnancy. J Matern Fetal Neonatal Med. 2019;32(23):3923–30. PubMed PMID: 29772936. Epub 2018/05/19.

158. Couper S, Clark A, Thompson JMD, Flouri D, Aughwane R, David AL, et al. The effects of maternal position, in late gestation pregnancy, on placental blood flow and oxygenation: an MRI study. J Physiol. 2020. PubMed PMID: 33369732. Epub 2020/12/29.

159. Stone PR, Burgess W, McIntyre J, Gunn AJ, Lear CA, Bennet L, et al. An investigation of fetal behavioural states during maternal sleep in healthy late gestation pregnancy: an observational study. J Physiol. 2017;595(24):7441–50. PubMed PMID: 29023736. PMCID: PMC5730849. Epub 2017/10/13.

160. Anderson NH, Gordon A, Li M, Cronin RS, Thompson JMD, Raynes-Greenow CH, et al. Association of supine going-to-sleep position in late pregnancy with reduced birth weight: a secondary analysis of an individual participant data meta-analysis. JAMA Netw Open. 2019;2(10):e1912614. PubMed PMID: 31577362. PMCID: PMC6777255. Epub 2019/10/03.

161. Silver RM, Hunter S, Reddy UM, Facco F, Gibbins KJ, Grobman WA, et al. Prospective evaluation of maternal sleep position through 30 weeks of gestation and adverse pregnancy outcomes. Obstet Gynecol. 2019;134(4):667–76. PubMed PMID: 31503146. PMCID: PMC6768734. Epub 2019/09/11.

162. O'Brien LM, Warland J, Stacey T, Heazell AEP, Mitchell EA, Consortium S. Maternal sleep practices and stillbirth: findings from an international case-control study. Birth. 2019;46(2):344–54. PubMed PMID: 30656734. Epub 2019/01/19.

163. O'Brien LM, Warland J. Typical sleep positions in pregnant women. Early Hum Dev. 2014;90(6):315–7. PubMed PMID: 24661447. PMCID: PMC4005859. Epub 2014/03/26.

164. Cronin RS, Chelimo C, Mitchell EA, Okesene-Gafa K, Thompson JMD, Taylor RS, et al. Survey of maternal sleep practices in late pregnancy in a multi-ethnic sample in South Auckland, New Zealand. BMC Pregnancy Childbirth. 2017;17(1):190. PubMed PMID: 28623890. PMCID: PMC5474014. Epub 2017/06/19.

165. Coleman J, Okere M, Seffah J, Kember A, O'Brien LM, Borazjani A, et al. The Ghana PrenaBelt trial: a double-blind, sham-controlled, randomised clinical trial to evaluate the effect of maternal positional therapy during third-trimester sleep on birth weight. BMJ Open. 2019;9(4):e022981. PubMed PMID: 31048420. PMCID: PMC6502032. Epub 2019/05/03.

166. Kember AJ, Scott HM, O'Brien LM, Borazjani A, Butler MB, Wells JH, et al. Modifying maternal sleep position in the third trimester of pregnancy with positional therapy: a randomised pilot trial. BMJ Open. 2018;8(8):e020256. PubMed PMID: 30158217. PMCID: PMC6119420. Epub 2018/08/31.

167. Warland J, Dorrian J, Kember AJ, Phillips C, Borazjani A, Morrison JL, et al. Modifying maternal sleep position in late pregnancy through positional therapy: a feasibility study. J Clin Sleep Med. 2018;14(8):1387–97. PubMed PMID: 30092890. PMCID: PMC6086963. Epub 2018/08/11.

Chapter 22
Sleep in Older Patients

Armand Michael Ryden and Cathy Alessi

Keywords Human sleep with aging · Central sleep apnea · REM sleep behavior disorder · Behavioral therapies for insomnia · Syndromes of aging

Learning Points
1. There are well-established changes in sleep with aging, including worsening sleep fragmentation and decreasing slow-wave sleep.
2. Changes in sleep have been linked to the pathophysiology of Alzheimer's disease.
3. Sleep-disordered breathing is a common condition in older patients, with a marked increase in central sleep apnea due to comorbidities.
4. Older patients, even those who have mild to moderate dementia, can benefit from treatment of obstructive sleep apnea.

A. M. Ryden (✉)
Pulmonary, Critical Care and Sleep Medicine Division, Veterans Affairs Greater Los Angeles Healthcare System, Los Angeles, CA, USA

David Geffen School of Medicine at University of California, Los Angeles, Los Angeles, CA, USA
e-mail: armand.ryden@va.gov

C. Alessi
David Geffen School of Medicine at University of California, Los Angeles, Los Angeles, CA, USA

Geriatric Research, Education and Clinical Center, Veterans Affairs Greater Los Angeles Healthcare System, Los Angeles, CA, USA
e-mail: Cathy.Alessi@va.gov

5. Behavioral therapies are first-line treatment for insomnia in all adults, particularly in those who are older.
6. Optimizing iron stores is a key first step in the treatment of restless legs syndrome.
7. REM sleep behavior disorder is tied to the development of alpha-synucleinopathy related neurodegenerative disorders, such as Parkinson's disease, Lewy body dementia, and multisystem atrophy.

Introduction

Sleep disorders in older adults offer unique challenges. With advancing age many patients accrue increasing numbers of comorbidities. More than two-thirds of those with multiple comorbidities report sleep problems. These problems can include difficulty falling asleep, difficulty staying asleep, or sleepiness during the day. This chapter will explore age-related changes in sleep and the effects of sleep disorders on selected syndromes of aging. It will also explore the epidemiology, clinical presentations, and management decisions that are unique to sleep disorders commonly encountered in older adults.

Sleep and Aging

There is strong evidence that there are changes in sleep efficiency and sleep stage architecture with aging. Advancing age is generally associated with advanced (i.e., earlier) sleep timing, longer sleep-onset latency, shorter sleep duration, increased sleep fragmentation, and decreased slow-wave sleep [1]. The reduction in non-REM stage 3 (N3) sleep with age is more prominent in men than women. It is less clear if there are significant changes in REM sleep with aging. There is evidence that excessive daytime sleepiness increases with aging. Naps, including unplanned naps, are more frequent in older people. However, napping and excessive daytime sleepiness are associated with comorbidities such as depression, pain, and nocturia [2]. Thus, increased napping may not be a part of normal aging per se. Using the multiple sleep latency test as a measure of sleep propensity in healthy subjects of different ages showed that older adults (age 66–83 years) had a decreased sleep propensity, possibly related to a weakened homeostatic drive to sleep [3]. It is reasonable to conclude that excessive daytime sleepiness in older people may be due to comorbidities rather than being part of the natural aging process.

It is not clear whether changes in sleep with age are due to a decreased ability to sleep or a decreased need to sleep. However, there are several lines of evidence that suggest that short sleep duration and disturbed sleep are associated with adverse health and cognitive outcomes. Decreased sleep efficiency and higher amount of wake after sleep onset have been associated with greater cognitive decline in older people. There is emerging evidence that sleep disruption is associated with β-amyloid (Aβ) protein accumulation and tau neurofibrillary tangles that are characteristic of Alzheimer's disease (AD). Experimental evidence in animal models has shown that sleep plays a crucial role in the clearance of Aβ through the glymphatic system [4]. Aβ cerebrospinal fluid levels have been associated with poor sleep efficiency and increased napping [5]. Excessive daytime sleepiness has been longitudinally associated with the development of Aβ positivity [6, 7]. There is preliminary evidence that acute sleep deprivation can increase Aβ deposition in healthy adults [8]. These findings support a hypothesis that sleep disruption with aging may lead to a decline in cognitive function by promoting the deposition of pathological proteins. However, most of the data are still cross-sectional in nature. Since neuronal systems in the brain crucial to sleep-wake homeostasis are impacted by deposition of these abnormal proteins, it is reasonable to conclude that these pathological changes may be a cause of sleep disruption and excessive daytime sleepiness (EDS) [1]. It is reasonable to conclude that there is likely a bidirectional relationship between sleep disturbance and neurodegenerative disease.

Sleep and sleep disruption have an impact on the body as well as the brain. Numerous prospective studies have shown a U-shaped relationship between sleep duration and mortality, with both short and long sleep durations conferring an increased risk of death [9]. Whether short or long sleep directly causes excess death is difficult to prove given all of the potential confounders, despite attempts to mathematically control for known comorbidities. Sleep may be short or long due to known or unknown health factors. However, there is strong evidence that sleep quality and quantity are associated with overall health. Changes in sleep stage distribution with age may contribute to the age-related changes in metabolism. N3 sleep is associated with growth hormone secretion. The reduction in N3 sleep with aging may be partly responsible for the decrease in growth hormone in older men [10]. Sleep deficiencies have also been linked to metabolic dysregulation that may contribute to diseases that impact healthy aging such as obesity and diabetes [11]. Given the link between insufficient and fragmented sleep on quality of life and health outcomes, there is a need for awareness, evaluation, and treatment of the sleep disorders that commonly affect older adults.

Sleep-Disordered Breathing

Sleep-disordered breathing comprises both obstructive and central sleep apnea syndromes. Obstructive sleep apnea (OSA) occurs when the airway is obstructed during sleep, which is determined by the persistence of respiratory effort during the apneas on a sleep study. If there are no detectable efforts during the apneas, the disorder is classified as central sleep apnea (CSA) because there is a momentary defect in the central control of breathing. Approximately 40% of adults who have CSA have Cheyne-Stokes respiration (CSR), which is a periodic cycling between hypoventilation and hyperventilation [12]. Congestive heart failure is the most commonly recognized cause of CSA and is associated with CSR. Other common causes of CSA include cerebrovascular accidents, chronic kidney disease, atrial fibrillation, and opioid use. OSA is by far the most common sleep-related breathing disorder; however there can be overlap between obstructive and central sleep apnea. The consequences of respiratory events during sleep include arousals from sleep and cyclical drops in the blood oxygen level. This ultimately leads to sleep fragmentation and nocturnal hypoxemia, which may lead to insomnia symptoms, excessive daytime sleepiness and may have potential health consequences.

Many of the risk factors for OSA increase with age. Estimates of the prevalence of OSA have varied widely and are dependent on the populations studied. Results from a US cohort studied between 2007 and 2010 have estimated moderate to severe OSA to occur in 6% of women and 13% of men between ages 30 and 70 years [13]. Evidence suggests that OSA is underdiagnosed in the general population, particularly in women. Less is known about the epidemiology of OSA in an older population; there is a suggestion that the risk of OSA increases with advancing age until 70 years after which there is a plateau [14]. Male gender is clearly a risk factor for OSA. However, this gender gap lessens significantly after menopause in women.

The risk of having CSA also increases with older age. CSA has been found to be 2–3 times more common in people aged 65–90 than in those aged 39–64 years. This is likely due to the increased prevalence of conditions associated with CSA such as congestive heart failure, atrial fibrillation, chronic kidney disease, and chronic pain syndromes treated with opioids [12]. For instance, it is estimated that upward of 50% of patients with stable heart failure have some form of sleep-disordered breathing (SDB). The majority of these patients have a form of CSA; however, many have OSA or a combination of the two disorders.

The major symptoms of OSA include excessive daytime sleepiness, sleep disruption, and snoring. The classic patient with OSA is an obese male with snoring, gasping, and daytime sleepiness. However, these associations are less predictive in an older population. Other important symptoms of SDB include nocturia, insomnia, morning headaches, nocturnal confusion, and daytime impairments in mood and cognition. Snoring is indicative of a partially collapsed airway and is a useful predictor of the presence of OSA or future development of the condition. The lack of classic symptoms and findings should not preclude further evaluation for OSA, particularly in older patients.

The primary modalities for testing for OSA include an in-laboratory attended polysomnogram (PSG) or a home sleep apnea test (HSAT). PSG is generally considered the gold standard for the diagnosis of OSA; however HSAT has been shown to be a reasonable diagnostic modality in patients with symptoms suggestive of moderate to severe OSA without significant comorbidities [15]. HSAT can be performed at much lower costs than PSG, which can dramatically improve access to OSA testing, and some patients may be more comfortable sleeping at home than in a sleep laboratory. In an older population, there are concerns that the usability of the

HSAT equipment may be compromised by impairments in dexterity or cognition. One study showed that self-assembled HSAT combined with symptoms was able to accurately diagnose OSA in an older patient population [16]. A smaller study also showed a high degree of correlation between HSAT and PSG in older patients [17]. However, HSAT in older populations appears to be an area that has been understudied.

Continuous positive airway pressure (CPAP) therapy is the gold standard treatment for OSA. CPAP devices essentially use air to stent open the upper airway in order to combat airway obstruction. The vast majority of trials of CPAP therapy have focused on patients who are middle-aged. Only recently have there been randomized controlled trials focused on CPAP therapy in older individuals. The PREDICT trial comprised of 231 patients and found that CPAP improved subjective sleepiness and was cost-effective in patients aged greater than 65 years [18]. A similarly sized study in Spain among patients with severe OSA over the age of 70 years found that CPAP improved quality of life, mood, and some indices of neurocognitive function [19]. A smaller pilot study found that CPAP improved episodic and short-term memory as well as executive functioning with a suggestion of increased connectivity on neuroimaging [20]. A larger study to extrapolate these results to moderate OSA failed to show the same neurocognitive benefits but did show that sleepiness and quality of life were improved on CPAP in those older than 70 years of age [21]. Observational studies have suggested that CPAP is well-tolerated and may have a mortality benefit in older patients including in those over the age of 80 [22]. Studies on whether CPAP adherence is better or worse in an older population have had mixed results, and any changes in CPAP adherence with age may be due to factors other than advancing age [23]. CPAP has been found to be well-tolerated and beneficial in patients with mild to moderate Alzheimer's disease [24]. Age alone should not be a barrier to the testing for and treatment of OSA. Even the presence of dementia should not preclude using CPAP for OSA.

The impact of the treatment of OSA on cardiovascular outcomes has shown mixed results, with observational studies generally showing benefit of CPAP in reducing cerebrovascular events, while randomized controlled trials have largely been negative. The observational studies have shown stronger links between OSA and stroke than between OSA and coronary events [25]. It is hypothesized that those with severe OSA who survive to older age may have ischemic preconditioning of the heart protecting them to some extent from myocardial infarction. One large randomized controlled trial of 2717 patients aged 45 to 75 years followed on average for 3.7 years showed no reduction in cardiovascular events with CPAP therapy [26]. A meta-analysis of studies including this one also showed no cardiovascular benefit in largely middle-aged patients [27]. The major limitation of these studies is that adherence to CPAP was fairly low among participants. Furthermore, significant excessive daytime somnolence was an exclusion criterion in many studies. In a population of older adults, the diagnosis and treatment of OSA may not be a potent strategy to reduce cardiovascular events relative to other strategies, particularly in the absence of excessive daytime sleepiness. However, in an individual who is adherent to therapy, CPAP may confer some cardiovascular benefit although this remains unproven.

Oral appliances that shift the jaw forward (mandibular advancement or mandibular repositioning devices) are a viable treatment alternative to positive airway pressure for many patients with OSA. The principle behind this therapy is that moving the jaw forward pulls the tongue away from the oropharynx, which may also beneficially reconfigure the soft palate. The American Academy of Sleep Medicine recommends the use of oral appliances, rather than no treatment, for those who are intolerant of CPAP therapy or who have a strong preference for an alternative to PAP therapy [28]. It is generally thought that oral appliances are more effective in those with mild OSA; however there is not strong data to support this assumption. If adherence to oral appliance therapy were higher, this would mitigate the fact that reduction in AHI is generally less than the reduction achieved with PAP. Oral appliances generally require good dentition to hold the device in place, which would present a barrier to use in individuals missing teeth or who require dentures. Oral appliance therapy specifically in older patients has not been studied extensively. One small postal study in older veterans showed that only one-third were confident in the use of the device and felt that it was an effective treatment [29].

As previously discussed, CSA syndromes are increasingly common in older patients. CSAs can sometimes be treated with CPAP, but more advanced bilevel modalities such as adaptive servoventilation (ASV) are sometimes also used to treat CSA. ASV treats CSA by increasing ventilatory support during hypopneas, breathing for the patient during apneas, but decreasing ventilatory support during periods of excessive ventilation. This helps "smooth out" the overall breathing pattern. The SERVE-HF trial revealed significant safety concerns for the use of ASV in CSA among patients with symptomatic heart failure and a reduced ejection fraction (EF) ($\leq$ 45%), where the ASV group had an increased all-cause and cardiac mortality [30]. ASV is therefore not recommended to be used in the presence of reduced systolic function. It is still considered a therapeutic option in patients who have CSA due to heart failure with a preserved EF or from other causes. A review looking at the efficacy of ASV in older patients with central or combined central and obstructive sleep apnea in patients with preserved EF was only able to identify 6 studies with sample sizes ranging from 45 to 126 patients and mean ages in the mid to late 60s [31]. These studies demonstrated an improvement in sleep-related symptoms and daytime functional status. ASV use for CSA not due to heart failure does not seem to have been systematically studied in older patients. In general, ASV is an option in older patients with CSA who do not respond to CPAP alone; however long-term benefits have not been established.

Insomnia

Insomnia is a highly prevalent sleep disorder with advanced age, affecting 30–48% of older adults [32]. This high prevalence may be related to age-related changes in sleep and the accumulation of comorbidities and medications with older age that are associated with insomnia. In addition, the higher prevalence of insomnia in women compared to men seen in younger adults appears to continue into old age, with a meta-analysis showing that the greater relative risk of insomnia in women compared with men increases with age, from 1.28 in young adults to 1.73 in those aged 65 years and older [33]. Several epidemiologic studies have linked sleep disturbances to worse health-related quality of life, nursing-home placement, and even death in older people [32]. Late-life insomnia is often a chronic problem, and without treatment, symptoms often persist for years.

Several age-related changes in sleep may contribute to insomnia in older adults. Common changes include a decreased sleep efficiency (time spent asleep divided by total time spent in bed), decreased total sleep time, and increased sleep latency (time to fall asleep). An earlier bedtime and earlier morning awakening, more awakenings, more total wakefulness during the night, and more daytime napping are also common. As described above, older age, especially among men, is associated with less N3 sleep, whereas the percentage of stages N1 and N2 increases with age [34]. Many age-related changes in sleep occur by middle age, with sleep parameters remaining relatively stable among healthy people after age 60 [34]. There is some question of the clinical significance of these age-related changes in sleep in healthy people. For example, with sleep deprivation, older adults may actually show less daytime sleepiness, less evidence of decline in performance measures, and a quicker recovery than younger adults [35]. In studies comparing good sleepers with poor sleepers, poor sleepers were found to take more medications, make more clinician visits, and have poorer self-ratings of health, suggesting that some age-related changes in sleep may reflect poor health, rather than aging per se.

Many comorbidities and medications are associated with insomnia in older adults. Depression is perhaps the most common and strongly associated psychiatric comorbidity associated with insomnia in older people [36]. Anxiety is also a common risk factor for developing insomnia. Many medical conditions that are common in older adults also contribute to insomnia. For example, the prevalence of insomnia is higher in individuals with hypertension, heart disease, arthritis, lung disease, gastrointestinal reflux, stroke, and neurodegenerative disorders. Symptoms such as pain, paresthesia, cough, dyspnea, gastroesophageal reflux, and nocturia also contribute to insomnia. Medications can also impair sleep or alter sleep architecture. Sleep can be disturbed if stimulating medications (e.g., caffeine, sympathomimetics, bronchodilators, activating psychiatric medications) are taken too near to bedtime, and sedating medications taken during the daytime can lead to more daytime sleeping and a decrease in nighttime sleep drive. Caregiving for others (such as loved ones with dementia) is also a common factor contributing to insomnia in older adults [37].

PSG is not routinely indicated in the evaluation of older patients presenting with insomnia, unless another comorbid sleep condition is suspected or the patient has not responded to first-line therapy for insomnia disorder [38]. Sleep diaries with daily entries over 1 to 2 weeks can be very helpful in determining the severity of the insomnia as well as identifying possible perpetuating factors such as extended daytime napping or irregular bedtimes. Wrist actigraphy in conjunction with a sleep diary can be used to obtain a more objective measure of the patient's overall sleep-wake pattern, and use of actigraphy has been recommended in patients with insomnia when objective estimates of sleep parameters will aid clinical decision-making [39]. Wrist actigraphy can also be used in identifying circadian rhythm disorders and for use in nursing-home residents unable to complete detailed sleep diaries and for whom other forms of sleep monitoring (e.g., PSG) can be difficult to obtain.

Behavioral therapies, particularly cognitive-behavioral therapy for insomnia, CBT-I, are recommended as first-line treatments for insomnia in all adults [40]. Evidence for use of behavioral treatments is particularly compelling in older adults where the potential adverse effects of sedative-hypnotic medications are particularly worrisome, such as increased risk of falls and fractures and increased risk of cognitive decline. In addition to low likelihood of adverse effects, behavioral treatments are preferred by most patients and have better long-term efficacy than sedative-hypnotics [41]. Behavioral therapies for insomnia have also been demonstrated to be effective in older adults with comorbid conditions, such as depression.

Several randomized trials and systematic reviews provide strong evidence for CBT-I [38, 40, 42], including among older adults [43]. CBT-I may include stimulus control, sleep restriction, and cognitive therapy, often with other components such as sleep hygiene and relaxation techniques [44]. Stimulus control is designed to break the negative associations patients have with their sleep environment, which have come about from maladaptive behaviors. Examples of stimulus control include using the bed for sleep or intercourse, only, and to only go to bed when tired enough to fall asleep. Sleep restriction limits the amount of time the patient spends in bed, usually guided by their actual sleep time from the sleep diary, to help the patient fall asleep more quickly and have more consolidated sleep. Cognitive therapy addresses the maladaptive thoughts or dysfunctional beliefs patients have about their sleep. Sleep hygiene is also commonly provided, including education on general guidelines to maintain a healthy sleep-wake routine. Other components of CBT-I may include various relaxation techniques, scheduled worry time during the day, and other interventions. These components can be used with older adults, sometimes with adaptations for safety, including developing alternatives to getting out of bed at night for those at high risk for falls.

CBT-I has reliably been shown to improve sleep efficiency, decrease nighttime wakefulness, and increase satisfaction with sleep [38, 40, 42]. In trials comparing CBT-I with a prescription sedative-hypnotic agent, participants reported better improvement in sleep and more satisfaction with the CBT-I therapy [45]. As noted above, studies that compare CBT-I with pharmacologic therapy typically show that the improvements with CBT-I are more sustained. In addition, newer delivery models that involve the use of the Internet and/or phone applications [46], nonspecialist providers [43], and telehealth-based CBT-I have demonstrated evidence for effectiveness, suggesting a variety of options may be used to provide this therapy to older people.

Studies have found variable effects of bright light, either provided from natural sunlight or light boxes, on insomnia symptoms in older adults [47, 48]. Effects of bright light on circadian rhythm problems are more clearly established [49]. For example, light therapy has been recommended in adults with an advanced sleep phase and in older adults with dementia [49]. Evidence suggests that aerobic exercise (combined with sleep hygiene education) improves sleep in older adults with insomnia [50]. Tai chi has also been demonstrated to improve sleep quality in individuals with insomnia, including older adults [51].

In general, older adults are more likely than younger adults to experience adverse side effects of sedative-hypnotics, such as an increased risk of falls and fractures, and cognitive decline. In one meta-analysis of sedative-hypnotics in older adults with insomnia, the number of individuals needed to treat for improved sleep quality was more than twice as high as the number needed to harm for any adverse event, suggesting these agents were more likely to cause harm than benefit [52]. If a sedative-hypnotic is used in an older adult, the smallest dose of the agent with the least risk of adverse events should be chosen for the shortest duration necessary.

Benzodiazepines bind nonselectively to the gamma-aminobutyric-acid-benzodiazepine (GABA-A) receptor subunits, resulting in sedative, anxiolytic, and amnestic effects. Temazepam, lorazepam, and estazolam are intermediate-acting benzodiazepines that are most commonly used for insomnia; triazolam is a shorter-acting agent that is also used for insomnia. Longer-acting benzodiazepines (e.g., flurazepam, quazepam) should not be used in older adults due to a long half-life that can result in significant daytime effects. In addition to falls and fracture, other side effects associated with benzodiazepines in older adults include confusion, rebound insomnia, tolerance, and withdrawal symptoms on discontinuation [53]. There is also evidence for an increased risk of pneumonia in older people with Alzheimer's disease [54]. These agents are all on the Beer's list of potentially inappropriate medications for older adults [55].

Nonbenzodiazepine-benzodiazepine receptor agonists (NBRAs, e.g., zolpidem, zaleplon, eszopiclone) bind selectively to the GABA-type A receptors and generally produce sedation and amnestic effects without the anxiolytic properties. These agents likely have similar efficacy to benzodiazepines but with a somewhat better side effect profile, in part due to their relatively short duration of action. Zolpidem and zaleplon should only be taken immediately before bed because of their rapid onset of action. Eszopiclone has a longer duration of action than the other NRBAs and is better for sleep maintenance but may cause drowsiness in the morning. Evidence suggests that the NBRAs also increase risk of falls and fractures in older adults [56]. The emergence of complex sleep-related behaviors such as sleep driving and sleep eating that has been reported with NBRAs [57] has led to a black box warning for these agents. NBRAs are also all included on the Beer's list of potentially inappropriate medications for older adults [55].

Melatonin receptor agonists (e.g., ramelteon) act at MT1/MT2 melatonin receptors. Ramelteon has been shown to reduce self-reported sleep latency in older adults [58], with few side effects, but somnolence, dizziness, headache, and fatigue can occur. Evidence suggests ramelteon does not lead to significant rebound insomnia or withdrawal effects [58].

Other agents are available for treatment of insomnia. The tricyclic antidepressant doxepin is available in an ultralow-dose formulation (3–6 mg) that selectively antagonizes H1 receptors, which is believed to have sleep-promoting effects. Data suggest that this low-dose doxepin does not have more significant anticholinergic side effects compared to placebo [59]. A newer class of medications that antagonize the orexin system has been developed. These dual orexin receptor antagonists include suvorexant and lemborexant. A trial of 277 participants with mild to moderate probable Alzheimer's disease showed an improvement in polysomnographic total sleep time of 28 minutes with suvorexant. There were increases in daytime sleepiness but no apparent changes in cognitive function testing [60]. Low-dose trazodone has also been used for insomnia, with some evidence for effectiveness in decreasing sleep latency and increasing sleep duration; the most common side effects appear to be daytime sleepiness, headache, and orthostatic hypotension [61]. There is a lack of evidence to support use of atypical antipsychotics for insomnia in the absence of other serious psychiatric illness and significant concern for harm [62].

Almost half of all older adults report the use of nonprescription over-the-counter (OTC) sleeping agents, commonly sedating antihistamines, melatonin, or herbal products. The sedating antihistamines (e.g., diphenhydramine) are the most common ingredients in OTC drugs marketed for sleep [63]. Diphenhydramine is sedating through its potent anticholinergic effect and tolerance to its sedating effect develops rapidly. The long half-life of diphenhydramine may result in next-day sedation. Side effects can be quite problematic in older adults (e.g., dry mouth, urinary retention, delirium, decreased cognition, constipation, increased ocular pressure), so diphenhydramine is not recommended for insomnia in older patients. Other supplements are available OTC, such as melatonin and valerian, but recent guidelines do not recommend use of these agents for insomnia [64].

Restless Legs Syndrome/Periodic Leg Movements

Restless legs syndrome (RLS) is defined by the urge to move one's legs. The other defining features of RLS are an improvement with movement, worsening with relaxation, and an evening onset. More rarely RLS can also affect and may even be limited to the arms. This urge to move is often described as an uncomfortable sensation in the limbs. The prevalence of RLS does increase with age with up to an 8% prevalence in older patients [65]. A similar prevalence has been found in patients with cognitive impairment and dementia [66]. The pathophysiology of RLS is thought to involve low levels of iron stores in the brain. Increasing prevalence of iron deficiency may in part explain why older patients have an increase in RLS symptoms. Other comorbidities such as chronic kidney disease, neuropathy, and the use of antidepressants and neuroleptics are also associated with RLS [67]. The accrual of these comorbidities may explain why RLS is more common in older patients. In older individuals it is difficult to distinguish "primary RLS," i.e., RLS without comorbidities, from comorbid RLS.

The diagnosis of RLS is made solely on clinical evaluation. The International Classification of Sleep Disorders-Third Edition (ICSD-3) recommends that the diagnosis be based on an urge to move the legs that worsens during rest, is at least partially relieved by movement, and occurs most predominately in the evening [68]. The presence of periodic leg movements can help support the diagnosis of RLS. The diagnosis is challenging in older patients due to the need to rule out other conditions such as neuropathy and radiculopathy. Patients may attribute complaints about their legs to leg cramps, edema, and arthritis which are all prevalent in older individuals. Another challenge is that patients with significant cognitive impairment may have difficulty describing their symptoms. It has been suggested that behaviors such as rubbing or kneading the legs be considered as evidence for RLS in patients with dementia. Excessive motor activity such as pacing, kicking, rubbing feet together, foot tapping, and cycling movements can all be used as signs of RLS [69]. This approach was used to create an instrument validated in cognitively intact patients with and without RLS. Using iron deficiency, symptom of discomfort in legs and a behavioral observational tool among other factors can be used to predict the presence of RLS [70].

The presence of RLS in older patients may adversely impact their quality of life. The presence of RLS was found to be associated with a subsequent decline in physical function [71]. Severity of RLS has been linked to decreased quality of life scores, including daily and social functioning [72]. Abnormal nocturnal behaviors are a risk factor for the institutionalization of patients with dementia. It stands to reason that a condition causing the urge to walk around at night could worsen such behaviors and contribute to a risk of falls. Indeed, in 1 study in a sample of 59 patients, probable RLS was found to predict nocturnal agitation behaviors along with OSA [73]. There has been a link between RLS symptoms in patients with dementia and the presence of apathy, which is hypothesized as due to a common problem in the dopaminergic system [74].

Periodic leg movements of sleep (PLMS) are stereotypical extensions of the great toe with dorsiflexion of the ankle occasionally including flexions of the knee and hip that occur repeatedly. PLMS have been shown to increase substantially with age in healthy adults [75]. In healthy individuals it is controversial what the impact of PLMS have on sleep. PLMS have been correlated with increased nocturnal blood pressure, autonomic activity, and incident cardiovascular disease [76]. The diagnosis of periodic limb movement disorder (PLMD) requires a frequency of at least 15 leg movements per hour and that the patient have sleep disturbance or impaired daytime functioning that is not better explained by another current sleep disorder [68]. Therefore, patients who have RLS by definition cannot have PLMD. Also, other medical or neurologic disorders have to be excluded as the cause of the patients' symptoms in order to make a PLMD diagnosis. Given that comorbidities are common in older adults, it can be challenging to diagnose PLMD in this population.

The treatments for RLS and PLMD are similar. The first step of therapy is to ensure adequate iron stores. Iron supplementation should be given if the ferritin level is below 75 ng/ml. Supplemental iron has been found to be an effective therapy for RLS without significant adverse effects [77]. The mainstay of pharmacologic therapy has traditionally been non-ergot dopamine agonists such as ropinirole and pramipexole. These therapies have been effective for the treatment of RLS symptoms, but are not without potential side effects, such as sleep attacks and gastrointestinal side effects. The most worrisome side effects of these agents include behavioral disinhibition such as impulsive gambling. It would stand to reason that older adults may have more difficulty tolerating these agents. However, a study of patients treated with this class of medication in those with Parkinson's disease did not find a significant difference in tolerability between older and younger patients, with 90% tolerating this therapy [78]. Another potential adverse outcome stemming from the use of dopaminergic therapy is the risk for augmentation, which is an earlier timing of symptoms, spread of symptoms to previously unaffected limbs, and/or increased intensity of symptoms. Augmentation is thought to occur at around 9% per year among patients on pramipexole [79]. Many experts feel that this is an unacceptable risk of augmentation and suggest that an alternative class of therapeutic agents should be considered for first-line therapy.

The major alternative class of therapeutic agents are the alpha-2-delta calcium channel ligands such as gabapentin and pregabalin. Of these agents only gabapentin enacarbil is FDA approved for the treatment of RLS. There is strong evidence that pregabalin is as effective as dopamine agonists and confers a decreased risk for augmentation [80]. As with many drugs in older people, these agents should be used with caution since there is significant variability in the pharmacokinetics of drugs such as gabapentin, in part due to changes in renal function [81]. The accumulation of these medications can theoretically cause somnolence, dizziness, and gastrointestinal disturbances. However, the safety and efficacy of these medications in an older patient population for RLS have not been specifically studied.

Opioids can be an effective therapy for the treatment of refractory RLS [69]. However, this class of medications comes with significant safety concerns including constipation, somnolence, impaired cognition, and a potential for drug overdose. The American Geriatrics Society recommends avoidance of opioids in combination with other central nervous system depressants in older adults and in those with a history of falls [55].

Non-pharmacologic therapies should also be considered in the treatment of RLS. The majority of non-pharmacologic advice is the recommendation that patients avoid substances that provoke RLS symptoms. Such exacerbating factors include antidepressants, alcohol, caffeine, and sleep deprivation. Alternative therapies that include exercise, massage, transcutaneous stimulation, pneumatic compression, and yoga have been shown to have benefit in low-quality studies [82]. Additional controlled trials on alternative or complementary therapies for RLS in older adults are needed.

REM Sleep Behavior Disorder

REM sleep behavior disorder (RBD) involves dream enactment behavior with a failure to inhibit muscle tone as normally occurs during REM sleep. RBD can potentially cause injury to the patient or a bed partner due to acting out dream actions such as punching, kicking, or running while unconscious. The prevalence of RBD in adults over the age of 40 has been estimated to be around 1% [83]. Clinical samples of patients have shown that patients typically present for evaluation of RBD in their mid-60s while having had approximately 5 years of symptoms [84]. Indeed, the prevalence of RBD was found to be 2% among those older than 60 years [85]. Therefore, RBD is essentially a disease of aging.

This strong predilection for older adults is likely due to the connection of RBD to neurodegenerative disorders of aging, in particular alpha-synucleinopathies [86]. There is a high prevalence of RBD in those with Parkinson's disease, Lewy body dementia, and multisystem atrophy. However, RBD may be a precursor to the development of these disorders. Over the course of 15 to 20 years of observation, up to 90% of patients with RBD will ultimately develop a neurodegenerative disorder associated with alpha-synuclein [87]. It is thought that this relationship is due to a shared pathophysiology with early deposition of alpha-synuclein in areas of the brain stem that inhibit muscle tone during REM sleep.

The diagnosis of RBD requires both a history of dream enactment and findings of abnormally increased muscle tone during REM sleep during polysomnography making it the only parasomnia that explicitly requires confirmatory findings on PSG to make a diagnosis [67]. Conditions that confound the diagnosis of RBD are significant sleep-disordered breathing and PTSD, which can both present with apparent dream enactment behavior. There is some evidence that REM sleep tone is also increased in sufferers of PTSD making the distinction diagnostically challenging. There is also further evidence that the presence of PTSD may be a risk factor in the development of RBD [88].

The primary goal of treating RBD is to avoid nocturnal injury and to prevent sleep disruption. The first priority should be to ensure that the patient is sleeping in a safe environment and that they are not a danger to themselves or others. The two major pharmacological treatments of RBD are low-dose clonazepam and melatonin. In older patients it is preferable to avoid benzodiazepines when possible making melatonin the primary first choice for therapy. There is evidence from small randomized trials and two retrospective studies that melatonin reduces both REM sleep without atonia and the clinical manifestations of RBD [89]. The mechanism of action for melatonin in RBD is not known. Often very high doses (up to 18 mg) of melatonin are sometimes required. Clonazepam also has evidence from case series at improving RBD behaviors; however caution must be used in those with dementia or gait instability [90]. A single-center retrospective review of RBD patient experiences with melatonin and clonazepam showed that both medications improved dream enactment behaviors. However, only melatonin was associated with reduced injuries and falls, while clonazepam was associated with increased adverse effects such as sleepiness, unsteadiness, dizziness, and trouble thinking [91].

Sleep Disturbance among Residents in Long-Term Care Settings

Sleep problems are common among older people in long-term care settings, such as nursing homes (NHs) [92]. Many older NH residents have an irregular sleep-wake rhythm, with fragmented nighttime sleep and excessive daytime napping [93]. In addition to older age, other common factors associated with poor sleep in these residents include medical and psychiatric comorbidities, polypharmacy, a disruptive nighttime environment, limited physical activity and lack of exposure to bright light during the daytime, and increased time spent in bed during the day. Sleep disturbance in NH residents is associated with lower quality of life, less involvement in social activities, and other adverse consequences. Evidence suggests that sleep disturbance in NH residents is also associated with distress in NH staff, resident agitation, and prescription of psychotropic medications [94]. In addition to identifying and treating primary sleep disorders, the management of sleep disturbance in NH residents usually requires a multidimensional treatment approach to improve the nighttime sleeping environment and increase daytime physical activity (as appropriate) as well as bright light exposure. A recent meta-analysis suggested the most promising approaches were increased daytime light exposure, nighttime use of melatonin, and acupressure [95]. Sedating medications may have limited benefit in improving sleep of NH home residents, particularly given the complex factors in metabolism of these drugs in frail older adults and adverse consequences, including increased risk of hip fracture [96].

References

1. Mander BA, Winer JR, Walker MP. Sleep and Human Aging. Neuron. 2017;94(1):19–36.
2. Foley DJ, Vitiello MV, Bliwise DL, Ancoli-Israel S, Monjan AA, Walsh JK. Frequent napping is associated with excessive daytime sleepiness, depression, pain, and nocturia in older adults: findings from the National Sleep Foundation '2003 sleep in America' poll. Am J Geriatr Psychiatry. 2007;15(4):344–50.
3. Dijk DJ, Groeger JA, Stanley N, Deacon S. Age-related reduction in daytime sleep propensity and nocturnal slow wave sleep. Sleep. 2010;33(2):211–23.
4. Xie L, Kang H, Xu Q, Chen MJ, Liao Y, Thiyagarajan M, et al. Sleep drives metabolite clearance from the adult brain. Science. 2013;342(6156):373–7.
5. Ju YE, McLeland JS, Toedebusch CD, Xiong C, Fagan AM, Duntley SP, et al. Sleep quality and preclinical Alzheimer disease. JAMA Neurol. 2013;70(5):587–93.

6. Spira AP, An Y, Wu MN, Owusu JT, Simonsick EM, Bilgel M, et al. Excessive daytime sleepiness and napping in cognitively normal adults: associations with subsequent amyloid deposition measured by PiB PET. Sleep. 2018;41(12).
7. Carvalho DZ, St Louis EK, Knopman DS, Boeve BF, Lowe VJ, Roberts RO, et al. Association of Excessive Daytime Sleepiness with Longitudinal β-amyloid accumulation in elderly persons without dementia. JAMA Neurol. 2018;75(6):672–80.
8. Shokri-Kojori E, Wang GJ, Wiers CE, Demiral SB, Guo M, Kim SW, et al. β-Amyloid accumulation in the human brain after one night of sleep deprivation. Proc Natl Acad Sci U S A. 2018;115(17):4483–8.
9. Kripke DF, Langer RD, Elliott JA, Klauber MR, Rex KM. Mortality related to actigraphic long and short sleep. Sleep Med. 2011;12(1):28–33.
10. Van Cauter E, Leproult R, Plat L. Age-related changes in slow wave sleep and REM sleep and relationship with growth hormone and cortisol levels in healthy men. JAMA. 2000;284(7):861–8.
11. Van Cauter E, Spiegel K, Tasali E, Leproult R. Metabolic consequences of sleep and sleep loss. Sleep Med. 2008;9(Suppl 1):S23–8.
12. Donovan LM, Kapur VK. Prevalence and characteristics of central compared to obstructive sleep apnea: analyses from the sleep heart health study cohort. Sleep. 2016;39(7):1353–9.
13. Peppard PE, Young T, Barnet JH, Palta M, Hagen EW, Hla KM. Increased prevalence of sleep-disordered breathing in adults. Am J Epidemiol. 2013;177(9):1006–14.
14. Young T, Shahar E, Nieto FJ, Redline S, Newman AB, Gottlieb DJ, et al. Predictors of sleep-disordered breathing in community-dwelling adults: the sleep heart health study. Arch Intern Med. 2002;162(8):893–900.
15. Kapur VK, Auckley DH, Chowdhuri S, Kuhlmann DC, Mehra R, Ramar K, et al. Clinical practice guideline for diagnostic testing for adult obstructive sleep apnea: An American Academy of sleep medicine clinical practice guideline. J Clin Sleep Med. 2017;13(3):479–504.
16. Morales CR, Hurley S, Wick LC, Staley B, Pack FM, Gooneratne NS, et al. In-home, self-assembled sleep studies are useful in diagnosing sleep apnea in the elderly. Sleep. 2012;35(11):1491–501.
17. Polese JF, Santos-Silva R, de Oliveira Ferrari PM, Sartori DE, Tufik S, Bittencourt L. Is portable monitoring for diagnosing obstructive sleep apnea syndrome suitable in elderly population? Sleep Breath. 2013;17(2):679–86.
18. McMillan A, Bratton DJ, Faria R, Laskawiec-Szkonter M, Griffin S, Davies RJ, et al. Continuous positive airway pressure in older people with obstructive sleep apnoea syndrome (PREDICT): a 12-month, multicentre, randomised trial. Lancet Respir Med. 2014;2(10):804–12.
19. Martínez-García M, Chiner E, Hernández L, Cortes JP, Catalán P, Ponce S, et al. Obstructive sleep apnoea in the elderly: role of continuous positive airway pressure treatment. Eur Respir J. 2015;46(1):142–51.
20. Dalmases M, Solé-Padullés C, Torres M, Embid C, Nuñez MD, Martínez-Garcia M, et al. Effect of CPAP on cognition, brain function, and structure among elderly patients with OSA: a randomized pilot study. Chest. 2015;148(5):1214–23.
21. Ponce S, Pastor E, Orosa B, Oscullo G, Catalán P, Martinez A, et al. The role of CPAP treatment in elderly patients with moderate obstructive sleep apnoea: a multicentre randomised controlled trial. Eur Respir J. 2019;54(2).
22. López-Padilla D, Alonso-Moralejo R, Martínez-García M, De la Torre CS. Díaz de Atauri MJ. Continuous positive airway pressure and survival of very elderly persons with moderate to severe obstructive sleep apnea. Sleep Med. 2016;19:23–9.
23. Sawyer AM, Gooneratne NS, Marcus CL, Ofer D, Richards KC, Weaver TE. A systematic review of CPAP adherence across age groups: clinical and empiric insights for developing CPAP adherence interventions. Sleep Med Rev. 2011;15(6):343–56.
24. Chong MS, Ayalon L, Marler M, Loredo JS, Corey-Bloom J, Palmer BW, et al. Continuous positive airway pressure reduces subjective daytime sleepiness in patients with mild to moderate Alzheimer's disease with sleep disordered breathing. J Am Geriatr Soc. 2006;54(5):777–81.

25. Posadas T, Oscullo G, Zaldívar E, Garcia-Ortega A, Gómez-Olivas JD, Monteagudo M, et al. Treatment with CPAP in elderly patients with obstructive sleep apnoea. J Clin Med. 2020;9(2).
26. McEvoy RD, Antic NA, Heeley E, Luo Y, Ou Q, Zhang X, et al. CPAP for prevention of cardiovascular events in obstructive sleep apnea. N Engl J Med. 2016;375(10):919–31.
27. Yu J, Zhou Z, McEvoy RD, Anderson CS, Rodgers A, Perkovic V, et al. Association of Positive Airway Pressure with Cardiovascular Events and Death in adults with sleep apnea: a systematic review and meta-analysis. JAMA. 2017;318(2):156–66.
28. Ramar K, Dort LC, Katz SG, Lettieri CJ, Harrod CG, Thomas SM, et al. Clinical practice guideline for the treatment of obstructive sleep apnea and snoring with Oral appliance therapy: An update for 2015. J Clin Sleep Med. 2015;11(7):773–827.
29. Carballo NJ, Alessi CA, Martin JL, Mitchell MN, Hays RD, Col N, et al. Perceived effectiveness, self-efficacy, and social support for Oral appliance therapy among older veterans with obstructive sleep apnea. Clin Ther. 2016;38(11):2407–15.
30. Cowie MR, Woehrle H, Wegscheider K, Angermann C, d'Ortho MP, Erdmann E, et al. Adaptive servo-ventilation for central sleep apnea in systolic heart failure. N Engl J Med. 2015;373(12):1095–105.
31. Baniak LM, Chasens ER. Sleep disordered breathing in older adults with heart failure with preserved ejection fraction. Geriatr Nurs. 2018;39(1):77–83.
32. Patel D, Steinberg J, Patel P. Insomnia in the elderly: a review. J Clin Sleep Med. 2018;14(6):1017–24.
33. Zhang B, Wing YK. Sex differences in insomnia: a meta-analysis. Sleep. 2006;29(1):85–93.
34. Edwards BA, O'Driscoll DM, Ali A, Jordan AS, Trinder J, Malhotra A. Aging and sleep: physiology and pathophysiology. Semin Respir Crit Care Med. 2010;31(5):618–33.
35. Zitting KM, Münch MY, Cain SW, Wang W, Wong A, Ronda JM, et al. Young adults are more vulnerable to chronic sleep deficiency and recurrent circadian disruption than older adults. Sci Rep. 2018;8(1):11052.
36. Miner B, Gill TM, Yaggi HK, Redeker NS, Van Ness PH, Han L, et al. Insomnia in community-living persons with advanced age. J Am Geriatr Soc. 2018;66(8):1592–7.
37. McCurry SM, Gibbons LE, Logsdon RG, Vitiello MV, Teri L. Insomnia in caregivers of persons with dementia: who is at risk and what can be done about it? Sleep Med Clin. 2009;4(4):519–26.
38. Schutte-Rodin S, Broch L, Buysse D, Dorsey C, Sateia M. Clinical guideline for the evaluation and management of chronic insomnia in adults. J Clin Sleep Med. 2008;4(5):487–504.
39. Smith MT, McCrae CS, Cheung J, Martin JL, Harrod CG, Heald JL, et al. Use of Actigraphy for the evaluation of sleep disorders and circadian rhythm sleep-wake disorders: an American Academy of sleep medicine clinical practice guideline. J Clin Sleep Med. 2018;14(7):1231–7.
40. Qaseem A, Kansagara D, Forciea MA, Cooke M, Denberg TD. Physicians CGCotACo. Management of Chronic Insomnia Disorder in adults: a clinical practice guideline from the American College of Physicians. Ann Intern Med. 2016;165(2):125–33.
41. Belanger L, LeBlanc M, Morin C. Cognitive behavioral therapy for insomnia in older adults. Cognitive Behavioral Practice. 2012;19:101–15.
42. Morin CM, Bootzin RR, Buysse DJ, Edinger JD, Espie CA, Lichstein KL. Psychological and behavioral treatment of insomnia: update of the recent evidence (1998-2004). Sleep. 2006;29(11):1398–414.
43. Alessi C, Martin JL, Fiorentino L, Fung CH, Dzierzewski JM, Rodriguez Tapia JC, et al. Cognitive behavioral therapy for insomnia in older veterans using nonclinician sleep coaches: randomized controlled trial. J Am Geriatr Soc. 2016;64(9):1830–8.
44. Morgenthaler T, Kramer M, Alessi C, Friedman L, Boehlecke B, Brown T, et al. Practice parameters for the psychological and behavioral treatment of insomnia: an update. An American academy of sleep medicine report. Sleep. 2006;29(11):1415–9.
45. Mitchell MD, Gehrman P, Perlis M, Umscheid CA. Comparative effectiveness of cognitive behavioral therapy for insomnia: a systematic review. BMC Fam Pract. 2012;13:40.

46. Zachariae R, Lyby MS, Ritterband LM, O'Toole MS. Efficacy of internet-delivered cognitive-behavioral therapy for insomnia - a systematic review and meta-analysis of randomized controlled trials. Sleep Med Rev. 2016;30:1–10.
47. Friedman L, Zeitzer JM, Kushida C, Zhdanova I, Noda A, Lee T, et al. Scheduled bright light for treatment of insomnia in older adults. J Am Geriatr Soc. 2009;57(3):441–52.
48. Gammack JK. Light therapy for insomnia in older adults. Clin Geriatr Med. 2008;24(1):139–49, viii.
49. Auger RR, Burgess HJ, Emens JS, Deriy LV, Thomas SM, Sharkey KM. Clinical practice guideline for the treatment of intrinsic circadian rhythm sleep-wake disorders: advanced sleep-wake phase disorder (ASWPD), delayed sleep-wake phase disorder (DSWPD), Non-24-hour sleep-wake rhythm disorder (N24SWD), and irregular sleep-wake rhythm disorder (ISWRD). An update for 2015: An American Academy of sleep medicine clinical practice guideline. J Clin Sleep Med. 2015;11(10):1199–236.
50. Reid KJ, Baron KG, Lu B, Naylor E, Wolfe L, Zee PC. Aerobic exercise improves self-reported sleep and quality of life in older adults with insomnia. Sleep Med. 2010;11(9):934–40.
51. Raman G, Zhang Y, Minichiello VJ, D'Ambrosio CM, Wang C. Tai chi improves sleep quality in healthy adults and patients with chronic conditions: a systematic review and meta-analysis. J Sleep Disord Ther. 2013;2(6).
52. Glass J, Lanctôt KL, Herrmann N, Sproule BA, Busto UE. Sedative hypnotics in older people with insomnia: meta-analysis of risks and benefits. BMJ. 2005;331(7526):1169.
53. McIntosh B, Clark M, Spry C. Benzodiazepines in older adults: a review of clinical effectiveness, cost-effectiveness, and guidelines. 2011.
54. Taipale H, Tolppanen AM, Koponen M, Tanskanen A, Lavikainen P, Sund R, et al. Risk of pneumonia associated with incident benzodiazepine use among community-dwelling adults with Alzheimer disease. CMAJ. 2017;189(14):E519–E29.
55. American Geriatrics Society 2019 Updated AGS Beers Criteria® for Potentially Inappropriate Medication Use in Older Adults. J Am Geriatr Soc. 2019;67(4):674–94.
56. Treves N, Perlman A, Kolenberg Geron L, Asaly A, Matok I. Z-drugs and risk for falls and fractures in older adults-a systematic review and meta-analysis. Age Ageing. 2018;47(2):201–8.
57. Dolder CR, Nelson MH. Hypnosedative-induced complex behaviours: incidence, mechanisms and management. CNS Drugs. 2008;22(12):1021–36.
58. Roth T, Seiden D, Sainati S, Wang-Weigand S, Zhang J, Zee P. Effects of ramelteon on patient-reported sleep latency in older adults with chronic insomnia. Sleep Med. 2006;7(4):312–8.
59. Rojas-Fernandez CH, Chen Y. Use of ultra-low-dose (≤6 mg) doxepin for treatment of insomnia in older people. Can Pharm J (Ott). 2014;147(5):281–9.
60. Herring WJ, Ceesay P, Snyder E, Bliwise D, Budd K, Hutzelmann J, et al. Polysomnographic assessment of suvorexant in patients with probable Alzheimer's disease dementia and insomnia: a randomized trial. Alzheimers Dement. 2020;16(3):541–51.
61. Jaffer KY, Chang T, Vanle B, Dang J, Steiner AJ, Loera N, et al. Trazodone for insomnia: a systematic review. Innov Clin Neurosci. 2017;14(7–8):24–34.
62. Thompson W, Quay TAW, Rojas-Fernandez C, Farrell B, Bjerre LM. Atypical antipsychotics for insomnia: a systematic review. Sleep Med. 2016;22:13–7.
63. Abraham O, Schleiden L, Albert SM. Over-the-counter medications containing diphenhydramine and doxylamine used by older adults to improve sleep. Int J Clin Pharm. 2017;39(4):808–17.
64. Sateia MJ, Buysse DJ, Krystal AD, Neubauer DN, Heald JL. Clinical practice guideline for the pharmacologic treatment of chronic insomnia in adults: An American Academy of sleep medicine clinical practice guideline. J Clin Sleep Med. 2017;13(2):307–49.
65. Allen RP, Walters AS, Montplaisir J, Hening W, Myers A, Bell TJ, et al. Restless legs syndrome prevalence and impact: REST general population study. Arch Intern Med. 2005;165(11):1286–92.

66. Guarnieri B, Adorni F, Musicco M, Appollonio I, Bonanni E, Caffarra P, et al. Prevalence of sleep disturbances in mild cognitive impairment and dementing disorders: a multicenter Italian clinical cross-sectional study on 431 patients. Dement Geriatr Cogn Disord. 2012;33(1):50–8.
67. Figorilli M, Puligheddu M, Ferri R. Restless legs syndrome/Willis-Ekbom disease and periodic limb movements in sleep in the elderly with and without dementia. Sleep Med Clin. 2015;10(3):331–42, xiv-xv.
68. American Academy of Sleep Medicine. The international classification of sleep disorders -Third Edition (ICSD-3). 2nd ed. Westchester, Ill: American Academy of Sleep Medicine; 2014. p. xviii, 297.
69. Allen RP, Picchietti D, Hening WA, Trenkwalder C, Walters AS, Montplaisi J, et al. Restless legs syndrome: diagnostic criteria, special considerations, and epidemiology. A report from the restless legs syndrome diagnosis and epidemiology workshop at the National Institutes of Health. Sleep Med. 2003;4(2):101–19.
70. Richards KC, Bost JE, Rogers VE, Hutchison LC, Beck CK, Bliwise DL, et al. Diagnostic accuracy of behavioral, activity, ferritin, and clinical indicators of restless legs syndrome. Sleep. 2015;38(3):371–80.
71. Zhang C, Li Y, Malhotra A, Ning Y, Gao X. Restless legs syndrome status as a predictor for lower physical function. Neurology. 2014;82(14):1212–8.
72. Cuellar NG, Strumpf NE, Ratcliffe SJ. Symptoms of restless legs syndrome in older adults: outcomes on sleep quality, sleepiness, fatigue, depression, and quality of life. J Am Geriatr Soc. 2007;55(9):1387–92.
73. Rose KM, Beck C, Tsai PF, Liem PH, Davila DG, Kleban M, et al. Sleep disturbances and nocturnal agitation behaviors in older adults with dementia. Sleep. 2011;34(6):779–86.
74. Talarico G, Canevelli M, Tosto G, Vanacore N, Letteri F, Prastaro M, et al. Restless legs syndrome in a group of patients with Alzheimer's disease. Am J Alzheimers Dis Other Dement. 2013;28(2):165–70.
75. Pennestri MH, Whittom S, Adam B, Petit D, Carrier J, Montplaisir J. PLMS and PLMW in healthy subjects as a function of age: prevalence and interval distribution. Sleep. 2006;29(9):1183–7.
76. Koo BB, Blackwell T, Ancoli-Israel S, Stone KL, Stefanick ML, Redline S, et al. Association of incident cardiovascular disease with periodic limb movements during sleep in older men: outcomes of sleep disorders in older men (MrOS) study. Circulation. 2011;124(11):1223–31.
77. Trotti LM, Becker LA. Iron for the treatment of restless legs syndrome. Cochrane Database Syst Rev. 2019;1:CD007834.
78. Rizos A, Sauerbier A, Falup-Pecurariu C, Odin P, Antonini A, Martinez-Martin P, et al. Tolerability of non-ergot oral and transdermal dopamine agonists in younger and older Parkinson's disease patients: an European multicentre survey. J Neural Transm (Vienna). 2020;127(6):875–9.
79. Silver N, Allen RP, Senerth J, Earley CJ. A 10-year, longitudinal assessment of dopamine agonists and methadone in the treatment of restless legs syndrome. Sleep Med. 2011;12(5):440–4.
80. Allen RP, Chen C, Garcia-Borreguero D, Polo O, DuBrava S, Miceli J, et al. Comparison of pregabalin with pramipexole for restless legs syndrome. N Engl J Med. 2014;370(7):621–31.
81. Conway JM, Eberly LE, Collins JF, Macias FM, Ramsay RE, Leppik IE, et al. Factors in variability of serial gabapentin concentrations in elderly patients with epilepsy. Pharmacotherapy. 2017;37(10):1197–203.
82. Xu XM, Liu Y, Jia SY, Dong MX, Cao D, Wei YD. Complementary and alternative therapies for restless legs syndrome: an evidence-based systematic review. Sleep Med Rev. 2018;38:158–67.
83. Haba-Rubio J, Frauscher B, Marques-Vidal P, Toriel J, Tobback N, Andries D, et al. Prevalence and determinants of rapid eye movement sleep behavior disorder in the general population. Sleep. 2018;41(2).
84. Olson EJ, Boeve BF, Silber MH. Rapid eye movement sleep behaviour disorder: demographic, clinical and laboratory findings in 93 cases. Brain. 2000;123(Pt 2):331–9.

85. Kang SH, Yoon IY, Lee SD, Han JW, Kim TH, Kim KW. REM sleep behavior disorder in the Korean elderly population: prevalence and clinical characteristics. Sleep. 2013;36(8):1147–52.
86. Boeve BF, Silber MH, Ferman TJ, Lin SC, Benarroch EE, Schmeichel AM, et al. Clinicopathologic correlations in 172 cases of rapid eye movement sleep behavior disorder with or without a coexisting neurologic disorder. Sleep Med. 2013;14(8):754–62.
87. Iranzo A, Fernández-Arcos A, Tolosa E, Serradell M, Molinuevo JL, Valldeoriola F, et al. Neurodegenerative disorder risk in idiopathic REM sleep behavior disorder: study in 174 patients. PLoS One. 2014;9(2):e89741.
88. Elliott JE, Opel RA, Pleshakov D, Rachakonda T, Chau AQ, Weymann KB, et al. Posttraumatic stress disorder increases the odds of REM sleep behavior disorder and other parasomnias in Veterans with and without comorbid traumatic brain injury. Sleep. 2020;43(3).
89. McGrane IR, Leung JG, St Louis EK, Boeve BF. Melatonin therapy for REM sleep behavior disorder: a critical review of evidence. Sleep Med. 2015;16(1):19–26.
90. Aurora RN, Zak RS, Maganti RK, Auerbach SH, Casey KR, Chowdhuri S, et al. Best practice guide for the treatment of REM sleep behavior disorder (RBD). J Clin Sleep Med. 2010;6(1):85–95.
91. McCarter SJ, Boswell CL, St Louis EK, Dueffert LG, Slocumb N, Boeve BF, et al. Treatment outcomes in REM sleep behavior disorder. Sleep Med. 2013;14(3):237–42.
92. Zhu X, Hu Z, Nie Y, Zhu T, Chiwanda Kaminga A, Yu Y, et al. The prevalence of poor sleep quality and associated risk factors among Chinese elderly adults in nursing homes: a cross-sectional study. PLoS One. 2020;15(5):e0232834.
93. Martin JL, Webber AP, Alam T, Harker JO, Josephson KR, Alessi CA. Daytime sleeping, sleep disturbance, and circadian rhythms in the nursing home. Am J Geriatr Psychiatry. 2006;14(2):121–9.
94. Webster L, Costafreda Gonzalez S, Stringer A, Lineham A, Budgett J, Kyle S, et al. Measuring the prevalence of sleep disturbances in people with dementia living in care homes: a systematic review and meta-analysis. Sleep. 2020;43(4).
95. Capezuti E, Sagha Zadeh R, Pain K, Basara A, Jiang NZ, Krieger AC. A systematic review of non-pharmacological interventions to improve nighttime sleep among residents of long-term care settings. BMC Geriatr. 2018;18(1):143.
96. Berry SD, Lee Y, Cai S, Dore DD. Nonbenzodiazepine sleep medication use and hip fractures in nursing home residents. JAMA Intern Med. 2013;173(9):754–61.

Index

© Springer Nature Switzerland AG 2022
M. S. Badr, J. L. Martin (eds.), *Essentials of Sleep Medicine*,
Respiratory Medicine, https://doi.org/10.1007/978-3-030-93739-3